Joseph T. OConnor

The American homoeopathic pharmacopoeia

Joseph T. OConnor

The American homoeopathic pharmacopoeia

ISBN/EAN: 9783742815651

Manufactured in Europe, USA, Canada, Australia, Japa

Cover: Foto ©Lupo / pixelio.de

Manufactured and distributed by brebook publishing software (www.brebook.com)

Joseph T. OConnor

The American homoeopathic pharmacopoeia

THE

AMERICAN

HOMŒOPATHIC

PHARMACOPŒIA.

SECOND EDITION.

THOROUGHLY REVISED AND AUGMENTED,

BY

JOSEPH T. O'CONNOR, M.D.,

LATELY PROFESSOR OF MATERIA MEDICA AND TOXICOLOGY, AND FORMERLY PROFESSOR OF CHEMISTRY AND TOXICOLOGY IN THE NEW YORK HOMŒOPATHIC MEDICAL COLLEGE.

COMPILED AND PUBLISHED

BY

BOERICKE & TAFEL,

NEW YORK, PHILADELPHIA, CHICAGO.

1883.

TO THE

HOMŒOPATHIC PROFESSION OF AMERICA,

IN WHOSE SERVICE OUR BEST EFFORTS HAVE EVER BEEN ENLISTED,
WE RESPECTFULLY DEDICATE

This Work.

BOERICKE & TAFEL.

REVISER'S PREFACE.

A homœopathic pharmacopœia should give all the directions needed to enable the pharmacist or physician to prepare or to obtain the exact article or substance used by the prover or provers of any drug.

In the present work the attempt is made to do so, and to this end all sources of information attainable have been laid under contribution. While endeavoring to compress the work within somewhat narrow limits, no necessary detail either of description for identification, or of manipulation in the pharmaceutical or chemical processes, has been consciously omitted, and special scope has been given to the desire to furnish as full a list of tests and their applications to the various drugs, as could be in general desired.

The homœopathic chemist should have a practical knowledge of at least qualitative analysis, and should have a fair working acquaintance with botany and zoology. It is needless to add that he ought to be well versed in the drug business as such. In addition to these qualifications he should be possessed of honest purpose to supply the various preparations used in homœopathy, not only in the strictest purity, but also in the exact form or quality that will logically be called for from a knowledge of the specific substance used in the proving.

A pharmacopœia can only be a compilation, and the writer lays claim to but little in the present work as being original. In preparing the pages for the press a small part only of the former edition was allowed to stand. The chemical articles have been with few exceptions entirely rewritten, botanical descriptions have been in some cases materially condensed, in others much expanded; some descriptions which could not be compared with authorities have been allowed to remain, notably of those drugs introduced into our Materia Medica by Dr. Mure, of Brazil, and a few have been taken from the *British Homœopathic Pharmacopœia.*

The reviser desires to express here his obligation to his friend, Prof. T. F. Allen, for material assistance in the department of botany.

For the modes of preparing medicines for homœopathic use as given within these pages, the publishers assume all responsibility; that portion of the book is the result of their many years' experience, and the reviser has felt that in this part of the subject, anything more than a suggestion from him would be uncalled for.

A feature in the book which may call for criticism is the attempt to give credit under each article, to the first prover or introducer of the remedy; the writer has used as references the list of authorities placed at the beginning of each remedy in *Allen's Encyclopedia of Pure Materia Medica*, and *Kleinert's Quellen-Nachweis der Physiologischen Arzneiprüfungen.* In many cases it was impossible to settle satisfactorily to the writer's mind the question of priority, and in most of such instances no credit has been given; in others the provings, as we have them, are from poisoning cases, and here no mention of names could be made; in still others information on the subject was not at hand. In no article, however, has credit been given or omitted without what appeared to be good reason for such action.

The terminology used in this work is that of the *Pharmacopœia Germanica* adopted by Hahnemann in his *Materia Medica Pura;* occasional lapses from this standard appear, however, where such variations have received the sanction of long usage, but terms accepted in other pharmacopœias are given as subtitles in the synonyms.

In conclusion, the reviser ventures to express a hope that the book may be accepted as a standard in its department by the homœopathic pharmacist, physician and undergraduate.

PUBLISHERS' ANNOUNCEMENT.

THE present work was undertaken by the publishers to meet the decided demand for a homœopathic pharmacopœia, especially adapted to the wants of the homœopathic profession and the homœopathic pharmacists in America.

The various European pharmacopœias have done excellent service in their time. The "British Homœopathic Pharmacopœia, 1882," published under the direction of the British Homœopathic Society, is the accepted authority in England, while Dr. Schwabe's "Pharmacopœia Homœopathica Polyglottta" 1880, occupies a similar position with the majority of the profession in Germany.

Neither of these, however, is exactly adapted to meet the requirements of the practitioners in this country for various reasons. The former adopts the innovation of prescribing that the tinctures should contain in ten parts the soluble matter of one part of the dry plant. This rule if adopted, would necessitate a careful drying of all fresh plants in order to calculate their percentage of water. This, in our estimation, would needlessly complicate the process, it looks well enough in theory but is tedious and difficult of practical execution. In other respects this is a work of great merit and bears evidence of very careful preparation and of high scholarship. In Dr. Schwabe's "Polyglotta" on the other hand the rules laid down by *Hahnemann* for the preparation of the remedies are closely followed, and remedies introduced after his time are brought under the same rules as far as practicable; however, no descriptions of plants are given, or of the chemical processes.

The *American Homœopathic Pharmacopœia* has been planned

to include all medicinal substances used in homœopathy, either fully or partially proved, as well as others in actual use or occasional demand, to identify them accurately and concisely after the highest authorities, to give reliable working formulas for the preparation of the chemicals, and finally, to convert them into remedial agents in accordance with the rules laid down by *Hahnemann*.

No trouble or expense has been spared to secure this object.

The revision of the work in its second edition was entrusted to Dr. J. T. O'Connor, of Amenia, New York, formerly Professor of Chemistry at the New York Homœopathic College, who also saw the book through the press; and we take this opportunity of expressing our sincere thanks and acknowlment for the prompt and faithful manner in which he has performed this difficult task.

PART I.

GENERAL

HOMŒOPATHIC PHARMACEUTICS.

In the manufacture and preservation of Homœopathic medicines, care must be taken to avoid everything that can in the least affect their purity. Such influences as light, smoke, strong odors, etc., must be guarded against. Strong-smelling substances used for homœopathic purposes, which could contaminate the others, must, therefore, be kept separate. All homœopathic remedies, tinctures as well as potencies, should be protected from sunlight.

UTENSILS.

Bottles and Glasses.—For neutral substances as well as for remedies, only new, well-cleansed bottles and glasses should be used. They should be of white (so-called), *i. e.*, colorless, flint glass. For remedies sensitive to light, vials covered with black varnish should be used.

Glass-stoppered Bottles should only be used for substances which corrode cork—such as acids, iodine and bromine preparations, etc.

Note.—Yellow or amber-colored bottles were introduced some years ago, it being claimed that they afforded protection against the chemical rays of light. However, such protection is afforded to but few chemicals, and as it is claimed by several writers that non-medicinal substances exposed for some time to yellow light acquire medicinal properties, it follows that amber-colored bottles are inadmissible as receptacles of homœopathic remedies. Besides this, it practically prevents a proper examination of the contents of the bottles.

Weights.—Unless otherwise specified, the United States apothecaries' weight is understood.

Corks.—The corks used must be of the best quality, and as free from pores as possible.

Measuring Glasses.—Measuring glasses, properly graduated, are used for measuring the liquid vehicles used in preparing potencies or attenuations, but they should never be used for measuring any medicinal substance.

Mortars.—For pulverizing very hard substances, a highly-polished iron mortar and pestle of the same material are employed; other metallic mortars must not be used. For softer substances porcelain mortars are suitable.

Triturating Mortars.—Triturating mortars and pestles must be made either of porcelain, the inside of the mortar and the face of the pestle being ground or unglazed, or of wedgewood-ware, or of agate. Mortars made of metal are not to be used for triturating. Special mortars must be used for each separate remedy, with the name of the remedy marked on each mortar.

Sieves.—Only hair or silk sieves can be used; the former for the coarser powders in the preparation of tinctures, the latter for the finer, in making triturations. Sieves designed for sugar of milk must not be used for other purposes.

Spatulas and Spoons.—Spatulas and spoons must be made of horn, bone, or porcelain.

Funnels.—Only glass or porcelain funnels may be used; never metallic ones.

Chopping Board.—The chopping board must be made of sound, well-seasoned maple, free from knots.

Chopping Knife.—The chopping knife, used for cutting up plants, must be made of good steel, and always kept well-polished.

Presses.—Presses used for plants must be well made, and so constructed that they can readily be taken apart, and thoroughly cleansed.

THE CLEANSING OF UTENSILS.

In making homœopathic preparations, the utmost cleanliness must be observed. Accordingly, utensils, even when used for the first time, must be thoroughly cleansed.

Glasses and bottles are to be washed several times with rain water, then rinsed with distilled water, and after draining, are to be dried at a high temperature.

Porcelain vessels must be scalded with boiling water, and dried at a high temperature.

The press is taken apart, and washed first with cold, then with hot water, and then dried thoroughly.

All utensils should be cleansed immediately after use.

Glasses and bottles which have been used for a particular tincture or potency, however well cleansed, must not be used for another preparation.

NEUTRAL SUBSTANCES OR VEHICLES.

AQUA DESTILLATA.

Distilled Water.—Formula H_2O. Molecular weight 18.

Preparation of Distilled Water.—Rain water collected some time after the commencement of a storm, as the portion falling earlier contains particles of dust and various organic and inorganic matters, which had been suspended or dissolved in the air, is subjected to distillation in an apparatus expressly designed for that purpose. A copper still and block-tin condenser are generally used, but it is best to use a still that is gold or nickle-plated throughout, as Silica is dissolved out by steam from an ordinary glass retort, and porcelain stills are objectionable for the same reason. The distilled water must be filled at once into glass-stoppered bottles, that it may not become contaminated by dust or spores floating in the air. Water prepared and preserved in this manner will remain pure for years.

Properties.—Distilled water is a transparent, colorless, odorless, tasteless liquid, whose density at the temperature of 15° or 15. 5° C. (59° or 60° F.) is taken as unity for the determination of specific gravity of liquid and solid bodies; but the weight of 1 CC. of water at its maximum density (given below) is called 1 gramme, and thus furnishes the starting point of the metric system of weights. Water is at its maximum density at the temperature 4° C.; below that temperature it expands gradually till the freezing point 0° C. (32° F.) is reached, when it becomes solid, forming ice whose specific gravity is .916—thus showing an expansion at the moment of solidification, of $\frac{1}{11}$ of its bulk. Above 4° C. water expands slightly for every degree of heat added, till at 100° C. (212° F.) at the sea level, it is converted into vapor, at the same time being violently agitated or boiling.

Tests of Purity.—Distilled water should have the physical characteristics noted above; it should leave no residue after evaporation, should be indifferent to test papers, and should give no precipitate when treated with barium chloride, silver nitrate, ammonium oxalate, or hydrogen sulphide.

The presence of carbonic oxide will be proven by a white precipitate when agitated with lime water.

ALCOHOL.

Spirit of Wine.—In commerce, there is now obtainable everywhere, pure alcohol, free from fusel oil, containing 90 per cent. of anhydrous alcohol. Hence, it is scarcely ever necessary for the pharmacist to rectify the raw spirit. In homœopathic pharmacy especially, particular care should be exercised not to use alcohol which had been used in making medicinal preparations, and which had been recovered by distillation. Should it be necessary to rectify the raw spirit containing fusel oil, the following method is offered: Dilute raw spirit with distilled water until its specific gravity is 0.86 or 0.87. Macerate with fresh burned charcoal, broken in small pieces, for one or two days with frequent stirring, and finally pour the liquid into a retort and distil by the heat of a water bath.

Alcohol entirely free from fusel oil, is to be subjected to redistillation in an apparatus especially adapted for the purpose. The product should be reduced to 87 per cent. (Tralles), or a specific gravity of 0.83, by adding distilled water; (95 per cent. alcohol [Tralles] may be reduced to 87 per cent. [Tralles] by adding to seven parts of the former one part of distilled water). This is the standard officinal strength of so-called homœopathic alcohol.

NOTE.—When a stronger alcohol is employed to prepare a tincture, the strength (according to Tralles) is expressed.

Dilute Alcohol.—Consists of seven parts alcohol, specific gravity 0.83, and three parts distilled water, the mixture having specific gravity 0.89.

Properties.—Absolute alcohol is a colorless, transparent, very mobile, volatile liquid, whose specific gravity at 15.5° C. (60° F.) is 0.7938. It boils at 78.4° C. (173° F.), but the temperature of the boiling point is higher, if diluted with water, according to the degree of dilution.

It mixes in all proportions with distilled water and remains clear. Its odor and taste are purely alcoholic, warm, fragrant and agreeable. It is very inflammable, burning with a faint, bluish flame and without smoke. Its solvent power extends over a wide range.

Tests.—Diluted with distilled water in equal proportions, alcohol should yield no foreign odor, nor, when a few drops are rubbed between the hands, should any foreign odor be perceptible. Treated with a few drops of solution of silver nitrate and exposed to bright light, it remains unchanged if pure.

Add slowly to the alcohol its own weight of pure concentrated sulphuric acid. If the alcohol is pure, it remains colorless; if fusil oil is present, a reddish color will be developed, from the formation of amyl-sulphuric acid.

SACCHARUM LACTIS.

Formula, $C_{12}H_{22}O_{11}, H_2O$.
Molecular Weight, 360.
Common Name, Sugar of Milk.
Synonym, Lactose.

Sugar of Milk.—This sugar is one of the constituents of milk. In the vegetable kingdom it is very rarely found.

Pure lactose is in odorless, white, hard, four-sided rhombic prisms. Its taste is faintly sweet, and between the teeth it gives a sandy or "gritty" feeling. It is soluble in two and one-half parts of boiling water, but requires six parts of water at ordinary temperatures. It is insoluble in alcohol, or even a 60 per cent. alcohol, in ether and chloroform.

Its watery solution does not form a syrup.

By heating to 150° C. (302° F.) it gives up its water of crystallization. By long boiling in a weak watery solution it becomes changed into galactose. The same transformation is effected more rapidly by digestion with dilute mineral acids or with strong solutions of organic acids. Galactose, under the influence of beer yeast undergoes vinous fermentation.

Preparation.—The general outlines of the method are as follows: Fresh milk is allowed to stand till its cream rises—then skimmed, and treated with rennet to coagulate the casein. The latter is removed and the residue is a solution of milk sugar and the salts of milk, but is not wholly free from casein and butter-fat. Upon evaporation of this liquid, called whey, the milk sugar is obtained in crystals as above described. It is a constant by-product in the manufacture of cheese. The crystals so obtained are redissolved in water, treated with animal charcoal and recrystallized after filtration.

It is extremely difficult to free milk sugar from slight amounts of foreign substances by repeated crystallization from watery solution, for the water does not surrender all of the sugar.

To overcome the difficulty, Stapf devised the following method: Dissolve a pound of the finest milk sugar in four pounds of boiling distilled water; filter the solution while yet warm, through the finest Swedish filter paper, and thoroughly mix the filtrate in a glass or porcelain dish, with four pounds of pure absolute alcohol. The vessel is then to be covered tightly and set aside in a cool place so that the sugar may crystallize out.

At the end of three or four days there will be found on the bottom and sides of the vessel a crust about one-sixth of an inch in thickness, crystalline and glistening, whose weight will be found to very nearly equal that of the milk sugar dissolved in the beginning of the process. The crystalline mass is then to be collected, washed with distilled water, to which has been added some alcohol, dried between folds of bibulous paper and preserved for use.

Character and Tests.—Milk sugar must be entirely free from fat or the other constituents of milk, which freedom will be shown by its perfect whiteness; it should not be hygroscopic, nor should it have any rancid, musty, sour, or other foreign smell or taste.

Milk sugar may be adulterated with cane sugar; in this case the increased sweetness as well as the more ready solubility in water will serve to detect the falsification. If alum be present, a white precipitate will be thrown down on adding to the solution of milk sugar an alkaline hydrate not in excess.

If copper, from copper vessels in the preparation of the sugar, be present, a reddish-brown precipitate will occur on the addition of potassium ferro-cyanide solution. Chloride of sodium, or phosphates, will be detected by silver nitrate solution, nitric acid dissolving the phosphate of silver formed but not the chloride. Sulphuric acid will be detected by barium nitrate or chloride.

If a solution of milk sugar redden blue litmus paper, the fact is due to free acid, and shows, in all probability, that the sugar was prepared from milk that had become sour.

GLOBULES OR PELLETS.

Globules are prepared from pure cane sugar. They must be white, of uniform size for each number as given below, perfectly globular, not too hard, and entirely soluble in distilled water. When freshly made they are somewhat soft, but become harder by age. Addition of flour, glucose, glycerine, or starch, to make them soft, or to keep them so, is an adulteration. They are assorted according to size and designated by numbers from 8 to 80.

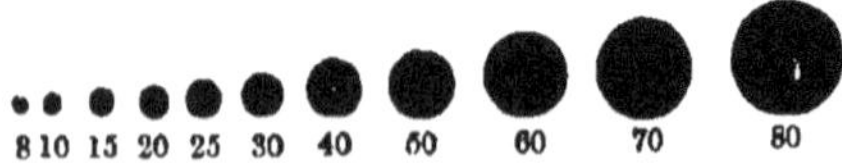

Measure of Globules.—The number given to any size of globules is determined by laying ten of equal size in a line and in close contact with each other; the space so occupied, given in millimetres, is the number by which that particular size is designated.

THE PROCURING OF MEDICINAL SUBSTANCES.

Fresh Plants.—As to the time when the fresh plant is to be gathered, the directions to be followed are, with few exceptions, given under the remedy. If such directions are wanting, it is to be assumed that the plants have been collected by the prover at the season in which their medicinal virtue is greatest, *e. g.*, narcotic plants while in bloom, others shortly before, or when coming into bloom.

Only such plants should be collected as are healthy, strongly developed, faultless, and free from dust and caterpillar's nests, and when growing wild in a locality known to be most favorable to their development. Cultivated flowers are employed only in cases where the prover has expressly prescribed their use. Plants should be gathered when the weather has previously been sunny and dry, and after the morning-dew has disappeared from them. The collected specimens must not be packed too closely in carrying, and should be quickly subjected to manipulation, that they may yield their full strength unchanged.

Fresh Portions of Plants.—The same principles apply to the collection of fresh portions of plants.

Fruits and Seeds ought to be collected in their fully ripe condition (unless the unripe is prescribed).

Woods are collected before the beginning of spring, ere the buds are developed.

Herbs should be cut above the root-leaves.

Barks are collected from resinous trees and shrubs at the time of, or before the development of the leaves: from the non-resinous, in autumn.

Roots are dug, unless specially directed otherwise, as follows: Of annual plants, before the ripening of the seed; of biennials, in the spring of the second year; of perennials, in autumn.

Twigs are to be used only when of the present year's growth.

Drugs, Metals, Minerals, Chemicals, Etc.—The genuineness and purity of drugs, metals, minerals, chemicals, etc., must be tested according to the stated rules, before being employed for any homœopathic purposes.

PRELIMINARY MANIPULATIONS.

Fresh Plants and Parts of Plants.—The fresh plant, or part of it, is re-examined as to its undoubted identity, then carefully freed from any impurities that might have accidentally escaped notice in gathering it. Only those parts are taken for use which are specified under the respective remedy. The operation must be carried on as quickly and uninterruptedly as possible in the following manner: The plant should be cut up with a well polished steel knife, free from rust, on a well cleansed chopping board; then divided as finely as possible with an equally well cleansed chopping knife. The finely divided mass is then to be treated in the manner more minutely described under Class I or II or III, according to which the tincture is to be prepared. Fresh fruits and seeds, if they can be cut up, are treated as above; if not, they are simply crushed in a mortar.

Dried Plants and their Parts.—For the preparation of tinctures, they are pulverized coarsely; for the preparation of triturations, as finely as possible.

Metals, Minerals and Chemical Preparations.—The rule for this class is to reduce the crude substance to a state so finely divided, that, if it is to be triturated, such can be done uniformly. This we accomplish with a part of these substances by pounding, but with most metals by precipitation.

NOTE.—Hahnemann employed metallic foil or filings, or comminuted the metals on a whet-stone. Later microscopic examinations have shown, however, that this method of subdividing is very imperfect, and renders the purity of the metal very doubtful, particles of the iron or whet-stone becoming mingled with it. The uniform distribution of the crude substance, on the other hand, has been shown to have been accomplished only in triturations prepared from precipitates. For this reason we employ precipitates, since we consider this departure from Hahnemann's rules to be in no wise subversive of Homœopathy. Moreover, the triturations prepared from precipitates have been used for re-provings, and it is only by the use of precipitates that we can obtain preparations of constant uniformity.

PREPARATION OF POTENCIES OR ATTENUATIONS.

Two scales are employed in potentizing, viz., the *centesimal* and the *decimal.*

The Centesimal Scale.—This scale was introduced by Hahnemann, and is still retained in making the higher potencies, while the lower potencies are now more generally made on the decimal scale. The centesimal scale is based on the principle that the first potency must contain the $\frac{1}{100}$ part of the drug power, and each following potency the $\frac{1}{100}$ part of the one preceding it. However, as tinctures and solutions are prepared by different rules, the drug power varies, and hence the quantity of the mother-tincture or solution and of the neutral vehicle must be so proportioned that the first potency represents the $\frac{1}{100}$ part of the drug power. In preparing the second, and following potencies, to one minim or part by weight of the preceding potency, ninety-nine minims or parts by weight of the neutral vehicle are added. The respective "classes" which prescribe the relative proportions for the different potencies give the necessary information.

The Decimal Scale.—During Hahnemann's lifetime another method, the decimal scale, introduced by Dr. Constantine Hering, found many adherents among homœopathic physicians. In preparing remedies according to this scale, it is the rule that the first potency should contain the $\frac{1}{10}$ of the drug power, while the following potencies are prepared with one minim or part, by weight, of the preceding potency to nine minims or parts, by weight, of the neutral vehicle. (Compare the classes.)

ATTENUATIONS.

Potentiation of Liquid Substances.—Potentiation must be carried on in an apartment free from all odors, dust and direct sunlight. The vials used for this purpose must be round, and their capacity should be such that the quantity of preparation to be succussed therein shall only two-thirds fill them. The name of the remedy with the number of the potency is marked both on the cork and on the vial, using the simple numeral for the potencies on the centesimal scale, and affixing an x to the numeral for potencies on the decimal scale.

Potentiation on the Centesimal Scale.—Into the duly marked vial intended for the first potency, the proper proportion of mother-tincture or solution is poured and the vehicle added—as mentioned under the class according to which the tincture has been prepared (see pp. 11-18),—then the vial is carefully corked and shaken by ten powerful downward strokes of the arm.

The second potency is made by adding to one minim of the first potency ninety-nine minims of the vehicle, the vial being shaken again as directed above. All subsequent potencies are made in like manner, *i. e.*, by adding to one part of the preceding potency ninety-nine minims of the vehicle, and giving the mixture ten succussive strokes.

In this manner potencies may be carried up to the one thousandth or higher; attenuations above the thirtieth are termed *High Potencies.*

Potentiation on the Decimal Scale.—Into the duly marked vial intended for the first decimal potency the proper proportion of mother-tincture or solution is poured and the vehicle added—as mentioned under the class according to which the tincture or solution has been prepared (see page 19–25)—the vial is then well corked, and the contents shaken with ten vigorous downward strokes of the arm. All following potencies are made in the same manner, except that for each new potency, one minim or part of the preceding potency and nine minims or parts of the vehicle are measured into the vial, and then shaken as directed above.

NOTE.—We are explicit in directing the proper proportion of the substance being first put into the vial, and the vehicle afterwards, because this is a rule which all careful pharmacists should follow, to prevent the possibility of mistakes.

TRITURATIONS.

Potentiation of Dry Substances.—Dry substances, *i. e.*, those whose medicinal power, according to homœopathic principles, must first be developed by trituration with sugar of milk, ought to be manipulated in a warm and dry atmosphere. Before beginning the work we must satisfy ourselves that the apparatus to be used is perfectly clean. Mortars should be washed first with cold water, then with hot water, and carefully wiped dry, and lastly, a small quantity of alcohol is to be burned in the mortar. This must be done for every subsequent trituration.

TRITURATIONS ON THE CENTESIMAL SCALE.—Hahnemann so lucidly gives the technical directions to be observed in triturating, in his *Chronic Diseases*, Vol. 1, p. 183, that we give here a careful translation: "First add one grain of the substance to about one-third of ninety-nine grains of sugar of milk in a porcelain mortar, unglazed or ground to an unpolished surface by rubbing with wet sand; mix the medicine and the sugar of milk together for a moment with a porcelain spatula, then after triturating the mixture vigorously for six minutes, scrape the trituration together for four minutes from the bottom of the mortar and from the face of the (also unglazed) porcelain pestle, in order that the trituration may be uniformly mixed, and again triturate the scraped-up mass (without further addition of sugar of milk) a second time for six minutes with the same force. To this powder, again scraped up for four minutes, in which the first third of ninety-nine grains has been used, we add now the second third, mixing both together with a spatula for a moment, and again triturating for six minutes with the same force, and then again scraping up the trituration for four minutes, triturate vigorously six minutes a second time, and having scraped this mass together for four minutes, incorporate the third portion of sugar of milk by stirring with the spatula so that the whole mixture after six minutes vigorous trituration and four minutes scraping together may for the last time be triturated six minutes and then scraped together carefully." This is the first (1) trituration. To prepare the second (2) trituration, one grain of the first trituration is added to the one-third part of ninety-nine grains of sugar of milk mixed in a mortar with the spatula, and so treated that each third is twice well triturated for six minutes, and scraped together for four minutes, and then put into a well-stoppered bottle. In the same way one grain of the second (2) trituration is treated in preparing the third (3). The trituration must be done energetically, but not so much so that the sugar of milk shall cleave so strongly to the bottom of the mortar that it cannot in four minutes be scraped together. To make any higher trituration, one grain of the preceding trituration to that desired is triturated with ninety-nine grains of sugar of milk as directed above.

CONVERSION OF THE THIRD CENTESIMAL (3) TRITURATION INTO

LIQUID POTENCIES.—The substances triturated according to the centesimal scale to the third (3), are brought by this continuous process to such a degree of attenuation that they dissolve in or combine with a liquid vehicle, such as alcohol or water, and can thus be carried to a still higher degree of subdivision. This method of conversion, Hahnemann describes as follows:

"In order to convert the potent trituration into the liquid state, and still further develop its power, we avail ourselves of the experience, hitherto unknown to chemistry, that all medicinal substances triturated to the third (3), are soluble in water and alcohol. Fifty minims of distilled water are added with the measuring glass to one grain of the third (3) trituration, and this by agitation is readily dissolved; then fifty minims of alcohol are added, and the stoppered vial, only two-thirds filled with the mixture, is shaken ten times; this is the fourth (4) potency. Of this, one minim is added to ninety-nine minims of alcohol, and the well corked vial shaken ten times; this is the fifth (5) potency. The following potencies are each prepared with one minim of the preceding potency to ninety-nine minims of alcohol, and each shaken ten times."

TRITURATIONS ON THE DECIMAL SCALE.—For the triturations to be prepared according to the decimal scale, we follow the same method in triturating as is given under the centesimal scale, except that first ten parts by weight of the crude substance are triturated with thirty grains of sugar of milk for twice six minutes, and each time scraped together for four minutes. We then add thirty grains more of sugar of milk, triturate again twice six minutes and each time scrape together for four minutes, finally adding thirty grains more of sugar of milk, and triturating the mixture in the same manner. This is the first decimal (1x) trituration. Ten parts by weight of this preparation, triturated with three times thirty parts by weight of sugar of milk in precisely the same manner, gives the second decimal (2x) trituration. Of this, ten parts by weight with three times thirty parts by weight of sugar of milk gives the third decimal (3x), and in this way, the trituration each time of ten parts by weight of the preceding trituration, with ninety parts by weight of sugar of milk is continued for any higher trituration desired on the decimal scale.

CONVERSION OF THE SIXTH DECIMAL (6x) TRITURATION INTO LIQUID POTENCIES.—We dissolve one grain of the 6x trituration in fifty minims of distilled water in a vial, adding thereto fifty minims of alcohol, and shaking the vial ten times; this is the 8x potency. (The 7x, according to the rule governing this scale cannot be prepared in the proportion of one to nine.) One drop of the 8x potency with nine minims of dilute alcohol, shaken ten times, gives the 9x potency. One minim of the 9x potency with nine minims of alcohol, and shaken ten times gives the 10x potency. All following potencies are each prepared with one minim of the preceding potency to nine minims of alcohol, and each shaken ten times.

NOTE.—Hahnemann directs *drops* of drug and vehicle to be used, but as there is no uniformity in the measure of a drop of the different liquids, we have adopted the more exact measure of *minims*.

MEDICATED GLOBULES.

Medication of Globules.—Moisten the globules with the requisite potency, in a bottle two-thirds filled, cork the bottle, and shake it so that all the globules shall become uniformly moistened. Then invert the bottle, standing it on the cork, and let it remain in that position from nine to ten hours. Then loosen the cork a little, and let the liquid that may have collected within the neck of the bottle drain out. In a few days the pellets will be entirely dry, and ready for dispensing. It is not proper to dispense medicated globules until they have become perfectly dry.

Potencies prepared with dilute alcohol cannot be used for medicating globules, as the globules become disintegrated by the solvent power of the water contained in the dilute alcohol.

Medicated pellets, like all other homœopathic medicines, require to be kept well corked, and protected from heat and sunlight. Carefully kept they retain their virtue many years.

NOTE.—Hahnemann gives another method in his *Chronic Diseases*, Vol. 1, page 187: "The globules are poured into a clean porcelain bowl, rather deep than broad, and enough of the required potency dropped upon them to moisten completely every globule in the space of one minute. The contents of the bowl are then emptied on a piece of clean, dry filtering paper, so that any excess of liquid may be absorbed, and the globules spread out that they may soon dry. The dry globules are then poured into a vial duly marked with the name and potency, and securely corked."

PROPORTIONS OF MEASURE AND WEIGHT IN THE PREPARATION OF TINCTURES, SOLUTIONS, POTENCIES AND TRITURATIONS.

The proportion of measure and weight, employed in the preparation of tinctures, solutions, potencies and triturations, are for the sake of more convenient reference, arranged in nine classes, to which attention is called under each medicine.

CLASS I.

TINCTURES.

Tinctures prepared with equal parts by weight of juice and alcohol.

The fundamental rule for this class is contained in Hahnemann's *Mat. Med. Pura*, under Belladonna.

The freshly-gathered plant, or part thereof, chopped and pounded to a pulp, is enclosed in a piece of new linen and subjected to pressure. The expressed juice is then, by brisk agitation, mingled with an equal part by weight of alcohol. This mixture is allowed to stand eight days in a well-stoppered bottle, in a dark cool place, and is then filtered.

Amount of drug power of tincture, ½.

POTENTIATION.

a. Centesimal Scale.

2 minims of tincture and 98 minims of dilute alcohol give the 1st potency.

1 minim of the 1st potency and 99 minims of alcohol give the 2d potency.

All the following potencies are prepared with one minim of the preceding potency to ninety-nine minims of alcohol.

b. Decimal Scale.

2 minims of tincture and 8 minims of dilute alcohol give the 1x potency.

1 minim of the 1x potency and 9 minims of dilute alcohol give the 2x potency.

1 minim of the 2x potency and 9 minims of dilute alcohol give the 3x potency.

All following potencies are prepared with one minim of the preceding potency to nine minims of alcohol.

CLASS II.

TINCTURES.

Tinctures expressed by the aid of two parts of alcohol added to three parts of plant, or part thereof.

The fundamental rule for this class is contained in Hahnemann's *Mat. Med. Pura*, under Thuya.

The finely chopped, fresh plant, or part thereof, is weighed. To every three parts, two parts by weight of alcohol are taken. Then the chopped plant is moistened with as much alcohol as is necessary to bring the mass to a thick pulp, and is well stirred. Adding the rest of the alcohol, the whole is mixed together and strained through a piece of new linen. The tincture thus obtained is allowed to stand eight days in a well-stoppered bottle, in a dark, cool place, and then filtered.

Amount of drug power of tincture, ½.

POTENTIATION.

a. Centesimal Scale.

2 minims of tincture and 98 minims of dilute alcohol give the 1st potency.

1 minim of the 1st potency and 99 minims of alcohol give the 2d potency.

All following potencies are prepared with one minim of the preceding potency to ninety-nine minims of alcohol.

b. Decimal Scale.

2 minims of tincture and 8 minims of dilute alcohol give the 1x potency.

1 minim of the 1x potency and 9 minims of dilute alcohol give the 2x potency.

1 minim of the 2x potency and 9 minims of alcohol give the 3x potency.

All following potencies are prepared with one minim of the preceding potency to nine minims of alcohol.

CLASS III.

TINCTURES.

Tinctures prepared with two parts by weight of alcohol to one part of plant, or part thereof.

The fundamental rule for this class is contained in Hahnemann's *Mat. Med. Pura*, under Scilla.

The fresh plant, or part thereof, is pounded to a fine pulp and weighed. Then two parts by weight of alcohol are taken, and after thoroughly mixing the pulp with one-sixth part of it, the rest of the alcohol is added. After having stirred the whole, and having filled it into a well-stoppered bottle, it is allowed to stand eight days, in a dark, cool place. The tincture is then separated by decanting, straining and filtering.

Amount of drug power of tincture, $\frac{1}{6}$.

POTENTIATION.

a. Centesimal Scale.

6 minims of tincture and 94 minims of dilute alcohol give the 1st potency.

1 minim of the 1st potency and 99 minims of alcohol give the 2d potency.

All following potencies are prepared with one minim of the preceding potency to ninety-nine minims of alcohol.

b. Decimal Scale.

6 minims of tincture and 4 minims of dilute alcohol give the 1x potency.

1 minim of the 1x potency and 9 minims of dilute alcohol give the 2x potency.

1 minim of the 2x potency and 9 minims of alcohol give the 3x potency.

All following potencies are prepared with one minim of the preceding potency to nine minims of alcohol.

CLASS IV.

TINCTURES.

Tincture prepared with five parts by weight of alcohol.

The fundamental rule for this class is contained in Hahnemann's *Mat. Med. Pura*, under Spigelia and Staphisagria.

Weigh the finely divided substance (dried vegetable and animal substances are pulverized, fresh animal substances are pounded) and pour over it five parts by weight of alcohol, then let the mixture remain eight days (provided that for the particular medicine a longer maceration is not required), at ordinary temperature in a dark place, shaking it twice a day; then pour off, strain and filter.

Amount of drug power of tincture, $\frac{1}{10}$.

POTENTIATION.

a. Centesimal Scale.

10 minims of tincture and 90 minims of alcohol give the 1st potency.

1 minim of the 1st potency and 99 minims of alcohol give the 2d potency.

All following potencies are prepared with one minim of the preceding potency to ninety-nine minims of alcohol.

b. Decimal Scale.

As the tincture contains $\frac{1}{10}$ drug power, it corresponds to the 1x potency.

1 minim of tincture and 9 minims of alcohol give the 2x potency.

All following potencies are prepared with one minim of the preceding potency to nine minims of alcohol.

CLASS V—*a*.

AQUEOUS SOLUTIONS.

One part by weight of the medicinal substance is dissolved in nine parts by weight of distilled water.

Amount of drug power of solution, $\frac{1}{10}$.

POTENTIATION.

a. Centesimal Scale.

10 minims of the solution and 90 minims of distilled water give the 1st potency.

1 minim of the 1st potency and 99 minims of alcohol give the 2d potency.

All following potencies are prepared with one minim of the preceding potency to ninety-nine minims of alcohol.

b. Decimal Scale.

As the solution contains $\frac{1}{10}$ drug power, it corresponds to the 1x potency.

1 minim of the solution and 9 minims of distilled water give the 2x potency.

1 minim of the 2x potency and 9 minims of dilute alcohol give the 3x potency.

1 minim of the 3x potency and 9 minims of alcohol give the 4x potency.

All following potencies are prepared with one minim of the preceding potency to nine minims of alcohol.

CLASS V—β.

AQUEOUS SOLUTIONS.

One part by weight of the medicinal substance is dissolved in ninety-nine parts by weight of distilled water.

Amount of drug power of solution, $\frac{1}{100}$.

POTENTIATION.

a. Centesimal Scale.

As the solution contains $\frac{1}{100}$ drug power, it corresponds to the 1st potency.

1 minim of the solution and 99 minims of dilute alcohol give the 2d potency.

All following potencies are prepared with one minim of the preceding potency to ninety-nine minims of alcohol.

b. Decimal Scale.

As the solution contains $\frac{1}{100}$ drug power, it corresponds to the 2x potency.

1 minim of the solution and 9 minims of dilute alcohol give the 3x potency.

1 minim of the 3x potency and 9 minims of alcohol give the 4x potency.

All following potencies are prepared with one minim of the preceding potency to nine minims of alcohol.

CLASS VI—*a*.

ALCOHOLIC SOLUTIONS.

One part by weight of the medicinal substance is dissolved in nine parts by weight of alcohol.

Amount of drug power of solution, $\frac{1}{10}$.

POTENTIATION.

a. Centesimal Scale.

10 minims of the solution and 90 minims of alcohol give the 1st potency.

1 minim of the 1st potency and 99 minims of alcohol give the 2d potency.

All following potencies are prepared with one minim of the preceding potency to ninety-nine minims of alcohol.

b. Decimal Scale.

As the solution contains $\frac{1}{10}$ drug power, it corresponds to the 1x potency.

1 minim of the solution and 9 minims of alcohol give the 2x potency.

All following potencies are prepared with one minim of the preceding potency to nine minims of alcohol.

CLASS VI—*β*.

ALCOHOLIC SOLUTIONS.

One part by weight of the medicinal substance is dissolved in 99 parts by weight of alcohol.

Amount of drug power of solution, $\frac{1}{100}$.

POTENTIATION.

a. Centesimal Scale.

As the solution contains $\frac{1}{100}$ drug power, it corresponds to the 1st potency.

1 minim of the solution and 99 minims of alcohol give the 2d potency.

All following potencies are prepared with one minim of the preceding potency to ninety-nine minims of alcohol.

b. Decimal Scale.

As the solution contains $\frac{1}{100}$ drug power, it corresponds to the 2x potency.

1 minim of the solution and 9 minims of alcohol give the 3x potency.

All following potencies are prepared with one minim of the preceding potency to nine minims of alcohol.

CLASS VII.

TRITURATION OF DRY MEDICINAL SUBSTANCES.

The fundamental rule for this class is contained in Hahnemann's *Mat. Med. Pura*, under Arsenicum.

For the trituration and potentiation of dry medicinal substances the following proportions of weight and measure form the basis:

a. Centesimal Scale.

One part by weight of the medicinal substance to 99 parts by weight of sugar of milk gives the 1st trituration.

All following triturations are prepared with one grain of the preceding trituration to ninety-nine grains of sugar of milk.

Conversion into Liquid Potencies.

One grain of the 3d trituration dissolved in 50 minims of distilled water and mixed with 50 minims of alcohol gives the 4th potency.

1 minim of the 4th potency to 99 minims of alcohol gives the 5th potency.

All following potencies are prepared with one minim of the preceding potency to ninety-nine minims of alcohol.

b. Decimal Scale.

One part by weight of the medicinal substance to 9 parts by weight of sugar of milk gives the 1x trituration.

All following triturations are prepared with one grain of the preceding trituration to nine grains of sugar of milk.

Conversion into Liquid Potencies.

One grain of the 6x trituration dissolved in 50 minims of distilled water and mixed with 50 minims of alcohol, gives the 8x potency.

1 minim of the 8x potency to 9 minims of dilute alcohol gives the 9x potency.

1 minim of the 9x potency to 9 minims of alcohol gives the 10x potency.

All following potencies are prepared with one minim of the preceding potency to nine minims of alcohol.

CLASS VIII.

TRITURATION OF LIQUID SUBSTANCES.

The rule for this class is contained in Hahnemann's *Chronic Diseases*, under Petroleum.

For the trituration of these substances the following proportions of weight and measure form the basis:

a. Centesimal Scale.

1 minim of the substance to 99 grains of sugar of milk gives the 1st trituration.

1 part by weight of the 1st trituration to 99 parts by weight of sugar of milk gives the 2d trituration.

All following triturations are prepared with one grain of the preceding trituration to ninety-nine grains of sugar of milk.

Conversion into Liquid Potencies.

One grain of the 3d trituration dissolved in 50 minims of distilled water and mixed with 50 minims of alcohol, gives the 4th potency.

1 minim of the 4th potency to 99 minims of alcohol gives the 5th potency.

All following potencies are prepared with one minim of the preceding potency to ninety-nine minims of alcohol.

b. Decimal Scale.

1 minim of the substance to 9 grains of sugar of milk gives the 1x trituration.

1 part by weight of the 1x trituration to 9 parts by weight of sugar of milk gives the 2x trituration.

All following triturations are prepared with one grain of the preceding trituration to nine grains of sugar of milk.

Conversion into Liquid Potencies.

One grain of the 6x trituration dissolved in 50 minims of distilled water and mixed with 50 minims of alcohol, gives the 8x potency.

1 minim of the 8x potency to 9 minims of dilute alcohol gives the 9x potency.

1 minim of the 9x potency to 9 minims of alcohol gives the 10x potency.

All following potencies are prepared with one minim of the preceding potency to nine minims of alcohol.

CLASS IX.

TRITURATION OF FRESH VEGETABLE AND ANIMAL SUBSTANCES.

For this class, the lower triturations of which cannot be preserved, the rule is found in Hahnemann's *Chronic Diseases*, under Agaricus.

Fresh vegetables and animals are first pounded or grated to a fine pulp, then triturated and potentized according to the following proportions by weight and measure:

a. Centesimal Scale.

Two parts* by weight of the substance and 99 parts by weight of sugar of milk gives the 1st trituration.

One part by weight of the first trituration to 99 parts by weight of sugar of milk gives the 2d trituration.

All following triturations are prepared with one part by weight of the preceding trituration to ninety-nine parts by weight of sugar of milk.

Conversion into Liquid Potencies.

One grain of the 3d trituration dissolved in 50 minims of distilled water and mixed with 50 minims of alcohol gives the 4th potency.

1 minim of the 4th potency to 99 minims of alcohol gives the 5th potency.

All following potencies are prepared with one minim of the preceding potency to ninety-nine minims of alcohol.

a. Decimal Scale.

Two parts by weight of the substance and 9 parts by weight of sugar of milk give the 1x trituration.

1 part by weight of the 1x trituration to 9 parts by weight of sugar of milk gives the 2x trituration.

All following triturations are prepared with one part by weight of the preceding trituration to nine parts by weight of sugar of milk.

Conversion into Liquid Potencies.

One grain of the 6x trituration dissolved in 50 minims of distilled water and mixed with 50 minims of alcohol gives the 8x potency.

1 minim of the 8x potency to 9 minims of dilute alcohol gives the 9x potency.

1 minim of the 9x potency to 9 minims of alcohol gives the 10x potency.

All following potencies are prepared with one minim of the preceding potency to nine minims of alcohol.

---

* Two parts are taken because of loss by evaporation during trituration.

NOMENCLATURE.

In homœopathy the old Latin nomenclature of Hahnemann's time, still used at this date in the official Pharmacopœia of the German Empire, has been retained, and adopted by all the text books of the school. In all cases where only one species of a genus of plants is officinal, the medicine bears the name of the genus or species, thus instead of saying Aconitum Napellus, we say *Aconitum;* instead of Atropa Belladonna, *Belladonna.* If later, another plant of the same genus is proved, as for example, Aconitum Lycoctonum, its name receives the distinctive addition *Lycoctonum,* while by the name *Aconitum* alone we always understand Aconitum Napellus. To avoid mistakes, we give under the officinal name, in Part II, treating of Special Homœopathic Pharmaceutics, the name of the species and its synonyms.

θ is used to denote Mother Tinctures.

Dil. (Dilutions) is used to denote Liquid Potencies or Attenuations.

Trit. is used to denote Triturations.

The simple numeral, 1, 2, 3, etc., added to the name of a remedy, signifies that the preparation has been potentized on the *Centesimal* scale.

The Latin numeral ten (x) added to the simple numeral, viz.: 1x, 2x, 3x, etc., signifies that the preparation has been potentized on the *Decimal* scale.

PART II.

SPECIAL

HOMŒOPATHIC PHARMACEUTICS.

ABELMOSCHUS.

Synonym, Hibiscus Abelmoschus, *Wight and Arnott.*
Nat. Ord., Malvaceæ.
Common Name, Musk Seed.

A shrub growing in Egypt, and in the East and West Indies. The seeds are known under the names of *Semen Abelmoschi, Alceæ Ægyptiacæ,* and *Grana Moschata.* They are kidney-shaped, three to four millimetres long and about two millimetres wide; are characterized by many brown concentric striæ, with grayish furrows between the striæ. They have an agreeable odor like that of musk, and an aromatic taste.

Preparation.—The dried seeds are powdered and covered with five parts by weight of alcohol. After mixing well, and pouring it into a well-stoppered bottle, it is allowed to stand eight days in a dark, cool place, shaking it twice a day. The tincture is then poured off, strained and filtered.

Drug power of tincture, $\frac{1}{10}$.

Dilutions must be prepared as directed under Class IV.

ABIES CANADENSIS, *Michaux.*

Synonym, Pinus Canadensis, *Willd.*
Nat. Ord., Coniferæ.
Common Names, Hemlock Spruce, Canada Pitch.

A well known evergreen tree found in rocky woods in British America and the United States as far south as the Alleghenies. It is commonly from 70 to 80 feet high. The trunk is straight and from two to three feet in diameter. The leaves are linear, small, flat, obscurely denticulate, spreading in two directions, making apparently two rows. The cones are ovoid, slightly longer than the leaves, terminal and pendulous.

The first provings were made under direction of Dr. Gatchell.

Preparation.—The fresh bark and young buds are pounded to a pulp and weighed. Then two parts by weight of alcohol are taken, and after mixing the pulp thoroughly with one-sixth part of it, the rest of the alcohol is added. After having stirred the whole well, and having poured it into a well-stoppered bottle, it is allowed to stand eight days in a dark, cool place. The tincture is then separated by decanting, straining and filtering.

Drug power of tincture, $\frac{1}{6}$.

Dilutions must be prepared as directed under Class III.

ABIES NIGRA, *Poiret.*

Nat. Ord., Coniferæ.

Common Name, Black or Double Spruce.

A tree found growing in swamps and cold mountain woods in northern United States and Canada. Its leaves are short, being six or eight lines long, either dark green or glaucous-whitish. Cones ovoid, being one to one and one-half inches long, mostly recurved, persistent, the scales with a thin, often erosely-dentate edge.

The first provings were made under direction of Dr. Leaman.

Preparation.—Two parts by weight of the gum are dissolved in nine parts by weight of 95 per cent. alcohol and designated as mother tincture.

Drug power of tincture, $\frac{1}{10}$.

Dilutions must be prepared as directed under Class VI—*a*.

ABROTANUM.

Synonym, Artemisia Abrotanum, *Linn.*

Nat. Ord., Compositæ.

Common Name, Southernwood.

A shrub, native of southern Europe and the Levant. It is about three feet in height, leaves bi-pinnatifid, the young leaves covered with whitish silky hairs. The taste is burning, sharp and bitter; the odor aromatic mixed with that of lemons.

Preparation.—The fresh leaves gathered in July and August are chopped and pounded to a pulp and weighed. Then two parts by weight of alcohol are taken, and having mixed the pulp thoroughly with one-sixth part of it, the rest of the alcohol is added. After having stirred the whole well, and having poured it into a well-stoppered bottle, it is allowed to stand eight days in a dark, cool place. The tincture is then separated by decanting, straining and filtering.

Drug power of tincture, $\frac{1}{6}$.

Dilutions must be prepared as directed under Class III.

ABSINTHIUM.

Synonyms, Artemisia Absinthium, *Linn.* Absinthium Vulgare, *Lamarck.*

Nat. Ord., Compositæ.

Common Name, Common Wormwood.

A shrub three or four feet high, growing wild in Europe in dry, stony places; naturalized in New England. Leaves bi and tri-pinnatifid; the uppermost ones undivided, all silky-hairy.

The flower heads are yellow, nodding, hemispherical. Taste very bitter; odor strong and root-like.

The first proving was made under Dr. Gatchell's directions.

Preparation.—The fresh young leaves and blossoms are chopped and pounded to a pulp and weighed. Then two parts by weight of alcohol are taken, and having mixed the pulp thoroughly with one-sixth part of it, the rest of the alcohol is added. After having stirred the whole well, and having poured it into a well-stoppered bottle, it is allowed to stand eight days in a dark, cool place. The tincture is then separated by decanting, straining and filtering.

Drug power of tincture, $\frac{1}{6}$.

Dilutions must be prepared as directed under Class III.

ACALYPHA INDICA, *Linn.*

Nat. Ord., Euphorbiaceæ.

Common Name, Indian Acalypha.

This plant, growing one or two feet high, is found in the East Indies. In appearance it resembles the Nettle or Amaranth.

Preparation.—The fresh plant is pounded to a pulp and weighed. Then two parts by weight of alcohol are taken, and after thoroughly mixing the pulp with one-sixth part of it, the rest of the alcohol is added. After having stirred the whole well, and having poured it into a well-stoppered bottle, it is allowed to stand eight days in a dark, cool place. The tincture is then separated by decanting, straining and filtering.

Drug power of tincture, $\frac{1}{6}$.

Dilutions must be prepared as directed under Class III.

ACIDUM ACETICUM GLACIALE.

Present Name, Glacial Acetic Acid.

Formula, $C_2 H_4 O_2$.

(Concentrated Acetic Acid, corresponding to at least 84 per cent. of anhydrous acid. Br.)

Preparation of Glacial Acetic Acid.—Of pure crystallized sodium acetate ten parts are taken and by heat deprived of its water of crystallization. The residue, less than six parts, is upon cooling, broken up and placed in a glass tubulated retort upon a sand-bath and warmed to a temperature of 120° F. Then eight parts of pure concentrated sulphuric acid are added, the retort connected with a receiver by suitable apparatus, and the contents submitted to distillation.

The sulphuric acid unites with the sodium of the sodium acetate, forming acid sodium sulphate, and pure anhydrous acetic acid is distilled over into the receiver, which should be kept cool. If the heat be too great, and especially toward the last of the process, sulphurous oxide, carbonic oxide and carbonaceous compounds will be apt to come over and contaminate the product.

Properties.—Glacial acetic acid crystallizes near the freezing-point of water (34° F.), and remains crystalline until the temperature rises to above 9° C. (48° F.); it contains, then, about one per cent. of water, or not less than 84 per cent. of acetic anhydrid. At the ordinary temperatures it is a colorless liquid with a pungent acetous odor, and vesicates the skin. When heated to boiling (248° F.), the vapor is inflammable and burns with a blue flame. Its specific gravity is 1.065. As it is hygroscopic it should be kept in well-stoppered bottles.

Tests.—Pure acetic acid should leave no residue on evaporation. Empyreumatic matter is best detected by neutralizing the acid with sodium carbonate and then adding a small quantity of a solution of potassium permanganate. If the latter loses its color, and afterward a brown precipitate deposits, empyreumatic matter is present. Hydrogen sulphide, solution of silver nitrate and solution of barium nitrate must not color or cloud the acid when diluted. Solution of indigo must not lose its color when heated with the acid.

Preparation for Homœopathic Use.—One part by weight of pure glacial acetic acid is dissolved in nine parts by weight of distilled water.

Amount of drug power, $\frac{1}{10}$.

Dilutions must be prepared as directed under Class V—*a*.

ACIDUM BENZOICUM.

Present Name, Benzoic Acid.

Formula, $HC_7H_5O_2$.

Molecular Weight, 122.

Preparation of Benzoic Acid.—Take of benzoin in coarse powder any quantity. Spread it in a layer not thicker than three centimetres upon the bottom of a shallow iron pan, covered with filtering paper luted or pasted to the outside. Over the whole is placed a long cone of white card-board. Upon the application of heat by means of a sand-bath, the benzoic acid sublimes and condenses upon the inner surface of the cone.

Properties.—Benzoic acid exists in permanent, white feathery, soft light plates, or occasionally six-sided needles. When prepared as above it has the odor of gum benzoin from a small portion of volatile oil which has been condensed with the crystals. It fuses at 121° C. (249.5° F.) but under water at 100° C. (212° F.), its vapor coming off readily with the steam. The vapor irritates the air-passages.

Tests.—If carefully heated on platinum foil, benzoic acid melts to a colorless or yellowish fluid, finally vaporizing with combustion and leaving no residue. The presence of hippuric acid is indicated by the reddish color when fused on platinum, or by a slight carbonaceous residue. If the latter be considerable, sugar or a tartrate has been present. Non-carbonaceous residue shows mineral matters. If one-fifth of a gramme be well shaken with ten centimetres of distilled water and the mixture then tinged a dark red with solution of potassium permanganate, the color will not change inside of five minutes, but it will do so immediately if hippuric acid or benzoic acid made from urine, or cinnamic acid be present.

It was first proven by Dr. Jeanes.

Preparation for Homœopathic Use.—One part by weight of pure benzoic acid is dissolved in nine parts by weight of alcohol.

Amount of drug power, $\frac{1}{10}$.

Dilutions must be prepared as directed under Class VI—*a*.

Triturations of the pure benzoic acid are prepared as directed under Class VII.

ACIDUM BORACICUM.

Present Name, Boracic Acid. Boric Acid.

Formula, $H_3 BO_3$.

Molecular Weight, 62.

Preparation of Boracic Acid.—It is prepared by decomposing borax in a hot solution by adding thereto hydrochloric acid.

Properties.—It crystallizes out on evaporation in small white, silky-looking, six-sided scales, which feel greasy to the touch, without odor and having a scarcely perceptible acid taste; when heated it melts in its own water of crystallization and leaves a hard, glass-like mass. The acid is soluble in three parts of boiling water, in twenty-six parts at ordinary temperatures, and in six parts of alcohol.

Tests.—Its alcoholic solution burns with a green flame; a solution in water imparts a brown color to turmeric paper, and faintly reddens blue litmus paper, and is precipitated by nitrate of silver or chloride of barium, the precipitates redissolving if a large amount of water be added.

Preparation for Homœopathic Use.—The pure boracic acid is prepared by trituration, as directed under Class VII.

ACIDUM BROMICUM.

Present Names, Hydrogen Bromide. Hydrobromic Acid.

Formula, HBr.

Molecular Weight, 81.

Preparation of Hydrobromic Acid.—By the action of sulphuric acid upon bromides of the alkalies the bromine is liberated and unites with the hydrogen of the acid, thus forming hydrogen bromide; at the same time is formed a sulphate of the base. A solution of equal parts of potassium bromide and water is made, and there is added to it gradually and cautiously a little more than one part of strong sulphuric acid. Heat materially assists the reaction. The mixture is suffered to cool, when if water be not in excess, crystals of potassium sulphate will crystallize out in a few days. The supernatant liquid is then poured into a glass retort and submitted to distillation, nearly to dryness. The distillate is a solution of hydrobromic acid in water, and its strength must be determined by the usual methods. The solution may be standardized by dilution with water to a specific gravity of 1.203.

Properties.—Pure hydrobromic acid is a colorless, highly acid, pungent gas; it fumes in moist air and is freely soluble in water. The solution as prepared under the above given directions is a colorless, transparent liquid without odor, and has a strongly acid reaction. It should be kept in dark bottles and examined occasionally to see if any decomposition has taken place, which will be indicated by its acquiring a yellow color.

Tests.—It should leave no residue upon evaporation. Silver nitrate produces a white precipitate which is insoluble in dilute nitric acid and somewhat sparingly soluble in ammonia, but freely in potassium cyanide.

Preparation for Homœopathic Use.—One part by weight of pure hydrobromic acid is dissolved in nine parts by weight of distilled water.

Amount of drug power, $\frac{1}{10}$.

Dilutions must be prepared as directed under Class V—*a*.

ACIDUM CARBOLICUM.

Synonyms, Phenic Acid, Phenylic Alcohol, Phenol.
Present Name, Carbolic Acid.
Formula, $HC_6 H_5 O$.
Molecular Weight, 94.

Origin.—Carbolic acid occurs in coal tar products, in the urine of man and herbivorous animals, and by the dry distillation of Salicin, Salicylic acid, Benzoin, and many organic bodies.

Preparation of Carbolic Acid.—When coal tar (one of the secondary products of gas manufacture) is subjected to distillation, there first comes over a mixture of hydro-carbons which are lighter than water; as the process continues and the temperature rises, a yellow oil distils over, which is heavier than water, and is commonly called *dead oil.*

The *dead oil* is submitted to distillation, and the product which comes over between the temperatures 300° and 400° F. contains carbolic acid. In order to extract the acid from the distillate, the latter is shaken with a hot concentrated solution of potassium hydrate and some of the solid hydrate. A white crystalline mass is deposited which is separated from the liquid portion and treated with a little water, thus forming a solution of so-called carbolate of potash; this is separated from a quantity of oil which floats above it, and decomposed with hydrochloric acid, when the carbolic acid appears as an oily layer upon the surface of the liquid. The latter is drawn off, digested with a little fused calcium chloride to remove the water, and distilled.

The distilled liquid, when exposed to a low temperature, solidifies to a mass of long, colorless needles which may be again liquefied at the temperature of the hand.

Properties.—Absolutely pure carbolic acid has no smell of creosote; its odor is described as peculiar and slightly aromatic. The crystals liquefy at about 40° C. (104° F.); the acid boils at about 181° C. (357.8° F.). The presence of a small amount of water hinders the crystallization by cold. It is soluble in fifteen parts of water; is freely soluble in alcohol, ether, glacial acetic acid, chloroform, carbon disulphide, and the ethereal and fatty oils.

Tests.—It is indifferent to litmus paper. A slip of deal wood dipped in it and afterward into hydrochloric acid and dried, acquires a greenish-blue color. Upon treating the acid with a little aniline and then adding solution of sodium hypochlorite, a fine blue color is produced, and one of the best tests is by the use of bromine water in excess, when a yellow-white, flocky precipitate of tri-brom-phenol is thrown down.

Preparation for Homœopathic Use.—One part by weight of pure crystallized carbolic acid is dissolved in nine parts by weight of alcohol.

Amount of drug power, $\frac{1}{10}$.

Dilutions must be prepared as directed under Class VI—*a*.

ACIDUM CHROMICUM.

Present Name, Chromic Anhydride. Improperly termed Chromic Acid.

Formula, $Cr\,O_3$.

Molecular Weight, 100.5.

Preparation of Chromic Acid.—Dissolve ten parts of potassium bichromate in seventeen parts of boiling distilled water; add gradually and cautiously, with constant stirring by means of a glass rod, twenty-five parts of pure concentrated sulphuric acid; let stand for one day, and remove the crystals of potassium disulphate which will have formed. Warm the liquid over a water-bath and add carefully fifteen parts of concentrated sulphuric acid, and put aside for twenty-four hours. The crystals of chromic anhydride may now be collected in a funnel partly filled with broken glass or with glass-wool. The crystals may be rendered perfectly free from water by suffering them to drain upon unglazed earthenware plates in a drying-room. They are then to be transferred to dry bottles and hermetically sealed.

Properties.—Chromic anhydride comes in fine crimson needles, which are very deliquescent and extremely soluble in water and alcohol; the solutions have the color of the crystals, but this is fainter, according to the degree of dilution.

Upon heating they darken in color, becoming almost black, but upon cooling again the original color returns. They melt at a temperature of 300° C. (572° F.), and if the heat be increased, they are decomposed into chromic oxide and free oxygen.

Chromic anhydride is an energetic oxidizer, giving up oxygen readily, especially upon contact with organic matter. With anhydrous alcohol, the action is so intense that flame is produced. In all these cases the anhydride is reduced as above stated.

Tests.—The only impurities likely to be present in the crystals are potassium bichromate and sulphuric acid. The former will be determined by its not dissolving in cold dilute alcohol; the latter, by first boiling the chromic anhydride with a large excess of dilute hydrochloric acid, and gradually adding dilute alcohol till all the chromic anhydride is reduced to chromic oxide. The fluid is then to be treated with two volumes of water and tested with barium chloride. If sulphuric acid be present, a white precipitate will occur which may be only in sufficient amount to cause mere cloudiness.

Preparation for Homœopathic Use.—One part by weight of pure chromic acid is dissolved in nine parts by weight of distilled water.

Amount of drug power, $\frac{1}{10}$.

Dilutions must be prepared as directed under Class V—*a*.

ACIDUM CHRYSOPHANICUM.

Present Name, Chrysophanic Acid.

Formula, $C_{15} H_{10} O_4$.

Molecular Weight, 254.

Source.—Chrysophanic acid is the chief constituent of *Goa powder*, in which it exists to the amount of eighty-four per cent. It is also found in *Rumex crispus*, in the root of *Rheum officinale*, and in the yellow lichen, *Parmelia parietina*.

Preparation of Chrysophanic Acid.—As the acid is almost insoluble in cold water, Goa powder is first treated with the latter, to remove all substances soluble therein; the residue is then treated with benzol and from the benzol solution chrysophanic acid crystallizes out.

Properties.—Pure chrysophanic acid, from benzol solution, is in pale or orange-yellow monoclinic prisms; from alcoholic solution, in orange-yellow matted needles. The crystals are without odor and almost without taste. They melt at 162° C. (323. 6° F.), but crystalize again on cooling; at a higher temperature a small portion sublimes in golden-yellow needles, but the greater part is carbonized; the acid is very slightly soluble in cold water; somewhat more so in boiling water, to which it gives a yellow color. It dissolves in 1125 parts of alcohol at 30° C. (86° F.), but in 224 parts of boiling alcohol. It is readily soluble in benzol, ether, glacial acetic acid and amyl alcohol.

Tests.—Concentrated sulphuric acid dissolves it with a red color, from which solution it separates out in yellow flocks upon the addition of water. A solution of a caustic alkali dissolves it with a beautiful dark red color, the solution upon evaporation changing in color to violet-blue. By the addition of an acid to the alkaline solution the chrysophanic acid precipitates in yellow flocks.

Preparation for Homœopathic Use.—The pure chrysophanic acid is prepared by trituration as directed under Class VII.

ACIDUM CITRICUM.

Present Name, Citric Acid.

Formula, $C_6 H_8 O_7$.

Molecular Weight, 210.

Citric acid occurs in lemons, oranges and most acidulous fruits and vegetables. It is in these cases generally accompanied by other organic acids. It is in large amount in the juice of the lemon, oranges and allied species.

Preparation of Citric Acid.—Take hot lemon juice and add gradually to it powdered chalk till the acid is neutralized. The resulting calcium citrate is thrown on a filter and washed with hot water till the washings run clear. The filtrate is then mixed with enough cold water to give bulk, and then is added a mixture of one part sulphuric acid with twelve of water, until the calcium has all become a sulphate. The mixture is then boiled, filtered, evaporated to specific gravity 1.210, and finally set aside to crystallize. Iron vessels, or those made in part of iron, should be avoided in the preparation of citric acid.

Properties.—Citric acid is in rhombic prisms with dihedral ends, the surfaces of the latter being trapezoidal; by the latter circumstance the crystals are distinguished from those of tartaric acid. They are permanent in dry air, colorless, odorless and of an intensely acid taste. At the ordinary temperature they are soluble in their own bulk of water, and in half that amount of boiling water; in their own volume of 90 per cent. alcohol and not at all in absolute ether. A watery solution decomposes readily, producing acetic acid and developing a mouldy growth. At 100° C. (212° F.) the crystals dissolve in their water of crystallization; at about 175° C. (347° F.) they are decomposed into water, carbonous and carbonic oxides, acetone and aconitic acid. When heated to carbonization, citric acid, unlike tartaric acid, develops no caramel odor.

Tests.—The usual impurities found in citric acid are, sulphuric acid, lime and traces of lead. A systematic method of testing the purity of the acid is as follows: Dissolve a large crystal and a few small ones with some fragments of broken crystals, in ten times their bulk of distilled water. One part of the solution is treated with hydrogen sulphide; no alteration of color or no precipitate shows absence of lead. Should, however, lead be present in mere traces, the reaction will not be manifest till after the solution has been treated with caustic ammonia in excess. A second portion tested with lead acetate will give a precipitate which, however, will not be dissolved by nitric acid if sulphuric acid be present. Lime is best detected by incinerating some crystals of the acid and testing the ash in the usual way. The presence of tartaric acid, which is not infrequently used as an adulterant in citric acid, will be shown by adding to a solution of the suspected acid a small quantity of potassium acetate, when a white crystalline precipitate of cream of tartar will be thrown down. Lime water added in excess to a solution of citric acid produces no precipitate in the cold, but upon boiling for some time a white precipitate is formed.

Preparation for Homœopathic Use.—The pure citric acid is prepared by trituration, as directed under Class VII.

ACIDUM FLUORICUM.

Present Names, Hydrogen Fluoride. Hydrofluoric Acid. Fluoric Acid.

Formula, HF.

Molecular Weight, 20.

Preparation.—When powdered fluor spar is mixed with twice its weight of concentrated sulphuric acid and heated in a leaden retort whose neck fits tightly into a leaden condensing tube kept cool by a mixture of ice and salt around it, a colorless liquid distils over, and only calcium sulphate is found in the retort. The distillate is the so-called hydrofluoric acid, but as yet not quite pure. It combines eagerly with fluorides of potassium and sodium and upon this fact its further purification depends. By heating dry potassium hydrofluorate to redness in a platinum still, there is obtained a colorless liquid, which boils at 19.5° C. (67° F.) and at about 12.8° C. (55° F.) has specific gravity 0.988. It unites with water with great violence; dissolves all ordinary metals except gold, platinum, silver, mercury and lead, and has a remarkable affinity for silica, uniting with it in even its most refractory form.

Test.—A piece of glass thinly coated with beeswax, and from which the beeswax has been in parts removed, will, when "flowed" with an aqueous solution of the acid, be etched or "eaten in" wherever the glass has been exposed to its action. Caution is required when experimenting with it or using it in any way. Its vapors are extraordinarily injurious to the air passages, and the liquid, if dropped upon the skin, causes long lasting, very painful, almost incurable sores.

The first provings were made under direction of Dr. C. Hering.

Preparation for Homœopathic Use.—One part by weight of pure fluoric acid is dissolved in 99 parts by weight of distilled water, and must be preserved in gutta-percha vials.

Amount of drug power, $\frac{1}{100}$.

Dilutions must be prepared as directed under Class V—β, except that distilled water must be used for all dilutions to the 3 or 6x, gutta-percha vials being employed for diluting as well as for preserving.

ACIDUM FORMICICUM.

Present Name, Formic Acid.

Formula, $CH_2 O_2$.

Molecular Weight, 46.

Origin.—The name "formic acid" is derived from that of the red ant (*Formica rufa*), from which the acid was first obtained; it also exists in the hairs of a caterpillar (*Bombyx processionea*), in some other insects, in the needles of the pine, in stinging nettles, in old oil of turpentine; it is found in minute quantity in sweat and urine, and can be produced by the oxidation of many organic substances.

Preparation.—Preferably, by heating oxalic acid with glycerine. Pure concentrated glycerine is added to crystallized oxalic acid in a retort. Upon heating a little above 100° C. (212° F.) decomposition ensues, with the production of carbonic oxide, which escapes, and dilute formic acid which distils over. When the production of the gas ceases, more oxalic acid is added and the heating continued, upon which a stronger formic acid passes over, and on further addition of oxalic acid, an acid of constant strength is obtained. The dilute acid may be rendered water-free by heating dried oxalic acid in it and allowing the solution to crystallize. The oxalic acid retains the water, and by decanting the liquid from the crystals and redistilling, pure formic acid is obtained.

Properties.—In the pure state it is a clear, colorless liquid, fuming slightly in the air, and having a very penetrating odor; it is corrosive, and upon the skin it raises blisters and causes wounds similar to those produced by burns. It boils at 100° C. (212° F.) and at 0° C. (32° F.) it solidifies to a white crystalline mass, whose specific gravity is 1.235. It mixes with water, alcohol and ether, in all proportions, but the alcoholic solutions will be found to contain some ethyl formate.

Preparation for Homœopathic Use.—One part by weight of pure formic acid is dissolved in nine parts by weight of distilled water.

Amount of drug power, $\frac{1}{10}$.

Dilutions must be prepared as directed under Class V—*a*.

ACIDUM GALLICUM.

Present Name, Gallic Acid.

Formula, $C_7\,H_6\,O_5,\,H_2O$.

Molecular Weight, 188.

Origin.—Gallic acid is found in nut-galls, sumach, hellebore root, tea, pomegranate root, and in many other plants.

Preparation of Gallic Acid.—Powdered galls are moistened with water to a thin magma, and set aside for five or six weeks in a warm place; fermentation occurs and an impure gallic acid is one of the results. This is treated with three times its weight of water, boiled to dissolve the gallic acid, filtered, and the solution set aside to cool; the deposited gallic acid is collected, drained, pressed between folds of bibulous paper to remove any mother liquor, and if necessary, purified by recrystallization from water, or by solution in hot water with animal charcoal. On filtering and cooling, most of the acid separates in the form of slender acicular crystals, which are white or fawn-colored.

Properties.—Gallic acid is in silky acicular crystals, whose taste is astringent and weakly acid. They are without odor.

The acid is soluble in 100 parts of cold water and in ten parts of 90 per cent. alcohol. At the temperature of boiling water, the crystals give up their water of crystallization, amounting to 9.58 per cent.

When heated to about 215° C. (419° F.) they break up into pyrogallic acid and carbonic oxide.

Solution of gallic acid when exposed for some time to the air decomposes, evolving carbonic oxide and precipitating a blackish substance.

The solution of gallic acid reddens blue litmus paper.

Tests.—Gallic acid is distinguished from tannin by its crystalline structure; tannin is entirely amorphous; gallic acid does not precipitate either albumen or gelatine from their solutions, as does tannin.

Preparation for Homœopathic Use.—The pure gallic acid is prepared by trituration, as directed under Class VII.

ACIDUM HYDROCYANICUM.

Present Name, Hydrogen Cyanide, Hydrocyanic Acid.

Common Name, Prussic Acid.

Formula, HCN or HCy.

Molecular Weight, 27.

Origin.—Hydrocyanic acid can be obtained from many members of the vegetable kingdom; in some it exists free, in others—and probably the greater number—it cannot be found till after the plant, or part of it used for this purpose, has been crushed and treated with water.

In these cases a nitrogenous body, Amygdalin, is decomposed under the influence of a ferment, such as Emulsin or Synaptase, present in the organic structure.

The acid is known to exist ready formed in the juice of the bitter cassava; it is obtainable from the bitter almond, the kernels of plums and peaches, seeds of the apple, the cherry laurel, etc.

Preparation of Hydrocyanic Acid.—The usual method of preparing the acid is as follows: In a small, tubulated retort dissolve two ounces of potassium ferro-cyanide in powder in ten ounces of water and add one fluid ounce of sulphuric acid previously diluted with four ounces of water and cooled. Transfer the solution to a glass retort with condenser and receiver attached. Place in the receiver eight ounces of distilled water (condenser and receiver must be kept cold). Apply heat by means of a sand bath, and distil slowly till the liquid in the receiver has increased to seventeen fluid ounces. Add to this three ounces of distilled water, or as much as may be required to bring the acid to the standard strength, in which 100 grains of the acid, precipitated with a solution of silver nitrate, will yield 10 grains of dry silver cyanide. So prepared and so diluted it is the standard hydrocyanic acid used in medicine.

Properties of the Medicinal Acid.—The officinal hydrocyanic acid is a volatile liquid perfectly clear and colorless. It reacts weakly acid to test paper and only temporarily. The acid has a peculiar odor, resembling that of bitter almonds, and somewhat pungent. It is apt to decompose after being kept some time, and should in all cases be carefully excluded from light.

Tests.—As the acid is, even when dilute, very unstable, it should be tested first as to its identity. To the liquid supposed to contain HCy, is added a few drops of a solution of ferrous sulphate, and then potassium hydrate in excess. After exposure to the air for fifteen minutes with frequent agitation, hydrochloric acid is added in excess, which dissolves the already precipitated ferrous-ferric hydrate, leaving undissolved the ferric ferro-cyanide or Prussian blue. If the amount of the HCy be minute, the solution so tested will, after the addition of HCl in excess, only appear green, the blue precipitate not settling down for some time.

If a specimen of the acid reddens litmus paper strongly or permanently, showing the presence of other acid, it should be rejected. Sulphuric or hydrochloric acid, if present, may be detected by the barium chloride or the silver nitrate test, in the usual way.

The first provings were made by Dr. Jörg and his pupils.

Preparation for Homœopathic Use.—The officinal hydrocyanic acid (containing about 2 per cent. of the anhydrous acid) is mixed with equal parts by weight of distilled water.

Amount of drug power, $\frac{1}{100}$.

Dilutions must be prepared as directed under Class VI—β.

ACIDUM LACTICUM.

Present Name, Lactic Acid.

Formula, $C_3 H_6 O_3$.

Molecular Weight, 90.

Origin.—The acidity of sour milk depends upon the presence of an acid produced by the transformation of sugar of milk into lactic acid by the influence of the decomposing casein, the chief albuminous body contained in milk.

The acid may also be produced from other sugars by the same ferment, and is found free in many vegetable substances in a state of decomposition.

Preparation of Lactic Acid.—Dissolve eight parts of cane sugar in fifty parts of water, and to the mixture add one part of poor cheese and three parts of chalk. The whole is then set aside and allowed to stand for five or six weeks at a temperature of 26.6° C. (80° F.). The lactic acid formed from the cane sugar under the influence of the changing casein in the cheese, combines with the lime of the chalk, forming crystals of calcium lactate and disengaging carbonic oxide. At the end of the process, the crystals are collected, dissolved in boiling water and recrystallized, and digested with one-third their weight of sulphuric acid, thus converting the lime into sulphate and setting free the lactic acid. Upon the addition of alcohol, the whole of the calcium sulphate is precipitated and the lactic acid dissolved; upon evaporating the alcohol, the lactic acid remains behind.

Properties.—Lactic acid is a colorless, or very slightly yellowish, odorless, transparent liquid, of syrupy consistency. It is strongly acid to the taste and to litmus paper. It is soluble in all proportions in water and alcohol, less so in ether.

Tests.—The best means of determining the identity of lactic acid is by producing some of its salts and examining their form under the microscope. Zinc lactate when deposited quickly from its solutions shows under the microscope needles aggregated in spherical masses. For impurities the following may be used: When mixed with equal volumes of alcohol and ether, a clear solution is evidence of the absence of lactates, mannite, sugar and gum. Treated with zinc oxide in excess and heated, and then extracted with absolute alcohol and the filtrate evaporated, a sweet residue is, if present, glycerine. When treated with solutions of hydrogen sulphide, barium chloride, silver nitrate and ammonium oxalate, it should give no precipitate; and when heated, it should give neither the odor of acetic nor of butyric acid.

Preparation for Homœopathic Use.—One part by weight of pure lactic acid is dissolved in 99 parts by weight of alcohol.

Amount of drug power, $\frac{1}{100}$.

Dilutions must be prepared as directed under Class VI—β.

ACIDUM MOLYBDÆNICUM.

Present Name, Molybdic tri-oxide, Molybdic Acid.

Formula, $Mo\,O_3$.

Molecular Weight, 144.

Preparation of Molybdic Acid.—To obtain this acid, calcine sulphide of molybdenum at a red heat in an open vessel, and neutralize the acid by means of caustic ammonia. To free it from this combination, precipitate it by nitric or acetic acid, or expose the compound to a high heat, and wash the acid obtained in water, dry and melt it in a glass vessel or a platinum crucible.

Properties.—This is a white porous, light mass, fusible, volatile, becoming yellow at a high temperature, and white again on cooling, of a metallic taste, soluble in 570 parts of cold water.

Test.—For identification dissolve molybdic acid in ammonia, dilute with water and dilute solution of phosphoric acid. A yellow precipitate indicates molybdic acid.

Preparation for Homœopathic Use.—The pure molybdic acid is prepared by trituration, as directed under Class VII.

ACIDUM MURIATICUM.

Synonyms.—Hydrogen Chloride. Hydrochloric Acid. Acidum Hydrochloridum. Muriatic Acid.

Present Name, Hydrochloric Acid.

Common Name, Spirit of Salt.

Formula, HCl.

Molecular Weight, 36.5.

Ordinary muriatic acid is a solution of HCl *gas* in water. It is, at times, erroneously called *liquid* muriatic acid, but *aqueous* muriatic acid would be a better term.

Origin.—Hydrochloric acid occurs free among the gases emanating from active volcanoes, and sometimes in the spring and river waters of volcanic districts. Commercially it is always prepared by the decomposition of sodium chloride and of ammonium chloride.

Preparation of Muriatic Acid.—"Take of chloride of sodium, dried, forty-eight ounces (avoirdupois); sulphuric acid, forty-four fluid-ounces; water, thirty-six fluid-ounces; distilled water, fifty fluid-ounces. Pour the sulphuric acid slowly into thirty-two fluid-ounces of the water, and when the mixture has cooled, add it to the chloride of sodium previously introduced into a flask having the capacity of at least one gallon (imp. measure). Connect the flask by corks and a bent glass tube with a three-necked wash-bottle, furnished with a safety tube, and containing the remaining four fluid-ounces of the water; then, applying heat to the flask, conduct the disengaged gas through the wash-bottle, into a second bottle containing the distilled water, by means of a bent tube dipping about half an inch below the surface; and let the process be continued until the product measures sixty-six fluid-ounces, or the liquid has acquired a specific gravity of 1.16. The bottle containing the distilled water must be kept cool during the whole operation." (Br. P.)

Properties of the Pure Acid.—Officinal muriatic acid, when pure, is a transparent colorless liquid, having a suffocating odor and extremely corrosive properties. It fumes in the air. The strongest hydrochloric acid, specific gravity 1.21, contains 43 per cent. of HCl gas, and upon heating evolves the latter till specific gravity is reduced to 1.10 and the liquid contains 20 per cent. of the gas. After this the liquid distils over unchanged.

Tests.—Chiefly to determine the presence or absence of arsenic, sulphurous and sulphuric acids, free chlorine, nitrous oxides, zinc and iron chlorides. The test for arsenic and for sulphurous acid may be done by Hager's method in one operation. 4 or 5 CC. of hydrochloric acid are placed in a test tube, and diluted with an equal volume of distilled water. A piece of chemically pure zinc is dropped into the test tube and the latter loosely closed by a cork, into the internal face of which have been inserted two strips of filtering paper, one moistened with lead acetate solution, the other with silver nitrate solution. Should the latter be blackened, the presence of arsenic is indicated; if the lead paper shows a darkening, sulphurous acid is present.

Dilute with two volumes of distilled water and test for sulphuric acid, by means of barium chloride solution; a white precipitate, insoluble in nitric acid, shows sulphuric acid; for free chlorine or nitrous oxides, by means of starch and potassium iodide solution, a blue coloration shows either free chlorine or nitrous oxides present, or perhaps both. Iron may be detected by potassium sulphocyanide solution, a slight addition of which will cause a red coloration. Upon evaporating a few drachms of the acid in a platinum dish, the absence of any residue shows absence of salts, including those of the above metals.

The first provings were made under Hahnemann's directions.

Preparation for Homœopathic Use.—One part by weight of pure muriatic acid (specific gravity 1.16) is dissolved in two parts by weight of distilled water.

Amount of drug power, $\frac{1}{10}$.
Dilutions must be prepared as directed under Class V—*a*.

ACIDUM NITRICUM.

Synonym, Aqua Fortis.
Present Names, Hydrogen Nitrate. Nitric Acid.
Formula, HNO_3.
Molecular Weight, 63.
Nitric acid, of the specific gravity 1.420.

Nitric acid is never found free in nature, except in very minute amount. But in combination with a base, it is found in the vegetable and in great abundance in the mineral kingdom. When nitrogenous animal substances undergo decomposition, ammonia is formed, and in the presence of water and a base, oxidation ensues, with the production of water and nitric acid; the latter uniting with the base, a nitrate results. By treating the nitrate with sulphuric acid, nitric acid is displaced and set free, and at the same time a sulphate is formed.

Preparation of Nitric Acid.—On a small scale, in the laboratory, nitric acid is prepared by distilling potassium nitrate with an equal weight of concentrated sulphuric acid. The capacity of the retort should be such that the mixture will not more than two-thirds fill it. As soon as the acid has well soaked into the nitre, a gradually increasing heat may be applied by means of the sand-bath, when the acid will distil over. At the beginning and towards the end of the operation the retort becomes filled with a red vapor. This is due to the decomposition, by heat, of a portion of the colorless vapor of nitric acid, into water, oxygen and nitrogen tetroxide.

General Properties.—The strongest nitric acid obtainable has a specific gravity 1.52, and is not entirely water-free, containing about 15 per cent. The officinal nitric acid of the United States and British pharmacopœias has specific gravity 1.42; it is a colorless, transparent liquid and at the ordinary atmospheric pressure, has a definite boiling point, 120.5° C. (249° F.).

The acid is strongly corrosive. Under the influence of light it suffers decomposition from the liberation of oxygen and the formation of the lower oxides of nitrogen, which latter impart a yellow color to it. Animal tissues are stained permanently yellow by it, from the picric acid produced. Many vegetable matters are transformed by it into violently explosive bodies.

The first provings were made under Hahnemann's directions.

Tests.—The acid, diluted with two volumes of distilled water, should give no precipitate when treated with barium nitrate or silver nitrate in solution, otherwise the presence of sulphuric or hydrochloric acid, respectively, is shown. When agitated in a test tube with chloroform and afterward treated with hydrogen sulphide it should remain colorless; a reddening in the first case indicates the presence of iodine, in the latter of iodic acid. It should evaporate without residue.

Preparation for Homœopathic Use.—One part by weight of pure nitric acid (specific gravity 1.42) is dissolved in nine parts by weight of distilled water.

Amount of drug power, $\frac{1}{10}$.

Dilutions must be prepared as directed under Class V—*a*.

ACIDUM OXALICUM.

Present Names, Hydrogen Oxalate. Oxalic Acid.

Formula, $H_2C_2O_4$, $2H_2O$.

Molecular Weight, 126.

Origin and Formation.—Oxalic acid is found in combination with iron in the mineral Humboldtite, in the vegetable kingdom, combined with potassium in *Oxalis*, *Rumex* and their allies, with sodium in *Salicornia* and *Salsola* and their relatives, and with calcium in rhubarb and many lichens. It is also found in considerable quantity in guano, in combination with ammonia and calcium. It can be produced artificially by the oxidation of many organic non-nitrogenous bodies.

Preparation.—Oxalic acid is manufactured on a large scale by oxidizing saw-dust with a mixture of potassium hydrate and sodium hydrate. It is found that the latter will not produce oxalic acid without the presence of the former, and to use this alone would be too expensive. A mixture is made of one part, by their molecular weights, of the potassium to two parts of the sodium hydrate. The solution should have specific gravity 1.35. It is then made into a thick paste with saw-dust, and heated upon iron plates for several hours. The water in the alkaline hydrate is decomposed, hydrogen is given off, and the oxygen converts the wood into oxalic acid. On treating the mass with cold water a quantity of sodium oxalate is left undissolved; this is boiled with calcium hydrate, thus forming sodium hydrate and calcium oxalate, the latter being insoluble. The calcium oxalate is now decomposed with dilute sulphuric acid, the sparingly soluble calcium sulphate being produced. This is removed, and the solution on evaporation yields crystals of oxalic acid.

Properties.—Oxalic acid separates from a hot aqueous solution in colorless transparent crystals derived from an oblique rhombic prism. They are easily soluble in water and alcohol; are without odor and have an intensely acid taste. With a slight increase of temperature they lose their water of crystallization and crumble to a white powder. At a high temperature, a part decomposes into carbon monoxide, carbon di-oxide and water, another part into carbon di-oxide and formic acid, and a third part sublimes unchanged.

The remedy was first introduced by Dr. Koch, Sr.

Tests.—The dryness of the crystals will show the absence of sulphuric, nitric and saccharic acids; upon incinerating in a platinum dish the absence of ash will indicate freedom from mineral salts; a special test for nitric acid, if present, is indigo solution; for sulphuric acid, barium chloride; extraneous organic matters, will be evidenced by their carbonization when the crystals are heated with sulphuric acid.

Preparation for Homœopathic Use.—The pure oxalic acid is prepared by trituration, as directed under Class VII.

ACIDUM PHOSPHORICUM.

Present Names, Glacial Phosphoric Acid. Mono-Hydrogen Phosphate. Meta-Phosphoric Acid.

Formula, HPO_3.

Molecular Weight, 80.

Preparation of Phosphoric Acid.—It is usually obtained by treating bones burned to whiteness, with an equal weight of sulphuric acid. The bone ash is decomposed into calcium sulphate which is insoluble, and calcium and magnesium phosphates and phosphoric acid, which are left in solution. After filtration the liquid is neutralized with ammonium carbonate or hydrate, which unites with any sulphuric acid that may be present, and precipitates the phosphates above mentioned, and also forms with the phosphoric acid ammonium phosphate. After removing the precipitated phosphates the liquid is evaporated to dryness and heated to redness in a platinum vessel. Ammonium sulphate is driven off, ammonium phosphate is deprived of its ammonia, and meta-phosphoric acid is left. The product still contains some ammonia, and a better process for obtaining the acid perfectly pure is as follows: Burn phosphorus, found free from sulphur, in a two-necked glass globe, through which a current of dry air is passed continuously. The oxide resulting is converted into the glacial acid by addition of water and subsequent fusion in a platinum vessel.

Properties.—Glacial phosphoric acid is in colorless, ice-like, transparent masses, which are very hygroscopic, and soluble in water and in alcohol; the solution has a strongly acid reaction and taste.

Tests.—After saturation with hydrogen sulphide no precipitate should occur even after a long time (absence of arsenic and metals). Treated with indigo solution and with potassium permanganate solution, no decoloration should take place (absence of nitric and phosphorus acids). Upon heating some fragments of the fused acid in a strong solution of potassium hydrate, the odor of ammonia will reveal the presence, if any, of that body. Boiled with six volumes of distilled water, and adding strong nitric acid, upon adding in excess strong ammonium hydrate a white precipitate indicates magnesium or aluminium. If a fresh portion of the above solution be treated with absolute alcohol in large excess, no turbidity should occur.

The drug was first proven under Hahnemann's direction.

Preparation for Homœopathic Use.—One part by weight of purified glacial phosphoric acid is dissolved in ninety parts by weight of distilled water, and then are added ten parts of alcohol.

Amount of drug power, $\frac{1}{100}$. Mark 2x.

Dilutions must be prepared as directed under Class V—*a*.

ACIDUM PICRICUM.

Present Name, Picric Acid.
Synonyms, Carbazotic acid. Tri-nitrophenol.
Formula, $HC_6 H_2 (NO_2)_3 O$.
Molecular Weight, 229.

Preparation.—Picric acid is an oxidation-product resulting from the action of nitric acid upon certain organic substances, such as indigo, silk, salicin, coumarin, phlorizdin, the resin of *Xanthorrhœa hastilis*, aloes, storax, benzoin, etc. It is most economically prepared from carbolic acid. One part of the latter is gradually added to strong nitric acid, and when the reaction, which is violent, subsides, three parts of fuming nitric acid are added and the whole boiled till nitrous fumes are no longer given off. Upon cooling, the picric acid will be found in crystals, and after being removed they may be further purified by redissolving and recrystallizing from a solution in alcohol after a preliminary washing in cold water.

Properties.—Picric acid exists in bright yellow, glistening, crystalline scales. It is without odor, but has an intensely bitter taste. Upon gradual heating the crystals melt to a yellow fluid, which, on cooling, becomes crystalline again. When rapidly heated they sublime with the formation of yellow suffocating fumes. They are sparingly soluble in cold water, more readily in boiling water, and easily in alcohol, ether, chloroform, benzol, etc. The solution in benzol is colorless; in all the others named the color is a bright yellow and is imparted permanently to silk, wool, the skin and other animal tissues.

First proven by Parisel, of Paris, in 1868, later in America by Dr. L. B. Couch.

Tests.—Its identity may be determined from the above-mentioned characteristics, and by dropping into a hot solution of it a solution of potassium cyanide, when the liquid becomes of a deep red color from the formation of isopurpurate of potassium. Picric acid may be adulterated with different salts, especially nitre and sodium picrate; also with oxalic acid and boracic acid. All these substances will remain as a residue from a solution of dried and powdered picric acid in 150 volumes of benzine.

Preparation for Homœopathic Use.—One part by weight of pure picric acid is dissolved in ninety-nine parts by weight of distilled water.

Amount of drug power, $\frac{1}{100}$.

Dilutions must be prepared as directed under Class V—β.

Triturations of the pure picric acid are prepared as directed under Class VII.

ACIDUM SALICYLICUM.

Present Name, Salicylic Acid.
Formula, $C_7 H_6 O_3$.
Molecular Weight, 138.

Origin.—Salicylic acid is found free in the flowers of *Spiræa ulmaria*, and as methylsalicylic acid, in the ethereal oil of *Gaultheria procumbens;* it can be formed by the oxidation of salicin, cumarin, indigo.

Preparation.—Salicylic acid is made on a large scale synthetically, by causing a rearrangement of the elements of a molecule of carbonic oxide and one of carbolic acid, so as to form a new molecule, thus, $C_6 H_6 O + C O_2 = C_7 H_6 O_3$. The presence of sodium seems to be necessary, and the process is practically as follows: Dry sodium carbolate is placed in a retort and dry carbonic oxide is caused to pass through it, not too rapidly; as soon as this is begun the temperature is raised to 100° C. (212° F). The passage of the gas still continuing, the temperature is raised very slowly so that in the course of several hours 180° C. is reached, and finally from 220° to 250° C. (426°–486° F.). The operation is ended when no more carbolic acid comes over. The residue in the retort contains sodium carbonate and impure sodium salicylate. It is dissolved in water, decomposed with hydrochloric acid, recrystallized, and then further purified by re-solution and treatment with animal charcoal.

Properties.—Pure salicylic acid is in loose masses of small, fine, colorless needles, white and lustrous. They fuse at 159° C. (318.2° F.). By carefully heating they sublime unchanged, but if heated rapidly they decompose into carbolic acid and carbon di-oxide. They are soluble in 700 parts of cold water, readily in boiling water, alcohol and ether, and have a sweetish sour taste, and redden blue litmus paper.

First proven by Dr. Lewi, in Germany.

Tests.—Salicylic acid in watery solution, when treated with ferric chloride solution, gives rise to an intense violet color. The purity of the acid is shown by its difficult solubility in cold water, its ready and complete solution in alcohol, and the behavior of the dry acid when gently and carefully heated in a test tube. Even before the melting point is reached the acid begins to sublime in beautiful needles, and at a higher temperature is dissipated without residue. Carbolic acid, if present, will be detected by the bromine-water test. It is unaffected by barium chloride.

Preparation for Homœopathic Use. The pure salicylic acid is prepared by trituration, as directed under Class VII.

ACIDUM SUCCINICUM.

Present Name, Succinic Acid.
Formula, $C_4 H_6 O_4$.
Molecular Weight, 118.

Origin.—Succinic acid is found ready-formed in amber, from which by heating in iron retorts, it may be readily obtained. It is also found in some of the resins of coniferous trees, in *Artemesia, Lactuca*, etc. It is among the products of the action of nitric acid upon most fatty and waxy substances; it is found in small quantity in various animal fluids, and in wines and fermented liquors, being formed during the production of sugar. It is also obtainable from calcium malate in the presence of decomposing casein, as well as from tartrates, etc.

Preparation.—In a short-necked glass retort is placed dry amber, broken to a coarse powder, until the retort is half filled; the latter after being connected with a large receiver, is deeply buried in a sand-bath and the heat gradually raised till 280° C. (536° F.) is reached. The temperature is kept at this point as long as white vapors are given off. The white vapors condense in the well cooled receiver to a dark yellow acid fluid, which consists of succinic acid, some acetic acid and water, upon the surface of which floats oil of amber. The greater part of the succinic acid condenses in crystals within the neck of the retort. After the apparatus has become cool, the crystals are collected, dissolved in hot water, the solution filtered through filtering paper, to separate any adhering oil of amber, and the filtrate evaporated, when the acid crystallizes out.

Properties.—The officinal succinic acid is not pure; it forms yellow or greyish-yellow crystals, permanent in the air. They have the odor of oil of amber and an empyreumatic acid taste. Except that their solutions in water and alcohol are not colorless, they behave as do the crystals of the pure acid. The pure acid is odorless and is in colorless transparent, or white crystals. They melt at 180° C. (356° F.), are soluble in 20 parts of water at ordinary temperatures, and in 2 parts of boiling water; they are readily soluble in alcohol, but with difficulty in ether.

Tests.—A solution of succinic acid, neutralized with ammonia and treated with ferric chloride, gives a brown-red precipitate. If acetic acid be present, it may be detected by the white precipitate produced in concentrated solution, by potassium acetate; oxalic acid, by the white precipitate when treated with calcium chloride; sulphuric acid by barium chloride. Upon incineration no residue should be left.

Preparation for Homœopathic Use.—The pure succinic acid is prepared by trituration, as directed under Class VII.

ACIDUM SULPHURICUM.

Present Name, Hydrogen Sulphate. Sulphuric Acid.
Common Names, Sulphuric Acid. Oil of Vitriol.
Formula, $H_2\,SO_4$.
Molecular Weight, 98.

Origin.—Sulphuric acid does not exist in nature in the free state, except in the waters of some springs and in the Rio Vinagre in South America; but as sulphate it is found in many minerals, and in both vegetable and animal organisms.

Preparation.—When sulphur is burned in the air or in oxygen, it combines with two atoms of oxygen, forming sulphurous oxide; upon solution in water and exposure to the air, the sulphurous oxide takes up an additional atom of oxygen, producing sulphuric oxide. In the presence of water each of these oxides becomes an acid. The process above outlined is complicated when the need of oxidizing sulphurous oxide rapidly, is brought into the problem. For this purpose nitric acid, which gives up readily a part of its oxygen, is used, and in the form of one of the lower oxides of nitrogen acts as the oxygen carrier. The whole process is substantially as follows: In a furnace sulphur is burned, or iron pyrites is roasted; the product of the combustion of the sulphur is led into a leaden chamber connected with the furnace, together with atmospheric air and the nitrogen tetroxide gas resulting from the decomposition of a nitrate placed in a part of the furnace. The $N_2 O_4$ gives up two atoms of O to two molecules of $S O_2$, thus forming two molecules of $S O_3$. A current of atmospheric air is drawn slowly through the chamber, from which the $N_2 O_2$ takes two atoms of oxygen and is thereby reconverted into $N_2 O_4$ and is ready to oxidize anew two fresh molecules of $S O_2$. And so the process continues. To transform the $S O_3$ into $H_2 S O_4$ steam is blown into the chamber at various points, and from it the required H_2O is obtained. Special arrangements are used by which loss of the nitrogen oxides is avoided. The sulphuric acid as it is formed falls to the floor of the chamber, or condensing on its walls trickles down, and is allowed to accumulate till its specific gravity is 1.5; then it is drawn off, concentrated in leaden pans until the specific gravity is 1.7, and is further concentrated in vessels of glass or platinum until its maximum specific gravity, 1.85, is reached.

Properties.—Sulphuric acid is a dense, oily, colorless liquid, and when of specific gravity 1.85, contains forty parts of sulphuric anhydride and nine of $H_2 O$. It has a remarkable affinity for water, with which it unites, with the evolution of great heat; it takes the elements forming water, from any substance containing them and hence its destructive action upon all organized bodies, most of which it chars, *i. e.*, leaving only their carbon behind. At the temperature —20° C. (4° F.) it solidifies, and at 327° C. (620° F.) it boils and may be distilled. Its salts are called sulphates; the normal sulphates are all soluble in water, except those of the alkaline earths. In order to obtain it chemically pure it must be redistilled, and the process is not suitable to the pharmaceutical laboratory.

The acid was first proven by Hahnemann.

Tests.—Commercially pure sulphuric acid should always be tested for arsenic, sulphurous acid, the lower acids of the nitrogen series and lead. Sulphates of the alkalies, of the earths and of metals are proven absent, if upon mixing the acid with four volumes of alcohol and setting the mixture aside for an hour, no precipitate occurs—the mixture remaining perfectly clear; sulphurous acid is absent if the diluted acid, upon treatment with indigo solution, or solution of potassium permanganate, does not discharge the color of the test. Arsenic and lead will be detected by the yellow precipitate in the first named, by the blackish one in the second, when the acid largely diluted is treated with hydrogen sulphide.

Preparation for Homœopathic Use.—One part by weight of pure sulphuric acid, specific gravity 1.843, is dissolved in nine parts by weight of distilled water.

Amount of drug power, $\frac{1}{10}$.
Dilutions must be prepared as directed under Class V—*a*.

ACIDUM TANNICUM.

Synonyms, Di-Gallic Acid. Gallo-Tannic Acid. Tannin.
Present Name, Tannic Acid.
Formula, $C_{14}\ H_{10}\ O_{9}$.
Molecular Weight, 322.

Origin and Varieties.—The tannins are the astringent principles of plants and are widely distributed throughout the vegetable kingdom. Most of them are glucosides of gallic acid. The officinal tannin, or gallo-tannic acid U. S. P., is properly, when pure, di-gallic acid. All the tannins have the power of precipitating gelatin and albumen from their solutions, and ferric salts are thrown down by them as a dark precipitate. With the ferric salts the tannins from kino, catechu and the tea plant give greenish precipitates, while tannin from galls produces a blue-black precipitate. Gallo-tannic acid or di-gallic acid is obtained in large quantity from nut-galls, and to this source the pharmacist looks for the officinal preparation.

Preparation.—"Expose the powdered galls to a damp atmosphere for two or three days, and afterwards add sufficient ether to form a soft paste. Let this stand in a well closed vessel for twenty-four hours, then having quickly enveloped it in a linen cloth, submit it to strong pressure in a suitable press so as to separate the liquid portion. Reduce the pressed cake to a powder, mix it with sufficient ether, to which one-sixteenth of its bulk of water has been added, to form again a soft paste, and press this as before. Mix the expressed liquids and expose the mixture to spontaneous evaporation until, by the aid subsequently of a little heat, it has acquired the consistence of a soft extract; then place it on earthen plates or dishes, and dry it in a hot-air chamber at a temperature not exceeding 212° F."—Br. P.

Properties.—Officinal tannic acid is in pale yellow amorphous masses, faintly lustrous and without odor; is readily soluble in water and alcohol; insoluble in absolute ether. The solutions redden blue litmus paper. A not too dilute solution gives precipitates with phosphorous, sulphuric and hydrochloric acids, with the salts of the alkali metals and of the heavy metals. Its well known coagulating power upon albumen, gelatin and allied animal substances, and also the blue-black precipitate produced by it with ferric salts, need only to be mentioned.

Tests.—It should be completely soluble in five parts of cold distilled water, forming a yellow-brown solution tolerably clear; it should make a clear solution in ten parts of 90 per cent. alcohol, and when to this solution is added half its volume of ether no noteworthy turbidity, or at least no precipitate, should occur.

Preparation for Homœopathic Use.—The pure tannic acid is prepared by trituration, as directed under Class VII.

ACIDUM TARTARICUM.

Present Name, Tartaric Acid.

Formula, $C_4 H_6 O_6$.

Molecular Weight, 150.

Origin.—It occurs in grapes, pine apples, tamarinds and several other fruits. The tartaric acid of commerce is prepared from crude tartar, an impure acid-potassium-tartrate, which is precipitated from fermenting grape-juice by the alcohol produced in the process.

Preparation of Tartaric Acid.—"Take of acid tartrate of potash forty-five ounces; distilled water a sufficiency; prepared chalk, twelve and a half ounces; chloride of calcium, thirteen and a half ounces; sulphuric acid, thirteen fluid ounces. Boil the acid tartrate of potash with two gallons of the water, and add gradually the chalk, constantly stirring. When the effervescence has ceased, add the chloride of calcium dissolved in two pints of the water. When the tartrate of lime has subsided pour off the liquid, and wash the tartrate with distilled water until it is rendered tasteless. Pour the sulphuric acid, first diluted with three pints of the water, on the tartrate of lime; mix thoroughly, boil for half an-hour with repeated stirring, and filter through calico. Evaporate the filtrate at a gentle heat until it acquires the specific gravity of 1.21, allow it to cool, and then separate and reject the crystals of sulphate of lime which have formed. Again evaporate the clear liquor till a film forms on its surface, and allow it to cool and crystallize. Lastly, purify the crystals by solution, filtration (if necessary) and recrystallization."—Br. P.

Properties.—Tartaric acid is in oblique rhombic prisms, transparent and colorless. They are soluble in three-quarters of their own weight of cold water, and in three parts of alcohol; insoluble in ether, chloroform and benzin. The solutions are strongly acid in reaction, and if kept, unless they are very strong, deposit a fungous growth and are found to contain acetic acid.

The substance was first proven by Dr. Nenning, a contemporary of Hahnemann.

Tests.—Several crystals of the acid are to be dissolved in twice their weight of distilled water, by repeated agitation; a similar amount of the acid is to be treated with four times its weight of 97 or 98 per cent. alcohol. In both cases the solutions should be clear and complete. The watery solution is to be diluted with its own volume of distilled water, and portions of it are to be tested by hydrogen sulphide for metals, by ammonium oxalate solution for calcium compounds, and for sulphuric acid by the barium nitrate test. By heating, the acid carbonizes, giving off the odor of burnt sugar, and the carbonaceous matter is finally consumed without residue.

Preparation for Homœopathic Use.—The pure tartaric acid is prepared by trituration as directed under Class VII.

ACIDUM URICUM.

Synonym, Lithic Acid.

Present Name, Uric Acid.

Formula, $C_5 N_4 H_4 O_3$.

Origin.—This acid is a product of the animal organism, being next to the last of a succession of oxidation processes whose final outcome is urea.

Preparation of Uric Acid.—It may be prepared from human urine by concentration and addition of hydrochloric acid; it crystallizes out after some time in the form of small, reddish, translucent grains, very difficult to purify. It is more readily obtained from the solid white excrement of serpents, which can be easily procured, and which consists almost entirely of uric acid and ammonium urate. This is reduced to powder, and boiled in dilute solution of caustic potash; the liquid, filtered from the residue of feculent matter and earthy phosphates, is mixed with excess of hydrochloric acid, boiled for a few minutes, and left to cool. The product is collected on a filter, washed until free from potassium chloride, and dried by gentle heat.

Properties.—Uric acid, thus obtained, is a glistening, snow-white powder, tasteless, inodorous, and very sparingly soluble. It is seen under the microscope to consist of minute, but regular crystals. It dissolves in concentrated sulphuric acid without apparent decomposition, and is precipitated by dilution with water. By destructive distillation, uric acid yields cyanic acid, hydrocyanic acid, carbon dioxide, ammonium carbonate, and a black coaly residue, rich in nitrogen. By fusion with potassium hydrate, it yields potassium carbonate, cyanate and cyanide. Uric acid is remarkable for the facility with which it is altered by oxidizing agents, and the great number of definite and crystallizable compounds obtained in this manner, or by treating the immediate products of oxidation with acids, alkalies, reducing agents, etc.

Tests.—Uric acid is perfectly well characterized, even when in very small quantity, by its behavior with nitric acid. A small portion mixed with a drop or two of nitric acid in a small porcelain capsule dissolves with copious effervescence. When this solution is cautiously evaporated nearly to dryness, and, after the addition of a little water, mixed with a slight excess of ammonia, a magenta-red tint called murexide is immediately produced.

Preparation for Homœopathic Use.—The pure uric acid is prepared by trituration, as directed under Class VII.

ACONITUM.

Synonym, Aconitum Napellus, *Linn.*

Nat. Ord., Ranunculaceæ.

Common Names, Monkshood. Wolfsbane. Aconite.

The genus Monkshood is spread all over Europe, either growing spontaneously in the mountain districts, or cultivated in gardens for decoration. Though all species possess more or less narcotic powers, it is, notwithstanding, by no means indifferent from which we draw our exceedingly important medicine. Experience has declared itself for the above stated species and *exclusively* for the plant *growing wild*, which is indigenous to the Swiss, Carinthian and Styrian Alps, the Pyrenees, the Dauphiny, the mountains of Silesia, Bavaria and the Hartz. The herbaceous annual stem of aconite starts from an elongated conical tuberous root two to four inches long, and sometimes an inch in thickness. This root tapers off in a long tail with numerous branching rootlets from its sides. The dried root is more or less conical or tapering, enlarged and knotty at the summit, which is crowned with the base of the stem; it is from two to four inches long, and from a half to one inch thick. The tuber-like portion of the root is more slender, much shrivelled longitudinally, and beset with the prominent bases of rootlets. The stem is upright, three to four feet high, roundish-angulate and in its upper half clothed with spreading dark green leaves, which are paler on their under side, long-petioled and five-lobed, the lobes deeply two to five cleft. The uppermost leaves are more simple than the lower. The stem is crowned with the beautiful raceme of dark violet helmet-shaped flowers. The root is dark brown, and when dry breaks with a short fracture, showing a white and farinaceous, or brownish or grey inner substance, sometimes hollow in its centre. A transverse section of a sound root shows a pure white central portion, somewhat star-shaped and having seven or eight rays or points. By this it may be differentiated from the root of Aconitum cammarum, whose central portion is more distinctly five-pointed.

Introduced into our Materia Medica by Hahnemann.

Preparation.—In the flowering time, June and July, the entire plant, except the root, is chopped and pounded to a pulp, enclosed in a piece of new linen and subjected to pressure. The expressed juice is then, by brisk agitation, mingled with an equal part by weight of alcohol, the mixture is poured into a well-stoppered bottle, allowed to stand eight days in a dark, cool place, and then filtered. It is also recommended to prepare a tincture according to Class II.

Drug power of tincture, ½.

Dilutions are prepared as directed under Classes I and II

ACONITUM CAMMARUM, *Jacquin.*

Synonym, Aconitum Variegatum, *Linn.*

Nat. Ord., Ranunculaceæ.

This is a species of aconite found growing in the same localities as the aconitum napellus, and sometimes improperly substituted for or mixed with the same. The roots are smaller than in aconitum napellus, and the generally clearly-shaped star of five points shown on section will distinguish it from the eight-rayed irregular star in the centre of the latter.

Preparation.—The fresh root is chopped and pounded to a pulp and weighed. Then two parts by weight of alcohol are taken, the pulp mixed thoroughly with one-sixth part of it, and the rest of the alcohol added. After stirring the whole well, and pouring it into a well-stoppered bottle, it is allowed to stand eight days in a dark, cool place. The tincture is then separated by decanting, straining and filtering.

Drug power of tincture, $\frac{1}{6}$.

Dilutions must be prepared as directed under Class III.

ACONITUM FEROX, *Wallich.*

Nat. Ord., Ranunculaceæ.

This is the most poisonous species of aconite known; it is found growing on the Himalaya mountains, the roots supplying the famous Indian (Nipal) poison called Bikh, Bish, or Nabee. This species is considered by *Hooker* and *Thompson* as a variety of *Aconitum napellus.* In commerce the roots are simple tubers, elongated-conical in form, and dark brown; but as they are dried by fire-heat and often steeped in cow's urine to protect them against the ravages of insects, it can be readily seen that no trustworthy data for their identification can be given. In India the roots of allied and nearly equally poisonous aconites, viz., *uncinatum, palmatum, luridum* and *napellus* are gathered together, and such collections indiscriminately used under the name Bikh or Bish.

Preparation.—The root is finely powdered and covered with five parts by weight of alcohol, and having poured it into a well-stoppered bottle, it is allowed to stand eight days in a dark, cool place, shaking it twice a day. The tincture is then separated by decanting, straining and filtering.

Drug power of tincture, $\frac{1}{10}$.

Dilutions must be prepared as directed under Class IV.

ACONITUM LYCOCTONUM, *Linn.*

Nat Ord., Ranunculaceæ.

This is a yellow-flowered species of aconite found growing in the same localities as the aconitum napellus. The yellow flowers and the soft hairy covering of the leaves distinguish it from *aconitum napellus.*

Preparation.—The fresh herb, gathered when coming into bloom, is chopped and pounded to a pulp, enclosed in a piece of new linen and subjected to pressure. The expressed juice is then, by brisk agitation, mingled with an equal part by weight of alcohol. This mixture having been poured into a well-stoppered bottle, is allowed to stand eight days in a dark, cool place and then filtered.

Drug power of tincture, $\frac{1}{2}$.

Dilutions must be prepared as directed under Class I.

ACONITUM RADIX.

Root of Aconitum Napellus.

Preparation.—The fresh root of the uncultivated plant is chopped and pounded to a pulp and weighed. Then two parts by weight of alcohol are taken, the pulp mixed thoroughly with one-sixth part of it, and the rest of the alcohol added. After stirring the whole well, and pouring it into a well-stoppered bottle, it is allowed to stand eight days in a dark, cool place. The tincture is then separated by decanting, straining and filtering.

Drug power of tincture, $\frac{1}{6}$.

Dilutions must be prepared as directed under Class III.

ACTÆA.

Synonym, Actæa Spicata, *Linn.*

Nat. Ord., Ranunculaceæ.

Common Names, Common Herb Christopher. Bane-berry.

This elegant perennial herb, growing from one to two feet high, is found all over Germany, though not frequently; it likes a stony ground in mountain forests and shady humid woods.

On naked, smooth, stiff, ramose above, geniculated stems stand the petiolate, ternate-manifold compound leaves, with ovate-cordate, serrato-dentate leaflets. The white flowers with caducous petals, appear in loose racemes, on long peduncles, growing out of the axils. The fruit is a smooth berry, subovate, and shining black, when ripe. The perennial root forms a strong ramose-fibrous stock of dark brown, and when dried, black color; the long, fine ramifying rootlets show on section a stellate quadri-partite medullary substance.

Introduced into the Homœopathic Materia Medica by Dr. Petroz, of Spain.

Preparation.—The fresh root, gathered in May, before the plant is in flower, is chopped and pounded to a pulp and weighed. Then two parts by weight of alcohol are taken, the pulp mixed thoroughly with one-sixth part of it, and the rest of the alcohol added. After stirring the whole well, and pouring it into a well-stoppered bottle, it is allowed to stand eight days in a dark, cool place.

The tincture is then separated by decanting, straining and filtering.

Drug power of tincture, $\frac{1}{6}$.

Dilutions must be prepared as directed under Class III.

ADELHEIDSQUELLE.

Mineral spring at Heilbrunn, contains among other substances, iodine, bromine, alumina, soda, etc.

Analysis (*Pettenkofer*).

Sod. Iod.,	.22	Carbonate of Soda,	.216	Free Carb. gas,	13.18 c.c.
" Brom.,	.367	" Lime,	.584	Carburetted H.,	8.02
" Chlor.,	38.068	" Magn.,	.144	Oxygen,	1.38
" Sulph.,	.048	" Iron,	.072	Nitrogen,	6.54
Potass. Chlor.,	.020	Alumina,	.142		
		Silica,	.147		
		Organic,	.165		

Preparation.—Never proven in potencies, but if required, prepare first and second dilutions with distilled water, third and higher potencies with alcohol.

ÆSCULUS GLABRA, *Willd.*

Synonyms, Æ. Carnea. Æ. Ohioensis. Pavia Glabra.
Nat. Ord., Sapindaceæ.
Common Names, Fetid or Ohio Buckeye. Buckeye Tree.

This is a large tree, growing abundantly in rich alluvial lands of Ohio and other states watered by the Ohio river. The bark exhales an unpleasant odor, as in the rest of the genus. Leaves opposite, pointing out. Leaflets fine, with a serrate or toothed edge, and straight veins, like a chestnut leaf. Flowers small, not showy; stamens curved, much longer than the corolla, which is of a pale yellow, and consists of four upright petals. Fruit prickly when young. The fruit is said to be actively poisonous, producing symptoms analogous to those caused by strychnia.

It was first systematically proven by Dr. E. M. Hale.

Preparation.—The fresh hulled nut is chopped and pounded to a pulp and weighed. Then two parts by weight of alcohol are taken, the pulp mixed thoroughly with one-sixth part of it, and the rest of the alcohol added. After stirring the whole well, and pouring it into a well-stoppered bottle, it is allowed to stand eight days in a dark, cool place. The tincture is then separated by decanting, straining and filtering.

Drug power of tincture, ⅙.

Dilutions must be prepared as directed under Class III.

Triturations are prepared from the whole dried fruit, as directed under Class VII.

ÆSCULUS HIPPOCASTANUM, *Linn.*

Synonym, Hippocastanum Vulgare.
Nat. Ord., Sapindaceæ.
Common Name, Horse Chestnut.

The horse chestnut is a native of middle Asia, but flourishes well in temperate climates. It was introduced into Europe in the year 1576. It is now extensively cultivated as an ornamental tree, in both Europe and America. Leaves opposite, digitate; leaflets serrate, straight veined. Flowers in a terminal thyrsus or dense panicle, often polygamous, the greater portion with imperfect pistils and sterile. Pedicels jointed. Corolla spreading, white, spotted with purple and yellow, of five petals. Stamens declined; leaflets seven. Its nuts are ovoid, mahogany-colored, perfectly smooth and shining, with a large oval hilum, which is paler-colored and rough.

The first proving was recorded by Dr. Cooley, of New York State.

Preparation.—The ripe, fresh, hulled nut is chopped and pounded to a pulp and weighed. Then two parts by weight of alcohol are taken, the pulp mixed thoroughly with one-sixth part of it, and the rest of the alcohol added. After stirring the whole well, and pouring it into a well-stoppered bottle, it is allowed to stand eight days in a dark, cool place. The tincture is then separated by decanting, straining and filtering.

Drug power of tincture, 1/6.

Dilutions must be prepared as directed under Class III.

ÆTHUSA.

Synonym, Æthusa Cynapium, *Linn.*

Nat. Ord., Umbelliferæ.

Common Names, Fool's Parsley. Dog Parsley. Dog Poison. Garden Hemlock. Lesser Hemlock.

This is a common weed, abundant throughout Europe, growing about a foot high, strongly resembling parsley in appearance, yet easily distinguished from it by its nauseous smell when rubbed, and its loathsome taste. Root spindle-shaped; stem erect and quite smooth, hollow, and sometimes violet-striped; leaves of a shining dark green, but lighter colored on their under surface, and ternate pinnate. The umbels are without involucre and with three-leaved pendulous involucels. Flowers white. Seeds globular and striated.

Introduced into our Materia Medica by Dr. Nenning, of Germany.

Preparation.—The whole fresh plant, when in flower, is chopped and pounded to a pulp and weighed. Then two parts by weight of alcohol are taken, the pulp mixed thoroughly with one-sixth part of it, and the rest of the alcohol added. After stirring the whole well, and pouring it into a well-stoppered bottle, it is allowed to stand eight days in a dark, cool place. The tincture is then separated by decanting, straining and filtering.

Drug power of tincture, 1/6.

Dilutions must be prepared as directed under Class III.

AGARICUS EMETICUS.

Proper Name, Russula Emetica, *Fr.*

Nat. Ord., Fungi.

Description.—Stem stout. Pileus fleshy, firm, obtuse, then depressed and infundibuliform, polished, two to three inches broad, blood-red, or growing pale about the margin. Flesh firm, cheesy, white. Gills very narrow and much crowded. Taste acrid and peppery.

Preparation.—The fresh mushroom is chopped and pounded to a pulp and weighed. Then two parts by weight of alcohol are taken, the pulp mixed thoroughly with one-sixth part of it, and the rest of the alcohol added. After stirring the whole well, and pouring it into a well-stoppered bottle, it is allowed to stand eight days in a dark, cool place. The tincture is then separated by decanting, straining and filtering.

Drug power of tincture, 1/6.

Dilutions must be prepared as directed under Class III.

AGARICUS MUSCARIUS, *Linn.*

Synonym, Amanita Muscarius.
Nat. Ord., Fungi.
Common Names, Toadstool. Bug Agaric. Fly Agaric.

This poisonous fungus grows, from August to October, in Europe, Asia, and America, and is found in dry pine and birch forests. Upon first appearing it is oval and enclosed in a soft, fleshy envelope; the young stem is short and thick, bulbous at the base, generally hollow when old, from four to six inches long, the part above the middle being provided with a white membranous ring; the cap is at first eminently vaulted, afterwards it becomes flatter, is scarlet-red, furnished with yellowish-white scales, which are sometimes wanting, with a white border, or a border with brown-yellow stripes; pulp yellowish, or white, or reddish, the lamellæ radiate from the middle to the margin; it has an offensive smell and a burning acrid taste.

It was first proven by Stapf, and afterward by Schreter and Hahnemann.

Preparation.—Select the younger specimens, which have convex cap, not yet hollow stem, and clean them from adherent earth by scraping; peel off the epidermis from the stem and cap, and then bruise the whole to a pulp and weigh. Then two parts by weight of alcohol are taken, and having mixed the pulp thoroughly with one-sixth part of it, the rest of the alcohol is added. After stirring the whole well, and pouring it into a well-stoppered bottle, it is allowed to stand eight days in a dark, cool place. The tincture is then separated by decanting, straining and filtering.

Drug power of tincture, $\frac{1}{6}$.

Dilutions must be prepared as directed under Class III.

AGAVE AMERICANA, *Linn.*

Nat. Ord., Amaryllidaceæ.
Common Names, American Aloe. Maguey. Century Plant.

This plant is a native of tropical America, but has been cultivated in the Southern States and in other warm regions. The leaves are mostly radical, thick and rigid, coriaceous, fleshy, lanceolate, spinous-dentate, with terminal spine. They are recurved and vary in length from three to six feet—sometimes reaching eight feet. In temperate climates the plant flowers rarely, and to this fact is due the name *century plant* which it has received. The flowers are yellow, in a pyramidal panicle at the top of the scape, which is often thirty feet high.

Preparation.—The fresh leaves are chopped and pounded to a pulp and weighed. Then two parts by weight of alcohol are taken, the pulp mixed thoroughly with one-sixth part of it, and the rest of the alcohol added. After stirring the whole well, and pouring it into a well-stoppered bottle, it is allowed to stand eight days in a dark, cool place. The tincture is then separated by decanting, straining and filtering.

Drug power of tincture, $\frac{1}{6}$.

Dilutions must be prepared as directed under Class III.

AGNUS CASTUS.

Synonym, Vitex Agnus Castus, *Linn.*
Nat. Ord., Verbenaceæ.
Common Name, Chaste Tree.

This shrub is indigenous in the south of Europe, on the shores of the Mediterranean; and is found growing on sandy spots at the foot of rocks. It is from three to five feet high, and much branched. Leaves opposite, petiolate, five to seven digitate; color dark green on upper, greyish on under surface, with a very strong smell. Flowers numerous, blue or purple, in long terminal spikes, having a strong, not disagreeable odor. Berries somewhat like peppercorns.

Introduced by Hahnemann.

Preparation.—The fresh, ripe berries, are pounded to a pulp and weighed. Then two parts by weight of alcohol are taken, the pulp mixed thoroughly with one-sixth part of it, and the rest of the alcohol added. After stirring the whole well, and pouring it into a well-stoppered bottle, it is allowed to stand eight days in a dark, cool place. The tincture is then separated by decanting, straining and filtering.

Drug power of tincture, $\frac{1}{6}$.

Dilutions must be prepared as directed under Class III.

AGROSTEMMA GITHAGO, *Linn.*

Synonym, Lychnis Githago, *Lamarck.*
Nat. Ord., Caryophyllaceæ.
Common Name, Corn Cockle.

This is a well-known weed, indigenous to Europe, growing in wheat-fields; the black seeds of cockle are injurious to the whiteness of the flour. It is an annual, clothed with long, soft appressed hairs; flowers long-peduncled; calyx lobes similar to the long and linear leaves, surpassing the broad and crownless purple-red petals, falling off in fruit.

Preparation.—The ripe, dried seeds, are coarsely powdered and weighed. Then five parts by weight of alcohol are poured upon the mass, and the whole is allowed to stand eight days in a well-stoppered bottle, in a dark, cool place, shaking it twice a day. The tincture is then poured off, strained and filtered.

Drug power of tincture, $\frac{1}{10}$.

Dilutions must be prepared as directed under Class IV.

AILANTHUS GLANDULOSA, *Desfontaines.*

Synonym, Rhus Chinense.
Nat. Ord., Simarubeæ.
Common Names, The Tree of Heaven. Chinese Sumach.

This tree is a native of China, but is well known in the United States, where it has within a few years been extensively cultivated as a shade tree, but although well adapted to this purpose, its extremely offensive odor at the time of flowering, as well as the injurious effects upon human beings from its emanations, according to some physicians, has excited such prejudice against it that in some portions of this country a determined effort towards its destruction has been made. In its general aspect and the character of its foliage, it appears like a gigantic sumach. It grows to a height of 60 feet and upwards. Its flowers are of a whitish-green color.

First provings made were under Drs. Hering and Lippe.

Preparation.—Equal parts of the fresh shoots, leaves, blossoms, and the young bark, are chopped and pounded to a pulp and weighed. Then two parts by weight of alcohol are taken, the pulp mixed thoroughly with one-sixth part of it, and the rest of the alcohol added. After stirring the whole well, and pouring it into a well-stoppered bottle, it is allowed to stand eight days in a dark, cool place. The tincture is then separated by decanting, straining and filtering.

Drug power of tincture, $\frac{1}{6}$.

Dilutions must be prepared as directed under Class III.

ALETRIS FARINOSA, *Linn.*

Synonym, Aletris Alba.
Nat. Ord., Hæmodoraceæ.
Common Names, Star Grass. Blazing Grass. Colic Root. Unicorn Root.

This is an indigenous perennial plant, the radical leaves of which spread on the ground in the form of a star. The leaves are sessile, unequal, lanceolate, entire, very smooth, longitudinally veined, thin and translucent and very sharp at the end. Stem one or two feet in height, nearly naked, or scapiform with remote scales, sometimes changing into leaves. It terminates in a slender spike, the flowers of which stand on very short pedicels, and with minute bracts at the base. The perianth is tubular, oblong, divided at the summit into six spreading segments, white, and when old, of a mealy or rugose appearance on the outside. The plant grows in almost all parts of the United States, in fields and about the borders of woods, and flowers in June and July.

Preparation.—The fresh bulb is chopped and pounded to a pulp and weighed. Then two parts by weight of alcohol are taken, the pulp mixed with one-sixth part of it, and the rest of the alcohol added. After stirring the whole well, and pouring it into a well-stoppered bottle, it is allowed to stand eight days in a dark, cool place. The tincture is then separated by decanting, straining and filtering.

Drug power of tincture, $\frac{1}{6}$.

Dilutions must be prepared as directed under Class III.

ALISMA PLANTAGO, *Linn.*

Synonym, Alisma Parriflora.
Nat. Ord., Alismaceæ.
Common Name, Water Plantain.

This is a herbaceous plant found in Europe and the United States, growing in streams, pools, ditches, and other standing water. Root perennial, leaves long petioled, ovate, oblong, or lanceolate, pointed, mostly rounded or heart-shaped at the base, three to nine nerved; panicle loose, compound, many-flowered, from one to two feet long; carpels obliquely obovate, forming an obtusely triangular whorl in fruit. The fresh root has the odor of Florentine orris, but the odor disappears on drying. It has an acrid and nauseous taste.

Preparation.—The fresh root is chopped and pounded to a pulp and weighed. Then two parts by weight of alcohol are taken, the pulp mixed thoroughly with one sixth part of it, and the rest of the alcohol added. After stirring the whole well, and pouring it into a well-stoppered bottle, it is allowed to stand eight days in a dark, cool place. The tincture is then separated by decanting, straining and filtering.

Drug power of tincture, $\frac{1}{6}$.

Dilutions must be prepared as directed under Class III.

ALLIUM SATIVUM, *Linn.*

Nat. Ord., Liliaceæ.

Common Name, Garlic.

This is a perennial bulbous plant, cultivated everywhere in civilized countries. Bulb compound; stem leafy to the middle, leaves linear-lanceolate; spathe one-leaved, long pointed, stem simple, two to three feet high; umbel bulbiferous. The bulb is composed of several oblong, pointed bulblets, enclosed in a three-layered membrane.

Introduced into our Materia Medica by Dr. Petroz, of France.

Preparation.—The fresh bulbs, gathered from June to August, and freed from their membranes, are chopped and pounded to a pulp and weighed. Then two parts by weight of alcohol are taken, the pulp mixed thoroughly with one-sixth part of it, and the rest of the alcohol added. After stirring the whole well, and pouring it into a well-stoppered bottle, it is allowed to stand eight days in a dark, cool place. The tincture is then separated by decanting, straining and filtering.

Drug power of tincture, $\frac{1}{6}$.

Dilutions must be prepared as directed under Class III.

ALNUS RUBRA.

Synonym, Alnus serrulata.

Nat. Ord., Betulaceæ.

Common Names, Red Alder. Tag Alder. Notch-leaved Alder.

This is the *Alnus Serrulata* of Willdenow. It is an indigenous shrub, growing in clumps on the borders of ponds and rivers, and in swamps. Its stems are numerous, from six to twelve feet high. Leaves obovate, acute at the base, sharply serrate with minute teeth, thickish, green both sides, smooth, or often downy beneath; flowers, which appear in April before the development of the leaves, are of a reddish-green color; stipules oval; fruit ovate. Its cones remain on the bush all winter.

Preparation.—The fresh bark is chopped and pounded to a pulp and weighed. Then two parts by weight of alcohol are taken, the pulp mixed thoroughly with one-sixth part of it, and the rest of the alcohol added. After stirring the whole well, and pouring it into a well-stoppered bottle, it is allowed to stand eight days in a dark, cool place. The tincture is then separated by decanting, straining and filtering.

Drug power of tincture, $\frac{1}{6}$.

Dilutions must be prepared as directed under Class III.

ALOE.

Synonym, Aloe Socotrina, *Lamarck.*

Nat. Ord., Liliaceæ.

Common Names, Aloes. Socotrine Aloes.

The aloes are natives of Southern and Eastern Africa. They are succulent plants of liliaceous habits, with persistent fleshy leaves, usually prickly at the margin, and erect spikes of yellow or red flowers. Many are stemless; others produce stems a few feet in height, which are woody or branching. In medicine, the inspissated juice from the leaves is used.

Socotrine aloes is imported in kegs and tin-lined boxes from Bombay, whither it has been carried by traders from the African coast. When of fine quality, it is dark, reddish-brown in color, and of a peculiar, rather agreeable odor. As imported, it is usually soft, at least in the interior of the mass, but it becomes harder by keeping. In thin fragments, its color is orange-brown; in powder, of a tawny red. It breaks with a conchoidal fracture.

It was first proven by Dr. Helbig, in Germany.

Preparation.—The inspissated juice is coarsely pulverized and covered with five parts by weight of alcohol. Having poured it into a well-stoppered bottle, it is allowed to stand eight days in a dark, cool place, shaking it twice a day. The tincture is then poured off, strained and filtered.

Drug power of tincture, $\frac{1}{10}$.

Dilutions must be prepared as directed under Class IV.

Triturations are prepared from the inspissated juice, as directed under Class VII.

ALSTONIA CONSTRICTA.

Nat. Ord., Apocynaceæ.

This is a tall shrub or small tree, indigenous to the colonies of New South Wales and Queensland.

Preparation.—The bark, in coarse powder, is covered with five parts by weight of alcohol, and having been poured into a well-stoppered bottle, is allowed to stand fourteen days in a dark place, being shaken twice a day. The tincture is then poured off, strained and filtered.

Drug power of tincture, $\frac{1}{10}$.

Dilutions must be prepared as directed under Class IV.

ALTHÆA.

Synonym, Althæa Officinalis, *Linn.*
Nat. Ord., Malvaceæ.
Common Name, Marshmallow.

A perennial herb, whose root is perpendicular and branching. Its stems, about three feet high, are branched and leafy. Leaves are alternate, with petioles, cordate above, oblong-ovate below, almost three-lobed above, irregularly serrate, pointed, and downy. The flowers, terminal and axillary, are on short peduncles, bearing one to three flowers. The five spreading, obcordate petals of the corolla are of a pale purplish color. The fruit consists of a united circle of capsules, each holding one seed.

The plant is found in the Eastern U. S., on borders of salt marshes.

Preparation.—The fresh root, collected in autumn from plants at least two years old, is chopped and pounded to a pulp and weighed. Then two parts by weight of alcohol are taken, the pulp mixed thoroughly with one-sixth part of it, and the rest of the alcohol added. After stirring the whole well, and pouring it into a well-stoppered bottle, it is allowed to stand eight days in a dark, cool place. The tincture is then separated by decanting, straining and filtering.

Drug power of tincture, $\frac{1}{6}$.

Dilutions must be prepared as directed under Class III.

ALUMEN.

Synonyms, Alumen crudum. Potassa Alum.
Common Names, Alum. Sulphate of Aluminium and Potassium.
Present Name, Potassio-aluminium Sulphate.
Formula, $K_2 Al_2 (SO_4)_4, 24H_2 O$.
Molecular Weight, 949.

The alums are double sulphates in which the hydrogen of two molecules of sulphuric acid is displaced by two atoms of a monad positive element and two of a triad one. In common alum, potassium is the univalent and aluminium the trivalent atom. But in place of potassium, any other of the alkali metals can be substituted, and instead of aluminium, chromium or iron. All the alums crystallize in cubes or octohedrons, and with the exception of chrome alum and iron alum are colorless. With each molecule are united twenty-four molecules of water of crystallization, which can be driven off by heat, and then there is left "burnt" or anhydrous alum. The word alum is used in ordinary language indifferently for the potassium or the ammonium compound.

Preparation.—The simplest mode of obtaining alum is by calcining pipe clay or some other clay containing very little iron, grinding it to powder and heating it on the hearth of a reverberatory furnace with half its weight of sulphuric acid, until it becomes a stiff paste. The mass is then exposed to the air for several weeks. During this time aluminium sulphate is formed, which can be dissolved out by treating the mass with water. Upon mixing this solution with one of potassium sulphate and evaporating, crystals of the composition given above are obtained.

Properties.—Alum has a sweetish taste followed by an astringent one. It is soluble in fifteen parts of cold and in one part of boiling water, and is insoluble in alcohol. At a red heat it is decomposed, sulphuric acid being given off and aluminium oxide and potassium sulphate remaining behind. The crystals effloresce slightly upon exposure to the air. Their solution is strongly acid to test paper.

Tests.—When treated with ammonium hydrate, the alum solution throws down a white precipitate, insoluble in excess of the reagent, but soluble in sodium hydrate.

A solution of alum should exhibit, if perfectly pure, no change upon treatment with hydrogen sulphide (absence of metals), nor upon the addition of potassium ferrocyanide (absence of iron). If sophisticated with ammonia alum, by adding to a solution of the suspected substance a caustic alkali and heating, the pungent odor of ammonia will be perceived.

It was first proven by Fr. Husemann.

Preparation for Homœopathic Use.—The pure potassa alum is prepared by trituration, as directed under Class VII.

ALUMINA.

Synonyms, Aluminium Tri-hydrate. Argilla Pura.

Common Name, Pure Clay.

Formula, $Al\,H_3\,O_3$.

Molecular Weight, 78.

Preparation of Alumina.—Alum free from iron is dissolved in pure boiling water, and decomposed by pure potassium carbonate, adding a little of the potash in excess. The whole is then digested gently for some time, to decompose a basic salt of alumina and sulphuric acid, which has been precipitated along with the alumina. The precipitate, now well washed and separated by filtering, is, while still moist, dissolved in muriatic acid, the solution filtered and the alumina precipitated anew by adding dilute caustic ammonium in excess. The obtained precipitate requires long continued washing to free it perfectly from retained sal ammoniac.

The preparation made by the above process—substantially that of Hahnemann, is the tri-hydrate whose formula is $Al\,H_3\,O_3$. When dried at a moderate heat, it is a soft friable mass which adheres to the tongue, and forms a stiff paste with water, but is not soluble therein. It dissolves readily in acids and in solutions of the permanent alkalies. Heated to redness it gives off water and contracts in volume.

The oxide, $Al_2\,O_3$, if such be wanted, may be readily obtained by heating the tri-hydrate to whiteness, after washing and drying. It is a white, tasteless, coherent mass, but little acted upon by acids, and is infusible except before the oxy-hydrogen blow-pipe.

The mineral called *corundum,* of which the ruby and sapphire are transparent varieties, consists of the nearly pure oxide in a crystallized state, with a little coloring oxide.

Properties and Tests.—Alumina is a fine white powder, soft to the touch, inodorous and tasteless, infusible, and insoluble in water.

Alumina was first proved under Hahnemann's directions.

Preparation for Homœopathic Use.—Alumina is prepared by trituration, as directed under Class VII.

ALUMINIUM METALLICUM.

Synonym, Metallic Aluminium.

Symbol, Al.

Atomic Weight, 27.

Origin.—This metal occurs very abundantly in nature in the state of silicate, as in felspar and its associated minerals; also in the various modifications of clay thence derived. It was first isolated by Wöhler (1828), who obtained it as a gray powder by decomposing aluminium chloride with potassium; and H. Sainte-Claire Deville (1854) by an improved process founded on the same principle, has succeeded in obtaining it in the compact form and on the manufacturing scale.

Manufacture of Metallic Aluminium.—The process consists in decomposing the double chloride of aluminium and sodium, $Al_2\ Cl_6$, $2Na\ Cl$, by heating it with metallic sodium, fluor-spar or cryolite being added as a flux. The reduction is effected in crucibles, or on a large scale on the hearth of a reverberatory furnace. Sodium is used as the reducing agent in préference to potassium: first, because it is more easily prepared; and, secondly, because it has a lower atomic weight, and, consequently, a smaller quantity of it suffices to do the same amount of chemical work.

Properties and Tests.—Metallic aluminium is silver-white, sonorous, unalterable in the air, having the specific gravity 2.56 only, that of iron being 7.7, and of lead 11.5. Its fusing point is somewhat lower than that of silver. It is not attacked by sulphuric or nitric acid, nor tarnished by sulphuretted hydrogen. Its proper solvent is muriatic acid. After silver, gold and platinum, it is the least alterable of the metals. By reason of its valuable properties, it will be applied to many purposes in the arts, if obtainable in sufficient quantities, and at a moderate cost.

Preparation for Homœopathic Use.—The pure metallic aluminium is prepared by trituration, as directed under Class VII.

AMBRA GRISEA.

Synonyms, Ambarum. Ambra Ambrosiaca. Ambra Vera. Ambra Maritima.

Common Name, Ambergris.

Origin.—Ambergris is found in the intestines and among the excreta of the sperm whale, *Physeter macrocephalus*. It is found floating upon the sea, and thrown upon the coast in tropical regions. It has many of the characteristics of concretions, and is considered to be of intestinal or biliary origin.

Properties.—It is fat-like in appearance, or more properly, waxy.

It comes in pieces of various sizes and shapes, of ashy-gray color, marbled, with whitish or dark streaks and spots. Although quite friable, it is with difficulty rubbed to powder. It is without taste, has a peculiar and agreeable odor. It becomes soft at the temperature of the hand, melts in boiling water, and at a higher temperature is dissipated with the production of white fumes, only a trace of ash remaining. It is soluble in alcohol, ether, and in fatty and volatile oils. Its specific gravity is 0.8–0.9.

Tests.—The description as given above will suffice for its identification or for differentiating a spurious or adulterated article from the genuine and pure one.

Preparation for Homœopathic Use.—The genuine, gray ambergris is prepared by trituration, as directed under Class VII.

AMMONIACUM.

Synonym, Dorema Ammoniacum, *Don.*

Nat. Ord., Umbelliferæ.

Common Name, Gum Ammoniac.

The *Dorema Ammoniacum* is a perennial plant, having a stout, erect flower-stem, six to eight feet high, which divides towards the upper part into numerous ascending branches, along which, at the time of flowering, are arranged the ball-like, simple umbels of very small flowers. The plant is widely distributed in Persia and neighboring countries, and makes the barren regions of the desert its habitat. The stem of the plant abounds in milky juice which flows out on the slightest puncture; the exudation speedily hardening, a part remains attached to the stem and a part falls to the ground. It is gathered by the peasants who sell it to the traders. It is found in commerce in "tears" and in irregular masses.

Properties.—The variety in masses is generally less pure than that in "tears." The latter are roundish, varying in size from that of a small pea to that of a cherry. Externally they are pale, creamy-yellow in color, opaque and milky-white within. By long keeping the outer part becomes somewhat brownish in color. Ammoniacum is brittle, breaking with a waxy fracture, but is easily softened by warmth. Its taste is bitter and acrid, its odor is peculiar and characteristic. It is partly soluble in alcohol, and when triturated with water produces a milky emulsion. Its specific gravity is about 1.2.

Introduced into our Materia Medica by Dr. Buchner, Germany.

Preparation.—The pure gum-resin in tears is prepared by trituration, as directed under Class VII.

AMMONIUM ACETICUM.

Synonyms, Liquor Ammonii Acetatis (Solution of Acetate of Ammonium). Spiritus Mindereri (Spirit of Mindererus).

Present Name, Ammonium Acetate.

Formula, $C_2 H_3 O_2 NH_4$.

Preparation of Acetate of Ammonium.—Take of diluted

acetic acid (acetic acid one part, distilled water seven parts) any quantity. Add ammonium carbonate gradually to the acid unto neutralization; then filter. This preparation should be freshly made when wanted. It is a colorless neutral liquid, of a somewhat pungent taste, having no odor. After being kept for some time, especially with exposure to the air and sunlight, it suffers partial decomposition, with the production of ammonium carbonate and acetic acid.

Tests.—It should evaporate completely over a water bath, leaving no residue; with hydrogen sulphide (for metals) it should give no precipitate or turbidity; nor with barium chloride solution (sulphuric acid); with silver nitrate a white precipitate insoluble in nitric acid shows the presence of HCl.

Preparation for Homœopathic Use.—One part by weight of pure "spirit of mindererus" is dissolved in nine parts by weight of distilled water.

Amount of drug power, $\frac{1}{10}$.

Dilutions must be prepared as directed under Class V—*a*.

AMMONIUM BENZOICUM.

Synonyms, Ammonii Benzoas. Benzoate of Ammonium.

Present Name, Ammonium Benzoate.

Formula, $NH_4\ C_7\ H_5\ O_2$.

Molecular Weight, 139.

Preparation of Benzoate of Ammonium.—"Take of solution of ammonia three fluid ounces or a sufficiency; benzoic acid two ounces; distilled water four fluid ounces. Dissolve the benzoic acid in three fluid ounces of solution of ammonia previously mixed with the water; evaporate at a gentle heat, keeping ammonia in slight excess, and set aside that crystals may form."—Br. P.

Properties.—Benzoate of ammonia is in minute, white, glistening, four-sided laminæ, having a bitter saline taste, whose odor is in some degree like that of benzoic acid; they are soluble in water and alcohol and decompose readily by heat, with the evolution of ammonia and the production of benzoic acid vapors, and without residue.

Tests.—The properties of the salt, as above stated, will suffice for determining its purity.

First proven by Dr. Wibmer, Germany.

Preparation for Homœopathic Use—The pure benzoate of ammonium is prepared by trituration, as directed under Class VII.

AMMONIUM BROMATUM.

Synonyms, Ammonii Bromidum. Bromide of Ammonium.

Present Name, Ammonium Bromide.

Formula, $NH_4\ Br$.

Molecular Weight, 98.

Preparation of Ammonium Bromide.—Pure ammonium bromide is best obtained by sublimation, as follows: In a retort, having a wide delivery tube, place 100 parts of thoroughly dried and powdered potassium bromide, together with 50 parts of dried and powdered ammonium sulphate. The retort is to be placed on a sand bath and buried in the sand so that the neck only protrudes; the neck of the retort is to be connected with a cooled receiver, and the temperature is to be gradually raised. The ammonium bromide comes over, condenses in the receiver and in the neck of the retort.

Properties.—Ammonium bromide is in colorless prismatic crystals or in a crystalline powder. It has a saline taste; is completely dissipated by heat. It is soluble in two parts of water, and in 15 or 20 parts of 90 per cent. alcohol, while it is almost insoluble in ether.

The first provings were by Dr. A. M. Cushing, U. S.

Tests.—It should give no precipitate with barium chloride (absence of sulphuric acid). Upon mixing it with starch solution and treating the mixture with a drop of chlorine water, no blue color should be developed (absence of iodine.) After its volatilization by heat, there should be no residue left.

Preparation for Homœopathic Use. The pure bromide of ammonium is prepared by trituration, as directed under Class VII.

AMMONIUM CARBONICUM.

Synonyms, Ammonii Carbonas. Ammoniæ Sesquicarbonas. Carbonate of Ammonium. Volatile Salt.

Present Name, Ammonium Carbonate.

Common Name, Sal Volatile.

Formula, $N_4 H_{16} C_3 O_8 = 2 NH_4 HCO_3 + (NH_3)_2 CO_3$.

Molecular Weight, 236.

Preparation.—Commercial carbonate of ammonia is prepared on the large scale by heating to redness, a mixture of one part of ammonium chloride with two parts of calcium carbonate in a retort to which a receiver is luted. Ammonium and calcium change places, and the ammonium carbonate thus formed condenses in the receiver. It consists of two molecules, the acid carbonate together with one of the normal carbonate, or it may be more properly considered as a mixture of the acid carbonate, $(NH_4) HCO_3$, with the carbamate of ammonium, $N_2 H_6 CO_2$, the latter, when dissolved in water, taking up the $H_2 O$ and becoming converted into normal carbonate, $(NH_4)_2 CO_3$. When the commercial carbonate is treated with water the half acid or sesquicarbonate, whose formula is given at the heading of this article, is dissolved. From a strong solution at 30° C. (86° F.) it may be crystallized out in large, transparent, rectangular prisms whose summits are truncated by octohedral faces. The sesquicarbonate can be separated into the normal carbonate, $(NH_4)_2 CO_3$, and the acid carbonate, $NH_4 HCO_3$, by treating it with a 90 per cent. alcohol, the latter taking up the normal carbonate while the acid carbonate remains undissolved.

Properties.—Commercial carbonate of ammonia is in masses, fibrous-crystalline in structure, white and translucent. Exposed to the air it suffers partial decomposition, giving off carbonic oxide and free ammonia, leaving behind the acid ammonium carbonate as a white powder having scarcely any odor of ammonia and reacting weakly alkaline to test paper. The ordinary carbonate of ammonia is soluble in three or four parts of water; hot water dissolves it with decomposition.

Tests.—The pure substance can be obtained by resublimation. It should be dissipated entirely when heated upon platinum foil. Its solution when over-neutralized by nitric acid should give no precipitate with barium chloride (absence of sulphate), nor with silver nitrate (absence of chloride), nor with hydrogen sulphide (absence of metals). If the acidified solution be now neutralized with ammonium hydrate and then treated with ammonium oxalate, a turbidity occurring after some moments, indicates the presence of calcium carbonate.

Introduced into our Materia Medica by Hahnemann.

Preparation for Homœopathic Use.—One part by weight of pure carbonate of ammonium is dissolved in nine parts by weight of distilled water.

Amount of drug power, $\frac{1}{10}$.

Dilutions must be prepared as directed under Class V—*a*.

Triturations of pure carbonate of ammonium, prepared as directed under Class VII., have been recommended, but the great volatility of the substance renders such preparations unsuitable.

AMMONIUM CAUSTICUM.

Synonyms, Aqua Ammoniæ. Liquor Ammonii Caustici. Liquor Ammoniæ Fortior.

Present Name, Ammonium Hydrate.

Formula, NH_4 HO (Ammonia Gas, NH_3).

Molecular Weight, 17, as NH_3.

Production.—By the destructive distillation of nitrogenous organic bodies, as well as by their slower decomposition known as putrefaction, ammonia is formed. This body is a gas, lighter than air, having a pungent odor and reacting strongly alkaline to test paper. It is soluble in water to an extraordinary degree, at ordinary temperatures one volume of water taking up over 700 volumes of the gas. This is more, however, than mere solution, for a definite chemical compound is formed by the union of one molecule of water with one of the gas, the atoms re-arranging themselves to form a new molecule, whose formula is NH_4 HO, and which is known as ammonium hydrate. Ammonium hydrate is a strong base, its radical ammonium, NH_4, readily displacing hydrogen from acids, to form true salts.

See article Ammonium Muriaticum.

Preparation.—Equal parts by weight are taken of ammonium chloride and fresh burnt lime. The former is to be reduced to powder and the latter must be slaked in a covered basin. The materials are then to be mixed, adding enough water to cause the mass to aggregate into lumps. The whole is then transferred to a roomy retort connected with a receiver, a wash-bottle containing water, through which the gas may pass, intervening. The receiver should contain water kept very cold. Upon applying heat very cautiously to the retort, ammonia is disengaged, uniformly and regularly, and condenses in the water in the receiver. The operation is to be continued till ammonia ceases to come over, when the liquid in the receiver is to be removed, and diluted with distilled water till its specific gravity is 0.959, at which density it contains ten per cent. of NH_3 gas.

Properties.—Water of ammonia is a transparent, colorless liquid, possessing the strong odor of ammonia gas; its density is lower than that of distilled water and decreases with its strength; its freezing point is below that of water, and is lowered as its strength increases. It is strongly alkaline to test paper, but the change of color so produced is evanescent. It gives up ammonia gas freely when the temperature is raised, and should be kept in well-stoppered bottles in a cool place.

Tests.—It should give no precipitate upon being treated with an equal volume of lime-water (absence of carbonate). When carefully neutralized with nitric acid, and then diluted with water, no empyreumatic odor should be observable, and it should give no precipitate with hydrogen sulphide (absence of metals), with ammonium oxalate (calcium), with silver nitrate (chloride), or with barium nitrate (sulphate). When heated to 100° C. (212° F.) it should evaporate without residue.

Preparation for Homœopathic Use.—The preparation, specific gravity 0.959, contains ten per cent. of ammoniacal gas, and therefore corresponds to the first decimal potency.

Dilutions must be prepared as directed under Class V—*a*.

AMMONIUM JODATUM.

Synonyms, Ammonii Iodidum. Iodide of Ammonium.

Present Name, Ammonium Iodide.

Formula, NH_4 I.

Molecular Weight, 145.

Preparation of Iodide of Ammonium.—One hundred parts of potassium iodide and forty-one parts of ammonium sulphate are to be dissolved each in eighty parts of distilled water, and the two solutions mixed. To the mixture is added one and a half times its volume of alcohol and the whole allowed to stand for a day in a cold place, and then filtered. The filtrate is then placed in a retort, the alcohol distilled off, the residue treated with stronger ammonia, with constant stirring, and is finally brought to dryness by means of a sand-bath. Towards the last of the operation the temperature may be raised to 110°–120° C. (230°–248° F.). As prepared above the ammonium iodide is not quite free from sulphate. To separate it from the latter, it is to be redissolved in alcohol, when the ammonium sulphate being insoluble may be filtered off and the filtrate evaporated or distilled to dryness.

Properties.—Ammonium iodide when quite pure is a white crystalline powder, without odor, and having a sharp saline taste. It is soluble in its own volume of cold water, and in eight or nine parts of alcohol. Its solutions are perceptibly acid to test paper. When exposed to the air it attracts moisture and undergoes partial decomposition, liberating iodine which gives a yellow color to the salt.

Tests.—The presence of fixed salts will be recognized by the residue left upon heating a portion of ammonium iodide on platinum foil. Upon adding to a solution of ammonium iodide, silver nitrate in excess, a precipitate will fall. As silver iodide is almost insoluble in caustic ammonia solution, if the latter be now added in excess the silver iodide may be removed by filtration. Upon adding nitric acid in excess to the filtrate, a merely opalescent turbidity should occur, a real precipitate indicating the presence of chloride or bromide. Such precipitate may be further tested by adding chlorine water and then some carbon di-sulphide; if the precipitate be a bromide, the bromine liberated by the chlorine water is taken up by the carbon di-sulphide, coloring the latter red; if it be a chloride no alteration of color ensues.

Sulphuric acid from sulphate may be known by a white precipitate, insoluble in nitric acid, occurring when barium nitrate is added to the acidified solution above mentioned.

Preparation for Homœopathic Use.—The pure iodide of ammonium is prepared by trituration, as directed under Class VII.

AMMONIUM MURIATICUM.

Synonyms, Ammonii Chloridum. Ammonium Chloratum. Muriate of Ammonia. Chloride of Ammonium.

Present Name, Ammonium Chloride.

Common Name, Sal Ammoniac.

Formula NH_4 Cl.

Molecular Weight, 53.5.

Preparation of Chloride of Ammonium.—Among the by-products of the destructive distillation of coal in the manufacture of illuminating gas, is the ammoniacal liquor, which is heavily charged with ammonium carbonate and sulphide. When coal-gas liquor is neutralized with hydrochloric acid ammonium chloride is formed, and carbonic oxide and hydrogen sulphide are liberated. The solution is partly evaporated and the impure ammonium chloride crystallizes out. The crystals are moderately heated in an iron pan, to deprive them of tarry matter with which they are contaminated, and finally are purified by sublimation in large iron vessels lined with clay and surmounted by domes of lead, as the vapors act readily upon iron. The purification of the salt in the pharmaceutical laboratory is not recommended, as the cost of a pure article is not high enough to warrant the slight expense of the process.

Properties.—Sublimed ammonium chloride is in white masses of fibro-crystalline texture; from its watery solutions it can be made to crystallize in cubes or octohedrons, the crystals being small and disposed in fern-like arrangement. The salt has a sharp saline taste, and is without odor; it is soluble in less than three parts of cold, and in one of boiling water. By its solution in water the temperature of the latter is considerably reduced. Heated on platinum foil it volatilizes in dense white fumes which remain for some time suspended in the air and upon cooling condense in small needle-like crystals.

Tests.—Fixed impurities will be shown by the residue left upon volatilizing the salt from platinum foil. Traces of iron are present in the best specimens of the commercial product, and sometimes ammonium sulphate is also found. Upon adding potassium ferro-cyanide to a not too dilute solution of ammonium chloride, a blue coloration will be developed if iron be present; a sulphate will be detected by the white precipitate, insoluble in nitric acid, occurring when a solution of barium chloride is added to one of the salt.

The first proving is by Neuning, in Germany.

Preparation for Homœopathic Use.—One part by weight of pure chloride of ammonium is dissolved in nine parts by weight of distilled water.

Amount of drug power, $\frac{1}{10}$.

Dilutions must be prepared as directed under Class V—*a*.

Triturations of the pure chloride of ammonium are prepared as directed under Class VII.

AMMONIUM NITRICUM.

Synonyms, Ammonii Nitras. Nitrum Flammans. Nitrate of Ammonium.

Present Name, Ammonium Nitrate.

Formula, $NH_4 NO_3$.

Molecular Weight, 80.

Preparation of Nitrate of Ammonium—By neutralizing ammonium hydrate with nitric acid, and evaporating the solution to crystallization, the salt is readily obtained.

Properties.—Ammonium nitrate forms permanent, odorless, transparent, hexagonal prisms, when the salt is obtained by slow evaporation of its solution; when the evaporation is done by heat unto complete dryness, the salt is in fibro-crystalline masses. It has a sharp saline and cooling taste. When in masses it is deliquescent. It is soluble in two parts of cold and in about its own volume of hot water and in twenty parts of alcohol. Its solution in water is accompanied by a notable decrease in temperature; when equal parts of the salt and water are taken the thermometer shows a falling of about 25° C. (45° F.). The salt fuses at 160° C. (320° F.), and at about 200° C. (392° F.) it is resolved into water and hyponitrous oxide or *laughing gas;* if the heat be applied too rapidly, or if it be raised to 320° C. (608° F.), it is decomposed suddenly with slight explosion into nitrogen, the lower oxides of nitrogen and ammonia.

Tests.—The usual impurities in ammonium nitrate are ammonium chloride and sulphate. Its watery solution should give no precipitate with silver nitrate or with barium nitrate solution. When heated upon platinum foil it should be completely dissipated, a residue indicating fixed salts.

Preparation for Homœopathic Use.—One part by weight of pure nitrate of ammonium is dissolved in nine parts by weight of distilled water.

Amount of drug power, $\frac{1}{10}$.

Dilutions must be prepared as directed under Class V—*a*.

AMMONIUM PHOSPHORICUM.

Synonyms, Ammonii Phosphas. Phosphate of Ammonium.

Present Name, Hydrogen-Diammonium Phosphate.

Formula, $(NH_4)_2\ HPO_4$.

Molecular Weight, 132.

Preparation of Phosphate of Ammonium.—"Take of diluted phosphoric acid, twenty fluid ounces; strong solution of ammonia, a sufficiency. Add the ammonia to the phosphoric acid until the solution is slightly alkaline, then evaporate the liquid, adding ammonia from time to time so as to keep it in slight excess, and when the crystals are formed, on the cooling of the solution, dry them quickly on filtering-paper placed on a porous tile, and preserve them in a stoppered bottle." —Br. P.

Properties.—Ammonium phosphate forms large, colorless, transparent crystals, having a cooling, saline taste. When exposed to the air, it effloresces slightly, losing ammonia. It is soluble in four parts of cold, and more readily in hot water; it is insoluble in alcohol and ether. When heated, or when its watery solution is boiled, it parts with ammonia. Its solutions are weakly alkaline to test paper. At a red heat it is converted, by the loss of all the ammonia, into metaphosphoric acid.

Tests.—A watery solution of ammonium phosphate should give no precipitate when treated with ammonium sulphide (absence of iron, lead, etc.), nor after acidification with nitric acid, with barium nitrate (absence of sulphuric acid), or with silver nitrate (absence of chloride). Ten parts by weight of the salt when heated to redness, as stated above, will, if pure, leave 6.06 parts of residue.

Preparation.—The pure phosphate of ammonium is prepared by trituration, as directed under Class VII.

AMMONIUM VALERIANICUM.

Synonyms, Ammonii Valerianas. Valerianate of Ammonium.

Present Name, Ammonium Valerianate.

Formula, $NH_4\ C_5\ H_9\ O_2$.

Molecular Weight, 119.

Preparation.—Ammonium valerianate is prepared by saturating valerianic acid with dry ammonia gas. The method given in the article ammonium causticum is to be used, except that the gas is to be first passed through a drying-tube or bottle filled with small pieces of freshly burnt lime. The gas is then led into the valerianic acid.

The complete saturation of the acid will be known by its ceasing to redden blue litmus paper, when the liquid may be set aside to crystallize. The crystals are to be collected, drained and finally dried by means of bibulous paper.

Properties.—Ammonium valerianate is in white four-sided tables, readily soluble in water and alcohol, having the odor of valerianic acid and a sharp, sweetish taste. The crystals effloresce in dry air, but in the presence of moisture they deliquesce. The salt is readily decomposed into ammonia and valerianic acid, and even in its solutions, it gives off ammonia and reacts acid to test paper after some time from the presence of free valerianic acid.

Tests. If a solution of a valerianate is rendered slightly alkaline to test paper, and then fully decomposed by solution of ferric chloride, and after a short time filtered, a red filtrate will indicate the presence of acetic acid. Its solution may be tested in the usual way with barium chloride and silver nitrate, for sulphuric and hydrochloric acids. After the addition of ammonia in excess, its solution will give a precipitate with magnesium sulphate, if phosphates are present. A residue left after heating to redness on platinum will show the presence of a fixed salt or compound.

Preparation for Homœopathic Use.—The pure valerianate of ammonium is prepared by trituration, as directed under Class VII.

AMPELOPSIS.

Synonym, Ampelopsis Quinquefolia, *Michaux.*
Nat. Ord., Vitaceæ.
Common Name, Virginian Creeper.

This is a common woody vine, growing in low or rich grounds throughout the United States, climbing extensively, sometimes by rootlets as well as by its disk-bearing tendrils. Tendrils fixing themselves to trunks of trees or walls by dilated sucker-like disks at their tips; leaves digitate, with five oblong-lanceolate, sparingly serrate leaflets; flower-clusters, cymose, of a greenish-white color. Calyx slightly five-toothed. Petals concave, thick, expanding before they fall. Its blossoms appear in July, and its small, blackish berries ripen in October. It is frequently called *American Ivy.* Its smooth dark green leaves turn crimson in autumn.

Preparation.—Equal parts of the fresh young shoots and the fresh bark are chopped and pounded to a pulp and weighed. Then two parts by weight of alcohol are taken, and having mixed the pulp thoroughly with one-sixth part of it, the rest of the alcohol is added. The whole is to be well stirred, and is then poured into a well-stoppered bottle, and allowed to stand eight days in a dark, cool place. The tincture is then separated by decanting, straining and filtering.

Drug power of tincture, $\frac{1}{6}$.

Dilutions must be prepared as directed under Class.

AMPHISBŒNA VERMICULARIS.

Synonym, Amphisbœna Flavescens.
Class, Reptilia.

Order, Sauria.
Family, Annulata.
Poison of a South American Snake.

This species of snake moves either backwards or forwards, as occasion may require, and is quite common in the woods of Brazil. Its body is cylindrical, from two to two and a half feet long, terminated by a very obtuse tail. It has no scales, properly speaking, but its skin is divided into quadrilateral compartments disposed in rings around the body; 228 on the trunk and 26 on the tail. The lower lip is divided into six long and narrow plates; the head is small, rather sharp, protected by scutellæ, and not distinguished from the neck. It has small eyes; the jaw is not dilatable, the teeth are conical, bent, unequal and distinct from each other; the nostrils are on the sides, and pierced in a single naso-rostral plate. The amphisbœna is of a brownish color above, and a pinkish-white under the belly.

Preparation.—The poison taken from the living animal is triturated as directed under Class IX.

AMYGDALÆ AMARÆ, *De Candolle.*

Synonyms, Amygdalus Communis. Prunus Amygdalus.
Nat. Ord., Amygdaleæ.
Common Name, Bitter Almond.

The almond-tree is probably a native of Persia, extending thence to Syria, and even to Algeria. It is very extensively cultivated in various parts in the south of Europe. The tree is fifteen or twenty feet in height, with spreading branches. Its leaves are lanceolate, serrate, and of a bright green color. The flowers are pale red in color, varying to white. The fruit is a drupe, with a velvety sarcocarp, and marked with a longitudinal furrow, where it opens when fully ripe. Within this covering is a rough shell, containing the kernel or almond.

The first proving seems to have been by Engler, in Germany.

Preparation.—The ripe kernel is finely chopped and pounded, covered with five parts by weight of alcohol, and allowed to stand eight days in a well-stoppered bottle, in a dark, cool place, shaking it twice a day. The tincture is then poured off, strained and filtered.

Drug power of tincture, $\frac{1}{10}$.

Dilutions must be prepared as directed under Class IV.

Triturations are prepared from the ripe kernel, as directed under Class VII.

AMYL NITRITE.

Synonyms, Nitrite of Amyl. Amyl Nitris.
Formula, $C_5 H_{11} NO_2$.
Molecular Weight, 117.

Preparation of Nitrite of Amyl.—Equal volumes of amyl alcohol, purified until it has a constant boiling point 132° C. (269.6° F.), and of nitric acid, are placed in a roomy glass retort, such that the mixture shall only occupy one-third of its capacity. Heat is applied and the temperature gradually increased till the mixture gives evidence of ebullition, when the source of heat may be removed, the chemical interchange no longer requiring its aid. The impure amyl nitrite condenses in a cooled receiver, but only that portion coming over below 100° C. (212° F.) should be retained. This should be washed with caustic soda to remove hydrocyanic acid and the lower oxides of nitrogen, and then rectified over fused potassium carbonate to separate water. Finally the product so obtained is to be redistilled and that part of the distillate which comes over between 95° and 100° C. (203°—212° F.) is to be preserved for medicinal use.

Properties.—Amyl nitrite is a yellowish ethereal liquid, having a peculiar odor resembling that of over-ripe pears, and a somewhat aromatic taste. The boiling point is about 95° or 96° C. (103°—104.6° F.), and its specific gravity from 0.877 to 0.900. When added drop by drop to caustic potash while fused by the application of heat, valerianate of potassium will be formed.

Tests.—The purity of a specimen of amyl nitrite is assured by its possessing the above described qualities.

Preparation for Homœopathic Use.—One part by weight of pure nitrite of amyl is dissolved in nine parts by weight of 95 per cent. alcohol.

Amount of drug power, $\frac{1}{10}$.

Dilutions must be prepared as directed under Class VI—*a*.

ANACARDIUM ORIENTALE.

Synonyms, Semecarpus Anacardium, *Linn.* Anacardium Officinarum.

Nat. Ord., Anacardiaceæ.

Common Names, Marking-nut Tree. Malacca Bean. Anacardium.

This is a small tree, growing in the West Indies and other parts of tropical America. The nut is heart-shaped; it consists of two shells, with a black caustic fluid between them, and of a sweet oily kernel. Great precaution is to be advised in handling these nuts, for the juice coming in contact with an irritable skin causes pustular eruptions, which are very painful and difficult to cure. Care must be taken to distinguish the marking-nut from the cashew nut, from *A. occidentale.* The latter is kidney-shaped and grayish-brown in color; the former is heart-shaped and is black and glossy.

Introduced by Hahnemann.

Preparation.—The crushed seed is covered with five parts by weight of 95 per cent. alcohol, and allowed to stand eight days in a well-stoppered bottle, in a dark, cool place, shaking it twice a day. The tincture is then poured off, strained and filtered.

Drug power of tincture, $\frac{1}{10}$.

Dilutions must be prepared as directed under Class IV.

Triturations are to be prepared from the black caustic fluid contained in the fruit, as directed under Class IX.

ANAGALLIS.

Synonyms, Anagallis Arvensis, *Linn.*
Nat. Ord., Primulaceæ.
Common Names, Scarlet Pimpernel. Poor Man's Weather-Glass.
This plant is a native of Europe, but has been naturalized in this country. The slender, mostly procumbent stems are smooth, branched, four-edged; the branches, opposite, diffused, the leaves, clasping, opposite, ovate-lanceolate, entire obtuse, with blackish translucent spots underneath. The small but beautiful flowers, scarlet, sometimes purple, blue or white, are on long pedicles in the axils. Calyx five-parted. Corolla wheel-shaped, with almost no tube, five-parted, longer than the calyx; the divisions broad. Petals obovate, obtuse, fringed with minute teeth or stalked glands. Stamens five; filaments bearded. Pod membranaceous, circumcissile, the top falling off like a lid, many seeded. The flowers' quickly closing at the approach of bad weather, gave origin to its common English name, Poor Man's Weather-Glass. The flowers appear in July and August.

Preparation.—The fresh plant (of the scarlet-flowered variety only), gathered before the development of the flowers, is chopped and pounded to a pulp, which is to be enclosed in a piece of new linen and subjected to pressure. The expressed juice is then, with brisk agitation, mingled with an equal part by weight of alcohol. This mixture is allowed to stand eight days in a well-stoppered bottle, in a dark, cool place, and then filtered.

Drug power of tincture, $\frac{1}{2}$.
Dilutions must be prepared as directed under Class I.

ANANTHERUM MURICATUM.

Synonyms, Andropogon Muricatus, *Retz.* Vetiveria Odorata, Virana.
Nat. Ord., Gramineæ.
Common Names, Bena. Cuscus. Vetiver. Viti-vayr.
A well known grass in the East Indies, cultivated on the Markarentas Islands for its medical use; the root is aromatic and stimulating or diaphoretic.

Preparation.—The root in coarse powder is covered with five parts by weight of alcohol, and then poured into a well-stoppered bottle, and allowed to stand eight days in a dark, cool place, shaking it twice a day. The tincture is then poured off, strained and filtered.

Drug power of tincture, $\frac{1}{10}$.
Dilutions must be prepared as directed under Class IV.

ANDIRA INERMIS, *Kunth.*

Synonyms, Andira Refusa. Geoffroya Inermis.
Nat. Ord., Leguminosæ.
Common Names, Bastard Cabbage Tree. Cabbage Tree Bark.
This tree, a native of Jamaica, and of other West India Islands,

branches only toward the top. Its leaves are pinnately divided, the leaflets being in pairs with one terminal; they are petiolate, ovate-lanceolate, pointed, smooth. The flowers are in terminal panicles. The bark is found in commerce in long pieces, somewhat thick, and fibrous, and frequently covered with growth of lichens; its color is brownish-gray externally, internally it is yellow. Its odor is disagreeable, and the taste is bitter-sweet and mucilaginous. It has a resinous fracture.

Properties.—The bark, in coarse powder, is covered with five parts by weight of alcohol, and having been poured into a well-stoppered bottle, is allowed to stand eight days in a dark, cool place, being shaken twice a day. The tincture is then poured off, strained and filtered.

Drug power of tincture, $\frac{1}{10}$.

Dilutions must be prepared as directed under Class IV.

ANEMONIN.

Formula, $C_{15} H_{14} O_7$.

Obtained from Anemone Pratensis.

Preparation of Anemonin.—By distilling water off the leaves or root, or indeed the whole herb, of *Anemone (Pulsatilla) pratensis, A. nemorosa, Ranunculus Sceleratus,* and other species of the Ranunculaceæ, the distillate is found to contain anemonin and anemonic acid.

Dobraschinky obtains anemonin by subjecting to distillation the fresh flowering herb *A. pratensis* and water, with one-tenth part of chloroform, and dissolving the residue of the chloroform extract in hot alcohol; the anemonin then separates in crystals.

Properties.—Anemonin is a camphor-like body, crystallizing in the tri-metric system. The crystals are transparent and colorless, without odor, and indifferent to test papers. In the cold they are sparingly soluble in alcohol. Ether and water dissolve but little, even at the boiling point. Chloroform dissolves it readily. The crystals soften at 150° C. (302° F.), giving off water and acrid vapors, forming, probably, a new body, for in this state the substance has a burning taste, and leaves the tongue numb for some days afterward.

Preparation for Homœopathic Use.—Anemonin is prepared by trituration, as directed under Class VII.

ANGELICA ARCHANGELICA, *Linn.*

Synonym, Archangelica Officinalis. *Hoffm.*

Nat. Ord., Umbelliferæ.

Common Name, Garden Angelica.

The root of garden angelica is long, thick, fleshy, supplied with numerous fibres, and sends up annually a round, hollow, smooth stem, purplish in color, rising five feet or more in height, and branching. The leaves are large, bi-pinnate, leaflets ovate-lanceolate, pointed, serrate. The flowers are greenish-white and small. The plant is cultivated in gardens in Europe, and occasionally in this country.

Preparation.—The dried root in coarse powder is covered with five parts by weight of alcohol. Having poured it into a well-stoppered bottle, it is allowed to stand eight days in a dark, cool place, and shaken twice a day. The tincture is then poured off, strained and filtered.

Drug power of tincture, $\frac{1}{10}$.

Dilutions must be prepared as directed under Class IV.

ANGUSTURÆ CORTEX.

Synonym, Galipea Cusparia, *St. Hilaire.*

Nat. Ord., Rutaceæ.

Common Name, Angustura or Cusparia Bark.

This is a small tree, irregularly branched, rising to the height of fifteen or twenty feet, with an erect stem from three to five inches in diameter, and covered with a smooth, gray bark. The tree grows abundantly on the mountains of Caroni, in Venezuela, between the 7th and 8th degrees of N. latitude. The bark is found in commerce in flattish or channeled pieces, in lengths varying from one to three inches, an inch or more wide and about one-eighth of an inch thick. Its outer side is covered with a cork-like layer, yellowish-gray in color, and easily removable. Beneath this layer is a dark brown resinous surface. Its fracture is short and resinous, and is dotted with sharply defined white points, these being aggregations of calcium oxalate crystals. The taste of the bark is bitter, and its odor is disagreeable.

It was first proven by Hahnemann.

Preparation.—The dried bark, reduced to a coarse powder, is covered with five parts by weight of alcohol. Having poured the mixture into a well-stoppered bottle, it is allowed to stand eight days in a dark, cool place, shaking it twice a day. The tincture is then poured off, strained and filtered.

Drug power of tincture, $\frac{1}{10}$.

Dilutions must be prepared as directed under Class IV.

ANISUM STELLATUM.

Synonym, Illicium Anisatum, *Linn.*

Nat. Ord., Magnoliaceæ.

Common Names, Star Anise-Seed. Badiane.

The fruit of a small tree, native of the southwestern provinces of China. It was introduced at an early period into Japan. The fruit is star-shaped, made up of eight one-seeded carpels. The seed is elliptical, somewhat flattened, truncated on one side; its upper edge is keeled, the lower rounded. Star anise has an agreeable, aromatic taste and smell, resembling fennel in these respects. When powdered it leaves a sub-acid after-taste. It must not be confounded with the ordinary anise of the United States and British Pharmacopœias.

It was first proved by Dr. Franz, Germany.

Preparation.—The dried, powdered fruit, is covered with five parts by weight of alcohol. Having poured the mass into a well-stoppered bottle, it is allowed to stand eight days in a dark, cool place, shaking it twice a day. The tincture is then poured off, strained and filtered.

Drug power of tincture, $\frac{1}{10}$.

Dilutions must be prepared as directed under Class IV.

ANTHEMIS.

Synonym, Anthemis Nobilis, *Linn.*

Nat. Ord., Compositæ.

Common Names, Common Chamomile. Roman Chamomile.

A small, creeping, perennial plant, putting forth in the latter part of the summer solitary flower-heads. It is abundant in Southern England, is found in Ireland, and is plentiful in Southern Europe. Stem prostrate, branching from the base; leaves finely incised, pinnatifid, segments linear, subulate. The flowers are like those of the compositæ in general. They are from one-half to three-fourths of an inch across, with a hemispherical involucre, made up of a number of equal bracts. Receptacle conical. The ray florets in the wild state number twelve or more, and are white, narrow, strap-shaped, and toothed at the end. The disk florets are yellow and tubular. In the cultivated plant the ligulate florets predominate over or replace entirely the tubular ones. Minute oil glands are sparingly scattered over the tubular parts of both kinds of florets. The whole plant has a strong aromatic odor and bitter taste.

Drs. Marcy and Peters seem to have first collected symptoms from provings of the whole plant.

Preparation.—The whole, fresh plant, gathered when coming into flower, is chopped and pounded to a pulp and weighed. Then two parts by weight of alcohol are taken, and after mixing the pulp thoroughly with one-sixth part of it, the rest of the alcohol is added. After stirring the whole well, and pouring it into a well-stoppered bottle, it is allowed to stand eight days in a dark, cool place. The tincture is then separated by decanting, straining and filtering.

Drug power of tincture, $\frac{1}{6}$.

Dilutions must be prepared as directed under Class III.

ANTHOXANTHUM ODORATUM, *Linn.*

Nat. Ord., Gramineæ.

Common Name, Sweet Vernal Grass.

This is a perennial, found growing in meadows, woods and on river banks, in Arctic Europe, Northern Africa, Siberia, Dahuria and Greenland; and has been introduced into North America. Its stem is from six to eighteen inches high, shining. Leaves flat, hairy; sheaths furrowed, often pubescent, mouth pilose. Panicle one to five inches long, pubescent or villous; branches short. Spikelets one-quarter to one-third inch long, fascicled, often squarrose, green; empty glumes ovate, acute, upper lanceolate, almost awned; two succeeding glumes two-lobed, pilose, awn in the sinus, slender, exserted; flower glume smaller, glabrous, obtuse, awnless. Paleæ one-nerved. Scales none. Stamens two, anthers large, linear, yellow; ovary glabrous, styles long, stigmas feathery. Fruit terete, acute, enclosed in the brown-shining flower glume and paleæ. Flowers appear in May and June.

Preparation.—The fresh herb, in flower, is chopped and pounded to a pulp and weighed. Then two parts by weight of alcohol are taken, the pulp mixed thoroughly with one-sixth part of it, and the rest of the alcohol added. After stirring the whole well, and pouring it into a well-stoppered bottle, it is allowed to stand eight days in a dark, cool place. The tincture is then separated by decanting, straining and filtering.

Drug power of tincture, ⅙.

Dilutions must be prepared as directed under Class III.

ANTHRACITE.

Vast masses of the vegetation of pre-historic times having been buried, subjected to pressure and probably to a mode of fermentation, are now found by man as coal. Of this there are three principal varieties, lignite, bituminous coal and anthracite. The latter contains about 90 per cent. of carbon, a little over 3 per cent. of hydrogen, and something less than 3 per cent. of oxygen, with less than 1 per cent. each of nitrogen and sulphur, while of ash it gives about 1.5 per cent., consisting chiefly of silica, alumina and ferric oxide.

Anthracite, or *stone coal*, is found in many parts of the world, but enormous deposits of it exist in Pennsylvania, U. S.

Preparation.—Anthracite is prepared by trituration as directed under Class VII.

ANTHRAKOKALI.

Synonym, Lithanthrakokali Simplex.

Preparation of Anthrakokali.—To seven parts of freshly prepared caustic potash in a state of fusion are added five parts of finely pulverized anthracite coal (which, for the originally proved preparation, was obtained from *Fünfkirchen*, a town in the Baranya district of Hungary); the vessel is taken from the fire, and the mixture triturated till a perfectly uniform black powder is formed, which is preserved in small, well-stoppered bottles.

Properties.—Rightly prepared anthrakokali is a black, very subtle, staining powder of alkaline taste; is inodorous and becomes moist in the air without deliquescing.

Tests.—Five grains of the preparation dissolved in an ounce of distilled water yield a darkish-brown solution, so dark indeed that after all insoluble matter has subsided the liquid is translucent only in thin layers.

Preparation for Homœopathic Use.—Anthrakokali is prepared by trituration as directed under Class VII. It must be preserved in well-stoppered bottles.

ANTIMONIUM CRUDUM.

Synonyms, Antimonii Sulphuretum. Stibium Sulphuretum Nigrum. Tersulphuret of Antimony. Sulphuret of Antimony. Black (Crude) Antimony.

Present Name, Antimonious Sulphide.

Formula, $Sb_2 S_3$.

Molecular Weight, 340.

Origin.—The crystallized tri-sulphide of antimony occurs as a natural mineral called stibnite, gray antimony or antimony glance. It is the source of all the antimony of commerce. It is found in various localities in Hungary, Germany, France, England and the United States.

Properties.—It is found in masses of aggregated needles, having a metallic lustre and of a lead-gray color, inclining to steel-gray, sometimes iridescent. It produces a streak of its own color. It is easily fusible, thin splinters melting even in the flame of a candle.

The crude substance should be used for homœopathic preparations, those pieces having the largest and most brilliant laminæ being selected. The pieces must be powdered, and ground with water, on a hard stone. This process will, after several repetitions, give a blackish powder, perfectly pure, without smell or taste, and insoluble either in water or alcohol.

Introduced into our Materia Medica by Hahnemann.

Preparation for Homœopathic Use.—The pure antimonium crudum is prepared by trituration, as directed under Class VII.

ANTIMONIUM IODATUM.

Synonyms, Antimonii Iodidum. Antimonious Iodide. Teriodide of Antimony.

Formula, $Sb\ I_3$.

Molecular Weight, 501.

Preparation of Iodide of Antimony.—Nicklès prepares this compound by treating pulverized antimony with iodine dissolved in carbon di-sulphide. The iodide dissolves in the liquid and crystallizes therefrom in red tabular hexagonal crystals.

Properties.—The crystals of antimonious iodide are permanent in the air, and dissolve slowly but completely in carbon di-sulphide, they are readily decomposed by water, forming an oxyiodide, and by alkaline hydrates and carbonates, yielding then pure antimonious oxide.

Preparation for Homœopathic Use.—Iodide of antimony is prepared by trituration, as directed under Class VII.

ANTIMONIUM OXYDATUM.

Synonyms, Antimonii Oxidum. Antimonious Oxide.

Present Name, Antimonious Oxide.

Formula, $Sb_2 O_3$.

Molecular Weight, 288.

Preparation of Oxide of Antimony.—The tri-oxide of antimony can be easily obtained by heating the tri-sulphide with strong hydrochloric acid, adding acid as long as hydrogen sulphide continues to be given off. The solution of tri-chloride thus formed is to be thrown into a large amount of water, when decomposition takes place and the so-called oxychloride (*powder of Algaroth*) is precipitated. This is to be repeatedly agitated with fresh supplies of water till free from acid reaction in each case, allowing the powder to settle and drawing off the supernatant water by a syphon. Finally, the oxychloride is to be treated with a strong solution of sodium carbonate, and the mixture allowed to stand, with occasional agitation for some hours. The resulting trioxide is removed by filtration, and repeatedly washed till the washings give no precipitate with a solution of silver nitrate acidulated with nitric acid.

Properties.—Antimonious oxide is a white or greyish-white heavy powder at ordinary temperatures, but turns yellow when heated, insoluble in water, but dissolving readily in hydrochloric or tartaric acid. It melts below a red heat, and sublimes when raised to a higher temperature in a closed vessel; when heated in the air it absorbs oxygen, becoming changed into the tetroxide. Its solution in hydrochloric acid yields a white precipitate with water, and an orange-red precipitate with sulphuretted hydrogen.

Tests.—Oxide of antimony dissolves completely when boiled with acid potassium tartrate in excess (absence of earthy impurities, etc.), and its solution in tartaric acid is not precipitated by silver nitrate (chlorides), barium chloride (sulphates), or potassium ferrocyanide (metals).

Preparation for Homœopathic Use.—The pure oxide of antimony is prepared by trituration, as directed under Class VII.

ANTIMONIUM SULPHURATUM AURATUM.

Synonyms, Antimonii Sulphuratum Aureum. Sulphurated Antimony. Golden Sulphuret of Antimony. Golden Sulphur.

Composition, $Sb_2 S_5$ and $Sb_2 S_3$ mixed with a small amount of $Sb_2 O_3$, the latter varying in quantity.

Preparation of Sulphurated Antimony.—One part of pure antimonious sulphide, obtained by fusing the native sulphide, the residue being treated by elutriation and afterward submitted to the action of ammonia water in the cold for some days, is added to twelve parts of a solution of soda containing 5.6 per cent. of pure sodium hydrate in distilled water. To the mixture is added thirty parts of distilled water, and the whole is boiled at a gentle heat for two hours, with constant stirring. Distilled water must be added from time to time to supply the loss by evaporation. The liquid is to be strained at once through a strainer of doubled cotton cloth, and into it before it cools at all, dilute sulphuric acid is to be dropped as long as the addition of the acid causes a precipitate. The precipitate must be washed with distilled water until the washings are no longer rendered turbid by the addition of barium chloride solution. Lastly, the precipitate is to be dried and reduced to powder.

Properties and Tests.—The golden sulphide of antimony is, when prepared by the above given process, a reddish-brown powder. It is insoluble in water and when treated with hydrochloric acid evolves hydrogen sulphide and forms a chloride. A solution of the golden sulphide made in boiling water should give no precipitate with barium chloride, or with ammonium oxalate. When sixty grains of the sulphide are dissolved in hydrochloric acid and the solution thrown into distilled water, a white precipitate falls which when dried weighs about fifty-three grains.

First proven by Dr. Mayerhofer, Germany.

Preparation for Homœopathic Use.—The pure sulphurated antimony is prepared by trituration, as directed under Class VII.

ANTIMONIUM TARTARICUM.

Synonyms, Antimonii Potassii-tartras. Tartarus Emeticus. Tartarus Stibiatus. Stibio-Kali Tartaricum. Tartrate of Antimony and Potassium. Tartarated Antimony.

Present Name, Potassio-antimonium Oxytartrate.

Common Name, Tartar Emetic.

Formula, $2\ C_4\ H_4\ K\ (Sb\ O)\ O_6 + H_2\ O$.

Molecular Weight, 664.

Preparation.—To eighteen fluid ounces of water at 100° C. (212° F.) in a glass vessel, add two ounces of oxide of antimony and two-and-a-half ounces of acid potassium tartrate. Both substances must be in the state of fine powder and mixed together before being added to the water. The mixture is to be boiled for an hour and filtered while hot. The filtrate is to be set aside to crystallize. The crystals are to be removed, and dried; they should be kept in a closely stoppered bottle. For further purification, they are redissolved in water, and precipitated from this solution by alcohol in the form of minute crystals.

Properties.—Tartar emetic is in colorless transparent rhombic octohedrons or tetrahedrons, which become opaque on exposure to the air. Their taste is sweetish and metallic. They are soluble in fourteen or fifteen parts of cold and in two parts of boiling water, and not at all in alcohol. The solution is acid to test paper, and becomes decomposed by most metallic salts, salts of the earthy metals, by tannic acid and by free alkalies.

Tests.—Dissolve one part of tartar emetic in fifteen parts of distilled water at the ordinary temperature; after shaking, the solution should be clear or very nearly so. Both acid and normal potassium tartrate will remain undissolved if present. Portions of the solution treated with solutions of barium chloride, silver nitrate, ammonium oxalate and potassium ferro-cyanide should suffer no change in color nor become turbid, otherwise the presence of sulphates, nitrates, calcium, copper or iron compounds is indicated (the silver solution should be added in a few drops only). For the detection of arsenic, Bettendorf's method may be used. A few grains of tartar emetic with nearly twice as much stannous chloride are placed in a test-tube with ten or twelve parts of a 25 per cent. hydrochloric acid, thoroughly agitated and then heated to boiling for three minutes, unless a reaction should appear sooner. If arsenic be present a brown precipitate occurs. If a 30 to 35 per cent. hydrochloric acid be used the change will occur immediately. The precipitate is to be collected, washed and dried, and when heated in a reduction-tube gives the well known arsenical mirror.

The drug appears first in Homœopathic Materia Medica in Hartlaub and Trinks.

Preparation for Homœopathic Use.—One part by weight of pure tartar emetic is dissolved in ninety-nine parts by weight of distilled water.

Amount of drug power, $\frac{1}{100}$.

Dilutions must be prepared as directed under Class V—β.

Triturations of pure tartar emetic are prepared as directed under Class VII.

ANTIRRHINUM LINARIUM, *Linn.*

Synonym, Linaria Vulgaris, *Miller* and *Lindley.*

Nat.Ord., Scrophulariaceæ.

Common Name, Common Toad-Flax.

This is a perennial herbaceous plant, between one and two feet high, with alternate, crowded, linear leaves, and a dense raceme of yellow spurred flowers. It is indigenous to Europe, but has been introduced into this country, and is found in great abundance along the roadsides and in old fields through the Middle States. It flowers from June to October. The plant when fresh has a somewhat disagreeable odor, which is in a great part dissipated by drying.

Preparation.—The fresh plant in flower is chopped and pounded to a pulp and weighed. Then two parts by weight of alcohol are taken and the pulp mixed thoroughly with one-sixth part of it, and the rest of the alcohol added. After stirring the whole well, and pouring it into a well-stoppered bottle, it is allowed to stand eight days in a dark, cool place. The tincture is then separated by decanting, straining and filtering.

Drug power of tincture, $\frac{1}{6}$.

Dilutions must be prepared as directed under Class III.

APHIS CHENOPODII GLAUCI.

Class, Insecta.

Order, Rhynchota.

Family, Aphidæ.

Common Name, Plant Louse from *Chenopodium Glaucum.*

These lice are found in great abundance upon the oak-leaved goosefoot (*Chenopodium Glaucum, Linn.*), from which they are gathered. The head is small and furnished with a long tubular beak, which is situated perpendicularly between the fore legs. The body is soft, oval, and provided at the posterior extremity with two slightly raised eminences, each of which is pierced by a tube or pore. From time to time there exudes through these orifices minute drops of a thick, sweetish fluid called "Honigthau." These insects feed upon the sap contained in the leaves, sucking up the circulating fluids with the greatest avidity, and when gorged with sap, the liquor passes out through the posterior pores as above described.

Dr. Meyer, of Germany, first proved it.

Preparation.—The live insects, bruised, are covered with five parts by weight of alcohol, poured into a well-stoppered bottle, and allowed to remain eight days in a dark, cool place, the whole being shaken twice a day. The tincture is then poured off, strained and filtered.

Drug power of tincture, $\frac{1}{10}$.

Dilutions must be prepared as directed under Class IV.

APIS MELLIFICA.

Class, Insecta.
Order, Hymenoptera.
Family, Apidæ.
Common Name, Honey Bee.

This well known insect lives in swarms in the wilds, and is also cultivated in proper establishments, to furnish honey and wax, two valuable products of its industry.

The first proving was by Dr. F. Humphreys, New York.

Preparation.—The live bees, put into a bottle, are irritated by shaking, and upon them is poured five times their weight of dilute alcohol. The whole is allowed to remain eight days, being shaken twice a day. The tincture is then poured off, strained and filtered.

Drug power of tincture, $\frac{1}{10}$.

Dilutions must be prepared as directed under Class IV., except that *dilute* alcohol be used for the 2x and 1 dilutions.

APIUM VIRUS.

Poison of the Honey Bee.

The proving of this preparation was first done by Dr. C. Hering.

Preparation.—Draw out the sting together with the poison bag from a bee freshly killed. Taking hold of the bag, insert the point of the sting into a small glass tube and squeeze the poison into it. Or, take a live bee with a pair of pincers and allow it to seize a small lump of sugar. It will immediately sting into the sugar, which will absorb the poison. Repeat this process until enough is accumulated to start a trituration. This poison is triturated as directed under Class VIII.

APOCYNUM ANDROSÆMIFOLIUM, *Linn.*

Nat. Ord., Apocynaceæ.
Common Name, Spreading Dog's Bane.

This perennial herb is two or three feet high, and abounds in a milky juice, which exudes upon wounding the plant. The smooth stem is erect, branched above, and of a red color on the side exposed to the sun. The leaves are petioled, opposite, ovate, acute, entire, and two or three inches long. The pale, rose-colored flowers are in loose, spreading cymes. The corolla tube is much longer than the calyx, with spreading border. The fruit consists of two long slender follicles, containing numerous imbricated seeds, attached to central receptacle, and each having a long tuft of silky down at the apex. The plant is found all over the United States north of the Carolinas. It flowers in June and July.

The first proving is by Dr. J. Henry, United States.

Preparation.—The fresh root is chopped and pounded to a pulp and weighed. Then two parts by weight of alcohol are taken, the pulp mixed thoroughly with one-sixth part of it, and the rest of the alcohol added. After stirring the whole well, and pouring it into a well-stoppered bottle, it is allowed to stand eight days in a dark, cool place. The tincture is then separated by decanting, straining and filtering.

Drug power of tincture, $\frac{1}{6}$.

Dilutions must be prepared as directed under Class III.

APOCYNUM CANNABINUM.

Nat. Ord., Apocynaceæ.

Common Name, American Indian Hemp, a faulty term; (better simply, American Hemp).

In general appearance and character, this species bears a close resemblance to the preceding. The stems are, however, more erect; the leaves are smaller and thicker than in the preceding; the cymes are paniculate; the corolla is small and greenish, with a tube not longer than the calyx, and an erect border; the internal parts of the flower are pinkish or purple. The plant grows in similar situations with *A. androsæmifolium*, flowers about the same period, and bears a similar fruit, except that the follicles are more slender; care must be taken not to confound these two varieties.

First proved by Dr. Black, of England.

Preparation.—The fresh root is chopped and pounded to a pulp and weighed. Then two parts by weight of alcohol are taken, and the pulp mixed thoroughly with one-sixth part of it, when the rest of the alcohol is to be added. After stirring the whole well, and pouring it into a well-stoppered bottle, it is allowed to stand eight days in a dark, cool place. The tincture is then separated by decanting, straining and filtering.

Drug power of tincture, $\frac{1}{6}$.

Dilutions must be prepared as directed under Class III.

APOMORPHIA.

Synonyms, Apomorphia Hydrochlorate. Apomorphiæ Hydrochloras. Muriate of Apomorphia. Apomorphine.

Formula, $C_{17}\ H_{17}\ NO_2$.

Molecular Weight, 267.

Preparation of Apomorphia.—By heating morphine in a sealed tube to 140°–150° C. (284°–302° F.) for two or three hours with a large excess of hydrochloric acid, the elements of one molecule of water are abstracted from the morphine and the resulting alkaloid is apomorphine. The reaction is exhibited as follows: $C_{17}\ H_{19}\ NO_3 - H_2\ O = C_{17}\ H_{17}\ NO_2$. The process is not so simple as the equation would indicate, for the product actually obtained is a compound of apomorphia with hydrochloric acid. The same body may be prepared by digesting morphia with excess of hydrochloric acid, under paraffin on the water-bath for some days. By decomposing the hydrochlorate with sodium bicarbonate the base may be obtained as a snow-white mass, which quickly turns green on exposure to the air. The hydrochlorate acts in a similar manner, as will be seen below.

Properties.—Hydrochlorate of apomorphine comes in commerce in amorphous masses or in the crystalline state, or as a mixture of both forms. It is soluble in about 30 parts of water at medium temperatures and in about 25 parts of alcohol. Its identity is determined by its behavior to the air, to certain solvents and reagents. Apomorphia itself is a colorless amorphous alkaloid; when exposed to the air it absorbs oxygen and quickly turns green, and is then less soluble in water, imparting to its solution in the latter an emerald-green color. It is then soluble in alcohol, producing a greenish-colored solution, while its solution in ether and benzol are purple-red, and in chloroform, violet. It is rarely found colorless, usually more or less greenish-gray. As in the process only about 10 parts of apomorphine are obtained from 100 parts of morphia and some special technical appliances are required to prevent its oxidation by exposure to the air, its production should be left to the manufacturing chemist.

Tests.—In addition to the properties mentioned above may be given some of the points of difference between its behavior and that of morphia under similar circumstances; first, its greater solubility in water and alcohol, but especially in ether, in which morphia is almost insoluble. The well known test, ferric chloride, which gives with morphia a greenish-blue coloration, produces in even 1 per cent. solutions of apomorphia a dark amethyst tint.

Preparation for Homœopathic Use.—The pure apomorphia is prepared by trituration, as directed under Class VII.

AQUILEGIA VULGARIS, *Linn.*

Nat. Ord., Ranunculaceæ.

Common Name, Common Garden Columbine.

This perennial herb is a native of Europe, where it grows in woody low grounds and forests; it is cultivated in our gardens as an ornamental flower. The stem is from one to three feet high, the leaves nearly smooth, glaucous, biternate, leaflets bifid and trifid, with rounded or ovoid lobes; the flowers at the edges of the stem and branches are pendant, blue or brown, rarely rosy, with incurved spurs.

Preparation.—The entire, uncultivated, fresh, blooming plant, is chopped and pounded to a pulp and then weighed. Then two parts by weight of alcohol are taken, the pulp mixed thoroughly with one-sixth part of it, and the rest of the alcohol added. After stirring the whole well, and pouring it into a well-stoppered bottle, it is allowed to stand eight days in a dark, cool place. The tincture is then separated by decanting, straining and filtering.

Drug power of tincture, $\frac{1}{6}$.

Dilutions must be prepared as directed under Class III.

ARALIA HISPIDA, *Michaux.*

Synonym, Aralia Mühlenbergiana.

Nat. Ord., Araliaceæ.

Common Names, Bristly Sarsaparilla. Wild Elder. Dwarf Elder.

This plant is found growing in rocky places in North America, common northward and southward along the mountains. Its stem is one to two feet high, bristly, leafy, terminating in a peduncle bearing several umbels; leaves twice pinnate; leaflets oblong-ovate, acute, cut-serrate. The flowers are white or greenish, more or less polygamous. Calyx-tube coherent with the ovary, the teeth very short or almost obsolete. Petals five, epigynous, oblong or obovate, lightly imbricated in the bud, deciduous. Stamens five, epigynous, alternate with the petals. Styles two to five, mostly distinct and slender, or in the sterile flowers short and united. Ovary two to five celled, with a single anatropous ovule suspended from the top of each cell, ripening into a berry-like drupe, with as many seeds as cells. Flowers in June.

Preparation.—The fresh root is chopped and pounded to a pulp and weighed. Then two parts by weight of alcohol are taken, the pulp mixed thoroughly with one-sixth part of it, and the rest of the alcohol added. After stirring the whole well, and pouring it into a well-stoppered bottle, it is allowed to stand eight days in a dark, cool place. The tincture is then separated by decanting, straining and filtering.

Drug power of tincture, $\frac{1}{6}$.

Dilutions must be prepared as directed under Class III.

ARALIA RACEMOSA, *Linn.*

Nat. Ord., Araliaceæ.

Common Name, American Spikenard.

This is an indigenous plant, growing in rich woodlands. Herbaceous; stem widely branched; leaflets heart-ovate, pointed, doubly serrate, slightly downy; umbels racemose; styles united. There are traces of stipules at the dilated base of the leaf-stalks. The plant is well known for its spicy, aromatic, large roots. Its greenish-white flowers appear in July.

First proven by Dr. S. A. Jones, U. S.

Preparation.—The fresh root is chopped and pounded to a pulp and weighed. Then two parts by weight of alcohol are taken, and after thoroughly mixing the pulp with one-sixth part of it, the rest of the alcohol is added. After stirring the whole well, and pouring it into a well-stoppered bottle, it is allowed to stand eight days in a dark, cool place. The tincture is then separated by decanting, straining and filtering.

Drug power of tincture, $\frac{1}{6}$.

Dilutions must be prepared as directed under Class III.

ARANEA DIADEMA, *Linn.*

Synonym, Epeira Diadema.
Class, Arachnida.
Order, Araneidea.
Family, Epeiridæ.
Common Names, Diadem Spider. Garden or Papal Cross Spider.

This spider is found all over Europe and America, in stables, on old walls, etc. It may be distinguished by its ovoid form of body, often as large as a small nut; a longitudinal line on the back, composed of yellow and white points, and traversed by three other similar lines.

First provings are recorded in A. H. Z., I, 122.

Preparation.—The live animal is crushed and covered with five parts by weight of alcohol. Having poured this into a well-stoppered bottle, it is allowed to remain eight days in a dark, cool place, being shaken twice a day. The tincture is then poured off, strained and filtered.

Amount of drug power, $\frac{1}{10}$.

Dilutions must be prepared as directed under Class IV.

ARANEA SCINENCIA.

Class, Arachnida.
Order, Araneidea.
Family, Epeiridæ.

Proven by Dr. Rowley, Louisville, Kentucky, who says: It is a grey spider found in the summer on walls and old places. I believe it does not spin a web; it is very quick in its movements, and takes its prey by a quick spring."

Preparation.—The live animal is covered with five parts by weight of alcohol and allowed to remain eight days in a well-stoppered bottle, in a dark, cool place, being shaken twice a day. The tincture is then poured off, strained and filtered.

Amount of drug power, $\frac{1}{10}$.

Dilutions must be prepared as directed under Class IV.

ARCTIUM LAPPA, *Linn.*

Synonyms, Lappa Major, *Gærtner.* Lappa Officinalis.
Nat. Ord., Compositæ.

Common Name, Burdock.

This is a coarse biennial weed, with a simple spindle-shaped root, about a foot in length, externally brown, internally white and spongy, giving off thread-like fibres. The stem is branching, pubescent, three or four feet high; leaves large, cordate, denticular, green on their upper surface, whitish and downy beneath, and on long petioles. The purple, globose flowers are in irregular terminal panicles. Imbricated scales of the involucre are furnished with hooked extremities, by which they adhere to clothes, and the coats of animals. This plant is common in the United States, on the roadsides, and in waste places.

The plant was first proven by Dr. Jacob Jeanes, U. S.

Preparation.—The fresh root, collected in spring, is chopped and pounded to a pulp and weighed. Then two parts by weight of alcohol are taken, and the pulp mixed with one-sixth part of it, and the rest of the alcohol added. After stirring the whole well, and pouring it into a well-stoppered bottle, it is allowed to stand eight days in a dark, cool place. The tincture is then separated by decanting, straining and filtering.

Drug power of tincture, $\frac{1}{6}$.

Dilutions must be prepared as directed under Class III.

ARGEMONE MEXICANA, *Linn.*

Nat. Ord., Papaveraceæ.

Common Name, Prickly Poppy.

This is an annual herbaceous plant, growing in the Southern and South-western States, and extending southwards through Mexico into the tropics. It is found also in similar climates in Asia and Africa. Varieties of it are cultivated in the Middle and Northern States as ornamental plants. The plant is from two to three feet high, erect, branching, bristly-spinous. Leaves sessile, long, sinuate-lobed, with prickly teeth on margin, and prickly on veins beneath. Flowers showy, axillary and terminal, on short peduncles. Sepals two or three, often prickly; petals four to six, yellow. Fruit an ovoid or oblong capsule, prickly, opening by valves on the top. The plant exudes a yellow juice when wounded.

Preparation.—The fresh plant just coming into bloom is pounded to a pulp and weighed. Then two parts by weight of alcohol are taken, the pulp mixed thoroughly with one-sixth part of it, and the rest of the alcohol added. After having stirred the whole well, pour it into a well-stoppered bottle, and let it stand eight days in a dark, cool place. The tincture is then separated by decanting, straining and filtering.

Amount of drug power, $\frac{1}{6}$.

Dilutions must be prepared as directed under Class III.

ARGENTUM.

Synonyms, Argentum Metallicum. Argentum Purificatum. Argentum Foliatum. Metallic Silver.

Common Name, Silver.
Symbol, Ag.
Atomic Weight, 107.7.

Origin.—Silver is found in the metallic state, but more often in combination with sulphur as sulphide, together with sulphides of other metals. The most important silver mines are those in the extreme western portion of the United States, in Mexico, Peru, and in the Hartz mountains in Germany.

The extraction of silver is done by methods which differ with the different characters of the ores. The sulphur-bearing silver ores are crushed to powder, mixed with common salt and roasted at a low red-heat in a suitable furnace, by which treatment the silver sulphide is converted into chloride. The mass is then placed in large cylinders with water and scraps of iron, and the whole agitated for some time: by this means the silver chloride becomes reduced to the metallic state. Mercury is now introduced, and the mass again agitated; the mercury dissolves the silver together with any gold or copper present, forming an amalgam. The latter is strained in a strong linen cloth, and the solid portion submitted to distillation in a retort, whereby the mercury is separated and recovered, and the silver in an impure state is left behind. The process is termed *amalgamation.* In the case of a lead-bearing silver ore, the whole is reduced to the metallic state; the alloy of silver and lead is then remelted and allowed to cool, when a portion of lead crystallizes, leaving in the liquid state the alloy referred to. This alloy is then melted in a reverberatory furnace whose hearth is composed of bone-ash, while a current of air, which is forced to pass over the lead, oxidizes the latter; the lead oxide fuses and is absorbed by the bone-ash, and the silver being unaffected is left in the pure state. This process is called *cupellation.*

Preparation.—Chemically pure silver may be obtained by boiling equal parts of silver chloride (precipitated from the purified nitrate), glucose and crystallized sodium carbonate, in three parts of water. The precipitated silver should first be washed with a very dilute hydrochloric acid solution, and finally with distilled water.

Properties.—Silver is a remarkably white metal, extremely brilliant and has specific gravity 10.5. It is harder than gold, but is extremely malleable and ductile. It is unaltered in the air at any temperature less than that of the oxyhydrogen *blast.* It fuses at 1000° C. (1832° F.), and under the oxyhydrogen blow-pipe it volatilizes. It unites readily with sulphur, chlorine and phosphorus, and dissolves easily in nitric acid. The ready tarnishing of silver in or near human habitations is due to the formation of a slight film of sulphide from the presence of free sulphur or of sulphur-bearing gases.

Metallic silver was first proven by Hahnemann.

Tests.—Chemically pure silver dissolves completely in pure nitric acid, forming a transparent colorless solution. From this solution diluted with distilled water, it may be precipitated as chloride; this being removed and the filtrate treated with hydrogen sulphide, any darkening in color will indicate the presence of other metal or metals. The filtrate on evaporation should leave no residue.

Preparation for Homœopathic Use.—Chemically pure silver, obtained in powder, as described above, is prepared by trituration, as directed under Class VII.

ARGENTUM NITRICUM.

Synonyms, Argenti Nitras. Nitrate of Silver.
Present Name, Argentic Nitrate.
Common Name, Lunar Caustic.
Formula, $Ag\ NO_3$.
Molecular Weight, 169.7.

Preparation of Nitrate of Silver.—When pure silver is treated with nitric acid free from chlorine, complete solution of the silver occurs with the formation of its nitrate. The solution is transparent and colorless, and in order to free it from excess of acid, it is placed in a porcelain dish upon a sand-bath, and, with constant stirring, heated to dryness; the heat is then raised till the substance fuses. After partial cooling a two-thirds volume of distilled water is added and the mass is dissolved, the solution placed in a shallow porcelain dish and set aside in a room free from dust, and whose temperature is from 30° to 40° C. (86°–104° F.). After some days the salt will have crystallized out. The crystals are to be removed, and drained in a glass funnel till dry.

Properties.—Crystallized silver nitrate forms colorless tables of the rhombic system. Their taste is bitter, caustic and metallic. They are soluble in their own weight of cold, and in half that amount of boiling water, and in four parts of boiling alcohol. The solutions are neutral in reaction.

The salt fuses easily on heating, and when cast into sticks is known as *lunar caustic*. It undergoes decomposition when in contact with organic matters in the presence of light, depositing a black substance, probably consisting of the suboxide. The crystals are anhydrous.

The first provings were under Hahnemann's directions.

Tests.—Those given under the article Argentum Metallicum. Ten grains of the salt when dissolved with distilled water, give with hydrochloric acid a precipitate which, when washed and thoroughly dried, weighs 8.44 grains.

Preparation for Homœopathic Use.—One part by weight of pure nitrate of silver is dissolved in nine parts by weight of distilled water.

Amount of drug power, $\frac{1}{10}$.

Dilutions must be prepared as directed under Class V—*a*, except that distilled water is used for the 1x, 2x and 3x and 1 dilutions, and dilute alcohol for the 4x and 2 dilutions, strong alcohol being used for all further attenuations.

Dilutions should be freshly made as required for use.

ARISTOLOCHIA CLEMATITIS, *Linn.*

Synonym, Aristolochia vulgaris.
Nat. Ord., Aristolochiaceæ.

Common Names, Long Birth-wort. Aristolochy.

The common aristolochia is a perennial, growing near hedges, ditches and vineyards, indigenous to Southern Europe. Its root is round, long, about the thickness of a goose-quill, irregularly contorted, in color grayish-brown. It has a bitter taste with some acridity and a disagreeable odor. The stems are erect, from two to four feet high, simple, smooth, striped, set with alternate, long petiolate, cordate, entire, vivid green above, gray-green below, leather-like leaves. The short-petiolate yellow flowers stand four to eight in the axils.

Preparation.—The fresh root, gathered in April or September, is chopped and pounded to a pulp and weighed. Then two parts by weight of alcohol are taken, and the pulp mixed thoroughly with one-sixth part of it; then the rest of the alcohol is added. After stirring the whole well and pouring it into a well-stoppered bottle, it is allowed to stand eight days in a dark, cool place. The tincture is then separated by decanting, straining and filtering.

Drug power of tincture, $\frac{1}{6}$.

Dilutions must be prepared as directed under Class III.

ARISTOLOCHIA MILHOMENS.

Synonyms, Aristolochia Grandiflora, *Gom.* Aristolochia Cymbifera, *Martius.*

Nat. Ord., Aristolochiaceæ.

Common Name, Brazilian Snake-Root.

A climbing plant with a glabrous stem; leaves alternate, uniformly cordate, pedati-nerved, with reticulate little veins between the nerves; they are supported by long petioles, furnished with a large, entire, reniform, amplexicaul stipule. Flowers solitary, upon a sulcate peduncle from four to five inches long. Perianth single, large, of a yellowish-brown color, tuberculated, curved, divided into two lips; the upper lip sharp, lanceolate, and somewhat bent outwards; the lower lip twice as long as the other, at first dilated at the base and expanding into a large oval disk with undulate borders. The whole flower is covered with prominent nerves. Stamens six, epigynous. Ovary glabrous, surmounted by a stigma with six short and rounded lobes.

Introduced into our Mat. Med. by Dr. Mure, Brazil.

Preparation.—The fresh flowers are pounded to a pulp and weighed. Then two parts by weight of alcohol are taken, and having mixed the pulp with one-sixth part of it, the rest of the alcohol is added. After stirring the whole well, and pouring it into a well-stoppered bottle, it is allowed to stand eight days in a dark, cool place. The tincture is then separated by decanting, straining and filtering.

Drug power of tincture, $\frac{1}{6}$.

Dilutions must be prepared as directed under Class III.

ARMORACIA.

Synonym, Cochlearia Armoracia, *Linn.*

Nat. Ord., Cruciferæ.

Common Names, Horse-radish. Crow-flowers.

The horse-radish is a native of Western Europe, growing wild in wet grounds. It is cultivated for culinary purposes, to which its root is applied. The root is perennial, and sends up many large leaves. The stem is round, smooth, erect, branching, two or three feet high. The radical leaves are lanceolate, waved, scalloped on the edges. The stem leaves are much smaller, often divided at the edges. The flowers are many, white, peduncled, in thick clusters.

The first provings appear in *Archiv. f. Hom.* 17, 3, 176.

Preparation.—The fresh root is taken out in autumn; after being cleaned is immediately comminuted with a grater and weighed. Then two parts by weight of alcohol are taken, and the pulp mixed thoroughly with one-sixth part of it; the rest of the alcohol is then added. After stirring the whole well, pour it into a well-stoppered bottle and let it stand eight days in a dark, cool place. The tincture is then separated by decanting, straining and filtering.

Drug power of tincture, $\frac{1}{6}$.

Dilutions must be prepared as directed under Class III.

ARNICA.

Synonym, Arnica Montana, *Linn.*

Nat. Ord., Compositæ.

Common Names, Arnica. Leopards-bane.

Description.—A perennial herb growing in mountainous districts of the Northern Hemisphere, with radical leaves, ovate, entire and obtuse; stem about one foot high, with lanceolate opposite leaves; radical leaves and stem, hairy. It produces large orange-yellow flowers, solitary, or at the summit of the stem. Involucral scales, hairy, and in a double row. Receptacle chaffy, one-quarter of an inch in diameter, with about twenty ligulate florets and a much larger number of tubular ones.

The root consists of a slender, brown, contorted root-stock, an inch or two in length, which sends down a number of slender fibres three or four inches long. It has a faintly aromatic smell and herby taste.

Preparation.—At the time of blooming, gather besides the root, which is the most important part, also the root-leaves, and full-blown flowers, which latter are to be taken out of the calyx, to remove the larvæ of the arnica fly (*Tripyta Arnicivora*) from the receptacle. Two parts of the root, one part of the herb, and one part of the flowers are pounded together to a fine pulp and weighed. Then two parts by weight of alcohol are taken, and after thoroughly mixing the pulp with one-sixth part of it, the rest of the alcohol is added. After stirring the whole well, and pouring it into a well-stoppered bottle, it is allowed to stand eight days in a dark, cool place. The tincture is then separated by decanting, straining and filtering.

Drug power of tincture, $\frac{1}{6}$.

Dilutions must be prepared as directed under Class III.

ARNICA E RADICE.

Root of Arnica Montana.

Preparation.—The fresh root carefully dried and pulverized, is covered with five parts by weight of alcohol, and allowed to remain eight days, in a well-stoppered bottle, in a dark, cool place, being shaken twice a day. The tincture is then poured off, strained and filtered.

Drug power of tincture, $\frac{1}{10}$.

Dilutions must be prepared as directed under Class IV.

ARSENICUM ALBUM.

Synonyms, Acidum Arseniosum. Arsenious Acid.

Present Name, Arsenious Oxide.

Common Name, White Arsenic.

Formula, As_2O_3.

Molecular Weight, 198.

Preparation of Arsenious Acid.—The greater part of the white arsenic of commerce is derived from the roasting of natural arsenides of iron, nickel and cobalt. The process is conducted in a reverberatory furnace, and the volatilized substance is condensed in specially arranged long chimneys. This crude product is freed from metallic arsenic and its sulphide by resublimation.

Properties.—When arsenious oxide is condensed at a temperature of 400°C. (752° F.), there is produced a transparent vitreous mass whose specific gravity is 3.738, and when deposited at a temperature slightly less than that just given, it crystallizes in right rhombic prisms. This form is known as vitreous arsenic, and upon keeping, becomes gradually changed into a white opaque mass resembling porcelain.

The second modification, obtained by condensing the sublimate at 200° C. (392° F.), is in brilliant octohedral crystals whose specific gravity is 3.69. The same crystalline form is obtained when a saturated aqueous solution is evaporated. The vitreous arsenic is slightly more soluble than the crystalline variety; one hundred parts of boiling water dissolve about twelve parts of the vitreous kind, but upon cooling, the greater portion separates, leaving about three parts in solution.

Owing to its comparative insolubility, arsenic has little or no taste, such as it has being described by some authorities as faintly sweet. Arsenic is soluble in hot hydrochloric acid, in solutions of the alkalies and of tartaric acid.

Tests.—For its identification in the commercial product, a few well known tests are here given. Heated in a reduction tube with charcoal, it is deoxidized, and metallic arsenic in the form of a dark metallic mirror is deposited in the cooler part of the tube, and at the same time the garlicky odor of volatilized metallic arsenic is perceived. If the portion of the tube containing the mirror be cut out, broken in fragments, placed in a test-tube and heated, the metallic arsenic is reoxidized and is deposited in the upper, cool part of the tube in octohedral crystals. By dissolving these crystals in water and adding a solution of hydrogen sulphide, there will be precipitated the bright yellow sulphide of arsenic, which is insoluble in dilute acids and is completely dissolved by the alkaline hydrates, their carbonates and sulphides.

Arsenious oxide may contain arsenious sulphide as an impurity; such specimens of arsenic will be more or less yellow in streaks or spots, and a small piece placed in a test-tube will not be entirely soluble in twenty-five parts of hydrochloric acid.

Preparation for Homœopathic Use.—One part of finely powdered, vitreous arsenious acid is boiled to complete solution in sixty parts of distilled water, and filtered. By the addition of distilled water the filtrate is increased to ninety parts, and then ten parts of 95 per cent. alcohol are added.

Amount of drug power, $\frac{1}{100}$.

Dilutions must be prepared as directed under Class VI—β.

Triturations are prepared of finely powdered, vitreous arsenious acid, as directed under Class VII.

Caution must be observed in handling arsenic, and especially in powdering it. In the latter case, it should be kept damp by alcohol, so that no dust may arise from it, and the nose and mouth should be protected by wearing a respirator arranged for the purpose of excluding the powder; in default of anything better, a moistened sponge will answer.

ARSENICUM CITRINUM.

Synonyms, Arsenicum Sulfuratum Flavum. Orpiment.

Present Name, Arsenious Sulphide.

Formula, $As_2 S_3$.

Molecular Weight, 246.

Origin and Preparation of Orpiment.—This substance is found in the native state as a mineral. It is prepared artificially by passing hydrogen sulphide through a solution of arsenious oxide in dilute hydrochloric acid, washing the precipitate thoroughly, and drying.

Properties and Tests.—The native trisulphide of arsenic consists of two equivalents of arsenic and three of sulphur. It is in masses of a fine lemon-yellow color, arranged in flexible laminæ, which are slightly translucent. It is insoluble in hydrochloric acid, but dissolves in sulphide of ammonium, and decomposes in boiling dilute nitric acid, with separation of sulphur. It melts easily and volatilizes at a higher temperature.

Preparation for Homœopathic Use.—The pure arsenious sulphide is prepared by trituration, as directed under Class VII.

ARSENICUM HYDROGENISATUM.

Synonym, Arsenetted Hydrogen. Arsine.

Present Name, Hydrogen Arsenide.

Formula, $As H_3$.

Preparation of Arsenetted Hydrogen.—This is prepared by

the action of sulphuric acid diluted with three parts of water, upon the arsenide of zinc, the latter being obtained by fusing equal weights of zinc and arsenic in an earthen retort. The alloy is to be granulated and introduced into a Woulf's two-necked bottle supplied with a thistle-tube passing through one neck nearly to the bottom of the bottle, while from the other neck passes a delivery tube. The diluted acid is then poured gradually down the thistle-tube until the layer of acid is higher than its lower end. The development of gas begins at once. The delivery-tube should be connected with a wash-bottle, from which the gas may be led to a receiver containing ice cold water, which will absorb one-fifth its own volume of gas. As the gas is extraordinarily poisonous, the whole proceeding, from the beginning, till the gas ceases to come over, should be conducted under a hood connected with a chimney having a good draught; or the receiver (a bottle or flask) may be fitted with a cork through which pass two tubes, one bringing the gas into the water, the other, or exit tube, bent and allowed to dip deeply into a strong solution of silver nitrate in a beaker. By this means the unused gas is decomposed, with the production of silver arsenide and free hydrogen.

Properties.—Hydrogen arsenide is a colorless gas, having a garlicky odor and specific gravity 2.7. When ignited in the air, it burns with a peculiar bluish-white flame, producing water and the fumes of arsenious oxide. A piece of porcelain held just at the extremity of the flame will receive a deposit of white arsenic, while if the porcelain be cold and held well in the flame so as to reduce its temperature below the combustion-point of arsenic, the latter will be deposited upon the porcelain as a dark metallic stain or spot.

Preparation for Homœopathic Use.—The provings were made by inhaling the gas diluted with atmospheric air. The saturated solution freshly prepared under the above directions, mixed with an equal quantity of distilled water, produces the 1x dilution.

Further dilutions must be prepared as directed under Class V—*a*.

ARSENICUM JODATUM.

Synonym, Arsenici Jodidum.
Present Name, Arsenious Iodide.
Common Name, Iodide of Arsenic.
Formula, $As\,I_3$.
Molecular Weight, 456.

Preparation of Iodide of Arsenic.—Arsenic and iodine unite when gently heated together, the combination being attended with considerable evolution of heat. Take one equivalent of arsenic and three equivalents of iodine, both in fine powder, and thoroughly mix them in a mortar by rubbing; place the mixture in a test tube, loosely corking the latter, and heat gently until the mass liquefies. After repeated agitation, pour the liquid iodide upon a porcelain tile; when cold, break it in pieces and dissolve in boiling alcohol, from which solution it may be re-crystallized on cooling.

Properties and Tests.—Obtained as directed above, arsenious iodide is in shining laminæ of a fine brick-red color, having specific gravity 4.39, which are soluble in alcohol and water, and sparingly so in hydrochloric acid. The aqueous solution strongly acidulated with hydrochloric acid, gives with hydrogen sulphide, the usual precipitate of arsenious sulphide.

First provings were by Dr. E. W. Beebe, U. S.

Preparation for Homœopathic Use.—The pure iodide of arsenic is prepared by trituration, as directed under Class VII.

ARSENICUM METALLICUM.

Synonym, Metallic Arsenic.

Symbol, As.

Atomic Weight, 75.

Origin and Preparation of Metallic Arsenic.—Arsenic is found in nature in the free state, but oftener combined with other metals, and especially with sulphur as sulphide. From arsenical pyrites or *mispickel*, it is readily obtained by roasting the ore and condensing the product in cooled receivers. On a small scale it may be obtained by heating a mixture of arsenious oxide with half its weight of fresh burnt charcoal in a crucible, the mixture being covered with two or three inches of charcoal in very small fragments, and the crucible so placed that this overlying layer of charcoal may be heated to redness first, to insure the reduction of any of the white arsenic which might escape from below. In order to collect the arsenic, another crucible, having a small hole drilled through the bottom, is cemented with fire-clay to the first in an inverted position. At a red heat, the charcoal simply abstracts the oxygen from the oxide, leaving the metallic arsenic condensed in the upper crucible.

Properties.—Metallic arsenic is a brittle substance, of a dark gray color and brilliant metallic lustre; upon exposure to the air its brilliancy is lost and the color deepens somewhat. Its specific gravity is 5.7 to 5.9. It volatilizes in the air when heated to 180° C (356° F.) with oxidation; heated in a sealed tube it fuses. It is not dissolved by water or any simple solvent, but when powdered and moistened, it is slowly converted into arsenious oxide. When placed in water the same result occurs from the presence of dissolved air.

It was first proven by Dr. Stevenson, U. S. (*N. A. J. of Homœopathy*, 1, 301).

Tests.—For tests and the detection of arsenic, see Arsenicum Album.

Preparation for Homœopathic Use.—The pure metallic arsenic is prepared by trituration, as directed under Class VII.

ARSENICUM RUBRUM.

Synonyms, Arsenicum Sulfuratum Rubrum. Arsenic Bisulphide.

Present Name, Arsenious Di-sulphide.

Common Names, Realgar. Sandarach.
Formula, $As_2 S_2$.
Molecular Weight, 214.
Description.—This compound occurs native as realgar, crystallized in oblique rhombic prisms, of an orange-red or ruby-red color, of a resinous lustre, and more or less translucent at the edges of its fracture, which is conchoidal and uneven; streak varies from orange-red to ruby-red; specific gravity 3.4 to 3.6. It is found accompanying ores of silver and lead in Transylvania, Hungary, Bohemia and Saxony.
Tests.—In addition to the above described properties, see Tests under Arsenicum Citrinum.
Preparation for Homœopathic Use.—The pure arsenious disulphide or realgar is prepared by trituration, as directed under Class VII.

ARTEMISIA VULGARIS, *Linn.*

Nat. Ord., Compositæ.
Common Names, Mugwort. Common Artemisia.
This perennial plant, growing wild in all parts of Europe, is rather well known; it differs from its next and most spread relation *Artemisia Absinthium*, by the dark green and quite smooth surface of its leaves and the mostly quite smooth and very stiff stalks, which are frequently of a dark violet-brown or purple color. It should not be mistaken for *Artemisia Campestris*, mingled with which it often occurs; the latter having a more spare growth, attenuated branches decumbent until the flowering time, and quite narrow, linear, setaceous leaves.
Introduced into our Materia Medica by Noack and Trinks.
Preparation.—The fresh root is chopped and pounded to a pulp and weighed. Then two parts by weight of alcohol are taken, the pulp mixed thoroughly with one-sixth part of it, and the rest of the alcohol added. After stirring the whole well, and pouring it into a well-stoppered bottle, it is allowed to stand eight days in a dark, cool place. The tincture is then separated by decanting, straining and filtering.
Drug power of tincture, $\frac{1}{6}$.
Dilutions must be prepared as directed under Class III.

ARUM MACULATUM, *Linn.*

Synonyms, Arum Vulgare. Aronis Communis.
Nat. Ord., Araceæ.
Common Names, Wake Robin. Spotted Arum.
This is a perennial herbaceous plant growing in leafy woods in Middle and Southern Europe. The arrow-shaped, long-petiolate, abruptly pointed leaves are smooth and not seldom sprinkled with grey-black irregular spots; the scape is naked, shorter than the petiole, and bears a large white sheath, from which a round, club-shaped, reddish spadix juts out. The white root, as large as a hazelnut, is roundish,

set with fibrils, fleshy, and has an extremely acrid smell, irritating the eyes and nose, especially when bruised, and a similar burning taste.

First proven by Dr. C. Hering.

Preparation.—The fresh root, gathered in early spring before the development of the leaves, is carefully chopped and pounded to a fine pulp, enclosed in a piece of new linen and subjected to pressure. The expressed juice is then, by brisk agitation, mixed with an equal part by weight of alcohol. This mixture is allowed to stand eight days in a dark, cool place, and then filtered.

Drug power of tincture, $\frac{1}{2}$.

Dilutions must be prepared as directed under Class I.

ARUM TRIPHYLLUM, *Linn.*

Synonyms, Arisæma Triphyllum, *Torrey.* Arum Atrorubens.

Nat. Ord., Araceæ.

Common Names, Indian Turnip. Jack in the Pulpit. Dragon's Root.

This plant is indigenous throughout the continent of America, and is found in moist, shady places. From its perennial root arises in the early spring a spathe, green without, variegated within by dark purple alternating with pale green stripes. Leaves trifoliate, generally in pairs, leaflets oval, acuminate. Spadix shorter than the spathe, varying from green to dark purple. Fruit, a bunch of bright scarlet berries. The root, a corm, is brown and wrinkled on the outside, internally white, fleshy. In the fresh state, it has a peculiar odor, and when chewed causes an unbearable acrid burning sensation in the mouth and throat.

The first proving is by Dr. J. Jeanes, U. S.

Preparation.—The fresh root, gathered in early spring before the development of the leaves, is carefully bruised (for its emanations irritate the eyes and nose) and weighed. Then two parts by weight of alcohol are taken, the pulp mixed with one-sixth part of it, and the rest of the alcohol added. After stirring the whole well, and pouring it into a well-stoppered bottle, it is allowed to stand eight days in a dark, cool place. The tincture is then separated by decanting, straining and filtering. It must be kept well protected against light and heat.

Drug power of tincture, $\frac{1}{6}$.

Dilutions must be prepared as directed under Class III.

Triturations. Dr. E. M. Hale recommends a rapid trituration of the expressed juice of the freshly gathered root, the preparation to be preserved in hermetically sealed bottles, guarded against light and heat.

ARUNDO MAURITANICA, *Desfontaines.*

Nat. Ord., Gramineæ.

Common Name, Reed.

An Italian grass.

Proved and introduced by Dr. F. Patti, Chazon a due de Sorentino; published in *Journ. de la Soc. Gall.*, Vol. VII, 1856.

Preparation for Homœopathic Use.—The fresh root-sprout is pounded to a fine pulp and weighed. Then two parts by weight of alcohol are taken, the pulp mixed thoroughly with one-sixth part of it, and the rest of the alcohol added. After stirring the whole well, and pouring it into a well-stoppered bottle, it is allowed to stand eight days in a dark, cool place. The tincture is then separated by decanting, straining and filtering.

Drug power of tincture, $\frac{1}{6}$.

Dilutions must be prepared as directed under Class III.

ASAFŒTIDA.

Synonyms, Narthex Asafœtida, *Falconer.* Ferula Asafœtida, *Linn.* Ferula Persica. Asafœtida Disgunensis.

Nat. Ord., Umbelliferæ.

Common Names, Asafœtida. Devil's Dung.

This is a native of Persia and neighboring countries. Is a large perennial herbaceous plant. The leaves are large, bi-pinnate and with large petioles. The stem rises from six to nine feet, and is crowned with a mass of umbels. Flowers pale yellow. The officinal drug is a gum resin obtained from the root.

Description.—Asafœtida comes in masses made up of "tears" varying in size, opaque and white on section, but after short exposure they become distinctly pink in color, and finally brownish. It has a strong garlicky odor and taste, with some acridity and bitterness. The tears become quite brittle when exposed to cold, and then they are readily powdered. When they are rubbed in a mortar with water, a milky emulsion is produced.

First provings are by Hahnemann, Stapf and Gross.

Preparation.—The gum-resin, obtained by incision, from the living root, from plants more than four years old, is covered with five parts by weight of 95 per cent. alcohol, and having poured it into a well-stoppered bottle, it is allowed to remain eight days in a dark, cool place, being shaken twice a day. The tincture is then poured off, strained and filtered.

Drug power of tincture, $\frac{1}{10}$.

Dilutions must be prepared as directed under Class IV, except that 95 per cent. alcohol is used.

ASARUM.

Synonyms, Asarum Europæum, *Linn.* Asarum Vulgare.

Nat. Ord., Aristolochiaceæ.

Common Names, Asarabacca. European Snake-Root. Fole's Foot. Hazel-wort. Wild Nard.

The hazel-wort grows all over Germany, also in all other parts of Europe, in shady, elevated forests, under small bushes, especially under hazel-bushes. The root is creeping, of the thickness of a straw, five to six inches long, geniculated, bent hither and thither, in some places knotty and set with thick fibres; the stalks, scarcely one inch high, villous, somewhat decumbent, end in two leaves, on petioles three to four inches long; the leaves are reniform, entire, shining dark green above, grayish-green below, run through with net-like veins, and sometimes set with slender hair; from the partition of the leaves the short petiolate, externally villous, green-red, internally dark purple flower arises.

Preparation.—The entire fresh plant, gathered when in flower, is chopped and pounded to a fine pulp, enclosed in a piece of new linen and subjected to pressure. The expressed juice is then, by brisk agitation, mixed with an equal part by weight of alcohol. This mixture is allowed to stand eight days in a well-stoppered bottle, in a dark, cool place, and then filtered.

Drug power of tincture, $\frac{1}{2}$.

Dilutions must be prepared as directed under Class I.

ASARUM CANADENSE, *Linn.*

Nat. Ord., Aristolochiaceæ.

Common Names, Wild Ginger. Canada Snake-root. Indian Ginger. Kidney-leaved Asarabacca.

This is an indigenous plant, inhabiting woods and shady places from Canada to the Carolinas. In appearance and botanical character this species very closely resembles *Asarum Europæum.* Its root is long, creeping, jointed, yellowish, fleshy. The stem is short, bearing two broad kidney-shaped leaves, light green above, veined and paler beneath. A single purple-brown flower grows in the fork of the stem.

Preparation.—The fresh root is chopped and pounded to a pulp and weighed. Then two parts by weight of alcohol are taken, the pulp mixed thoroughly with one-sixth part of it, and the rest of the alcohol added. After stirring the whole well, and pouring it into a well-stoppered bottle, it is allowed to stand eight days in a dark, cool place. The tincture is then separated by decanting, straining and filtering.

Drug power of tincture, $\frac{1}{6}$.

Dilutions must be prepared as directed under Class III.

ASCLEPIAS INCARNATA, *Linn.*

Synonym, Amœna.

Nat. Ord., Asclepiadaceæ.

Common Names, Flesh-colored Asclepias. Flesh-colored Swallow-wort. Rose-colored Silk Weed. Swamp Milk or Silk Weed. White Indian Hemp.

This species has a tall downy stem, branching above, two or three feet in height; leaves opposite, on short petioles, lanceolate, slightly hairy. Corollas deep purple, corona paler; umbels numerous, and two or more together at the top of stem or branches. It is found growing in wet places in the United States. Flowers from July to August. The plant exudes a milky juice when wounded.

Preparation.—The fresh root is chopped and pounded to a pulp and weighed. Then two parts by weight of alcohol are taken, the pulp mixed thoroughly with one-sixth part of it, and the rest of the alcohol added. After stirring the whole well, and pouring it into a well-stoppered bottle, it is allowed to stand eight days in a dark, cool place. The tincture is then separated by decanting, straining and filtering.

Drug power of tincture, $\frac{1}{6}$.

Dilutions must be prepared as directed under Class III.

ASCLEPIAS SYRIACA, *Linn.*

Synonym, Asclepias Cornuti, *Decaisne.*

Nat. Ord., Asclepiadaceæ.

Common Names, Silk Weed. Milk Weed. Virginia Swallow-wort.

Stem simple, leaves oblong-ovate, short acuminate on short petioles, downy beneath. Flowers large, pale purple, in globular umbels. Pods filled with seeds having long silky down. A common herb in the United States, growing in ditches and on roadsides.

Preparation.—The fresh root is chopped and pounded to a pulp and weighed. Then two parts by weight of alcohol are taken, the pulp mixed thoroughly with one-sixth part of it, and rest of alcohol added. After stirring the whole well, and pouring it into a well-stoppered bottle, it is allowed to stand eight days in a dark, cool place. The tincture is then separated by decanting, straining and filtering.

Drug power of tincture, $\frac{1}{6}$.

Dilutions must be prepared as directed under Class III.

ASCLEPIAS TUBEROSA, *Linn.*

Synonym, Asclepias decumbens.

Nat. Ord., Asclepiadaceæ.

Common Names, Pleurisy Root. Butterfly Weed. Colic Root. Orange Apocynum.

The root of the butterfly weed is large, fleshy, and from it arise numerous stems, two feet high, hairy, branching toward the top. Leaves alternate, oblong, lanceolate, upper surface dark green, paler beneath. Umbels numerous in a large terminal corymb. Flowers orange-red. Pods lanceolate-pointed, seeds having long silky down. The plant is found in dry fields in Canada and United States. It flowers in August.

Preparation.—The fresh root is chopped and pounded to a pulp and weighed. Then two parts by weight of alcohol are taken, the pulp mixed thoroughly with one-sixth part of it, and the rest of the alcohol added. After stirring the whole well, and pouring it into a well-stoppered bottle, it is allowed to stand eight days in a dark, cool place. The tincture is then separated by decanting, straining and filtering.

Drug power of tincture, $\frac{1}{6}$.

Dilutions must be prepared as directed under Class III.

ASCLEPIAS VINCETOXICUM, *Linn.*

Synonyms, Cynanchum Vincetoxicum, *Persoon.* Vincetoxicum Officinale, *Moench.*

Nat. Ord., Asclepiadaceæ.

Common Name, White Swallow-wort.

This plant is indigenous to Europe and is found there growing in rocky places. Stem two feet high, leaves cordate-ovate, acuminate, on very short petioles. Umbels small, axillary. The root-stock is about the thickness of a finger, knotty, and gives off many radicles. It is whitish or yellowish externally, internally yellowish. It has a disagreeable odor, somewhat similar to that of valerian, and a bitter, acrid taste.

Preparation.—The fresh leaves are chopped and pounded to a pulp and weighed. Then take two-thirds by weight of alcohol, and add it to the pulp, stirring and mixing the whole well together, and strain by the usual method through a piece of new linen. The tincture thus obtained is allowed to stand eight days in a well-stoppered bottle, in a dark, cool place, and then filtered.

Drug power of tincture, $\frac{1}{2}$.

Dilutions must be prepared as directed under Class II.

ASIMINA TRILOBA, *Dunal.*

Synonyms, Anona Triloba. Asimina Campaniflora. Parcelia Triloba. Uvaria Triloba.

Nat. Ord., Anonaceæ.

Common Name, Common Papaw.

This is a small tree from ten to twenty feet high, growing on the banks of streams in rich soil, from New York and Pennsylvania west to Illinois and southward. The young shoots and expanding leaves are clothed with a rusty down, but soon become glabrous. Leaves thin, obovate-lanceolate, pointed; petals dull purple, veiny, round-ovate, six in number, increasing after the bud opens, the outer ones three to four times as long as the calyx. Stamens numerous in a globular mass. Pistils few, ripening one to four large and oblong (three to four inches long), pulpy several-seeded fruits, yellowish in color, sweet and edible in autumn. Seeds horizontal, flat, enclosed in a fleshy aril. Flowers appear with the leaves in April and May.

Proven by E. H. Eisenboeg, U. S., Thesis, 1870.

Preparation.—The ripe seeds, coarsely powdered, are covered with five parts by weight of alcohol, and allowed to remain eight days, in a well-stoppered bottle, in a dark, cool place, being shaken twice a day. The tincture is then poured off, strained and filtered.

Drug power of tincture, $\frac{1}{10}$.

Dilutions must be prepared as directed under Class IV.

ASPARAGUS OFFICINALIS, *Linn.*

Nat. Ord., Liliaceæ.

Common Name, Asparagus.

This universally well known plant, cultivated in our gardens for culinary use, is a native of Europe, and is found in sandy places, near the sea-coast, in meadows, and along the borders of forests. The root is composed of a short shaft terminating in a cluster of round, long, white fibres. From this root spring up several herbaceous, round, glabrous stems, nearly three feet high; leaves in fascicles, about an inch long, glabrous; flowers small, greenish-yellow, solitary and axillary; fruit bacciform, scarlet-red, three-celled with two or three black seeds.

Introduced into our Materia Medica by Buchner's provings.

Preparation.—The young sprouts are chopped and pounded to a pulp and weighed. Then two parts by weight of alcohol are taken, the pulp mixed thoroughly with one-sixth part of it, and the rest of the alcohol added. After stirring the whole well, and pouring it into a well-stoppered bottle, it is allowed to stand eight days in a dark, cool place. The tincture is then separated by decanting, straining and filtering.

Drug power of tincture, $\frac{1}{6}$.

Dilutions must be prepared as directed under Class III.

ASPERULA ODORATA, *Linn.*

Nat. Ord., Rubiaceæ.

Common Names, Sweet-scented Wood-ruff. Wood Rowel.

This plant is a native of Europe, Northern Africa, Siberia, and Western Asia, growing in shaded hedgebanks, copses, etc. In Scotland it is found at a height of 1,200 feet. Rootstock is perennial, creeping, often stoloniferous. Stems are from six to eighteen inches high, subsimple, hairy beneath the nodes. Leaves are one to one and a half inches long, oblong-lanceolate, cuspidate, ciliate. Cymes subterminal, subumbellate. Corolla tube one-fourth of an inch in diameter, as long as the limb, with lobes obtuse. Fruit small, hispid, with hooked hairs. The lower leaves are six in a whorl, the upper seven to nine, shining, odoriferous in drying. Flowers appear in May and June.

Preparation.—The fresh herb, gathered shortly before coming into bloom, is chopped and pounded to a pulp and weighed. Then two parts by weight of alcohol are taken, the pulp mixed thoroughly with one-sixth part of it, and the rest of the alcohol added. After stirring the whole well, and pouring it into a well-stoppered bottle, it is allowed to stand eight days in a dark, cool place. The tincture is then separated by decanting, straining and filtering.

Amount of drug power, $\frac{1}{6}$.

Dilutions must be prepared as directed under Class III.

ASPLENIUM SCOLOPENDRIUM, *Linn.*

Synonym, Scolopendrium Officinarum, *Smith.*

Nat. Ord., Polypodiaceæ.

Common Name, Hart's Tongue.

This is a fern indigenous in Europe and America. It is found growing in shaded ravines and under limestone cliffs, near Chittenango Falls, and near Jamesville, Onondaga Co., New York. Frond oblong-lanceolate from an auricled heart-shaped base, entire or wavy-margined (seven to eighteen inches long, one to two inches wide), of a bright green color. Fruit-dots linear, elongated, almost at right angles to the midrib, contiguous by twos, one on the upper side of one veinlet, and the next on the lower side of the next superior veinlet, thus appearing to have a double indusium opening along the middle.

Preparation.—The fresh leaves are chopped and pounded to a pulp and weighed. Then two parts by weight of alcohol are taken, the pulp mixed thoroughly with one-sixth part of it, and the rest of the alcohol added. After stirring the whole well, and pouring it into a well-stoppered bottle, it is allowed to stand eight days in a dark, cool place. The tincture is then separated by decanting, straining and filtering.

Amount of drug power, $\frac{1}{6}$.

Dilutions must be prepared as directed under Class III.

ASTERIAS RUBENS.

Synonyms, Uraster Rubens. Asteracanthion Rubens.
Class, Echinodermata.
Order, Asteroidea.
Family, Asteriadæ.
Common Name, Star Fish.

This is a marine animal quite common along the various coasts of Europe, and occasionally found along the American coasts. It is shaped in exact resemblance to a five-pointed star, is garnet-red in color, and has the faculty of reproducing any member that has been accidentally lost. The central portion contains the mouth and stomach, the former being situated upon the under surface, and armed with hard papillæ in the place of teeth; the stomach is simply a globular sac. The nervous system is composed of a circular chain of ganglia from which nerve filaments are given off. An eye is situated at the extremity of each arm. The entire animal is supported by an external calcareous envelope or skeleton, covered with spines and tubercles. For locomotion, it is provided with numerous muscular, tube-like processes passing out through foramina in the shelly covering, and arranged in double rows on both surfaces. Each of these terminate in a disk, depressed in the centre.

Introduced into the Homœopathic Materia Medica by Dr. Petroz, Spain.

Preparation.—The live animal, cut up finely, is covered with five parts by weight of alcohol, poured into a well-stoppered bottle, and allowed to remain eight days in a dark, cool place, being shaken twice a day. The tincture is then poured off, strained and filtered.

Drug power of tincture, $\frac{1}{10}$.

Dilutions must be prepared as directed under Class IV.

ATRIPLEX OLIDUM.

Synonyms, Chenopodium Olidum, *Curt.* Chenopodium Vulvaria, *Linn.*

Nat. Ord., Chenopodiaceæ.

Common Name, Stinking Orache or Arach. Stinking Blite or Goosefoot.

This plant, a native of Europe, grows luxuriantly everywhere on ways, walls, heaps of rubbish, places for collecting manure; sprout stems from six to twelve inches long, erect or decumbent, with petiolate, rhombic-ovate, entire, gray-green leaves and flowers standing in the axils, and in glomerated naked racemes. During the flowering time the whole plant, especially the lower surface, looks as if dusted with flour, and when triturated, emits an exceedingly nauseous smell, similar to that of decayed cheese.

The drug was proven under direction of Dr. Berridge, England.

Preparation.—The fresh plant is chopped and pounded to a pulp and weighed. Then two parts by weight of alcohol are taken, the pulp mixed thoroughly with one-sixth part of it, and the rest of the alcohol added. After stirring the whole well, and pouring it into a well-stoppered bottle, it is allowed to stand eight days in a dark, cool place. The tincture is then separated by decanting, straining and filtering.

Drug power of tincture, $\frac{1}{6}$.

Dilutions must be prepared as directed under Class III.

ATROPINUM.

Synonyms, Atropia. Atropine.

Formula, $C_{17}H_{23}NO_3$.

Molecular Weight, 289.

An alkaloid obtained from Belladonna, especially from the root.

Preparation of Atropia.—Take of belladonna root, finely powdered, 48 ounces troy; chloroform *puriss.*, 4 ounces troy; dilute sulphuric acid, solution of potassium hydrate, alcohol, and water, of each a sufficiency. The powdered root is to be mixed with a pint of alcohol, then placed in a cylindrical percolator, and alcohol gradually added till 16 pints shall have passed through. The percolate is to be distilled till 12 pints of alcohol have come over. Dilute sulphuric acid is to be then added to the residue until its reaction is acid, and the liquid is to be evaporated till it measures one-half pint; then a half-pint of water is to be added and the whole filtered through fine filter-paper.

To the filtrate is added one and a half ounces troy of chloroform, and next the potassium hydrate till the reaction of the liquid is slightly alkaline; the whole is to be repeatedly agitated at intervals for at least half-an-hour. When the chloroformic layer has subsided, the upper lighter liquid is to be separated from it, and to the latter must be added one and a half ounces troy of the chloroform; repeat the agitation and separation of the two layers as before. To the lighter liquid add the remaining portion of the chloroform originally taken, with renewed agitation and separation. The three portions of heavier liquid are to be placed in a dish and set aside and the chloroform allowed to evaporate, when the atropia may be obtained in the dry state. The preparation so obtained may be crystallized by dissolving it in 7 or 8 volumes of boiling alcohol, which must be in the highest degree anhydrous, the so-called anhydrous alcohol of commerce not sufficing. The solution must then be placed in a flat dish and set aside in a room whose temperature is rather below the medium, that it may slowly evaporate.

Properties and Tests.—Pure atropine is in brilliant, well-defined, needle-shaped crystals. In commerce, the alkaloid is often found as a white or yellow-white powdery mass. It has a tolerably bitter, disagreeable taste, which remains for some time. The pure atropia is soluble in 350 parts of cold and in 60 of hot water, in 8 to 10 of alcohol, 30 to 35 of ether, 3 of chloroform. In watery solution it gradually undergoes decomposition. It fuses at 90° C. (194° F.), and when heated above 140° C. (284° F.), it is decomposed, leaving no residue; by careful heating it may be sublimed without change. When its watery solution is boiled, a minute portion of the alkaloid volatilizes with the vapor of water. Like all the true alkaloids, it has an alkaline reaction, neutralizes acids completely, forming then crystallizable salts, without, however, displacing the basic hydrogen of the acid. Air and moisture seem to produce some change in atropia, for exposure to them results in the alkaloid's becoming disagreeable in odor, yellow in color and losing its capability of crystallizing.

Tests.—Atropine dissolves slowly in concentrated sulphuric acid without change of color; if this solution be warmed till it becomes slightly brown, and then a few drops of water are added, an agreeable odor is evolved resembling that of the sloe blossom, or, according to some observers, that of the orange. On further heating, the odor is intensified.

When some drops of concentrated sulphuric acid are heated with a fragment of bichromate of potassium or molybdate of ammonia, and then some atropia, together with two or three drops of water, are added, the odor of oil of bitter almonds or of *Spiræa ulmaria* is produced. Picric acid does not precipitate the salts of atropia; hence, if a solution of atropia, after being acidified with dilute sulphuric acid, give a precipitate with this reagent, we must believe that some other alkaloid is present.

Daturia, an alkaloid from *Datura Stramonium*, has long been held by chemists to be identical with atropia, and is said to be frequently substituted for the latter; the physiological action of the two are known to be not identical, and as between the two, the picric acid test above given affords a ready means of distinguishing. The dilating power of atropia upon the pupil will not serve for its identification, for the alkaloid hyoscyamine possesses the same property, although the latter is somewhat slower in its action.

Preparation for Homœopathic Use.—Pure atropia is prepared by trituration, as directed under Class VII.

ATROPINUM SULPHURICUM.

Synonyms, Atropiæ Sulphas. Atropia Sulphurica.
Common Name, Sulphate of Atropia.
Formula, $(C_{17}\ H_{23}\ NO_3)_2,\ H_2\ SO_4$.
Molecular Weight, 676.

Preparation of Sulphate of Atropia.—Mix one part of atropia with two parts of distilled water; add dilute sulphuric acid, drop by drop, with constant stirring, till the alkaloid is dissolved and the solution made neutral. Evaporate to dryness in a room at a temperature not exceeding 37.7° C. (100° F.).

Properties.—Sulphate of atropia is a white crystalline powder, or forms small, colorless, silky prisms. It is soluble in three parts of cold water, and in ten parts of 90 per cent. alcohol; the solution should be neutral to test paper. It is insoluble in ether, chloroform and benzol. It has a disagreeable, bitter taste.

Tests.—If the alkaloid belladonnia be present, the fact may be determined by dissolving the salt in 200 parts of water and adding a few drops of sodium carbonate solution, when a distinct turbidity will occur. The salt, when burned on platinum foil, should leave no residue.

Preparation for Homœopathic Use.—The pure sulphate of atropia is prepared by trituration, as directed under Class VII.

AURUM.

Synonyms, Aurum Metallicum. Aurum Foliatum.
Common Name, Gold.
Symbol, Au.
Atomic Weight, 196.2.

Origin and Properties.—The metal gold is found in nature in the metallic state, generally alloyed with varying proportions of silver. It is found in veins in quartz or in the detritus of rock, as in river sand. From river sand it is obtained by simply washing and from the quartz by crushing and subsequent amalgamation with mercury.

Properties.—Gold is a brilliant, soft metal of an orange-yellow color. Its specific gravity is 19.33. It is very ductile and extraordinarily malleable. It fuses at 1250° C. (2282° F.). Is unalterable in the air and is not affected by any acid or alkali. It is soluble in chlorine, and liquids containing that element, such as nitro-muriatic acid, are used for dissolving the metal.

Precipitation of Gold.—Thirty grains of gold are dissolved in nitro-muriatic acid; to this solution six gallons of distilled water are added; then two ounces of ferrous sulphate are dissolved in one quart of distilled water, and the two solutions mixed together. Then is to be added chlorate of potassium in solution, and the whole is let stand until the ferrous sulphate is converted into a ferric salt, that is, until a drop of the solution no longer gives a blue precipitate with potassium ferri-cyanide (red prussiate of potash). Finally aqua ammonia is added in excess. The precipitated ferric hydrate carries down all the fine gold held in suspension. The ferric hydrate is now dissolved out with hydrochloric acid, the metallic gold collected on a filter, and after being thoroughly washed and dried is triturated, *secundum artem*.

It was introduced into our Materia Medica by Hahnemann.

Preparation for Homœopathic Use.—The precipitated metal is prepared by trituration, as directed under Class VII.

AURUM FULMINANS.

Proper Name, Ammonium Aurate. Composition not determined.

Preparation for Fulminating Gold.—This metallic substance, which at first was obtained by combining oxide of gold with ammonia, is more advantageously prepared by means of pure chloride of gold. It is thus procured by precipitating the chloride by ammonia in excess, after which the precipitate is well washed by boiling in a solution of ammonia. It is then, on drying, a yellowish-brown powder. It explodes at a temperature a little above that of boiling water or by the blow of a hammer, with a loud report and feeble flame.

Preparations for Homœopathic Use.—Only centesimal triturations are used, the first and second of which are prepared with starch moistened with diluted alcohol; all further triturations with sugar of milk, as directed under Class VII.

AURUM MURIATICUM.

Synonyms, Auri Chloridum. Muriate of Gold. Tri-chloride of Gold.

Present Name, Auric Chloride.

Common Name, Chloride of Gold.

Formula, $Au\ Cl_3$.

Preparation.—By digesting one part of pure gold in four parts of nitro-muriatic acid at a moderate heat, placing the solution in a flat porcelain vessel and heating on a glycerine bath at 115° C. (239° F.) until the vapor of hydrochloric acid ceases to come off. The mass is then dissolved in half its weight of distilled water and evaporated over concentrated sulphuric acid till it crystallizes.

Properties.—Chloride of gold is in yellow four-sided prisms or a crystalline yellow powder. It is very hygroscopic, and is easily soluble in water, alcohol and ether; its solutions are gradually reduced in the light. Heated above 150° C. (302° F.) it is decomposed with the evolution of chlorine and is reduced to the aurous state. Its taste is somewhat inky with a metallic after-taste.

The remedy was introduced into our Materia Medica by Hahnemann.

Preparation for Homœopathic Use.—The pure chloride of gold is dissolved in nine parts by weight of distilled water.

Amount of drug power, $\frac{1}{10}$.

Dilutions must be prepared as directed under Class V—*a*.

Triturations of the pure chloride of gold are prepared as directed under Class VII.

AURUM MURIATICUM NATRONATUM.

Synonyms, Auri et Sodii Chloridum. Auro-Natrium Chloratum. Sodium Chloro-Aurate.

Present Name, Auri-sodic Chloride.

Common Name, Chloride of Gold and Sodium.

Formula, Na Cl, Au Cl_3, $2H_2$ O.

Preparation of Chloride of Gold and Sodium.—This is prepared by mixing a solution of four parts of auric chloride in eight of water with one of four parts of sodium chloride in four of water and evaporating.

Properties.—The salt crystallizes in long four-sided prisms which are permanent in the air; they are of a golden-yellow color, dissolve readily and completely in water, but in alcohol only the gold chloride goes into solution.

It was first proven by Lembke, in Germany.

Preparation for Homœopathic Use.—The pure chloride of gold and sodium is prepared by trituration, as directed under Class VII.

AURUM SULPHURATUM.

Synonym, Sulphuretted Gold.

Present Name, Auric Sulphide.

Common Name, Yellow Sulphuret of Gold.

Preparation and Properties of Sulphuretted Gold.—Dissolve one part of auric chloride in ten volumes of cold water slightly acidulated with HCl; pass into the solution hydrogen sulphide until precipitation ceases to occur. The precipitate of auric sulphide is to be removed by filtration, thoroughly washed, and dried between folds of bibulous paper with the aid of a gentle heat. Auric sulphide is a flocculent substance of a strong yellow color, which becomes deeper by drying. It decomposes at a moderate heat by dissociation of its constituents.

Our authority for its use is Dr. Molin, France.

Preparation for Homœopathic Use. Sulphuretted gold is prepared by trituration, as directed under Class VII.

BADIAGA.

Synonyms, Spongia Palustris, *Linn.* Spongilla Lacustris, *Link.* Spongilla Fluviatilis.

Nat. Ord., Spongiæ.

Common Names, Badiaga. River Sponge. Fresh Water Sponge.

This beautiful green alga is to be found in stagnant waters and in ditches in Germany, but more especially in Russia. It is very similar in texture to the sea-sponge; appears in branching ramifications like stags' horns with rounded corners and roundish ends, from the thickness of a quill to that of a finger. It has a peculiar strong smell like that of putrescent crawfish.

Preparation.—The dried and pulverized sponge is covered with five parts by weight of alcohol; having poured it into a well-stoppered bottle, let it stand eight days in a dark, cool place, shaking twice a day. The tincture is then poured off, strained and filtered.

Drug power of tincture, $\frac{1}{10}$.

Dilutions must be prepared as directed under Class IV.

Triturations are prepared from the dried sponge, as directed under Class VI.

BALSAMUM PERUVIANUM.

Synonyms, Myrospermum Peruiferum, *De Candolle.* (Myroxylon Pereiræ, *Klotzsch.*)

Nat. Ord., Leguminosæ.

Common Names, Balsam of Peru. Quinquino.

Myrospermum Peruiferum is a handsome tree, growing to the height of fifty feet, and at six or ten feet from the ground throwing out spreading, ascending branches. It is found in San Salvador, Central America.

Description and Preparation of Balsam of Peru. The bark of the tree is bruised by beating with a blunt instrument; in a few days the injured bark either drops off or is removed, and the stem begins to exude the balsam. Balsam of Peru is a liquid, looking like molasses, but is somewhat less viscid. In thin layers it is deep orange-brown in color, and transparent. It has a balsamic odor which is also somewhat smoky, but when the liquid is smeared on paper and warmed the odor becomes fragrant and agreeable. Its specific gravity is 1.15. It is insoluble in water, but the latter abstracts from it a little cinnamic with traces of benzoic acid. It is soluble in absolute alcohol and chloroform.

It was first proven by Lembke, in Germany.

Preparation for Homœopathic Use.—The balsam is dissolved in the proportion of one part by weight to nine parts by weight of ninety-five per cent. alcohol, and designated mother-tincture.

Drug power of tincture, $\frac{1}{10}$.

Dilutions must be prepared as directed under Class V—*a*.

BAPTISIA.

Synonyms, Baptisia Tinctoria, *R. Brown.* Sophora Tinctoria, *Linn.* Podalyria Tinctoria, *Michaux.*

Nat. Ord., Leguminosæ.

Common Name, Wild Indigo.

This is an indigenous perennial herb growing abundantly throughout the United States, in dry and poor soil, in woods and on hills. Its stem is from two to three feet high, smooth and slender, very branchy, rather glaucous. Leaves small, three-foliate, wedge-obovate, bluish-green, almost sessile; stipules and bracts minute and deciduous; racemes few-flowered, terminal on the branches; corolla yellow; pods oval-globose, on a stalk. Flowers from July to September.

Preparation.—The fresh root, with its bark, is chopped and pounded to a pulp and weighed. Then two parts by weight of alcohol are taken, the pulp mixed thoroughly with one-sixth part of it, and the rest of the alcohol added. After stirring the whole well and pouring it into a well-stoppered bottle, it is allowed to stand eight days in a dark, cool place. The tincture is then separated by decanting, straining and filtering.

Drug power of tincture, $\frac{1}{6}$.

Dilutions must be prepared as directed under Class III.

BARTFELDER (Acid Spring).

Cold springs in Upper Hungary; temperature from 45° to 50° F.

Analysis (*Schultes*).

16 ounces furnished 11.59 grains of residue, containing

Sodium Carbonate,	6.07 grains.
Sodium Chloride,	3.03 "
Potassium Carbonate,	0.75 "
Potassium Chloride,	0.62 "
Ferrum Carbonate,	0.40 "
Silica,	0.35 "
Extractive matter,	0.37 "

Preparation.—Not proven in potencies, but if required, prepare first and second dilutions with distilled water, third and higher potencies with alcohol.

BARYTA ACETICA.

Synonym, Barium Acetate.

Present Name, Barium Acetate.

Common Name, Acetate of Barium.

Formula, $Ba\ (C_2H_3O_2)_2$.

Preparation of Acetate of Barium.—This salt is obtained by dissolving pure carbonate of barium in dilute acetic acid, with the aid of gentle heat, till it is neutralized. The liquid is diluted with an equal quantity of distilled water, filtered, evaporated to dryness, and preserved in well-stoppered bottles.

Properties and Tests.—Acetate of barium is a colorless salt, in oblique rhombic prisms, efflorescent in air and readily soluble in water, the solution giving an immediate white precipitate with a solution of sulphate of lime. If the salt itself is acted upon by sulphuric acid, acetic vapors are given off.

It was first proven by Dr. Gross, in Germany.

Preparation for Homœopathic Use.—One part by weight of acetate of barium is dissolved in nine parts by weight of distilled water.

Amount of drug power, $\frac{1}{10}$.

Dilutions must be prepared as directed under Class V—*a*.

Triturations of pure acetate of barium are prepared as directed under Class VII.

BARYTA CARBONICA.

Synonyms, Barium Carbonicum. Barii Carbonas.
Present Name, Barium Carbonate.
Common Name, Carbonate of Barium.
Formula, $Ba\ CO_3$.
Molecular Weight, 197.

Origin and Preparation of Carbonate of Barium.—Barium carbonate is found in nature as *witherite*, a yellowish or grayish, brilliant mineral, crystallizing in rhombic prisms, but oftener found in round or kidney-shaped masses. It may be prepared artificially by precipitating any soluble barium salt by a soluble carbonate, preferably of an alkali. The precipitate is to be collected by filtration, washed and dried.

Properties.—Barium carbonate, prepared as directed above, is a pure white, odorless, tasteless powder, almost insoluble in water. Its specific gravity is 4.2 to 4.3. It is soluble in water containing carbon dioxide; hydrochloric and nitric acids dissolve it with the formation of the salt of each.

Tests.—Barium carbonate should dissolve completely in dilute hydrochloric acid with evolution of $C\ O_2$ (an undissolved residue is barium sulphate). The filtrate precipitated from its solution by sulphuric acid in excess, is not affected by sodium carbonate (absence of metals of the earths). Ammonium sulphide or hydrogen sulphide produces no change in its solutions (absence of the metals).

It was first proven under Hahnemann's directions.

Preparation for Homœopathic Use.—The pure carbonate of barium is prepared by trituration, as directed under Class VII.

BARYTA JODATA.

Synonym, Barii Iodidum.
Present Name, Barium Iodide.
Common Name, Iodide of Barium.
Formula, $Ba\ I_2,\ 2H_2\ O$.
Molecular Weight, 427.

Preparation of Iodide of Barium.—To a solution of iodide of iron add barium carbonate in excess, boil the mixture and separate by filtration the ferrous carbonate. Set the filtrate aside to crystallize. Barium iodide crystallizes in colorless rhombic tables, soluble in water, and in alcohol containing water. It is very hygroscopic, and in contact with the air quickly decomposes with the separation of iodine and consequent yellowish-brown coloration of the salt. It is frequently found in commerce as a yellowish-white powder. Its taste is disagreeable and nauseating. It is very poisonous, as indeed are all the soluble compounds of barium.

Preparation for Homœopathic Use.—The pure iodide of barium is prepared by trituration, as directed under Class VII.

BARYTA MURIATICA.

Synonym, Barii Chloridum.
Present Name, Barium Chloride.
Common Name, Chloride of Barium.
Formula, $Ba\ Cl_2, 2H_2\ O$.
Molecular Weight, 244.

Preparation.—Take of barium carbonate, granulated, and of hydrochloric acid, each one part, and of water five parts. Add the water to the acid, and then gradually to the mixture add the carbonate. As soon as effervescence has nearly ceased, heat the liquid slightly, and after repeated stirrings filter. Set the filtrate aside to crystallize.

Properties.—Barium chloride is in colorless, transparent rhombic tables or plates, soluble in 4 parts of cold and in 1 of hot water, in 400 parts of cold and about 35 of hot alcohol; it is almost insoluble in absolute alcohol. It has the unpleasant, bitter, nauseating taste of the soluble barium compounds.

Tests.—Commercial barium chloride often contains small quantities of the chlorides of strontium and calcium; also aluminium chloride, ferric chloride, and occasionally traces of copper and lead. The strontium and calcium chlorides may be removed by washing the crystals with alcohol; after agitation of the powdered salt with alcohol and setting fire to a portion of the latter, its flame should show not the least tinge of red (absence of strontium). After precipitation by sulphuric acid and filtering, the filtrate should give no precipitate with sodium carbonate (absence of calcium). Its solution, when treated with hydrogen sulphide or ammonium sulphide, should show no change (absence of lead, iron and other metals). The complete solubility of the salt in water will prove the absence of sulphate and carbonate of barium. Its solution, when treated with sulphuric acid or a solution of a sulphate, gives a white precipitate insoluble in nitric acid. With silver nitrate solution a similar result occurs.

It was first proven by Hahnemann.

Preparation for Homœopathic Use.—One part by weight of pure chloride of barium is dissolved in nine parts by weight of distilled water.

Amount of drug power, $\frac{1}{10}$.

Dilutions must be prepared as directed under Class V—*a*.

Triturations of pure chloride of barium are prepared as directed under Class VII.

BELLADONNA.

Synonyms, Atropa Belladonna, *Linn.* Solanum Furiosum or Maniacum. Solanum Somniferum.

Nat. Ord., Solanaceæ.

Common Names, Deadly Nightshade. Common Dwale.

An herbaceous perennial plant, producing thick, smooth stems, four or five feet high. The stems are at first three-forked, afterwards two-forked, bearing above, bright green leaves in unequal pairs, pointed, oval and entire. The flowers are solitary, bell-shaped, pendulous and purple in color, and are followed by large purple-black berries. The root in a plant several years old is fleshy, creeping, a foot or more in length, between half an inch and one inch in thickness, and when dried, wrinkled longitudinally. The difference between the young and old roots is shown not only by the size but also by the fracture, which in old roots is woody, while in the young it is mealy or granulated. The plant is a native of Europe, extending east to the Caucasus, grows in shady places, flowers in July, and ripens its fruit in September.

It was first proven by Hahnemann.

Preparation.—The entire fresh plant, gathered when coming into flower, is chopped and pounded to a fine pulp, enclosed in a piece of new linen and submitted to pressure. The expressed juice is then, by brisk agitation, mingled with an equal part by weight of alcohol. This mixture is allowed to stand eight days in a well-stoppered bottle, in a dark, cool place, and then filtered.

Drug power of tincture, ½.

Dilutions must be prepared as directed under Class I.

BELLADONNA E RADICE.

Root of Atropa Belladonna, *Linn.*

Preparation.—The fresh root, gathered in autumn, is chopped and pounded to a fine pulp, enclosed in a piece of new linen, and submitted to pressure. The expressed juice is then, by brisk agitation, mingled with an equal part by weight of alcohol. This mixture is allowed to stand eight days in a well-stoppered bottle, in a dark, cool place, and then filtered.

Drug power of tincture, ½.

Dilutions must be prepared as directed under Class I.

BELLIS PERENNIS, *Linn.*

Nat. Ord., Compositæ.

Common Names, English Daisy. Garden Daisy. Hens and Chickens.

This is a perennial, found growing in pastures and meadows throughout Europe, and sparingly naturalized in some parts of the New England States. Rootstock short, fibres stout. Leaves long, fleshy, obovate-spatulate, obtuse or rounded at the crenate tip, midrib broad. Scape two to five inches high. Flower-head three-fourths to one inch in diameter, solitary; involucre of green bracts, obtuse, often tipped with black. Ray-flowers white or tipped with pink, disk bright yellow. Flowers in spring and summer.

It was proved by Dr. Thomas, of England.

Preparation.—The fresh plant, in flower, is chopped and pounded to a pulp, enclosed in a piece of new linen and submitted to pressure. The expressed juice is then, by brisk agitation, mingled with an equal part by weight of alcohol. This mixture is allowed to stand eight days in a dark, cool place, and then filtered.

Drug power of tincture, ½.

Dilutions must be prepared as directed under Class I.

BENZINUM NITRICUM.

Synonym, Nitrobenzolum.
Present Name, Nitro-benzol.
Common Names, Artificial Oil of Bitter Almonds.
Formula, $C_6\ H_5\ (NO_2)$.
Molecular Weight, 123.

Preparation of Nitro-benzol.—By adding benzol or benzine (not *gasoline,* sometimes called benzene, one of the distillation products of petroleum) in small quantities to warm concentrated nitric acid a reddish liquid is produced, which, when treated with water, throws down an oily precipitate of nitro-benzol. When the process is conducted at the boiling point there is a violent reaction, and there is also obtained some di-nitro-benzol. It is purified by washing with water and rectified over calcium chloride.

Properties.—Nitro-benzol is a transparent oily looking, yellowish liquid, whose specific gravity is 1.16 to 1.2. It is very slightly soluble in water, somewhat so in alcohol, but only with difficulty in aqueous alcohol. It mixes in all proportions with ether, chloroform, carbon disulphide and in the volatile and fatty oils. When cooled below 3° C. (37.2° F.) it crystallizes in needles. Its odor is similar to that of oil of bitter almonds and it has unfortunately been termed artificial oil of bitter almonds—unfortunately, because of the possibility of its being used for the genuine oil in culinary flavoring. It is extremely poisonous even by inhalation. It has a sweet taste.

Tests.—Nitro-benzol may be identified by its odor, together with its reaction with nascent hydrogen and the consequent production of anilin. A few drops are to be shaken with zinc and dilute sulphuric acid and digested for a little while. The mixture is to be filtered and the filtrate tested with potassium chlorate for anilin, when, if the latter be present, a violet color appears.

Preparation for Homœopathic Use.—One part by weight of nitro-benzol is dissolved in nine parts by weight of ninety-five per cent. alcohol.

Amount of drug power, $\frac{1}{10}$.

Dilutions must be prepared as directed under Class VI—*a.*

BERBERINUM.

Synonyms, Berberin. Berberia. Berberina.
Formula, $C_{20}\ H_{17}\ NO_4$.

Origin.—The alkaloid berberina exists in a number of plants belonging to different families—*e. g., Berberis vulgaris,* Calumba root, *Geoffroya Jamaicensis, Hydrastis Canadensis,* etc.

Berberina may be readily obtained from the root of hydrastis canadensis by making an extract with boiling water, treating this with hot alcohol, and after the addition of some water distilling off most of the alcohol. The residue is to be treated with nitric acid till the reaction is weakly acid, and the whole set aside to crystallize. After some days the nitrate of berberina can be removed and recrystallized from solution in hot water. The now purified nitrate can be decomposed by alkaline carbonate solution and the berberina crystallized out.

Properties.—Berberina is in permanent, small, glistening, yellow needles or prisms, of a bitter taste. They are soluble in about 500 parts of cold, and very readily in hot water; difficultly soluble in cold but easily in hot alcohol; insoluble in ether. The solutions are neutral. Heated upon a water-bath they lose 19.3 per cent. of water, at 120° C. (248° F.) they fuse to a yellow resinous mass, and at near 200° C. (392° F.) they decompose, giving off yellow odorous vapors. With the acids berberina forms golden-yellow, generally crystallizable, bitter tasting salts. When a solution of salt of berberina in hot alcohol is treated with a solution of iodine in potassium iodide, dark green scales rapidly form, having a metallic lustre, and which, when examined by transmitted light, are of a reddish-brown color.

Preparation for Homœopathic Use.—The pure berberina is prepared by trituration, as directed under Class VII.

BERBERIS.

Synonyms, Berberis Vulgaris, *Linn.* Spina Acida.

Nat. Ord., Berberidaceæ.

Common Names, Common Barberry. Pipperidge Bush.

This plant is indigenous to Europe, but is naturalized in New England. It is a bushy shrub three to eight feet high, whose branches are well supplied with thorns. Leaves obovate, bristly-serrate. The yellow flowers hang in clusters. The fruit is a small, oblong, scarlet berry, whose pleasant acid taste commends it for making a sweet preserve. The bark of the root is used in homœopathic pharmacy. It is of a grayish-brown color externally, and saffron-yellow within.

It was first proven by Hesse, in Germany.

Preparation.—The fresh bark from the root is coarsely powdered and weighed. Then two parts by weight of alcohol are added to it; the mixture is put into a well-stoppered bottle and allowed to stand eight days in a dark, cool place, shaking twice a day. The tincture is to be poured off, strained and filtered.

Drug power of tincture, $\frac{1}{3}$.

Dilutions must be prepared as directed under Class III.

BISMUTHUM METALLICUM.

Synonyms, Bismuthum. Metallic Bismuth.

Common Name, Bismuth.

Symbol, Bi.

Atomic Weight, 210.

Bismuth is found in nature in the metallic state in veins running through certain crystallized rocks. It chiefly occurs in Saxony and Bohemia. It is also found as *bismite* or oxide, as sulphide or *bismuthinite*, as sulpho-telluride and as carbonate.

Preparation of Metallic Bismuth.—The bismuth-bearing rock, broken up, is placed in iron tubes slightly inclined, and then heat is applied. The bismuth melts, and flowing out of the tubes, is caught in proper vessels and ladled into moulds.

Commercial bismuth contains arsenic, iron and other metals. It is freed from these by fusion with potassium nitrate, by which they are oxidized and form a slag, which is to be separated from the fused metal. Chemically pure bismuth may be obtained by reducing a pure specimen of the basic nitrate, by charcoal at a red heat.

Properties.—Bismuth is a hard, brilliant, reddish-white metal in crystalline laminæ. By melting a large amount of it, cooling it until a crust forms over it, breaking the crust and pouring out the liquid metal remaining, it may be obtained in large and beautiful rhombohedrons, which are often mistaken for cubes. Its specific gravity is 9.83. It melts at 264° C. (507.2° F.), and on solidifying expands $\frac{1}{32}$ of its volume. It is unaffected by dry air but tarnishes in the presence of moisture. At a red heat it burns with a bluish flame, forming the bismuthous oxide. At a white heat it is volatile. It is readily attacked by chlorine and by nitric acid, but is unaffected by hydrochloric and sulphuric acids in the cold.

Tests.—Digest the metal with a twenty per cent. nitric acid (tin and antimony remain undissolved); filter, and concentrate the filtrate to remove most of the nitrate by crystallization; filter again, and to this filtrate add water in large amount, when the remaining subnitrate will precipitate as a white powder; filter anew, and the filtrate when tested by sulphuric acid will give a white precipitate if lead be present; with potassium ferrocyanide, a blue, if iron, or a reddish-brown if copper be the impurity.

Preparation for Homœopathic Use.—The pure metallic bismuth is prepared by trituration, as directed under Class VII.

BISMUTHUM OXYDATUM.

Proper Name, Bismuthous Oxide.

Synonyms, Bismuthi Oxidum. Tri-oxide of Bismuth.

Common Name, Oxide of Bismuth.

Formula, $Bi_2 O_3$.

Molecular Weight, 468.

Preparation of Oxide of Bismuth.—When a bismuthous salt is treated with an alkaline hydrate, a white precipitate of bismuthous hydrate is thrown down; by boiling, the hydrate loses water and is converted into the oxide. A convenient process is as follows: Take of subnitrate of bismuth, one part; solution of soda (specific gravity 1.047), five parts; mix and boil for five minutes; then, having allowed the mixture to cool and the oxide to subside, decant the supernatant liquid, wash the precipitate thoroughly with distilled water, and finally dry it by the heat of a water-bath.

Properties.—Bismuth tri-oxide is a yellow powder, which becomes deeper in color when heated, but only transiently. It fuses at a red heat. It dissolves readily in hydrochloric, sulphuric and nitric acids, yielding the respective salts of bismuth.

Tests.—Silver and lead may be present as impurities. By dissolving a portion of the bismuthous oxide in hydrochloric acid, a white residue, insoluble in nitric acid, indicates silver; similarly, by using sulphuric acid a precipitate of white color and insoluble in dilute nitric acid, indicates lead.

It was first proven by Hahnemann.

Preparation for Homœopathic Use.—The pure oxide of bismuth is prepared by trituration, as directed under Class VII.

BISMUTHUM SUBNITRICUM.

Synonyms, Bismuthi Subnitras. Magisterium Bismuthi. Marcassita Alba.

Common Names, Pearl White. Subnitrate of Bismuth. White Oxide of Bismuth.

Formula, $[Bi\ (NO_3)_3] + [BiH_3O_3]_3$.

Molecular Weight, 1179.

Preparation of Subnitrate of Bismuth.—To 100 parts of pure nitric acid, specific gravity 1.185, in a capacious glass vessel, are to be gradually added twenty-five parts of coarsely powdered metallic bismuth, or as much of it as will dissolve at the temperature of the water-bath. Then add a small portion of the metal and heat the whole for about half an hour. The clear supernatant liquid is to be decanted and filtered through glass-wool, and to the filtrate is to be added, with constant stirring, forty to fifty parts of distilled water, or as much as may be required to produce a noticeable turbidity. This precipitate contains some arsenate of bismuth. The whole is to be allowed to stand in a cool place, when it is to be filtered through glass-wool, and the filtrate set aside to crystallize after being evaporated down to seventy or sixty-five parts. The crystals are to be collected on a filter of loosely arranged glass-wool, and the mother liquor evaporated to one-third of its volume, set aside, and the crystals obtained from it are to be added to those previously collected. The crystals are to be washed by dropping upon them a mixture of five parts of nitric acid with ten of distilled water. They are to be spread upon a porcelain tile and dried, at about 25° C. (77°F.). The preparation so obtained is the normal bismuthous nitrate, $[Bi\ (NO_3)_3]_2 + 9H_2O$.

From the normal nitrate, the basic salt or subnitrate is prepared in the following manner: 100 parts of crystallized bismuth tri-nitrate are powdered in a mortar and mixed with 400 parts of cold distilled water. The mixture is then added to 2100 parts of boiling distilled water in a glass vessel, and the whole stirred with a glass rod for some minutes. After the mixture has become cold, the precipitate is thrown upon a filter and washed, by pouring from a height 500 parts of cold distilled water; it is then spread upon porcelain tiles in thin layers, and dried at a temperature not exceeding 30° C. (86° F.). It should, while drying, be carefully protected from dust, sulphuretted hydrogen and ammonia gases. The methods as given above are, with slight changes, those of the Pharmacopœia Germanica.

Properties.—Subnitrate of bismuth is an odorless, almost tasteless, snow-white, crystalline powder, consisting of microscopic, colorless, rhombic prisms. With moistened litmus paper its reaction is acid. It is not changed by exposure to sunlight. Specimens of it becoming gray by such exposure, contain silver chloride. When heated to 100° C. (212° F.), it loses its water, and at a higher temperature it loses, without melting, its acid. The proportions of the constituents, bismuthous oxide, nitric acid and water, are rarely alike in any two preparations, and the oxide varies in amount between 79 and 81 per cent.

Tests.—The subnitrate of bismuth should dissolve without effervescence in five times its volume of pure nitric acid, specific gravity, 1.180, slightly warmed (absence of carbonate or sulphate). The strong acid solution is to be diluted with four to five volumes of distilled water and filtered. The filtrate is to be tested in successive portions. When treated with silver nitrate, barium nitrate and sodium sulphate solutions, no precipitate should occur (absence of chloride, sulphate and lead). Let a small quantity of the subnitrate be heated in a test-tube, with an equal amount of concentrated sulphuric acid, free from arsenic, until all the nitric acid is driven off, and to the solution add ten volumes of dilute sulphuric acid, arsenic-free, then add a small quantity of sodium chloride and a few pieces of pure zinc. The test-tube should be loosely corked, and there should project into it a piece of filter paper, moistened with silver nitrate solution. Upon heating the test-tube, the gray or darker staining of the silver nitrate indicates the presence of arsenic.

Preparation for Homœopathic Use.—The pure subnitrate of bismuth is prepared by trituration as directed under Class VII.

BLATTA AMERICANA, *Lamarck.*

Synonym, Kakerlac Americana, *Sars.*
Class, Insecta.
Order, Orthoptera.
Family, Blattina.
Common Name, Great American Cockroach.

The Blatta Americana, which is very common in Brazil, where it inhabits human dwellings, is an orthopterous insect, with an elongated, oval, rather flat body, from twelve to sixteen lines in length, of a brown-red color, which becomes paler under the belly. The prothorax is smooth, shining, of an ochre-yellow tint, with two large brown spots, which are sometimes united in one. In the male the elytra reach beyond the belly by a few lines; in the female they are a little shorter. They are marked with numerous longitudinal streaks which bifurcate near the dotted margin terminating the elytra. The wings are striate and reticular, of the length of the elytra. The antennæ which are longer than the body, exhibit at their base a small yellowish point. The feet are provided with black prickles and terminate in a tarsus with five articulations.

Preparation.—The live animal is crushed and triturated, as directed under Class IX.

BOLETUS LARICIS, *Linn.*

Synonyms, Agaricus Laricis. Fungus Laricis. Boletus Purgans. Polyporus Officinalis, *Fries.*

Nat. Ord., Fungi.

Common Names, Larch Agaric. Larch Boletus. Purging Agaric. White Agaric.

This is a fungus growing on the larch-tree of the old world, of various sizes. Pileus dirty-white, with livid stains, covered at first with dirty-yellow or brownish evanescent slime, subsquamose; stem cribrose above the ring, scrobiculate below, dirty-white; tubes adnate, subdecurrent, compound, at first nearly white. As found in commerce, it is deprived of its exterior coat, and consists of a light, white, spongy, somewhat farinaceous, friable mass, which, though capable of being rubbed into powder upon a sieve, is not easily pulverized in the ordinary mode, as it flattens under the pestle.

It was proved by Dr. W. H. Burt, U. S.

Preparation.—The dried fungus is covered with five parts by weight of alcohol, and after mixing well, the whole is poured into a well-stoppered bottle, and allowed to remain eight days in a dark, cool place, being shaken twice a day. The tincture is then poured off, strained and filtered.

Drug power of tincture, $\frac{1}{10}$.

Dilutions must be prepared as directed under Class IV.

Triturations of the dried fungus are prepared, as directed under Class VII.

BOLETUS SATANAS, *Lenz.*

Synonym, Satanic Boletus.

Nat. Ord., Fungi.

Common Name, Satan's Fungus.

Pileus pulvinate, smooth, somewhat viscid, brownish-tan color, then whitish, stem blunt, ovato-ventricose, reticulated above, blood-red; tubes free, minute, yellow, orifice from the first blood-red.

Preparation.—The fresh fungus is prepared by trituration, as directed under Class IX.

BONDONNEAU.

Bondonneau Mineral Water. (Saintes-Fontaines.)

Chemical Analysis.

In one liter, there was contained:

Free Sulphuric Acid, a trace, but it is very perceptible at the spring.

Free Carbonic Acid, ...	$\frac{5}{8}$ the volume of water.
Bicarbonate of Lime, ... }	0.390 grammes.
Bicarbonate of Magnesia, ... }	
Bicarbonate of Soda, ...	0.006 "
Potash salts, ...	a trace.

Sulphates (probably anhydrous) of	Soda, Lime, Magnesia,	0.043 grammes.
Chloride of Sodium,		0.030 "
Alkaline, Iodides and Bromides,		0.008 "
Arseniates,		a trace.
Sesquioxide of Iron with Manganese,		0.002 "
Silica and Alumina,		0.128 "
Earthy Phosphates,		a trace.
Nitrogenized organic matters,		an uncertain amount.

A proving by Dr. Espanet, France, is recorded.

Preparation.—If potencies are required, use distilled water for first and second dilutions, alcohol for third and higher potencies.

BORAX.

Synonyms, Natrum Biboracicum. Boras Sodicus. Sodii Boras. Borate of Sodium.

Present Name, Sodium Tetraborate.

Common Name, Borax.

Formula, $Na_2 B_4O_7, 10 H_2O$.

Molecular Weight, 382.

Origin and Preparation of Borax.—Borax is found native in several localities, in Transylvania, Peru, and Canada West, but more particularly in certain salt lakes in India, Thibet and California. The salt separated from these waters by evaporation, either naturally or by artificial aid, is known as crude borax or *tincal*. Crude borax is refined by treating it with either lime or soda, which removes a greasy substance with which the tincal is covered. The greater part of the borax used in the arts is now prepared in France by treating the native boracic acid found in lagoons in volcanic districts in Italy, notably in Tuscany, with sodium carbonate, both in boiling solution; insoluble matters settle down and the clear solution of borax is transferred to vessels in which it crystallizes. Artificial borax is for the most part purer than that obtained from tincal by the refining process, but the crystals often contain cracks, and this is a disadvantage when the borax is used for soldering. The refined borax is purified by recrystallization, and thus fitted for medicinal use.

Properties.—Borax is in large transparent prisms of the monoclinic system, generally combinations of a nearly rectangular prism having the acute and obtuse lateral edges truncated. When heated they melt in their water of crystallization, at the same time swelling up and solidifying to a loose spongy mass; at a red heat the salt fuses to a colorless transparent mass called borax-glass. Borax has a mild sweet cooling taste, with an alkaline after-taste; it is soluble in from twelve to fifteen parts of cold and in two of boiling water, in four or five parts of glycerine, and not at all in alcohol. It reacts slightly alkaline to test paper. It specific gravity is 1.7.

Tests.—Borax is frequently adulterated with alum and rock-salt. Several crystals should be dissolved and the solution tested; with hydrogen sulphide no change should occur (absence of metals); with sodium carbonate solution no precipitate (absence of the earthy metals); nor in very dilute solution, with barium chloride (absence of sulphate); nor with silver nitrate (absence of chloride).

It was first proven by Hahnemann.

Preparation for Homœopathic Use.—One part by weight of pure borax is dissolved in ninety-nine parts by weight of distilled water.

Amount of drug power, $\frac{1}{100}$.

Dilutions must be prepared as directed under Class V—β.

Triturations of pure borax are prepared as directed under Class VII.

BORRAGO OFFICINALIS, *Linn.*

Nat. Ord., Borraginaceæ.

Common Name, Borage.

This plant is found growing in waste grounds near habitations, in Europe. It is cultivated as a garden vegetable. It has ovate, alternate leaves, the lower ones on petioles. The sky-blue flowers are in cymes, which are terminal and axillary. The stem is about two feet high, erect; the whole plant is hairy.

Preparation.—The fresh leaves are chopped and pounded to a pulp, enclosed in a piece of new linen and submitted to pressure. The expressed juice is then, by brisk agitation, mingled with an equal part by weight of alcohol. This mixture is allowed to stand eight days, in a well-stoppered bottle, in a dark, cool place, and then filtered.

Drug power of tincture, $\frac{1}{2}$.

Dilutions must be prepared as directed under Class I.

BOVISTA.

Synonyms, Bovista Nigrescens. Fungus Ovatus. Lycoperdon Bovista, *Linn.*

Nat. Ord., Fungi.

Common Names, Puff-ball. Bull-fist. Puck-fist. Puck-ball. Puffin. Bunt. Devil's Snuff-box. Fuzz-ball.

Throughout the whole year, but especially in the beginning of autumn, the puff-ball is found on the pasture grounds and dry meadows of Europe. Nearly as round as a ball, it is at the base narrowed to form a thick, folded stalk. It is of variable size, its diameter from one inch to one foot; when young it is white, later of a dirty-yellow color, finally changing to umber-brown.

Proven by Hartlaub, in Germany.

Preparation.—The entire fungus collected in August or September is bruised and weighed. Then five parts by weight of dilute alcohol added to it, and having been put into a well-stoppered bottle, the whole is allowed to remain eight days in a dark, cool place, being shaken twice a day. The tincture is then poured off, strained and filtered.

Drug power of tincture, $\frac{1}{10}$.

Dilutions must be prepared as directed under Class IV., except that *dilute* alcohol is used for the 1x and 2x, and 1 dilutions.

Triturations are prepared from the ripe, brown-black powder, as directed under Class VII.

BRACHYGLOTTIS REPENS, *Forst.*

Common Name, Puka-Puka.

This is usually a shrub, though sometimes it has the appearance of a tree, twenty feet in height, growing in the northern island of New Zealand. It has broad, indented, glossy leaves, downy on the under surface. Its flowers are large, clustered and fragrant.

Preparation.—Equal parts of the fresh leaves and flowers are chopped and pounded to a pulp and weighed. Then two parts by weight of alcohol are taken, the pulp mixed thoroughly with one-sixth part of it, and the rest of the alcohol added. After stirring the whole well, and pouring it into a well-stoppered bottle, it is allowed to stand eight days in a dark, cool place. The tincture is then separated by decanting, straining and filtering.

Amount of drug power, $\frac{1}{6}$.

Dilutions must be prepared as directed under Class III.

BRANCA URSINA.

Synonyms, Heracleum Sphondylium, *Linn.* Acanthus Vulgaris.

Nat. Ord., Umbelliferæ.

Common Names, Bear's Breech. Cow-parsnip. Hogweed. Masterwort.

A plant found all over Europe. Stem three to six feet high, hairy, erect and branching toward the top. Flowers white, in umbels. Leaves pinnate with divided leaflets. The plant contains an acrid, irritating juice. The root is thick, fleshy, spindle-shaped and branching.

The remedy was proved by Dr. Rosenberg, in Germany.

Preparation.—The fresh plant, at the time of flowering, is chopped and pounded to a fine pulp and pressed out *lege artis* in a piece of new linen. The expressed juice is then, by brisk agitation, mingled with an equal part by weight of alcohol. This mixture is allowed to stand eight days in a well-stoppered bottle, in a dark, cool place, and then filtered.

Drug power of tincture, $\frac{1}{2}$.

Dilutions must be prepared as directed under Class I.

BRAYERA ANTHELMINTICA, *Kunth.*

Synonyms, Hagenia Abyssinica, *Willd.* Banksia Abyssinica, *Bruce.*

Nat. Ord., Rosaceæ.

Common Name, Koosso or Kousso. Kosbo Sika.

This is a handsome tree growing about twenty feet high, throughout the table-land of Abyssinia, at an elevation of from three to eight thousand feet. The plant is noted for its abundant foliage and fine panicles of flowers of a reddish tint, which at first are greenish. The leaves are mostly towards the ends of the branches; they are large, pinnate; leaflets lanceolate and serrated. The flowers have an herby, somewhat tea-like odor, and a bitter, acrid taste. Kousso, as seen in commerce, is of a light brown color, of a reddish tinge in the case of the female flowers. The latter are often obtainable separately under the name of *red kousso.*

Preparation.—The dried blossoms are coarsely powdered, covered with five parts by weight of alcohol, the mixture allowed to remain eight days in a well-stoppered bottle, in a dark, cool place, and shaken twice a day. The tincture is then poured off, strained and filtered.

Drug power, $\frac{1}{10}$.

Dilutions must be prepared as directed under Class IV.

Triturations are prepared from the dried blossoms, as directed under Class VII.

BROMIUM.

Synonym, Brominium.

Common Name, Bromine.

Symbol, Br.

Atomic Weight, 80.

A liquid non-metallic element.

Origin and Preparation of Bromine.—Bromine does not exist in nature in the free state. It is found in combination as bromide in the water of many salt springs, especially that of Theodorshall, near Kreuznach, in Prussia; it is found together with iodine in the ash of sea-weed, *varec;* it exists also in sponges and many marine animals. It is prepared from the mother-liquor of sea water or saline springs. These waters are first freed by crystallizing out the greater part of the chlorides and sulphates of sodium and potassium; the remaining liquid contains bromine, chiefly in the form of bromide of magnesium. This liquid is placed in a retort with peroxide of manganese and hydrochloric acid and distilled; chlorine gas is evolved in the liquid, displaces the bromine in the magnesium compound, and the bromine distils over. Bromine is produced by the above process at many salt works in the United States.

Properties.—Bromine is a dark red or brown-red liquid, whose specific gravity at 15° C. (59° F.) is between 2.98 and 2.99. It is extremely volatile, at ordinary temperatures giving off dark red vapors, and for this reason it is condensed under water from the retort in the process of its manufacture. Its vapor is 5.5 times as heavy as air, and is of a disagreeable, pungent odor, recalling in some degree that of chlorine. It boils at 63° C (145.4° F.). Lowig gives its boiling point as 45° C (113° F.). It dissolves sparingly in water, more readily in alcohol and in all proportions in ether. Like chlorine, it has a powerful affinity for hydrogen, although not to the same degree, and this explains its energetic action upon many organic substances. It corrodes wood and cork, first turning them yellow, and upon the skin, if in quantity, it produces immediate corrosion and violent inflammation. Its solutions are decomposed in the sunlight, bromine as such disappearing and hydrogen bromide being formed. Bromine should be preserved in bottles, with a layer of water over the bromine, the bottles securely closed with a glass stopper and kept in a cellar or other cool, dark place.

Tests.—The impurities most likely to be present in bromine are chlorine, iodine, bromide of carbon and of lead. The test for iodine as an impurity in bromine is as follows: Place 4 CC. of distilled water in a test-tube, add from five to ten drops of bromine, and then with slight agitation, caustic ammonia, drop by drop, till the fluid becomes clear and colorless; the liberation of free nitrogen occurs with effervescence, and the liquid contains ammonium bromide. The solution is now rendered acid with nitric acid, a few CC. of ferric chloride solution followed by about 2 CC. of chloroform are added and the whole shaken gently. In the bottom of the tube the chloroform collects, tinged violet if iodine be present, otherwise it remains colorless. This is a very delicate test, but where the iodine is in extremely small amount, the coloration will not show immediately.

For chlorine: In a small flask having a glass stopper shake thoroughly about 5 CC. of bromine with 15 CC. of distilled water; pour about 5 CC. of the liquid into a test-tube and shake thoroughly with its own volume of ether. The watery colorless layer is to be removed from the yellow ethereal layer by means of a separating funnel, shaken again with ½ volume of ether and the ethereal and watery layers separated as before. The watery solution is placed in a wide test-tube and heated to boiling or until no odor of ether is perceptible. Should the liquid react acid to test paper the presence of hydrogen chloride or of bromine chloride is probable. To about 3 CC. of the liquid are added five drops of silver nitrate solution and then 8 CC. of sesquicarbonate of ammonia solution; the whole is thoroughly shaken, boiled for two or three minutes, and should the fluid be not clear, placed aside for some time and the clear fluid decanted off. This is evaporated in a porcelain dish to a small volume, to which is then to be added 10 CC. of distilled water and the solution treated to excess with pure chlorine-free nitric acid. A precipitate, or rather dense turbidity, indicates the presence of chlorine in the original bromine. A weak opalescent turbidity, however, which does not deprive the liquid of translucency is due to the presence of a trace of silver bromide.

Tests.—The presence of bromide of carbon may be recognized by the separation and gathering of small drops in the bottom of the test-tube when the caustic ammonia is added during the process of testing for iodine. A few drops of bromine placed in flask or upon a watch glass should evaporate without residue. This is an easy test for bromide of lead, the only non-volatile impurity likely to be present.

Provings of Bromine were first made by Drs. Michaelis and Müller, Germany.

Preparation for Homœopathic Use.—One part of pure bromine is dissolved in ninety-nine parts by weight of distilled water.

Amount of drug power, $\frac{1}{100}$.

Dilutions must be prepared as directed under Class V—β, except that distilled water is used for dilutions to the 4x and 2, dilute alcohol for the next higher, and alcohol for all further dilutions.

BRUCEA ANTIDYSENTERICA.

Synonym, Angustura Spuria.

Common Name, False Angustura.

This is the bark of the tree Strychnos Nux Vomica, which is described under Nux Vomica.

Preparation.—The dried bark is pulverized and covered with five parts by weight of alcohol. Having poured it into a well-stoppered bottle, it is allowed to remain eight days in a dark, cool place, being shaken twice a day. The tincture is then poured off, strained and filtered.

Drug power of tincture, $\frac{1}{10}$.

Dilutions must be prepared as directed under Class IV.

BRUCINUM.

Synonym, Brucia.

Formula, $C_{23}H_{26} N_2 O_4, + 4 H_2 O$.

Preparation.—Brucia is an alkaloid, existing, together with strychnia, in nux vomica, in the St. Ignatius bean, and in several varieties of *Strychnos*. It is obtained from the mother liquors left after the preparation of strychnia from the seeds of *Strychnos Nux Vomica*, by concentrating them to the consistency of syrup and slightly supersaturating with dilute sulphuric acid. The mixture, if left to itself for a few days, deposits crystals of the sulphate of brucia, which are afterwards purified. The brucia is then separated by ammonia.

Properties.—Crystallized brucia is in transparent, oblique, rhombic prisms, or in star-like aggregations of acicular crystals, or is a white powder made up of crystalline scales. It dissolves with difficulty in cold, more readily in hot water. It dissolves freely in alcohol whether absolute or dilute, as it also does in amyl alcohol; in ether it is almost insoluble. When heated it fuses, parting with its water of crystallization; at a high temperature it is decomposed, leaving a bulky carbonaceous product.

Tests.—Concentrated nitric acid produces with brucia and its salts an intensely red fluid, which afterwards becomes orange-red, and upon heating, of a yellow color. If stannous chloride or ammonium sulphide be added to the heated fluid the faint yellow color becomes an intense violet. Strychnia is often present in ordinary specimens of brucia. To one part of brucia add twenty-five parts of absolute alcohol at the ordinary temperature; let the mixture stand for about an hour with occasional agitation. A perfectly clear solution should result, which is to be decanted from any undissolved portion if such be present. The latter is to be transferred to a watch-glass, evaporated to dryness and dissolved with a few drops of concentrated sulphuric acid. To it is added a small fragment of potassium bichromate and the fluid carefully moved about; a blue coloration passing successively through violet, red and green indicates the presence of strychnia.

Preparation for Homœopathic Use.—The pure brucia is pre-prepared by trituration, as directed under Class VII.

BRYONIA ALBA, *Linn*

Synonyms, Bryonia Vera. Vitis Alba.
Nat. Ord., Cucurbitaceæ.
Common Name, White Bryonia. Wild Hops.

Bryonia is a high climbing, perennial plant, growing in hedges and along fences, and is quite common in Germany and France. The perennial root of this plant is as thick as an arm, and at times even as large as the thigh; it is fleshy, succulent, branchy, of a yellowish-white color, circularly wrinkled without, acrid, bitter, disagreeable to the taste, and of a nauseating odor, which, however, disappears by desiccation. Its climbing stalk rises sometimes to the height of many feet; it is glabrous, creeping, channelled, and armed with spiral creepers; its leaves are alternate, angular, hispid, tuberculous on both sides, rough to the touch, palmated, five-lobed, the middle lobe trifid, elongated; flowers axillary, monœcious, in bunches; the male being supported on very long peduncles, the female larger than the male; calyx five-toothed, sharp; corolla in five divisions; stamens five, of which four are united two and two by the filaments and the anthers, the fifth free; berries round, black, polyspermous.

Bryonia Alba was the variety Hahnemann used in his experiments, and great care must be taken not to confound it with Bryonia Dioica, which grows in the same localities, but mostly in England.

Preparation.—The fresh root, gathered before the plant is in bloom, is chopped and pounded to a fine pulp, and pressed out *lege artis* in a piece of new linen. The expressed juice is then, by brisk agitation, mingled with an equal part by weight of alcohol. This mixture is allowed to remain for several weeks (to deposit amylum, with which it abounds), in a well-stoppered bottle, in a dark, cool place, and then filtered.

Drug power of tincture, ½.

Dilutions must be prepared as directed under Class I.

BUCHU.

Synonyms, Barosma Crenata, *Kunze.* Diosma Crenata, *Linn., De Candolle.*
Nat. Ord., Rutaceæ.
Common Name, Buchu.

Buchu leaves are afforded by three species of *Barosma.* These are erect shrubs several feet high, having smooth rod-like branches.

Leaves opposite, margins serrate, the margins and under surface furnished with oil-glands which are conspicuous. The flowers are white, five-parted; the fruit is in five erect carpels. The plants are indigenous to the Cape region of Southern Africa.

Description.—The leaves of *B. crenata* are oblong, oval or obovate, obtuse, narrowed toward the base into a distinct petiole; margin serrulate or crenulate; $\frac{3}{4}$ to $1\frac{1}{2}$ inches long, $\frac{3}{10}$ to $\frac{4}{10}$ of an inch wide.

Those of *B. serratifolia* are linear-lanceolate, equally narrowed toward either end, three-veined, apex truncate, always furnished with an oil cell; margin sharply serrulate; 1 to $1\frac{1}{2}$ inches long, about $\frac{2}{10}$ of an inch wide.

B. betulina: Leaves cuneate-obovate, apex recurved, margin sharply denticulate, teeth spreading; $\frac{1}{2}$ to $\frac{3}{4}$ inch long, $\frac{3}{10}$ to $\frac{5}{10}$ wide. Each of the three species can be obtained in commerce by itself; *B. betulina* is the least esteemed.

Preparation.—The dry leaves are coarsely powdered and covered with five parts by weight of alcohol; having poured this into a well-stoppered bottle, the mixture is to be allowed to remain eight days in a dark, cool place and shaken twice a day. The tincture is then poured off, strained and filtered.

Drug power of tincture, $\frac{1}{10}$.

Dilutions must be prepared as directed under class IV.

BUFO.

Synonyms. Cinereus. Rana Bufo.
Class, Amphibia.
Order, Anura.
Family, Bufonidæ.
Common Name, Toad.

This well-known animal is a native of North America, Europe, Southern Asia, and Japan.

It was proven by Dr. Carl Hencke, Germany.

Preparation.—The live animal is fastened to a slab of cork by four strong pins stuck through the webs of the feet. Then the poles of an induction apparatus in action are slowly drawn over the back of the animal, whereupon the poison very soon issues from the dorsal glands. This is removed with a small horn knife, and triturated according to Class VIII., but in the proportion of 1 part to 1000 parts sugar of milk, the preparation being equal to the 3x trituration.

BUFO SAHYTIENSIS.

Synonym, Bufo Agua.
Class, Amphibia.
Order, Anura.
Family, Bufonidæ.
Common Name, Toad of South America.

This toad is common in South America; it inhabits swamps and marshy regions. It is sometimes as large as two fists, though its size varies a good deal. It is readily known by its enormous rhomboidal parotids, whence it sends forth a large quantity of poison. Its head is flat, triangular, broader than long; it has a strong osseous edge, commencing at the tip of the muzzle, thence stretching towards the inner angle of the eye, round this organ, and finally terminating behind the lids. The eye and the tympanic wall are very large. The trunk, which is very large anteriorly in consequence of the large development of the parotids, is covered on each side of the dorsal spine with two irregular rows of large elliptical or conical bladders; sometimes there are such bladders on the sides. The anterior extremities do not reach to the end of the trunk; the posterior extremities reach beyond the muzzle by the length of the fourth toe. The toes are rather flattened; the first toe longer than the second. Its colors are various, consisting of a number of brown spots, which coalesce on the back and are separated on the abdomen by yellowish dots.

Introduced into our Materia Medica by Dr. Mure, Brazil.

Preparation.—The saliva, obtained by irritating the animal, is prepared by trituration, as directed under Class VIII.

BUXUS SEMPERVIRENS, *Linn.*

Nat. Ord., Euphorbiaceæ.

Common Name, Box.

An evergreen shrub, native of Western Asia, and much cultivated in this country as an edging plant to garden borders. It has opposite leaves, ovate, slightly wider near the base than at apex. The leaves have a disagreeable, bitter taste and a peculiar odor.

Preparation.—The fresh leaves are chopped and pounded to a pulp and weighed. Then two parts by weight of alcohol are taken, the pulp mixed thoroughly with one-sixth part of it, and the rest of the alcohol added. After stirring the whole well, and pouring it into a well-stoppered bottle, it is allowed to stand eight days in a dark, cool place. The tincture is then separated by decanting, straining and filtering.

Drug power of tincture, $\frac{1}{6}$.

Dilutions must be prepared as directed under Class III.

CACAO.

Synonym, Theobroma Cacao, *Linn.*

Nat. Ord., Sterculiaceæ.

Common Name, Cacao.

Origin.—Cacao seeds are furnished by Theobroma Cacao, T. angustifolium, *Sessé*, T. bicolor, *Humboldt*, and others of the same genus. The trees are found in the northern portion of South America, throughout Central America, and extend into Mexico, and are largely cultivated.

Description.—The seeds are ovoid, more or less appressed, about three-quarters to one inch long and nearly one half-inch broad. A well marked raphe extends along one edge in its whole length. The testa is red-brown to brown in color, fragile and papery. By prolongations of the inner seed-coat, the large, oily cotyledons of which the seed is mainly composed, are partitioned into a number of small irregular lobes, an arrangement which permits of the ready breaking up of the seed into a number of fragments.

Preparation.—Cacao seeds are prepared for use by removing them from the fruit and simply drying them, in which case they retain their astringent and bitter taste. These seeds are then prepared by trituration, as directed under Class VII.

CACTUS GRANDIFLORUS, *Linn.*

Synonym, Cereus Grandiflorus, *De Candolle.*

Nat. Ord., Cactaceæ.

Common Name, Night-blooming Cereus.

This well known flowering plant is a native of Mexico and the West India Islands. Its stems are nearly cylindrical, with five or six angles, beset with small radiating spines. Its flowers are large and white, opening in the evening and withering before sunrise, and have a powerful odor of benzoic acid and vanilla.

It was introduced into our Materia Medica by Dr. Rocco Rubini, of Italy.

Preparation.—The fresh flowers, together with the youngest and tenderest stems, gathered from plants growing in their native country, are chopped and pounded to a pulp and weighed. Then two parts by weight of alcohol are taken, the pulp mixed with one-sixth part of it, and the rest of the alcohol added. After stirring the whole well and pouring it into a well-stoppered bottle, it is allowed to stand eight days in a dark, cool place. The tincture is then separated by decanting, straining and filtering.

Drug power of tincture, $\frac{1}{6}$.

Dilutions must be prepared as directed under Class III.

CADMIUM METALLICUM.

Common Name, Cadmium.

Symbol, Cd.

Atomic Weight, 112.

Origin and Preparation of Cadmium.—Cadmium is found in nature associated with zinc in different ores of the latter metal, as the sulphide, carbonate or silicate. The only pure native compound of cadmium is the sulphide called *Greenockite*, found in Scotland.

In the process of reducing ores of zinc, the cadmium which they contain comes over among the first products of distillation, owing to its greater volatility. The impure product may be dissolved in dilute sulphuric acid, when upon the addition of metallic zinc, metallic cadmium is deposited. It may also be separated from the zinc by treating the solution with hydrogen sulphide, when cadmium sulphide is precipitated. This sulphide dissolved in concentrated hydrochloric acid yields chloride of cadmium, which, when treated with ammonium carbonate in excess, gives a precipitate of the carbonate of the metal. The latter is then mixed with carbon, placed in a retort and subjected to a red heat, and the metal distils over.

Properties.—Cadmium is a white metal with a tinge of blue. It is lustrous and takes a fine polish, but upon exposure to the air, it slowly acquires a whitish-gray tarnish. It is very malleable and ductile, and crackles like tin when bent. Heated to 82° C. (179.6° F.) it becomes brittle, and at 315° C. (599° F.) it melts, and on cooling crystallizes in regular octohedrons. It dissolves in hot hydrochloric or dilute sulphuric acid, forming the corresponding salt, but nitric acid is its best solvent. Most of its salts are colorless, and their solutions redden blue litmus paper.

Tests.—Cadmium may be readily identified by the precipitate of a yellow sulphide upon passing hydrogen sulphide into acid solutions containing the metal; the precipitate is insoluble in dilute acids and alkalies, the latter fact distinguishing it from the yellow sulphide of arsenic formed under similar circumstances. Cadmium is often accompanied by zinc and sometimes by copper. If the solution from which the precipitated sulphide has been filtered off be rendered alkaline by ammonium hydrate in excess, the precipitate of white sulphide of zinc will appear, or it may be made to do so by adding hydrogen sulphide. Copper may be detected by dissolving a small portion of cadmium in nitric acid, and adding ammonia, when if the former metal be present the blue coloration of ammonio-nitrate of copper will be seen.

Preparation for Homœopathic Use.—The pure metallic cadmium is prepared by trituration, as directed under Class VII.

CADMIUM SULPHURICUM.

Synonym, Cadmii Sulphas.
Present Name, Cadmium Sulphate.
Common Name, Sulphate of Cadmium.
Formula, $Cd\ SO_4, 4\ H_2\ O$.
Molecular Weight, 280.

Preparation of Sulphide of Cadmium.—Cadmium sulphate is easily obtained by dissolving the oxide or carbonate in dilute sulphuric acid; the solution is partly evaporated over a water-bath and then set aside to crystallize.

Properties and Tests.—Cadmium sulphate crystallizes in colorless monoclinic prisms which effloresce in air, are very soluble in water and insoluble in alcohol. They are without odor and have a metallic styptic taste. The impurities likely to be present in cadmium sulphate are arsenic and zinc; their presence may be detected by the methods given under cadmium metallicum.

The drug was introduced into our Materia Medica by Dr. Petroz, of Spain.

Preparation for Homœopathic Use.—The pure sulphate of cadmium is prepared by trituration, as directed under Class VII.

CAFFEIN.

Synonyms, Caffeia. Caffeinum.
Formula, $C_8 H_{10} N_4 O_2, H_2O$.
Molecular Weight, 212.

Origin.—Caffeine exists in the berries and leaves of the coffee plant, in the tea plant, in *Paullinia sorbilis* and in the leaves and twigs of *Ilex Paraguayensis*.

Preparation.—Exhaust ground coffee with boiling water; add acetate of lead in excess to precipitate the tannin present. Throw the whole upon a filter and carefully wash the precipitate with boiling water. The filtrate is then to be treated with hydrogen sulphide to free it from excess of lead, and after a second filtration ammonia is added to neutralize the liberated acetic acid, and the whole is evaporated at a gentle heat. On cooling, an abundant crystallization of nearly pure caffeine is produced. To purify it, it is redissolved in water, treated with animal charcoal and recrystallized.

Properties.—Caffeine crystallizes from its watery solutions in slender needles, having a silky lustre; they are quite flexible and often aggregated in star-shaped groups. Their taste is moderately bitter. They are soluble in 30 parts of water at medium temperatures, in 10 of boiling water, in 35 of 90 per cent. alcohol, in 550 of ether, and in 6 of chloroform. Although without alkaline reaction, caffeine forms a hydrochlorate and a sulphate and produces double salts with platinic chloride and silver nitrate. With acids of feeble power it does not unite; it sublimes at a high temperature without residue.

Tests.—In addition to the above-described properties, the following will be of service. Caffeine evaporated to dryness with a little chlorine-water yields a purple-red residue which becomes golden-yellow when more strongly heated, but it resumes the red color on the addition of ammonia.

Preparation for Homœopathic Use.—The pure caffein is prepared by trituration, as directed under Class VII.

CAHINCA.

Synonyms, Cainca. Chiococca Racemosa, *Jaquin*.
Nat. Ord., Rubiaceæ.
Common Name, Cluster-flowered Snowberry. David's Root.

This shrub grows in Brazil and the Antilles. Stem from five to ten feet high; leaves opposite, oval, pointed, entire; flowers pedunculated, whitish, axillary, in pendant bunches; fruit berriform; whitish, monospermous; root branchy, of a reddish-brown, consisting of cylindric pieces, from one and a half to two feet long, and of the thickness of a goose-quill or finger; it is fibrous, marked all along with furrows of a deep-color, covered with brown bark, annular, thin, fleshy, epidermis of a dirty white. Beneath this fleshy part is found a white wood, which is the axis of the root. The epidermis of the bark is of a resinous aspect when broken, of a disagreeable taste, bitter, a little acrid and slightly astringent, producing a roughness in the throat; the woody part has neither taste nor odor. The odor of the root is acrid, volatile, disagreeable, somewhat like that of valerian.

It was first proven by Dr. Koch, Sr.

Preparation.—The dried root-bark, is coarsely powdered, covered with five parts by weight of alcohol, and allowed to remain eight days in a well-stoppered bottle, in a dark, cool place, being shaken twice a day. The tincture is then poured off, strained and filtered.

Drug power of tincture, $\frac{1}{10}$.

Dilutions must be prepared as directed under Class IV.

CALADIUM.

Synonyms, Caladium Seguinum, *Vent.* Arum Seguinum, *Linn.*

Nat. Ord., Araceæ.

Common Names, Dumb Cane. Poisonous American Arum. Poisonous Pediveau.

This plant is a native of South America, growing on the wet prairies in the neighborhood of Paramaribo. Its stem is from five to six feet high, more than one inch thick, round, knotty, and abounding with milky juice. Its leaves are ovate-oblong, smooth, at the apex narrowed, petioles above canaliculate and clasping, sheath of the flowers pale green, its inner side purple, spadix yellow. The juice of this plant leaves an indelible stain on linen, and is so caustic that, if put upon the tongue or in the mouth, it produces swelling and inflammation.

The drug was introduced into the Homœopathic Materia Medica by Dr. Hering.

Preparation.—The fresh root is chopped and pounded to a pulp and weighed. Then two parts by weight of alcohol are taken, the pulp mixed thoroughly with one-sixth part of it, and the rest of the alcohol added. After stirring the whole well, and pouring it into a well-stoppered bottle, it is allowed to stand eight days in a dark, cool place. The tincture is then separated by decanting, straining and filtering.

Drug power of tincture, $\frac{1}{6}$.

Dilutions must be prepared as directed under Class III.

CALCAREA ACETICA.

Present Name, Calcium Acetate.

Common Name, Acetate of Lime.

Formula, $Ca\,(C_2\,H_3\,O_2)_2$.

Molecular Weight, 158.

Hahnemann's Preparation of Acetate of Lime.—Boil crude, well-washed oyster-shells for an hour in pure rain-water, then break into fragments, without using any metallic instrument, and dissolve in dilute acetic acid, heating up to the boiling point, until complete saturation is gradually effected. Filter and reduce to one-fifth by evaporation. The solution, of a dark yellow color, after a time precipitates a dark glutinous substance, whereby the color of the solution becomes paler. To this light-colored liquid add one-half its bulk of pure alcohol.

Amount of drug power, $\frac{1}{10}$.

Dilutions must be prepared as directed under Class V—*a*.

CALCAREA ARSENICICA.

Synonyms, Calcii Arsenias. Calcarea Arsenica.

Present Name, Tri-calcium Di-arsenate.

Common Name, Arsenate of Lime.

Formula, $3\ Ca\ O,\ 2\ As\ O_3 + 3\ H_2\ O$.

Preparation of Arsenate of Lime.—Distil four parts of powdered arsenious acid with a mixture of twelve parts nitric acid and one part muriatic acid, in a retort, to dryness. The residue is then to be brought to a faint red heat, and after cooling is dissolved in ten volumes of water, and neutralized by carbonate of potash, thus forming arsenate of potash in solution, which is to be decomposed by the addition of a solution of calcium chloride as long as a white precipitate is formed. This precipitate is to be carefully washed and dried.

Properties and Tests.—Arsenate of lime is a light, white amorphous powder, not soluble in water, but is readily so in dilute nitric acid. The solution remains clear when an excess of acetate of soda is added to it, but gives a white precipitate on the subsequent addition of ammonium oxalate. A small quantity boiled with an excess of caustic soda and filtered, gives, when exactly neutralized by nitric acid, a brick-red precipitate on the addition of solution of nitrate of silver.

Preparation for Homœopathic Use.—The pure arsenate of lime is prepared by trituration, as directed under Class VII.

CALCAREA CARBONICA.

Synonyms, Calcii Carbonas. Calcarea Ostrearum, *Hering*.

Present Name, Calcium Carbonate.

Common Names, Carbonate of Lime. Impure Carbonate of Lime.

Formula (of the c. p. salt), $Ca\ CO_3$.

Molecular Weight, 100.

Origin and Preparation of Hahnemann's Carbonate of Lime.—Cleaned, thick oyster-shells are broken into small pieces, and the inner snow-white portions carefully selected and powdered.

Preparation for Homœopathic Use.—The powdered oyster-shell (obtained as described above) is prepared by trituration as directed under Class VII.

CALCAREA CAUSTICA.

Synonym, Calcis Hydras.

Present Name, Calcium Hydrate.

Common Name, Slaked Lime.

Formula, $Ca\ (HO)_2$.

Molecular Weight, 74.

Preparation of Slaked Lime.—This is prepared by burning Carrara marble (carbonate of lime) in a covered crucible until a portion of product withdrawn for examination no longer effervesces on the addition of hydrochloric acid; when cold it is placed in a porcelain capsule, and slaked by the addition of half its weight of distilled water.

Properties.—Slaked lime forms a soft white powder of specific gravity 2.08, having a strong alkaline taste and reaction.

The first provings were made under direction of Dr. A. W. Koch.

Preparation for Homœopathic Use.—To one part of caustic (slaked) lime is added five parts of distilled water, in a warm bottle well stoppered, and left standing till cold. The mixture is then well shaken, and to it five parts of alcohol are added and the whole again well shaken. After several days, during which the mixture has been frequently shaken, the clear liquid is put into vials and well protected from air. As soon as it has absorbed carbonic acid, it must be rejected and a fresh preparation made.

Amount of drug power, $\frac{1}{10}$.

Dilutions must be prepared as directed under Class VI—*a*.

Triturations should not be prepared, as during trituration carbonic acid is absorbed from the atmosphere, forming carbonate of lime.

CALCAREA CHLORATA.

Synonyms, Calx Chlorinata. Calx Chlorata.

Common Names, Chlorinated Lime. Bleaching Powder.

Preparation and Composition of Chlorinated Lime.—Chlorinated lime or bleaching powder, is prepared by passing chlorine gas into boxes of lead or stone in which a quantity of calcium hydrate or slaked lime, in a very slightly moist state, is spread out upon shelves. The lime absorbs nearly half its weight of chlorine, and the result is a white powder which has a very peculiar smell, somewhat different from that of chlorine. The formula of the substance has not been accurately ascertained. Probably when produced under slightly different conditions of moisture in the calcium hydrate or with varying degrees of rapidity of saturation with the chlorine, it is not of exactly the same constitution. It has been held to consist of a mixture of calcium hypochlorite and chloride. Dr. Odling's formula is Cl—Ca—OCl, the substance being decomposed by water into the chloride and hypochlorite, Ca Cl, Ca ClO.

Properties.—Chlorinated lime is a white, dry or very slightly damp powder, in readily crumbling masses. In addition to its odor, already mentioned, it has a sharp, astringent, disagreeable taste. It is soluble in from ten to twelve parts of water, some unaltered hydrate remaining behind. Its solution is alkaline to test-paper. It is completely soluble in cold dilute hydrochloric acid, forming the chloride and liberating chlorine. It is hygroscopic, and gradually decomposes when exposed to the air. It should be kept in a cool, dry place.

Tests.—"Ten grains of chlorinated lime, mixed with thirty grains of iodide of potassium and dissolved in four fluid ounces of water, produce, when acidulated with two fluid drachms of hydrochloric acid, a reddish solution, which requires for the discharge of its color, at least 850 grain measures of the volumetric solution of hyposulphite of soda, corresponding to thirty per cent. of chlorine liberated by hydrochloric acid."—Br. P.

Good commercial bleaching powder contains about thirty-five per cent. of available chlorine. If insufficiently saturated with chlorine in the manufacture, the specimen examined will, on treatment with water, show an increase of the insoluble portion. Calcium chloride, if present in too great quantity, will cause the mass to become quite moist. Vegetable coloring matters are soon destroyed when treated with a solution of bleaching powder.

Preparation for Homœopathic Use.—One part by weight of chlorinated lime is dissolved in nine parts by weight of distilled water, and filtered through calico.

Amount of drug power, $\frac{1}{10}$.

Dilutions must be prepared as directed under Class V—*a*.

CALCAREA FLUORATA.

Synonyms, Calcii Fluoridum. Calcium Fluoride.

Present Name, Calcium Fluoride.

Common Name, Fluor-Spar.

Symbol, $Ca\ F_2$.

Origin and Properties of Calcium Fluoride.—It occurs in nature as the mineral fluor-spar, beautifully crystallized, of various colors, in lead-veins, the crystals having commonly the cubic, but sometimes the octohedral form, parallel to the faces of which latter figure they always cleave. Some varieties, when heated, emit a greenish, and some a purple phosphorescent light. The fluoride is quite insoluble in water, but is decomposed by sulphuric acid, generating hydrofluoric acid.

Preparation for Homœopathic Use.—Selected pieces of crystallized fluor-spar are prepared by trituration, as directed under Class VII.

CALCAREA HYPOPHOSPHOROSA.

Synonyms, Calcii Hypophosphis. Calcis Hypophosphis. Hypophosphite of Calcium.

Present Name, Calcium Hypophosphite.

Common Name, Hypophosphite of Lime.

Formula, $Ca\ (PH_2\ O_2)_2$.

Molecular Weight, 170.

Preparation of Hypophosphite of Calcium.—One hundred parts of freshly prepared calcium hydrate, and about 250 parts of distilled water, are placed in a deep stone-ware vessel; then forty parts of phosphorus (granulated under water) are added, and the whole is digested with frequent agitation and addition of water to supply the loss by evaporation, for a week or as long as the odor of phosphoretted hydrogen is perceptible. The mixture is then filtered, the residue washed on the filter and the washing added to the filtrate. Carbonic oxide is now passed through the filtrate as long as any precipitate of calcium carbonate occurs, the latter separated by filtration, and the filtrate evaporated to about ⅙ of its volume and set aside to crystallize.

Calcium hypophosphite occurs in either permanent, odorless, colorless crystals, or a white, crystalline powder of a pearly lustre. It is soluble in water, insoluble in alcohol; its taste is bitter and disagreeable.

Tests.—Calcium hypophosphite in watery solution gives, with silver nitrate solution, a white precipitate, which, by gently heating, becomes dark-colored, from a reduction of the hypophosphite of silver to the metallic state. A small quantity of the salt heated in a test-tube decrepitates and evolves the readily inflammable hydrogen phosphide. The absence of phosphate will be shown by its entire solubility in water (absence of carbonate also), and by its behavior with ammonium molybdate, which gives a blue precipitate.

Preparation for Homœopathic Use.—The pure hypophosphite of calcium is prepared by trituration, as directed under Class VII.

CALCAREA JODATA.

Synonyms, Calcarea Hydriodica. Calcii Iodidum. Calcium Iodatum. Iodide of Calcium.

Present Name, Calcium Iodide.

Common Name, Iodide of Lime.

Formula, CaI_2.

Molecular Weight, 294.

Preparation of Iodide of Calcium.—One part of amorphous phosphorus is treated with 30 parts of hot water, and finely powdered iodine is added gradually, with constant stirring, as long as it dissolves without color, the amount thus used being about 13½ parts. The colorless liquid is then decanted from the slight deposit and mixed with milk of lime prepared from 8 parts of lime, till the reaction is alkaline; the mixture is thrown upon a filter, and thereby are removed some phosphate, phosphite and excess of hydrate of calcium. The solution of calcium iodide thus obtained is concentrated by evaporation.

Properties.—Calcium iodide is a very soluble, deliquescent, white salt, which crystallizes with difficulty. It melts below a red heat, and if exposed to the air is decomposed, calcium oxide being formed and iodine liberated; its solution upon similar exposure precipitates calcium carbonate, the free iodine being held by the remaining iodide.

Tests.—Its identity is revealed by its behavior in solution with ammonium oxalate, a white precipitate showing the presence of calcium; and with mercuric chloride when a scarlet precipitate, soluble in excess of the reagent, demonstrates the presence of iodine. Upon treating its solution with sulphurous acid and then adding cupric sulphate in excess, the iodine unites with the copper, forming cuprous iodide; the precipitate is to be filtered off and the filtrate tested with silver nitrate solution, when a white precipitate is due, if present, to a chloride or bromide.

The first provings were made by Dr. W. James Blakely, U. S.

Preparation for Homœopathic Use.—The pure iodide of calcium is prepared by trituration, as directed under Class VII.

CALCAREA MURIATICA.

Synonyms, Calcii Chloridum. Chloride of Calcium. Muriate of Lime.

Present Name, Calcium Chloride.

Common Name, Chloride of Lime.

Formula, $Ca\ Cl_2$.

Molecular Weight, 111.

Chloride of Calcium prepared by fusion.

Preparation of Chloride of Calcium.—Calcium chloride is formed by neutralizing hydrochloric acid with calcium carbonate, adding a little of solution of chlorinated lime, filtering, evaporating until the resulting salt becomes solid and finally drying it at about 204° C. (nearly 400° F.).

Prepared as directed above, calcium chloride is in white, agglutinated masses, dry, but very deliquescent, containing nearly 25 per cent. of water, its formula being $Ca\ Cl_2 + 2\ H_2O$. It has a sharp, bitter, salty taste; is readily soluble in water and alcohol, the solutions being neutral. By carefully crystallizing it from its solutions, it can be obtained in four and six sided prisms, containing a little more than 49 per cent. of water. At a red heat it gives up its water of crystallization and fuses, becoming weakly alkaline in reaction; in this state it is in semi-translucent, whitish, friable masses.

Tests.—Calcium chloride should dissolve completely in twice its weight of water; its solution should not show any change upon treatment with lime water, caustic ammonia, barium chloride or hydrogen sulphide. Neither chlorine or hypochlorous acid should be evolved when hydrochloric acid is added to the salt.

Preparation for Homœopathic Use.—One part by weight of fused chloride of calcium is dissolved in nine parts by weight of distilled water.

Amount of drug power, $\frac{1}{10}$.

Dilutions must be prepared as directed under Class V—*a*.

CALCAREA OXALICA.

Synonyms, Calcii Oxalas. Calcium Oxalicum. Calcium Oxalate.

Common Name, Oxalate of Lime.

Formula, $Ca\ C_2\ O_4$.

Molecular Weight, 128.

Calcium oxalate is found in the juice of most plants, and in some in relatively large amount.

Preparation of Oxalate of Calcium.—It is formed whenever a strong solution of oxalic acid is added to a solution of a calcium salt; it falls as a white powder, which should be well washed with distilled water, and then dried on a water-bath.

Properties and Tests.—It is but little soluble in dilute hydrochloric, and quite insoluble in acetic acid. Nitric acid dissolves it easily. When dried at 37.7° C. (100° F.), it retains a molecule of water, which may be driven off by a rather higher temperature. Exposed to a red heat in a closed vessel, it is converted into calcium carbonate, with escape of carbon monoxide.

Preparation for Homœopathic Use.—The pure oxalate of calcium is prepared by trituration, as directed under Class VII.

CALCAREA PHOSPHORICA.

Synonyms, Calcii Phosphas Præcipitata. Calcis Phosphas. Precipitated Phosphate of Calcium.

Present Name, Calcium Phosphate.

Common Name, Phosphate of Lime.

Formula, $Ca_3 (PO_4)_2$.

Molecular Weight, 306.

Preparation of Precipitated Phosphate of Lime.—That used for the proving was a mixture of the basic and other phosphates of lime, obtained by Dr. Hering (Correspondenzblatt, 1837) by dropping dilute phosphoric acid into lime water, as long as a white precipitate was formed; this precipitate was washed with distilled water, and dried on a water-bath.

It was first proved by Dr. Hering.

Preparation for Homœopathic Use.—The phosphate of lime, obtained as described above, is prepared by trituration, as directed under Class VII.

CALCAREA SULPHURICA.

Synonyms, Calcii Sulphas. Sulphate of Calcium. Sulphate of Lime.

Present Name, Calcium Sulphate.

Common Names, Gypsum. Plaster of Paris.

Formula, $Ca SO_4, 2 H_2O$.

Molecular Weight, 172.

Origin and Preparation of Sulphate of Calcium.—The hydrated sulphate of calcium occurs native, forming gypsum, a transparent and regularly crystalline variety of which is called *selenite*.

Preparation.—It is prepared by precipitating a solution of calcium chloride with dilute sulphuric acid. The precipitate is to be washed with hot water and dried at about 30° C. (86° F.).

Properties.—Precipitated calcium sulphate is a fine, white crystalline powder. It is soluble in about 400 parts of cold, and with more difficulty in boiling water; in alcohol it is insoluble. Heated to 200° C. (392° F.) it parts with its water of crystallization.

The drug was proved by Dr. Clarence Conant, U. S.

Preparation for Homœopathic Use.—Sulphate of calcium is prepared by trituration as directed under Class VII.

CALENDULA.

Synonym, Calendula Officinalis, *Linn.*
Nat. Ord., Compositæ.
Common Name, Common Marigold.

This annual plant, originally from the south of Europe, is now cultivated in all our gardens. The root is pale yellow, cylindric, hairy; the stem erect, angular, hairy, branchy, from six to eighteen inches high; leaves inversely oval or lanceolate, spatula-shaped, entire or slightly sinuous, alternate, sessile, somewhat fleshy and downy; flowers large, yellow-red, broad, solitary, terminal, and have a disagreeable, slightly aromatic odor and a sourish, slimy, bitter taste. In sultry weather sparks, similar to electric sparks, have been seen issuing from these flowers; the seeds are curved, muricated, the inner seeds subulate, the outer ones boat-shaped, with a furrow on the back.

It was first proven by Dr. Franz, in Germany.

Preparation.—The fresh leaves at the top of the plant, together with the blossoms and buds, are chopped and pounded to a pulp, enclosed in a piece of new linen and subjected to pressure. The expressed juice is then, by brisk agitation, mingled with an equal part by weight of alcohol. This mixture is allowed to stand eight days in a well-stoppered bottle, in a dark, cool place and then filtered.

Drug power of tincture, ½.

Dilutions must be prepared as directed under Class I.

CALTHA PALUSTRIS, *Linn.*

Nat. Ord., Ranunculaceæ.
Common Names, Cowslip. Marsh Marigold.

This plant grows on marshes and ditch-banks in Arctic Europe, Northern and Western Asia to the Himalayas, and in North America. It is a coarse, glabrous, dark green, showy, very variable plant. Rootstock short, horizontal. Stem hollow, furrowed, eight inches to three feet long, sub-erect, prostrate, or procumbent and rooting from all the nodes. Leaves orbicular-reniform, deltoid-toothed. Stipules very large, membranous, glairy, quite entire in bud and enclosing the young leaf, as in magnoliaceæ (Dickson). Flowers terminal, few, one to two inches in diameter, bright golden-yellow. Sepals five or more, unequal, obovate or oblong. Petals none. Carpels several, sessile; ovules numerous, in two series. Follicles numerous, many-seeded. Seeds with a prominent raphe and thickened funicle. Flowers appear from March to May.

Preparation.—The fresh plant, gathered when in flower, is chopped and pounded to a pulp, enclosed in a piece of new linen and subjected to pressure. The expressed juice is then, by brisk agitation, mingled with an equal part by weight of alcohol. This mixture is allowed to stand eight days in a well-stoppered bottle, in a dark, cool place, and then filtered.

Drug power of tincture, ½.

Dilutions must be prepared as directed under Class I.

CAMPHORA.

A product of Camphora Officinarum, *Nees von Esenbeck.* (Laurus Camphora, *Linn.*)

Nat. Ord., Lauraceæ.

Common Name, Camphor.

Formula of Camphor, $C_{10} H_{16} O$.

The camphor tree or camphor laurel is widely spread through central China and the Japanese Islands. It is also found in the island of Formosa, and it is cultivated in a few sheltered spots in Italy. It is a large handsome tree; the leaves are on long petioles, are small, shining, and glaucous beneath. The flowers are small, white, and aggregated in clusters. All parts of the tree furnish camphor; in Formosa the wood is cut up into chips, exposed to the vapor of boiling water in vessels covered with a rude condensing apparatus. *Dryobalanops aromatica,* the camphor tree of Borneo and Sumatra, yields a different kind of camphor.

Description and Properties.—Camphor, as exported from Japan and Formosa, is in irregular friable masses, of grayish-white or pinkish hue. It is purified by sublimation. Purified camphor is in round bowls or convex cakes, colorless and translucent, traversed by numerous fissures which refract light so as to give a general white appearance to the mass. It breaks readily into irregular masses, but these are tough and not easily reduced to powder, yet if they be moistened with alcohol, ether, chloroform, glycerine or a volatile oil, their pulverization is readily accomplished. Camphor melts at 175° C. (347° F.), boils at 204° C. (399.2° F.) and volatilizes readily at ordinary temperatures. Between 0° C. (32° F.) and 6° C. (42.8° F.) its specific gravity is the same as that of water; at a higher temperature it expands more quickly, so that at 10° C. (50° F.) its specific gravity is 0.992. The taste and odor of camphor are peculiar; the taste is also warm, followed by a cool sensation. Camphor is very slightly soluble in water, about 1 part in 1500; but alcohol, ether, chloroform, carbon di-sulphide and the volatile and fixed oils dissolve it readily.

The drug was proven by Hahnemann.

Preparation.—One part by weight of refined camphor gum is dissolved in nine parts by weight of alcohol, and then filtered.

Drug power of tincture, $\frac{1}{10}$.

Dilutions must be prepared as directed under Class VI—*a*.

CANCER ASTACUS.

Synonym, Astacus Fluviatilis.
Class, Crustacea.
Order, Decapoda.
Family, Astacidæ.
Common Names, Craw-fish. Cray-fish. River Crab.

The common crab is a decapodous crustacean, which inhabits, in Europe, the borders of streams, small rivers and even lakes and ponds, where it stays in holes and under stones. Its body is oblong, generally cylindrical; the tail broad and long, covered with transverse scales, and furnished with swimming scales on the sides and at the extremity, turning in under themselves. The forepart of the body terminates in a short point jutting out between the eyes. It has ten claws, the two fore-claws terminating in strong and dentated pincers. Any member of its body, when destroyed or mutilated, is easily regenerated. The crabs change their calcareous coat every year, and at that time two hard, calcareous bodies, called crab's eyes, are found in their stomachs. These are intended to furnish the proper material towards the reproduction of the new coat. The female carries under her reverted tail, first her eggs, then her young, until they attain a certain size.

Dr. Buchner's provings in Germany introduced this remedy to homœopathic practice.

Preparation.—The live crab is crushed in a stone-mortar, to a fine paste, and covered with twice its weight of alcohol. After having been poured into a well-stoppered bottle, the mixture is allowed to remain eight days in a dark, cool place, and shaken twice a day. The tincture is then poured off and filtered.

Drug power of tincture, $\frac{1}{3}$.

Dilutions must be prepared as directed under Class I.

CANCHALAGUA.

Synonym, Erythræa Chilensis, *Persoon.*
Nat. Ord., Gentianaceæ.
Common Name, Centaury of Chili.

This plant is found growing in California and in some parts of South America. It is a small, grass-like plant, with lance-shaped leaves, and small, red blossoms, resembling in shape those of the forget-me-not.

It was first proven by Dr. Richter, U. S.

Preparation.—The whole plant, in flower, is carefully dried, powdered, and covered with five parts by weight of alcohol. Having poured this into a well-stoppered bottle, it is allowed to remain eight days in a dark, cool place, being shaken twice a day. The tincture is then poured off, strained and filtered.

Amount of drug power, $\frac{1}{10}$.

Dilutions must be prepared as directed under Class IV.

CANNABIS.

Synonym, Cannabis Sativa, *Linn.*
Nat. Ord., Urticaceæ.
Common Names, Hemp. Gallow Grass.

Common hemp is, an annual diœcious plant, indigenous to the western and central parts of Asia. It is cultivated in many temperate as well as tropical regions throughout the world. The plant is tall, erect. Leaves opposite, digitate, petiolate; leaflets lanceolate, serrate. Flowers small, green, solitary and axillary in the barren plant; spiked or racemed in the fertile one.

Cannabis sativa was first proven by Hahnemann.

Preparation.—The fresh blooming herb-tops, of both the male and the female herb, are chopped and pounded to a pulp and weighed. Then two parts by weight of alcohol are taken, the pulp mixed thoroughly with one-sixth part of it, and rest of the alcohol added. After stirring the whole well, and pouring it into a well-stoppered bottle, it is allowed to stand eight days in a dark, cool place. The tincture is then separated by decanting, straining and filtering.

Drug power of tincture, $\frac{1}{6}$.

Dilutions must be prepared as directed under Class III.

CANNABIS INDICA.

Synonym, Cannabis Sativa, *Linn.*, var. Indica.
Nat. Ord., Urticaceæ.
Common Names, Bhang. Ganja. Hashish. Indian Hemp.

The *Cannabis indica* is considered to be the same plant as *Cannabis sativa.* There is, however, a marked dissimilarity between the medicinal effects of the two plants. That grown in India is much more potent than the product of American or European culture, and in India certain narcotic products are not obtainable in quantity from plants grown at an altitude much less than 6,000 feet.

Elaborate provings were published by the American Prover's Union in Philadelphia, in 1839.

Preparation.—The dried herb-tops are bruised, covered with five parts by weight of alcohol, and allowed to remain eight days, in a well-stoppered bottle, in a dark, cool place, being shaken twice a day. The tincture is then poured off, strained and filtered.

Drug power of tincture, $\frac{1}{10}$.

Dilutions must be prepared as directed under Class IV.

CANNA GLAUCA, *Linn.*

Synonym, Canna Angustifolia, *Mure.*
Nat. Ord., Canniaceæ.
Common Name, (Brazilian) Imbiri.

This plant is a native of the West Indies, and inhabits damp regions, or the borders of brooks. Its stem is erect, cylindrical, growing to a height of about six feet out of a rhizome sending off numerous rootlets.

It is provided with knots, whence arise large alternate clasping leaves, lanceolate, having strong midribs, and sending off fine parallel transverse nerves. At its summit the stem produces the flower-bearing pedicles. Flowers alternate, on short peduncles, and accompanied by bracts. The corolla has a double perianth, with three divisions adhering to the triangular, greenish and glandular ovary; the stamens present the changing characters so common in this family.

Introduced into our Materia Medica by Dr. Mure, Brazil.

Preparation.—The fresh leaves are chopped and pounded to a pulp and weighed. Then two parts by weight of alcohol are taken, the pulp mixed thoroughly with one-sixth part of it, and the rest of the alcohol added. After stirring the whole well, and pouring it into a well-stoppered bottle, it is allowed to stand eight days in a dark, cool place. The tincture is then separated by decanting, straining and filtering.

Drug power of tincture, $\frac{1}{6}$.

Dilutions must be prepared as directed under Class III.

CANTHARIS.

Synonyms, Cantharis Vesicatoria, *De Geer.* Lytta Vesicatoria, *Fabricius.* Meloë Vesicatorius, *Linn.*

Class, Insecta.

Order, Coleoptera.

Family, Vesicantia.

Common Name, Spanish Fly.

This fly, of the middle and south of Europe, appears in the months of May and June, especially on the white poplar, privet, ash, elder, lilac, etc., upon the leaves of which they feed. The insect is about half an inch long, of a golden yellow-green; head inclined, almost cordiform; antennæ filiform, of twelve joints, black; antennulæ equally filiform, the posterior swollen at the extremity; eyes large, of a deep brown; mouth with an upper lip and two bifid jaws; body elongated, almost round and cylindric; two wings; elytræ soft, demi-cylindric, marked with longitudinal streaks; head and feet full of whitish hairs; the odor is sweetish, nauseous; taste very acrid, almost caustic. The larvæ of these insects have yellowish-white bodies, formed of three rings, six short feet, rounded head, two short filiform antennæ, two jaws and four feelers; they live in the ground, feed on roots, there undergo their metamorphosis, and do not come out till they are perfect insects. In May and June when the insects swarm upon the trees, they are collected in the mornings at sunrise, when they are torpid from the cold of the night, and easily let go their hold. Persons with their faces protected by masks and their hands with gloves, shake the trees or beat them with poles; and the insects are received as they fall, upon linen cloths spread underneath. They are then exposed in sieves to the vapor of boiling vinegar, and, having been thus deprived of life, are dried either in the sun or in apartments heated by stoves. The larger flies are much better for medical use than the smaller ones.

It was introduced into Homœopathic Medicine by Hahnemann.

Preparation.—Select perfect insects (large ones) that are not worm-eaten, rub them to a coarse powder and weigh. Then add five parts by weight of alcohol, and place the mixture in a well-stoppered bottle; let it stand eight days in a dark, cool place, shaking twice a day. The tincture is then poured off, strained and filtered.

Drug power of tincture, $\frac{1}{10}$.

Dilutions must be prepared as directed under Class IV.

Triturations are prepared from the powdered insect, as directed under Class VII.

CAPSICUM.

Synonym, Capsicum Annuum, *Linn.*

Nat. Ord., Solanaceæ.

Common Names, Cayenne Pepper. Red Pepper.

The *Capsicum* family seems to be indigenous to tropical America and Asia, and is cultivated in almost all parts of the world.

The *C. annuum* is an herbaceous plant, two or three feet high; stem branching above; leaves entire, glabrous, ovate and acuminate, on petioles. Flowers five-parted, corolla white and rotate. The fruit is an oblong berry, of a bright scarlet color, becoming darker on drying. The taste of the berry or pod is that of Cayenne pepper, which is well known. The flowers appear in July and August, and the fruit ripens in October. The variety that is long, conical, pointed, and generally recurved, whose base is not thicker than the finger, is chosen for our preparations.

It was proven under Hahnemann's direction.

Preparation.—The ripe, dried fruit, that has not been worm-eaten, is coarsely pulverized, covered with five parts by weight of alcohol and allowed to remain eight days in a well-stoppered bottle, in a dark, cool place, being shaken twice a day. The tincture is then poured off, strained and filtered.

Drug power of tincture, $\frac{1}{10}$.

Dilutions must be prepared as directed under Class IV.

CARBO ANIMALIS.

Synonyms, Animal Charcoal. Leather Charcoal.

Preparation of Animal Charcoal.—The preparation used by Hahnemann in his provings, and which ought, therefore, to be preferred to all others, was made as follows: Place a thick piece of ox-hide leather (neat's leather) on red-hot coals, where it must remain as long as it burns with a flame. As soon, however, as the flame ceases, lift off the red-hot mass, and extinguish it by pressing between two flat stones, and preserve it in well-stoppered bottles. If allowed to cool gradually in the air, most of the carbon would be consumed.

Preparation for Homœopathic Use.—The animal charcoal procured as described above, is prepared by trituration, as directed under Class VII.

CARBONEUM.

Common Name, Lampblack.

Preparation.—Carboneum is an amorphous carbon, produced by the imperfect combustion of oils or resins. That used for provings was obtained from the chimney of a coal-oil lamp; to obtain it, it is only necessary that the wick be turned up high while burning, thus causing imperfect combustion, when the lampblack is deposited upon the sides of the chimney.

It was proven by Dr. W. H. Burt, U. S.

Preparation for Homœopathic Use.—Lampblack, obtained as described above, is prepared by trituration, as directed under Class VII.

CARBONEUM CHLORATUM.

Synonyms, Carbon Tetrachloride. Carbonei Tetrachloridum. Chlorocarbon.

Formula, $C\,Cl_4$.

Molecular Weight, 154.

Preparation.—Carbon tetrachloride is produced by the action of chlorine on marsh-gas, by the action of chlorine on chloroform in the sunshine and by the action of chlorine on carbon di-sulphide. Chloroform is gently heated in a retort exposed to the sun, and a stream of dry chlorine gas is passed slowly and continuously through it, the liquid which distils over being repeatedly poured back till hydrochloric acid ceases to be evolved, after which the distillate is agitated with mercury to remove free chlorine, and then rectified by distillation on a water-bath.

Properties.—Carbon tetrachloride is a thin, colorless, oily-looking liquid having an agreeable aromatic odor. Its specific gravity is about 1.5; it boils between 77° and 80° C. (170.6° to 176° F.) It is insoluble in water, but soluble in alcohol and ether.

Preparation for Homœopathic Use.—One part by weight is dissolved in ninety-nine parts by weight of alcohol.

Amount of drug power, $\frac{1}{100}$.

Dilutions must be prepared as directed under Class VI—β.

CARBONEUM HYDROGENISATUM.

Proper Name, Hydrogen Di-Carbide.

Synonyms, Carburetted Hydrogen. Ethene. Ethylene.

Common Name, Olefiant Gas.

Formula, $H_4\,C_2$.

The chief illuminating constituent of coal-gas.

Preparation of Ethene or Olefiant Gas.—One volume of alcohol and four volumes of sulphuric acid are mixed with sand so as to form a thick paste, in a glass flask, the tube of which passes into a wash-bottle containing caustic potash. A second wash-bottle, partly filled with sulphuric acid is connected with the first, and furnished with a tube dipping into the water of the pneumatic trough over which the gas is to be collected. On the first application of heat to the contents of the flask, alcohol, and afterwards ether, make their appearance; but, as the temperature rises, and the mixture blackens, the ether-vapor diminishes in quantity, and its place becomes in great part supplied by a permanent inflammable gas; carbon dioxide and sulphurous oxide are also generated at the same time, besides traces of other products. The two last-mentioned gases are absorbed by the alkali in the first bottle, and the ether-vapor by the acid in the second, so that the olefiant gas is delivered tolerably pure.

Properties and Tests.—Olefiant gas thus produced is colorless, irrespirable, neutral, and but slightly soluble in water. Alcohol, ether, oil of turpentine, and even olive oil, as Faraday has observed, dissolve it to a considerable extent. It has a faint ethereal odor. On the approach of a kindled taper it takes fire, and burns with a splendid white light, far surpassing in brilliancy that produced by marsh gas. This gas, when mixed with oxygen, and fired, explodes with extreme violence. Its density is 0.978.

Ethene is decomposed by passing it through a tube heated to bright redness; a deposit of charcoal and tar takes place and the gas becomes converted into marsh gas, or even into free hydrogen and carbon, if the temperature be very high. This latter change is, of course, attended by increase of volume. Chlorine acts upon ethene in a very remarkable manner. When the two bodies are mixed, even in the dark, they combine in equal measures, and give rise to a heavy oily liquid, of sweetish taste and ethereal odor, to which the name of *ethene chloride*, or *Dutch liquid* (formula $C_2 H_4 Cl_2$), is given. It is from this peculiarity that the term *olefiant* gas is derived.

Preparation for Homœopathic Use.—A saturated solution in alcohol is made of the gas obtained as directed above, which will correspond to about the 1x dilution.

Dilutions must be prepared as directed under Class VI—*a*.

CARBONEUM OXYGENISATUM.

Synonyms, Carbon Monoxide. Carbonous Oxide.

Formula, CO.

Preparation of Carbonous Oxide.—Heat in a retort, finely powdered yellow potassium ferrocyanide with eight or ten times its weight of concentrated sulphuric acid. The salt is entirely decomposed, yielding a copious supply of perfectly pure carbonous oxide gas, which may be collected over water in the usual manner.

Properties and Tests.—Carbonous oxide is a combustible gas; it burns with a beautiful pale blue flame, generating carbon dioxide. It is colorless, has very little odor, and is extremely poisonous. Mixed with oxygen, it explodes by the electric spark, but with some difficulty. Its specific gravity is 0.973. Carbon monoxide unites with chlorine under the influence of light, forming a pungent, suffocating compound, possessing acid properties, called *phosgene gas*, or *carbonyl chloride*.

Preparation for Homœopathic Use.—Distilled water is saturated with carbonous oxide, and then diluted with an equal part by weight of distilled water.

Amount of drug power, $\frac{1}{100}$.

Dilutions must be prepared as directed under Class V—β.

CARBONEUM SULPHURATUM.

Proper Name, Carbon Disulphide.

Synonyms, Alcohol Sulphuris Lampadii. Sulphuret of Carbon. Carbonei Bisulphidum. Carbonic Sulphide.

Common Name, Bisulphide of Carbon.

Formula, $C S_2$.

Molecular Weight, 76.

Preparation.—Carbon disulphide is prepared by passing the vapor of sulphur over red-hot charcoal; the process is done in a retort and the distillate is condensed in a properly arranged receiver. The distillate is purified by agitating it with mercuric chloride or lead hydrate, and after mixing it with milk of lime it is redistilled over a water-bath. Carbon disulphide is a thin, colorless, mobile liquid, refracting light strongly. At 15° C. (59° F.) its specific gravity is about 1.269. It boils between 45° and 48° C. (113°–118.4° F.). It is extremely volatile, and its evaporation produces great cold; its vapor is very inflammable, burning with a blue flame, producing carbonic and sulphurous oxides. The vapor, when mixed with atmospheric air or oxygen forms an explosive compound. Ordinary carbon disulphide has a peculiar and very disagreeable odor, described as resembling that of decomposing cabbage, but when quite pure the odor is agreeable and chloroform-like. Its taste is sharp and aromatic. It is practically insoluble in water, but imparts to the latter its odor and taste; in absolute alcohol it is soluble as well as in ether. Its own solvent power over many substances is very great; of phosphorus and iodine it dissolves more than its own weight, while in the arts it is used to dissolve sulphur, caoutchouc, gutta-percha, paraffin, etc.

It was introduced into our Materia Medica by Dr. Buchner, Germany.

Preparation for Homœopathic Use.—One part by weight of pure bisulphide of carbon is dissolved in ninety-nine parts by weight of 95 per cent. alcohol.

Amount of drug power, $\frac{1}{100}$.

Dilutions must be prepared as directed under Class VI—β, except that 95 per cent. alcohol is used.

CARBO VEGETABILIS.

Common Names, Vegetable Charcoal. Wood Charcoal.

Preparation.—Vegetable charcoal may be readily obtained by placing wood in an iron retort and distilling, the residue being the carbon of the wood together with some mineral matter. On a large scale charcoal is made by the smothered combustion of a pile of wood partially covered with earth. Charcoal is a bluish-black, porous substance, having a peculiar glistening aspect and retaining minutely both the form and texture of the wood from which it was made. Its specific gravity is about 1.7. It has the property of absorbing gases and of condensing them within its porous mass; a good specimen of box-wood charcoal will absorb ninety volumes of ammonia gas. Hence charcoal contains a large amount of oxygen condensed from the air in which it was cooled from its heated state, and to this is due its valuable disinfecting and decolorizing powers. After continued exposure to gases it becomes saturated with them, but its absorbing powers are restored by heating it to redness out of contact with air.

It was proven by Hahnemann.

Preparation for Homœopathic Use.—We select the firmest piece of beech, or birch charcoal, of medium thickness, divested of the bark, clearly showing the texture of the wood, and allowing us to infer, from a certain bright lustre, that the carbonizing process was perfect. These pieces, after being divided into lumps of the size of a fist are again made red-hot, and then speedily extinguished in an earthen vessel provided with a well-fitting cover; having been allowed to cool, and the ashes which may have formed having been blown off, the pieces are pulverized very finely, and the powder is kept in well-stoppered bottles in a dry place.

This powder is prepared by trituration, as directed under Class VII.

CARDUUS BENEDICTUS.

Synonyms, Cnicus Benedictus, *Linn.* Centaurea Benedicta, *Linn.*

Nat. Ord., Compositæ.

Common Names, Blessed Thistle. Star Thistle.

An herbaceous annual, about two feet in height, indigenous to Southern Europe, but naturalized in the United States. Its leaves are long-lanceolate, deeply and irregularly dentate, the teeth furnished with thorny points. The fresh leaves are bright green and feel greasy; when dried they are greenish-gray and woolly. The upper leaves sessile, lower ones petiolate. The flowers are discoid, yellow, with dark stripes. The plant flowers in June.

Introduced into our Materia Medica by Noack and Trinks.

Preparation.—The fresh herb, gathered when the plant is in flower, is chopped and pounded to a pulp and weighed. Then two parts by weight of alcohol are taken, the pulp mixed thoroughly with one-sixth part of it, and the rest of the alcohol added. After stirring the whole well, and pouring it into a well-stoppered bottle, it is allowed to stand eight days in a dark, cool place. The tincture is then separated by decanting, straining and filtering.

Drug power of tincture, $\frac{1}{6}$.

Dilutions must be prepared as directed under Class III.

CARDUUS MARIANUS, *Linn.*

Synonyms, Cnicus Marianus. Silybum Marianum, *Gærtner.*
Nat. Ord., Compositæ.
Common Names, Milk Thistle. St. Mary's Thistle.

This is an annual or biennial, two or three feet high, not much branched, glabrous or with but very little cottony wool. Leaves are smooth and shining above, and variegated by white veins; the lower ones deeply pinnatifid, with broad, very prickly lobes; the upper ones clasping the stem by prickly auricles, but scarcely decurrent. Flower-heads large, drooping, solitary at the ends of the branches, with purple florets. Bracts of the involucre very broad at the base, with a stiff, spreading, leafy appendage, ending in a long prickle, and bordered with prickles at its base. Hairs of the pappus simple. The plant is a native of Southern Europe.

Proven by Dr. Reil, of Germany.

Preparation.—Take one part by weight of the ripe, whole seed, and cover with two parts by weight of dilute alcohol, and let it remain eight days in a well-stoppered bottle, in a dark, cool place, shaking it twice a day. The tincture is then poured off, strained and filtered.

Drug power of tincture, $\frac{1}{3}$.

Dilutions must be prepared as follows: the 1x with 30 drops of tincture to 70 drops of dilute alcohol; the 2x and 3x also with dilute alcohol. The 1 dilution, with 3 drops of tincture to 97 drops of dilute alcohol, the 2 with dilute alcohol; for higher potencies alcohol is used.

CARYA ALBA, *Nuttall.*

Nat. Ord., Juglandaceæ.
Common Names, Shag-Bark. Shellbark. Hickory Nut.

A large, handsome tree, yielding valuable wood and the greater portion of hickory nuts of the market; indigenous to North America. Bark of trunk shaggy, coming off in rough strips; inner bud-scales becoming large and conspicuous, persistent till the flowers are fully developed; leaflets five, when young minutely downy beneath, finely serrate, the three upper obovate-lanceolate, the lower pair much smaller and oblong-lanceolate, all taper-pointed; fruit globular or depressed; nut white, flattish-globular, barely mucronate, the shell thinnish and splitting when dry, into four, hard or woody valves. Nuts ripen and fall in October.

Preparation.—The ripe nuts are finely powdered, and covered with five parts by weight of alcohol. Having been poured into a well-stoppered bottle, the mixture is allowed to remain eight days in a dark, cool place, being shaken twice a day. The tincture is then poured off, strained and filtered.

Amount of drug power, $\frac{1}{10}$.

Dilutions must be prepared as directed under Class IV.

CASCARILLA.

Synonym, Croton Eleutheria, *Bennett.*
Nat. Ord., Euphorbiaceæ.
Common Name, Cascarilla.

The tree furnishing cascarilla is indigenous to the Bahama Islands. It is several feet high. The bark occurs in commerce in tubular or channelled pieces, rather rough and irregular and about four inches long; it is dull brown in color. It is often found in smaller pieces an inch or less in length, often nearly covered with a silvery-white lichen; the older bark is more rugose and crossed by many longitudinal cracks and fewer transverse ones. The fracture of the bark is short and resinous. Its odor is fragrant and its taste bitter and nauseous. When burned it gives an aromatic odor.

Introduced into our Materia Medica by Stapf, of Germany.

Preparation.—The dried bark, coarsely powdered, is covered with five parts by weight of alcohol, and allowed to remain eight days in a well-stoppered bottle, in a dark, cool place, being shaken twice a day. The tincture is then poured off, strained and filtered.

Drug power of tincture, $\frac{1}{10}$.

Dilutions must be prepared as directed under Class IV.

CASTANEA.

Synonyms, Castanea Edulis, *Gærtner.* Castanea Vesca, *Linn.*
Nat. Ord., Cupuliferæ.
Common Name, Chestnut.

The American chestnut is a large, fine tree. Leaves four to eight inches long and about two broad, oblong-elliptical, pointed, coarsely serrate, prominently straight-veined. When full-grown they are green and smooth on both sides. Sterile flowers are whitish, in long naked cylindrical catkins. The well known nuts are enclosed, two or three, in a prickly four-valved involucre or *burr.* The American chestnut is spread largely through the eastern and middle portions of the United States.

Provings have been made by Dr. H. C. Houghton, U. S.

Preparation.—The fresh leaves are chopped and pounded to a pulp and weighed. Then two parts by weight of alcohol are taken, the pulp mixed with one-sixth part of it, and the rest of the alcohol added. After stirring the whole well and pouring it into a well-stoppered bottle, it is allowed to stand eight days in a dark, cool place. The tincture is then separated by decanting, straining and filtering.

Drug power of tincture, $\frac{1}{6}$.

Dilutions must be prepared as directed under Class III.

CASTOR EQUORUM.

Synonyms, Castor Equi. Verrucæ Equorum.
Class, Mammalia.
Order, Equidæ.

Family, Equus Caballus.

This is the blackish excrescence, found on the inner side of the fore and hind legs of the horse, above the knee and below the hock joints, which readily exfoliates, and on rubbing emits a peculiar odor.

Proven by Dr. Bauer, Germany.

Preparation.—The substance is dried, pulverized and prepared by trituration, as directed under Class VII.

CASTOREUM.

Synonyms, Castoreum Sibiricum. Castor Fiber, *Linn.*
Class, Mammalia.
Order, Rodentia.
Family, Muridæ.
Common Names, Castor.

The castor beaver, an inhabitant of the northern portion of the Temperate Zone, is furnished with a certain odoriferous secretion from glands situated near the genital organs. In these animals a *cloaca* furnishes outlet for urinary and alvine excretions, and acts in the male as a sheath to its sexual organ, and in the female as a vestibule to the vagina. In both sexes the glands exist—in the male communicating with the preputial opening, in the female, with the vagina. The reservoirs or sacs in which the gland secretion is stored is brought into commerce under the name of castoreum. In the fresh state, the sacs are found massed together, the individual sacs being of an elongated pyriform shape, about two inches long, soft and somewhat flesh-colored. Upon drying, they become brownish, flattened and wrinkled. The contents of the fresh sacs are liquid, yellow in color, and odorous, and afterward dry to a reddish-brown, more or less hard mass. Castor has a fetid, peculiar, strong odor, and its taste is nauseating, acrid and bitter.

Hartlaub and Trinks give provings by Caspari and "N—g."

Preparation.—The dry substance is prepared by trituration as directed under Class VII, which is the preferable method in homœopathic practice, but "tincture" may be prepared by covering the dry substance with five parts by weight of alcohol, and allowing the mixture to remain eight days in a well-stoppered bottle, in a dark, cool place, and shaking twice a day. The tincture is then poured off, strained and filtered.

Drug power of tincture, $\frac{1}{10}$.

Dilutions, from tincture, must be prepared as directed under Class IV.

CATALPA.

Synonym, Catalpa Bignonioides, *Walt.*
Nat. Ord., Bignoniaceæ.
Common Name, Catalpa.

This fine, wide spreading tree, is a native of the Southern States, but is frequently cultivated farther north. It often reaches a height of fifty feet, and its trunk attains a diameter of two feet. Its bark is smooth externally and slightly glossy, grayish-brown in color and studded with round, wart-like elevations. Beneath this is a middle green layer, and lower still is a white layer of bast-fibres which, on drying, becomes yellow. Leaves opposite, petiolate, ovate, cordate, downy beneath, pointed. Flowers white, slightly tinged with violet, campanulate, dotted violet and yellow in the throat, in large, showy, terminal panicles. Corolla, four or five cleft, throat inflated. Fruit, a long, cylindrical pod, two-celled. Seeds, winged.

Preparation.—Equal weights of the fresh inner bark and of the fresh leaves are chopped and pounded to a pulp and weighed. Then two parts by weight of alcohol are taken, the pulp mixed thoroughly with one-sixth part of it, and the rest of the alcohol added. After stirring the whole well, and pouring it into a well-stoppered bottle, it is allowed to stand eight days in a dark, cool place. The tincture is then separated by decanting, straining and filtering.

Drug power of tincture, $\frac{1}{6}$.

Dilutions must be prepared as directed under Class III.

CAULOPHYLLUM.

Synonyms, Caulophyllum Thalictroides, *Michaux.* Leontice Thalictroides, *Linn.*

Nat. Ord., Berberidaceæ.

Common Names, Blue Cohosh. Pappoose Root. Squaw Root.

This is an indigenous, perennial herb, with matted, knotty rhizomes, stem smooth, about two feet high, near the summit sending out a large triternately compound leaf; flowers greenish-yellow, in a panicle, below which is often a smaller biternate leaf. It is the only known species of the genus. It is found in most parts of the United States, growing in rich woods. Its root has a sweetish, pungent taste. Flowers in April and May.

It was first proven by Dr. Burt, U. S.

Preparation.—The fresh root, gathered early in the season when growth begins, is chopped and pounded to a pulp and weighed. Then two parts by weight of alcohol are taken, the pulp thoroughly mixed with one-sixth part of it, and the rest of the alcohol added. After stirring the whole well and pouring it into a well-stoppered bottle, it is allowed to stand eight days in a dark, cool place. The tincture is then separated by decanting, straining and filtering.

Drug power of tincture, $\frac{1}{6}$.

Dilutions must be prepared as directed under Class III.

CAUSTICUM.

Synonym, Causticum Hahnemanni.

This is a preparation peculiar to homœopathy, and hence must be prepared exactly according to Hahnemann's directions.

It is probably a weak solution of Potassium hydrate.

Preparation of Causticum.—A piece of freshly burnt lime is put for one minute in distilled water, then placed in a dry vessel, where it crumbles to powder. Mix four parts of this powder with the same quantity of the bisulphate of potash (previously ignited, melted, and, after cooling, pulverized) dissolved in four parts of boiling water, in a heated porcelain mortar, and after stirring it to a stiff paste, put the mixture into a glass retort, the helm of which is connected with a receiver half immersed in cold water. Increase the heat gradually and distil to dryness. Mix the clear distilled liquid amounting to about three parts by weight, with an equal weight of strong alcohol.

Amount of drug power, $\frac{1}{2}$.

Dilutions must be prepared as directed under Class I.

CEANOTHUS AMERICANUS, *Linn.*

Synonym, Ceanothus Sanguinis.
Nat. Ord., Rhamnaceæ.
Common Names, New Jersey Tea. Red Root.

This is an indigenous shrubby plant, stems growing from one to three feet high, from a dark red root; branches downy; leaves ovate or oblong-ovate, three-ribbed, serrate, downy beneath, often heart-shaped at the base; common peduncles elongated; flowers in attractive white clusters at the top of naked flower branches, appear in July. The plant is found throughout the United States, growing in dry woodlands, barrens, etc. The leaves have been substituted for tea, to which they have a strong resemblance when dried, both in taste and odor.

Preparation.—The fresh leaves are chopped and pounded to a pulp and weighed. Then two parts by weight of alcohol are taken, the pulp mixed thoroughly with one-sixth part of it, and the rest of the alcohol added. After stirring the whole well, and pouring it into a well-stoppered bottle, it is allowed to stand eight days in a dark, cool place. The tincture is then separated by decanting, straining and filtering.

Drug power of tincture, $\frac{1}{6}$.

Dilutions must be prepared as directed under Class III.

CEDRON.

Synonym, Simaba Cedron, *Planchon.*
Nat. Ord., Simarubaceæ.
Common Name, Cedron.

A small tree, stem erect, six inches or less in diameter, with branching top. Leaves large, glabrous, pinnate; flowers pale brown, in long, branching racemes. The fruit is a drupe, containing a single seed. The fruit is of a yellowish-gray color, flat-ovate, with one edge convex and the other almost straight, the convex edge terminating in a blunt point. It is about two inches long, and its greatest width is about one and one-third inches. The seed is about an inch and a half long, five-sixths of an inch broad, and nearly half an inch thick. One side is convex, the other flat or slightly concave, and the flat side has an oval scar near one extremity. Though hard and compact, it is sectile. The seed is without odor, and has an intensely bitter taste. The tree is indigenous to tropical America.

It was introduced into our Materia Medica by Dr. Teste, of France, under whom the first provings were made.

Preparation.—The dried, powdered seed is covered with five parts by weight of alcohol, and allowed to remain eight days in a well-stoppered bottle, in a dark, cool place, being shaken twice a day. The tincture is then poured off, strained and filtered.

Drug power of tincture, $\frac{1}{10}$.

Dilutions must be prepared as directed under Class IV.

CEPA.

Synonym, Allium Cepa, *Linn.*
Nat. Ord., Liliaceæ.
Common Name, Onion.

The common onion is a bulbous, biennial plant, with a fistulous scape swelling towards the base. The scape appears in the second year, three or four feet high, and is surmounted by a large globular umbel of greenish-white flowers. The leaves are terete, fistulous and pointed. There are many varieties and the bulbs vary in size, shape and color accordingly. The plant is universally cultivated as a garden vegetable.

The first provings were by Dr. Hering.

Preparation.—The fresh, red, somewhat long bulb, is chopped and pounded to a pulp and weighed. Then two parts by weight of alcohol are taken, the pulp mixed thoroughly with one-sixth part of it, and the rest of the alcohol added. After stirring the whole well, and pouring it into a well-stoppered bottle, it is allowed to stand eight days in a dark, cool place. The tincture is then separated by decanting, straining and filtering.

Drug power of tincture, $\frac{1}{6}$.

Dilutions must be prepared as directed under Class III.

CEPHALANTHUS OCCIDENTALIS, *Linn.*

Nat. Ord., Rubiaceæ.
Common Names, Button Bush. Crane Willow.

An indigenous shrub about six feet high, found growing in moist places, as along streams, or on the borders of swamps. Stems are smooth or pubescent. Leaves on petioles, ovate, or oblong-lanceolate, pointed, opposite or in threes, with short intervening stipules. Flowers white, in dense, spherical, peduncled heads. The flowers appear in July and August.

Preparation.—The fresh bark is chopped and pounded to a pulp and weighed. Then two parts by weight of alcohol are taken, the pulp mixed thoroughly with one-sixth part of it, and the rest of the alcohol added. After stirring the whole well, and pouring it into a well-stoppered bottle, it is allowed to stand eight days in a dark, cool place. The tincture is then separated by decanting, straining and filtering.

Amount of drug power, $\frac{1}{6}$.

Dilutions must be prepared as directed under Class III.

CERASUS VIRGINIANA, *Michaux.*

Synonyms, Cerasus Serotina, DC. Prunus Virginiana.

Nat. Ord., Amygdaleæ.

Common Names, Wild Black Cherry.

The wild cherry is an indigenous forest tree, often attaining a height of from fifty to eighty feet, and not throwing out branches below twenty or thirty feet. Leaves lanceolate-oblong, with fine, sharp serratures, pointed and on petioles having from two to four glands. The flowers are white, in cylindrical clusters. Fruit purplish-black. The bark when deprived of epidermis is reddish-brown in color, brittle, and when in powder, of a much lighter tinge. When fresh, its odor resembles that of peach leaves. The taste is bitter and somewhat aromatic.

Preparation.—The fresh bark is chopped and pounded and weighed; then five parts of alcohol are added, and the mixture allowed to remain eight days in a well-stoppered bottle, in a dark, cool place, being shaken twice a day. The tincture is then poured off, strained and filtered.

Drug power of tincture, $\frac{1}{10}$.

Dilutions must be prepared as directed under Class IV.

CEREUS BONPLANDII.

Nat. Ord., Cactaceæ.

A variety of Cereus Grandiflorus.

Preparation.—The stems are chopped and weighed. Then two parts by weight of alcohol are taken, the pulp mixed thoroughly with one-sixth part of it, and the rest of the alcohol added. After stirring the whole well, and pouring it into a well-stoppered bottle, it is allowed to stand eight days in a dark, cool place. The tincture is then separated by decanting, straining and filtering.

Drug power of tincture, $\frac{1}{6}$.

Dilutions must be prepared as directed under Class III.

CERIUM OXALICUM.

Proper Name, Cerous Oxalate.

Synonym, Cerii Oxalas.

Common Name, Oxalate of Cerium.

Formula, $Ce\, C_2\, O_4 . 3H_2\, O$.

Molecular Weight, 283.

Preparation of Oxalate of Cerium.—Cerium is a somewhat rare metal which is not found in the free state. The chief source of the metal is *cerite*, a hydrated silicate of cerium containing also lanthanum and didymium. The mineral is found only in Sweden. Cerium forms three classes of compounds, viz.: cerous, ceric and ceroso-ceric, the latter being probably a compound of the other two. The only salt of cerium used in medicine is the oxalate.

Preparation.—To prepare cerium oxalate, there must be first obtained a cerous salt, free from lanthanum and didymium. The oxide may be used. Dissolve the oxide in hydrochloric acid, nearly neutralize the solution without allowing any permanent precipitate to form, add sodium acetate and sodium hypochlorite in excess, and boil for some time; lanthanum and didymium remain in solution and ceric oxide is precipitated. The ceric oxide is to be dissolved in sulphuric acid, and by boiling with sodium hyposulphite is reduced to cerous sulphate. From this the oxalate may be precipitated by ammonium oxalate or oxalic acid; the precipitate is to be well washed with water, pressed between folds of bibulous paper and dried at a heat not greater than 25° C. (77° F.).

Properties.—Cerous oxalate is a white powder insoluble in water and oxalic acid, it dissolves in a large amount of hydrochloric and in sulphuric acid. When strongly heated it leaves a black powder which takes fire in the air and burns till it is converted into yellow ceric oxide.

Tests.—Its solutions in acid should not effervesce (absence of carbonates), nor when treated with hydrogen sulphide should they give any precipitate (absence of heavy metals). When dissolved in boiling potassium hydrate, the solution should show no precipitate if treated with ammonium chloride in excess (absence of aluminium). A solution of the salt, when treated with calcium chloride or calcium sulphate, gives a white precipitate of calcium oxalate.

Preparation for Homœopathic Use.—The pure oxalate of cerium is prepared by trituration, as directed under Class VII.

CERVUS BRAZILICUS.

Synonym, Cervus Campestris.
Class, Mammalia.
Order, Artiodactyla.
Family, Cervina.
Common Names, Brazilian Stag. Guazouti.

This stag, whose form is extremely fine and graceful, inhabits the forests of Brazil. Its size is about the same as that of our stag. Its skin, the color of which never changes, is of a brownish-fallow, being rather lighter towards the abdomen, the posterior part of the thighs and the tail. The inferior surface of the lower jaw, the part above and below the eyes, the interior of the ears and the abdomen are white; a black line encircles the jaws and gradually disappears under the lower one. The eyes of the guazouti are black, it has no canine teeth; its mouth, which is very slender, tapers to a muzzle. The horns which, in every case, are not very high and extremely regular, are at first straight; they curve forward in the second year, send forth three antlers, the anterior being placed about two inches above the burr, which is turned a little inward, and the other two at the superior and posterior part of the staff. The horns become larger as they grow older, but the number of antlers remains the same.

Introduced into our Materia Medica by Dr. Mure, of Brazil.

Preparation.—A small piece of the fresh hide with the hair on, is triturated as directed under Class IX.

CHAMOMILLA.

Synonyms, Chamomilla Vulgaris. Matricaria Chamomilla, *Linn.*

Nat. Ord., Compositæ.

Common Names, Common Chamomile. Corn Fever-Few. German Chamomile.

This annual plant grows in uncultivated fields, among wheat and corn, especially in sandy regions, all over Europe.

From the fibrous root shoot up several stems, erect, striated, ramose, naked, from one to two feet long; the leaves are sparse, the lower double, the upper single, pinnate and dark green; the flowers are numerous, white, with yellow disk and in corymbs; calyx hemispherical, imbricated, scariose; the receptacle naked and conical; the stems are swollen at the top, the covering scales tiled, blunt, great, skinny at the margin, whitish or brownish.

The common chamomile is frequently confounded with the Roman chamomile, from which it is distinguished by its perennial stalk, its chaffy receptacle, its hollow peduncles, the green scales of the calyx, and by its rays being mostly turned in.

It was first proven by Hahnemann.

Preparation.—The whole fresh plant, when in flower, is chopped and pounded to a fine pulp, enclosed in a piece of new linen and subjected to pressure. The expressed juice is then, by brisk agitation, mingled with an equal part by weight of alcohol. The mixture is allowed to stand eight days in a well-stoppered bottle, in a dark, cool place, and then filtered.

Drug power of tincture ½.

Dilutions must be prepared as directed under Class I.

CHELIDONIUM.

Synonyms, Chelidonium Majus, *Linn.* Papaver Corniculatum Luteum.

Nat. Ord., Papaveraceæ.

Common Names, Celandine. Tetter-Wort.

This perennial plant grows all over Germany, as well as in France, in waste places, old walls, hedges, borders of highways, near habitations; the root is fusiform, of the thickness of a finger, reddish-brown without, yellowish within, containing, as do all parts of the plant, an acrid, yellow juice; stem ramose, hairy, one to two feet high;

leaves thin, winged, pinnatifid, bluish-green beneath, bright green above; flowers yellow, axillary, or terminal; peduncles in umbels; umbel simple, of four or five rays; calyx caduceous and two-leaved; corolla of four petals; petals ligulate, threads united with the anthers, imitating petals; silique polyspermous, unilocular, linear, thin.

It was first proven by Hahnemann.

Preparation.—The fresh plant is chopped and pounded to a pulp, enclosed in a piece of new linen and subjected to pressure. The expressed juice is then, by brisk agitation, mingled with an equal part by weight of alcohol. This mixture is allowed to stand eight days in a dark, cool place and then filtered.

Drug power of tincture, ½.

Dilutions must be prepared as directed under Class I.

CHELONE.

Synonyms, Chelone Glabra, *Linn.* Chelone Alba.

Nat. Ord., Scrophulariaceæ.

Common Names, Balmony. Snake-Head. Turtle-Head.

This is a common perennial herbaceous plant, found in wet situations throughout the United States. Its smooth, upright, branching stem rises to a foot or two in height. Leaves very short-petioled, lanceolate or lance-oblong, pointed, of varying width. Flowers are large, white, rose-colored or purple, nearly sessile in spikes or clusters, and closely imbricated with round-ovate concave bracts and bractlets. Calyx of five distinct imbricated sepals. Corolla inflated, tubular, with the mouth a little open; the upper lip broad and arched, keeled in the middle, notched at the apex; the lower woolly-bearded in the throat, three-lobed at the apex, the middle lobe smallest. Stamens four, with woolly filaments and very woolly heart-shaped anthers; and a fifth sterile filament smaller than the others. Seeds many, wing-margined. The shape of the flowers, resembling the head of a snake or tortoise, has given the common name to this plant. Flowers from July to September.

Preparation.—The fresh plant is pounded to a pulp and weighed. Then two parts by weight of alcohol are taken, the pulp mixed thoroughly with one-sixth part of it, and the rest of the alcohol added. After stirring the whole well, and pouring it into a well-stoppered bottle, it is allowed to stand eight days in a dark, cool place. The tincture is then separated by decanting, straining and filtering.

Drug power of tincture, ⅙.

Dilutions must be prepared as directed under Class III.

CHENOPODIUM ANTHELMINTICUM, *Linn.*

Synonyms, Ambrina Anthelmintica. Cina Americana.

Nat. Ord., Chenopodiaceæ.

Common Name, Wormseed.

A perennial plant, indigenous to tropical America, but naturalized in the United States. Stem two to five feet high, angular or furrowed, erect and branching. Leaves oblong-lanceolate, glandular, deeply serrate, and the lower ones at times almost laciniate-pinnatifid. Flowers small, greenish, in long, leafless, spiked panicles. It is usually found in waste places in the warmer portions of the United States. It flowers from July to September. The whole plant has an offensive yet slightly aromatic odor.

Proved by Dr. Jeanes, U. S.

Preparation.—The fresh herb, in flower, is chopped and pounded to a pulp and weighed. Then two parts by weight of alcohol are taken, the pulp mixed thoroughly with one-sixth part of it, and the rest of the alcohol added. After stirring the whole well, and pouring it into a well-stoppered bottle, it is allowed to stand eight days in a dark, cool place. The tincture is then separated by decanting, straining and filtering.

Drug power of tincture, $\frac{1}{6}$.

Dilutions must be prepared as directed under Class III..

CHENOPODIUM BOTRYS, *Linn.*

Nat. Ord., Chenopodiaceæ.

Common Names, Jerusalem Oak. Feather Geranium.

This variety is indigenous to Europe, but naturalized to a slight extent in North America. It is glandular-pubescent, leaves oblong sinuate-pinnatifid, flowers greenish, in leafless cymose racemes. The odor is aromatic.

Preparation.—The fresh herb is chopped and pounded to a pulp and weighed. Then two parts by weight of alcohol are taken, the pulp mixed thoroughly with one-sixth part of it, and the rest of the alcohol added. After stirring the whole well, and pouring it into a well-stoppered bottle, it is allowed to stand eight days in a dark, cool place. The tincture is then separated by decanting, straining and filtering.

Drug power of tincture, $\frac{1}{6}$.

Dilutions must be prepared as directed under Class III.

CHENOPODIUM GLAUCUM, *Linn.*

Nat. Ord., Chenopodiaceæ.

Common Name, Oak-leaved Goosefoot.

This plant is indigenous to Europe, where it is commonly found growing on rubbish, dung-heaps, or near stagnant, filthy water. It also grows in North America, though rarely, along the streets of towns. It is a low plant, stem from one foot to one foot and a half high, now erect, now decumbent, is often striped red and white-green, angular and naked. Leaves sinuately pinnatifid-toothed, oblong, obtuse, pale green above, and lighter, as if dusted with meal, beneath. The flower-racemes stand in the axils and at the end, consisting of green, densely accumulate florets without pedicels. Seeds sharp-edged, often vertical. Flowers appear from late summer through autumn.

Preparation.—The fresh herb and the flower, freed from an aphis living upon it, is chopped and pounded to a pulp and weighed. Then two parts by weight of alcohol are taken, the pulp mixed thoroughly with one-sixth part of it, and the rest of the alcohol added. After stirring the whole well, and pouring it into a well-stoppered bottle, it is allowed to stand eight days in a dark, cool place. The tincture is then separated by decanting, straining and filtering.

Drug power of tincture, $\frac{1}{6}$.

Dilutions must be prepared as directed under Class III.

CHIMAPHILA.

Synonyms, Chimaphila Umbellata, *Nuttall.* Chimaphila Corymbosa, *Pursh.* Pyrola Umbellata, *Linn.*

Nat. Ord., Ericaceæ.

Common Names, Pipsissewa. Prince's Pine.

A small, perennial evergreen plant, having a long running rootstock, from which arise several short stems. Leaves wedge-lanceolate, sharply serrate, thick, leathery, green and shining. Flowers, with petals flesh-colored and anthers violet, are in terminal, peduncled corymbs. The plant is small, and is found growing in the United States and Canada, in dry woods. The flowers appear in June and July.

The drug was introduced into our Materia Medica by Dr. S. A. Jones, U. S.

Preparation.—The fresh plant in flower is chopped and pounded to a pulp and weighed. Then two parts by weight of alcohol are taken, the pulp mixed thoroughly with one-sixth part of it, and the rest of the alcohol added. After stirring the whole well, and pouring it into a well-stoppered bottle, it is allowed to stand eight days in a dark, cool place. The tincture is then separated by decanting, straining and filtering.

Amount of drug power, $\frac{1}{6}$.

Dilutions must be prepared as directed under Class III.

CHINA.

Synonyms, China Regia. Cinchona Calisaya, *Weddell.*

Nat. Ord., Rubiaceæ.

Common Names, Calisaya Bark. Yellow Cinchona. Yellow Peruvian Bark.

The genus *Cinchona* is a member of the tribe *Cinchoneæ,* of the order *Rubiaceæ.* The tribe consists of shrubs or trees, with opposite leaves, two-celled ovary, capsular fruit and numerous minute seeds. The genus *Cinchona* is recognized by its deciduous stipules, terminal panicles of flowers, calyx superior, five-toothed, corolla tubular, five-lobed, with fringed margins. The corolla possesses a faint, agreeable odor, and in color is rosy, purplish or white. The cinchonas are evergreen, with fine-veined leaves having a strong midrib. The petiole is sometimes as long as the leaf, and at times colored red. The leaves are ovate, obovate, or nearly circular, but in some species lanceolate, rarely cordate, always entire and generally glabrous. The species of cinchona resemble each other so much that their definition is not easy. Bentham and Hooker, in 1873, estimated the number of the species as about thirty-six. The cinchonas are natives of South America, between 10° N. latitude and 22° S. latitude, and are found always growing in the mountainous regions, the average altitude of their habitat being from 5000 to 8000 feet above the sea. The bark is the portion of the tree used in medicine, and the most valuable kind is from *C. Calisaya*, a tall, stately tree growing in Bolivia and Southeastern Peru, at an altitude of from 5000 to 6000 feet above the sea-level. Calisaya bark is found in commerce in different shapes, depending upon modifications in the drying process to which the bark is subjected after being stripped from the tree. It comes in quills or in flat pieces. Quill calisaya is in tubes three-fourths to one and one-half inches thick, often rolled up at both edges, forming double quills. The quills vary in length. They are always covered with a rugged, thick, corky layer, marked with longitudinal and transverse cracks. This layer is easily detached, leaving its impression on the cinnamon-brown middle layer. The inner surface is dark brown and fibrous. The fracture is short and fibrous. Flat calisaya occurs in irregular flat pieces, often a foot or more in length, sometimes from three to four inches wide and from one-fifth to two-fifths of an inch thick. It is without the corky covering, is of a rusty orange-brown color, with dark stains on the outer side. The inner side has a wavy, fine fibrous texture. The kind prescribed in medicine previous to the use of quinine and for a long time afterward, is the pale cinchona bark, known as Loxa bark, and is chiefly afforded by C. officinalis. It comes in quills only, which are often double and from one-eighth to three-fourths inches in diameter. Their length varies greatly, from an inch, or even less, to, occasionally, twelve inches. The thinnest Loxa bark is about as thick as writing paper, and the thickest about one-tenth of an inch.

The drug has a special interest as being the one with which Hahnemann first experimented in proving medicines.

Preparation.—The dried bark is coarsely powdered and weighed. Then five parts by weight of alcohol are poured over it, and having put the mixture into a well-stoppered bottle, it is allowed to remain eight days in a dark, cool place, shaking it twice a day. The tincture is then poured off, strained and filtered.

Drug power of tincture, $\frac{1}{10}$.

Dilutions must be prepared as directed under Class IV.

Triturations are prepared from the powdered bark, as directed under Class VII.

CHININUM ARSENICUM.

Synonym, Arsenate of Quinia. Chininum Arsenicicum. Quiniæ Arsenias.

Common Name, Arsenate of Quinine.

Formula, $(C_{20}\ H_{24}\ N_2\ O_2)_3$ As $H_3\ O_4$, $2H_2\ O$.

Preparation of Arsenate of Quinia.—It is obtained in long prisms by saturating a solution of arsenic acid with quinia.

Properties and Tests.—It crystallizes in long, white prisms, is freely soluble in hot water and in alcohol, but sparingly soluble in cold water. The aqueous solution gives no precipitate with chloride of barium, but with nitrate of silver a brick-red precipitate is produced. When treated first with solution of chlorine and afterwards with ammonia, a splendid emerald-green color is produced.

Proven by Dr. Muhr, Germany.

Preparation for Homœopathic Use.—Arsenate of quinia is prepared by trituration, as directed under Class VII.

CHININUM MURIATICUM.

Synonyms, Chininum Hydrochloricum. Muriate of Quinia. Quiniæ Hydrochloras.

Common Names, Hydro-chlorate of Quinine.

Formula, $C_{20} H_{24} N_2 O_2$, HCl, $2H_2 O$.

Molecular Weight, 396.5.

Preparation of Muriate of Quinia.—By dissolving pure quinia in warm dilute hydrochloric acid unto neutralization. The solution is to be evaporated at a temperature not exceeding 30° C. (86° F.) and the crystals collected.

Properties and Tests.—It crystallizes in colorless needles of a silky appearance, aggregated in stars. They are neutral in reaction or faintly alkaline, without odor and of a very bitter taste. They are soluble in about thirty parts of cold and in two to three of boiling water, in three of alcohol and in nine of chloroform; (the sulphate is not soluble in chloroform). Heated on platinum foil it burns, leaving no residue. Barium chloride solution should give no precipitate with it (absence of sulphate).

Preparation for Homœopathic Use.—The pure muriate of quinia is prepared by trituration, as directed under Class VII.

CHININUM PURUM.

Synonym, Quinia.

Common Name, Pure Quinine.

Formula, $C_{20} H_{24} N_2 O_2$.

Molecular Weight, 324.

Preparation.—The alkaloid quinia is obtained by treating a cold solution of its sulphate with sodium carbonate unto neutralization, washing the precipitate with cold water and drying it at a temperature not exceeding 25° C. (77° F.).

Properties.—So prepared, quinia is a light, snow-white, flocky powder, without odor, possessing a very bitter taste and an alkaline reaction. It consists of microscopic prismatic crystals. It may be obtained in beautiful slender needles by the very slow evaporation of an ammoniacal solution. By heating it melts, and on cooling becomes a colorless, friable, amorphous mass. It is soluble in 364 parts of cold and in 200 of boiling water, and is readily soluble in alcohol, ether and chloroform.

Tests.—A characteristic test for quinia is as follows: One part of quinia is to be rubbed up with 200 parts of chlorine water and then treated with 25 parts of caustic ammonia. A dark green, resin-like precipitate is produced (*thalleiochin*) which is insoluble in water, ether and carbon disulphide; by dilute acids it is dissolved with a brown color, but upon treatment again with alkali it reprecipitates unchanged. Quinia may be adulterated with quinidia, cinchonia and cinchonidia. To determine such sophistication mix one part of precipitated quinia in a mortar with half its weight of ammonium sulphate, then add five parts of water and evaporate to dryness over a water-bath. To the residue, after complete cooling, is added ten parts by weight of cold water and the mixture thoroughly rubbed up for about a minute. After standing for half an hour the rubbing up is to be repeated and the whole thrown upon a filter. The process, from the beginning to the end, must be conducted at the same temperature, between 15° and 17° C. (50°–62.6° F.). Then to five parts of the filtrate, in a test-tube, are to be added seven parts of ammonia water whose specific gravity is at 15° C. (59° F.) 0.960. This amount of ammonia water is based on the assumption that the processes are conducted at 15° C.; if the temperature be higher a greater quantity of the alkali must be used, viz. at 16° C., 7½ parts, at 18° C., 8½ parts. The mixture in the test-tube is to be gently agitated for a minute, whereupon if the precipitated quinia was completely pure the mixture remains perfectly clear, while the presence of even minute quantities of quinidia, cinchonia or cinchonidia gives rise to a readily perceptible turbidity.

Preparation for Homœopathic Use.—The pure quinia is prepared by trituration, as directed under Class VII.

CHININUM SULPHURICUM.

Synonyms, Disulphate or Basic Sulphate of Quinia. Quiniæ Sulphas. Sulphate of Quinia. Sulphus Quinicus.

Common Name, Sulphate of Quinine.

Formula, $(C_{20}\,H_{24}\,N_2\,O_2)_2\,H_2\,SO_2,\,7H_2\,O$.

Molecular Weight, 872.

Preparation of Sulphate of Quinia.—All methods of extracting the alkaloids from cinchona barks consist in treating the bark with dilute acid and precipitating the alkaloids from the acid extract by means of lime or of sodium carbonate. The bark reduced to powder is boiled for an hour or less with eight or ten times its weight of water acidulated with twenty-five per cent. of hydrochloric acid, the decoction strained through a cloth and the residue boiled a second and sometimes a third time, with more and more dilute acid till the marc is completely exhausted. The extracts after cooling are mixed with a slight excess of milk of lime, added by small portions, to precipitate the alkaloids together with the coloring matter. The precipitate is left to drain and submitted to a gradually increasing pressure, the liquids which run off being collected in a single vessel; they yield after a while a fresh deposit. The pressed cake is now dried and macerated with alcohol in a closed vessel heated over a water-bath. The strength of the alcohol used depends upon the quality of the bark under treatment; for calisaya bark alcohol of seventy-five to eighty per cent. is sufficiently strong; but barks which contain a smaller proportion of quinia require alcohol of eighty-five to ninety per cent., since cinchonia is much less soluble in weak alcohol than is quinia. When the bark contains more quinia than cinchonia the alcoholic extract is treated with dilute sulphuric acid in excess and the alcohol recovered by distillation. The greater part of the quinia sulphate then separates in a crystalline mass, the rest, together with cinchonia sulphate, remaining in the mother liquor. Sodium carbonate is a better precipitant than lime for the alkaloids, because they are slightly soluble in lime-water and calcium chloride. Quinia sulphate is made in large amount by the manufacturing chemist, and it is advised to not prepare it in the pharmaceutical laboratory.

Officinal sulphate of quinia is in very white loose masses of fine, silky, flexible needles. They are without odor and have a permanently and extremely bitter taste. They are soluble in from 750 to 800 parts of water at medium temperatures, in from 25 to 30 of boiling water, in 65 of 90 per cent. alcohol, in 120 of dilute alcohol, slightly in ether and not at all in chloroform. The solutions are neutral in reaction. In water to which an acid has been added, the salt is easily soluble; in dilute sulphuric acid the solution is fluorescent with a blue tint. Upon exposure to the air, the salt effloresces; by heating it becomes phosphorescent, and at 120° C. (248° F.) it loses all of its water of crystallization.

Tests.—The purity of sulphate of quinine may be determined by the following tests: It dissolves in concentrated sulphuric acid without effervescence, and the solution remains clear and colorless. One part of the salt should dissolve in 100 parts of absolute alcohol, forming a transparent and colorless solution, and this solution, when treated with an equal amount of ether, should remain clear. One gramme of the salt selected from a large quantity is to be heated in a porcelain dish upon the water-bath for about twelve hours. In that time the amount of water driven off from the salt should be neither more nor less than 14 per cent. of the original weight taken, so that, in the case given, the residue will weigh .86 gramme. When heated upon platinum foil, it should first carbonize and then burn without leaving any residue (absence of fixed impurities). The above tests will serve to determine the purity of the salt. For its identification, the test given in the article *Chininum*, may be used. In addition, if treated with chlorine water and then with potassium ferro-cyanide and finally with ammonia, a deep red color is produced.

The drug was first proved by Dr. Piper, Germany.

Preparation for Homœopathic Use.—The pure sulphate of quinia is prepared by trituration, as directed under Class VII.

CHINOIDIN.

Synonyms, Amorphous Quinia. Quinoidine.

Preparation of Chinoidin.—Chinoidin is a mixture of several alkaloidal bodies, some of which exist in the chinchona bark and others are decomposition-products resulting from the chemical and physical influences to which the bark is subjected in the extraction of quinia. The chief constituents of chinoidin are amorphous quinidia, chinchonidia, cinchonia, chinicin and cinchonicin. It is obtained from the mother liquor left after the extraction of the sulphate of quinia, by precipitating with an alkali, washing and drying.

Properties.—Chinoidin is a dark brown, brittle mass, glistening-resinous in appearance, and breaking with a conchoidal fracture. It is without odor, and to the taste is only slightly bitter, but when dissolved in alcohol or dilute acids, the bitterness of the solution is extreme; it is more or less soluble in ether. The alcoholic solution is alkaline to test-paper. Its solution in boiling water is colorless, but upon cooling shows a white turbidity.

Tests.—When incinerated upon platinum foil, only a very small amount of ash should remain. When dissolved in dilute acid and then precipitated by ammonium hydrate, the weight of the washed and dried precipitate should about equal that of the original amount used in the test.

Preparation for Homœopathic Use.—One part by weight of chinoidin are dissolved in nine parts by weight of 95 per cent. alcohol.

Drug power of tincture, $\frac{1}{10}$.

Dilutions must be prepared as directed under Class VI—*a*.

Triturations are prepared of pure chinoidin as directed under Class VII.

CHIONANTHUS VIRGINICA, *Linn.*

Nat. Ord., Oleaceæ.

Common Names, Fringe-Tree. Snow-flower.

Chionanthus Virginica is a low tree or shrub, found growing on river banks in Southern Pennsylvania and southward. Its leaves are oval, oblong, or obovate-lanceolate; its snow-white flowers are on slender pedicels; the fruit is a drupe, purple, ovoid, six to eight lines long. The flowers, appearing in June, have petals one inch long, narrowly linear, acute, varying to five or six in number, which are barely united at the base. Calyx four-parted, very small, persistent, stamens two (rarely three or four), on the very base of the corolla, very short. Stigma notched.

Proven by Dr. Scudder, U. S.

Preparation.—The fresh bark is chopped, pounded to a pulp and weighed. Then two parts by weight of alcohol are taken, the pulp mixed thoroughly with one-sixth part of it, and the rest of the alcohol added. After stirring the whole well, and pouring it into a well-stoppered bottle, it is allowed to stand eight days in a dark, cool place. The tincture is then separated by decanting, straining and filtering.

Amount of drug power, $\frac{1}{6}$.
Dilutions must be prepared as directed under Class III.

CHLORALUM.

Synonyms, Chloral Hydrate. Chloral Hydras. Chloralum Hydratum Crystallisatum.

Common Names, Chloral. Hydrate of Chloral.

Formula, $C_2\ HCl_3\ O, H_2\ O$.

Molecular Weight, 165.5.

Formation and Preparation of Hydrate of Chloral.—When dry chlorine gas is passed into alcohol absolutely water-free, the chlorine abstracts hydrogen from the alcohol and aldehyde is formed. The following equation shows the action: $C_2\ H_6\ O + Cl_2 = C_2\ H_4O + (HCl)_2$. The passage of chlorine still continuing, the aldehyde yields three more atoms of hydrogen, their place being taken by three atoms of chlorine and the result is chloral; the reaction may be outlined as follows $(C_2\ H_4\ O) + (Cl_2)_9 = (C_2H\ Cl_3\ O)_3 + (H\ Cl)_9$, although in reality it is not as simple as the equation would show, for a secondary reaction takes place between the alcohol and the chlorine by which water is formed, and this uniting with the chloral produces chloral hydrate. Chloral hydrate is made on a large scale by the manufacturing chemist, and in commerce the article can be readily obtained in a state of undoubted purity.

Pure chloral hydrate is in dry, colorless, transparent, rhomboidal crystals having an aromatic, somewhat pungent odor and a disagreeable, somewhat caustic taste. It is soluble in one and a half parts of water. It dissolves in alcohol, ether, carbon disulphide and benzol. Heated to 58° C. (136.4 F.), it melts to a clear colorless fluid which, upon cooling to 30° C. (86° F.) begins to crystallize, and if further cooled becomes a solid, white, crystalline mass. At 94° C. (201.2° F.) it begins to boil and is dissipated without decomposition. At ordinary temperatures it volatilizes slightly, and when exposed to a damp atmosphere it attracts moisture. Its watery solution undergoes gradual decomposition from the separation of hydrochloric acid. When treated with caustic alkali it is decomposed into chloroform and a formate of the alkali.

Tests.—The impurity most to be feared in chloral hydrate is chloral alcoholate, an intermediate compound formed during the process of manufacture. Pure chloral hydrate should dissolve readily in water with no separation out of oily drops, thus showing that the specimen is neither chloral alcoholate nor a mixture with the same. The hydrate dissolves without changing its form, while the alcoholate is transformed into an oily-looking fluid before dissolving. The solution in dilute alcohol should not give any turbidity with silver nitrate, nor should it exhibit an acid reaction. The watery solution, however, has an acid reaction. The hydrate should not become damp in the air; if so, it indicates the presence of sulphuric acid. Heated in a silver spoon over the alcohol flame it melts but does not take fire even if the flame is brought quite close to it; and it finally dissipates completely. The alcoholate ignites easily under the above test, and burns with a yellow sooty flame. A cold watery solution of the hydrate will not decolorize a solution of potassium permanganate until after a long time; otherwise the alcoholate or other organic impurity is present.

It was proven by Dr. W. Eggert, U. S.

Preparation for Homœopathic Use.—One part by weight of pure chloral hydrate is dissolved in nine parts by weight of alcohol.

Amount of drug power, $\frac{1}{10}$.

Dilutions must be prepared as directed under Class VI—*a*.

CHLOROFORMUM.

Common Name, Chloroform.

Formula, $CH\,Cl_3$.

Molecular Weight, 119.5.

Origin and Preparation of Chloroform.—As was stated in the article Chloralum, that body is decomposed by a caustic alkali into chloroform and a formate; if, then, the process for making chloral be modified by the presence of a caustic alkali, chloroform and a formate will be the result. Such indeed is practically the mode in which chloroform is made on a large scale, the formate of the alkali being, however, decomposed into carbonate subsequently in the process. It is prepared by distilling one part of alcohol with six parts of chloride of lime and twenty-four parts of water, until about one and a half parts have come over. The distillate consists chiefly of chloroform and alcohol with some water, and separates into two layers, the heavier one being chloroform. The upper, aqueous layer is syphoned off and the chloroform is agitated with sulphuric acid to remove certain volatile oils which have distilled over; as soon as the two liquids separate the chloroform is drawn off and rectified by redistillation till it has a constant boiling point of 61° C. (142° F.).

Properties.—Chloroform is a thin colorless liquid of neutral reaction and having a peculiar, agreeable, ethereal odor. Its vapor when inhaled makes the impression of sweetness upon the sense of taste; the liquid when taken in the mouth has a burning, sweetish taste. Its sp. gr. at 0° C. (32° F.) is 1.525, and its vapor-density is 4.20. It is difficult to kindle and burns with a greenish flame. It dissolves slightly in water, imparting to that liquid its own sweet taste. It mixes in all proportions with alcohol, from which mixture it is partially precipitated by water. It dissolves readily in ether and is quite insoluble in sulphuric acid. It dissolves phosphorus, sulphur, iodine and many of the alkaloids and their salts. Its specific gravity at 15° C. (59° F.) is, according to Biltz, 1.502, but the addition of one-half per cent. of alcohol reduces the specific gravity at 15.2° C. (59.4° F.) to 1.4936, and if one per cent. of alcohol be added the specific gravity becomes 1.485. Pure chloroform under the influence of light suffers decomposition, but the addition of one-half per cent. of alcohol prevents such change.

Tests.—In addition to the specific gravity as given above and the physical properties there enumerated, chloroform, if pure, should evaporate without residue, and when shaken with half its volume of pure concentrated sulphuric acid should impart no color to the latter even after standing for twenty-four hours. To determine whether a pure chloroform has undergone partial decomposition a specimen of it is to be shaken with three volumes of water, and the latter tested with litmus and with silver nitrate solution; in neither case if it be unaltered should any change be observable.

It was proven by Lembke, in Germany.

Preparation for Internal Use.—One part by weight of pure chloroform is dissolved in nine parts by weight of alcohol.

Amount of drug power, $\frac{1}{10}$.

Dilutions must be prepared as directed under Class VI—*a*.

CHLORUM.

Synonym, Chlorinum.

Common Name, Chlorine.

Symbol, Cl.

Atomic Weight, 35.5.

Chlorine is one of the elements, but does not exist free in nature. It occurs in saline springs and in sea-water in combination with sodium, magnesium, potassium and calcium, and in the solid form there are found in the earth vast deposits of sodium chloride or common salt.

Preparation.—Chlorine is produced when a chloride is decomposed by an acid in the presence of some body whose attraction for the hydrogen of the acid is greater than that of chlorine. Inorganic bodies which easily part with their oxygen are used for this purpose. Hydrochloric acid and granulated manganese dioxide when heated together give off chlorine readily; the reaction is shown by the following equation: $(H\,Cl)_4 + Mn\,O_2 = Mn\,Cl_2 + (H_2\,O)_2 + Cl_2$. The gas is obtained more continuously when a mixture of two equivalents of sodium chloride, two of sulphuric acid and one of manganese dioxide are heated together in a flask. The reaction is exhibited as follows: $(Na\,Cl)_2 + (H_2SO_4)_2 + Mn\,O_2 = Mn\,SO_4 + Na_2SO_4 + (H_2\,O)_2 + Cl_2$. The process is conducted as follows: the materials are placed in a flask standing in a sand-bath over a gas furnace. The cork of the flask is provided with a safety-tube as well as a delivery-tube. From the delivery-tube passes a bent glass tube which is carried nearly to the bottom of a long bottle containing a few inches of strong sulphuric acid through which the gas bubbles as it comes over and by which it is rendered dry. From the bottle it is brought by another tube to a long receiver where it simply accumulates by its specific gravity, displacing the air; or if chlorine water be needed the gas is led into a partially closed receiver containing cold distilled water. The saturation of the water with the gas will be known by closing the bottle or receiver tightly and agitating it; until saturation is effected a partial vacuum is produced by the shaking.

Properties.—Chlorine is a yellowish-green gas possessing a peculiar suffocating odor and an astringent taste. It is wholly irrespirable. Its specific gravity is 2.46. At 11° C. (51.8° F.), one volume of water dissolves nearly three volumes of the gas. This solution is known as chlorine water and has essentially the properties of the gas. Chlorine water is a greenish-yellow, transparent liquid, which upon exposure to light begins to undergo decomposition, hydrochloric acid and oxygen being produced.

Chlorine decomposes many organic matters by its strong affinity for hydrogen, and secondarily, by the oxidizing power of the oxygen liberated at the same time; these facts explain its powerful action as a bleaching agent and its strong disinfecting properties.

Tests.—As it should only be used for homœopathic preparations when absolutely fresh, it is not necessary to offer any tests of its purity. If the gas have been made from hydrochloric acid some of the latter may have come over in the process. A small portion of the chlorine water may be shaken with mercury in excess as long as the odor of chlorine can be detected, when if hydrochloric acid be present blue litmus paper will be reddened by the liquid which remains.

It was first proven by Dr. Hering.

Preparation for Homœopathic Use.—The freshly prepared chlorine water, according to above formula, contains about three per cent. of chlorine gas; we take one part of it by weight and mix it with two parts by weight of distilled water.

Amount of drug power, $\frac{1}{100}$.

Dilutions must be prepared as directed under Class V—β.

CICUTA.

Synonyms, Cicuta Virosa, *Linn.* Cicuta Aquatica.

Nat. Ord., Umbelliferæ.

Common Names, Cow-bane. Water-hemlock. Water-parsnip.

This perennial plant inhabits the borders of ditches and rivulets, swamps, meadows, ponds, lakes, etc., all over Germany and the north and west of France; the root is thick, white, fleshy, elongated, transparent, hairy and hollow; its bark contains a yellow juice; its odor is strong and disagreeable, its taste acrid and caustic; stem straight, from one to two feet high, ramose, fistulous, glabrous, striated; leaves compound, bi- or trifid with lanceolate, incised-serrate leaflets; umbels loose, naked; involucels three or five-rayed; flowers white, uniform; fruit ovoid, furrowed, ten-ribbed. The whole plant is very poisonous, proving fatal to most animals which feed upon it, though it is said to be eaten with impunity by goats and sheep. Several instances are on record of children who have died from eating the root in mistake for parsnip.

First proved by Hahnemann.

Preparation.—The fresh root of the plant just coming into bloom is chopped and pounded to a fine pulp, enclosed in a piece of new linen and subjected to pressure. The expressed juice is then, by brisk agitation, mingled with an equal part by weight of alcohol. The mixture is allowed to stand eight days in a well-stoppered bottle, in a dark, cool place, and then filtered.

Drug power of tincture, $\frac{1}{2}$.

Dilutions must be prepared as directed under Class I.

CIMEX LECTULARIUS.

Class, Insecta.

Order, Heteroptera.

Family, Cimicidæ.

Common Name, Bed-Bug.

This insect is too well known to require a description.

It was first proved by Dr. Wahle, Germany.

Preparation.—The live insect, crushed, is covered with five parts by weight of alcohol. Having poured the mixture into a well-stoppered bottle, it is allowed to remain eight days in a dark, cool place, being shaken twice a day. The tincture is then poured off, strained and filtered.

Amount of drug power, $\frac{1}{10}$.

Dilutions must be prepared as directed under Class IV.

CIMICIFUGA.

Synonyms, Actæa Racemosa, *Linn.* Cimicifuga Racemosa, *Elliott.* Macrotys Racemosa.

Nat. Ord., Ranunculaceæ.

Common Names, Black Snake Root. Bugbane.

An indigenous perennial, whose stem is from three to eight feet high. The root is a knotted root-stock. Leaves large, bifid or trifid, with ovate leaflets having incised-serrate edges. Flowers small, white, with four to eight petals, minute and on claws. Racemes terminal, long and wand-like. The fruit is an ovoid pod, sessile, having many flat seeds. The plant flowers in June and July.

Preparation.—The fresh root is pounded to a pulp and weighed. Then two parts by weight of alcohol are taken, the pulp mixed thoroughly with one-sixth part of it, and the rest of the alcohol added. After stirring the whole well, and pouring it into a well-stoppered bottle, it is allowed to stand eight days in a dark, cool place. The tincture is then separated by decanting, straining and filtering.

Drug power of tincture, $\frac{1}{6}$.

Dilutions must be prepared as directed under Class III.

CINA.

Synonyms, Absinthium Santonica. Artemisia Cina, *Berg.* Artemisia Contra.

Nat. Ord., Compositæ.

Common Names, European Wormseed. Levant Wormseed. Tartarian Southernwood.

It is known that the drug brought to market under the name "wormseed" does not consist of seed, but of the undeveloped flowers, mixed with the scales of the calyx and the pedicels of different species of the genus artemisia. We prefer the sort brought us as *Semen Cinae* Levanticæ to all others; it consists of small, ovate-oblong, green-yellow flowerheads, becoming darker and more brownish by age, whose envelope is formed of tight recumbent, ovate, shining scales. They have a peculiar, nauseous, aromatic odor, which is somewhat like that of camphor, and a rough, loathsome, bitterish taste.

Cina was first proven by Hahnemann.

Preparation.—The dried flower, coarsely powdered, is covered with five parts by weight of alcohol, and allowed to stand eight days in a well-stoppered bottle, in a dark, cool place, being shaken twice a day. The tincture is then poured off, strained and filtered.

Drug power of tincture, $\frac{1}{10}$.

Dilutions must be prepared as directed under Class IV.

CINCHONINUM SULPHURICUM.

Synonym, Cinchoniæ Sulphas.

Common Name, Sulphate of Cinchonia.

Formula, $(C_{20}\ H_{24}\ N_2\ O)_2,\ H_2\ SO_4,\ 3H_2\ O$.

Molecular Weight, 768

Preparation of Sulphate of Cinchonia.—From the mother-liquor left after the crystallization out of sulphate of quinine, cinchonia is obtained by adding solution of soda in successive portions till the mother-liquor is slightly over-neutralized. The remaining alkaloids, including cinchonia, are thus precipitated and are to be thrown on a filter, washed with cold water and dried. The dried residue is to be washed several times with small amounts of cold alcohol, thus removing other alkaloids. The remaining portion is to be dissolved in eight or ten times its weight of water, the mixture heated, then neutralized with dilute sulphuric acid, and allowed to stand till a precipitate, if there be any, settles. Finally, animal charcoal is added and the whole boiled, filtered while hot, and the filtrate set aside to crystallize. The crystals are to be collected, drained and dried with bibulous paper.

Cinchonia-sulphate is in small, hard, white, or larger transparent oblique prisms, having a very bitter taste. They are soluble in sixty parts of water at medium temperatures, in five of ninety per cent. alcohol, in one and one-half of hot alcohol, and in thirty of chloroform; they are insoluble in ether.

Tests.—Sulphate of cinchonia when treated with chlorine water and afterward with caustic ammonia does not give the thalleiochin reaction as does quinia, nor does its solution in water show any fluorescence. When to a solution of a cinchonine salt, free from free acid or nearly so, is added potassium ferro-cyanide in excess, and the whole gently heated, there separates out on cooling, cinchonine ferro-cyanide in brilliant golden-yellow scales or in long needles, frequently arranged in the shape of a fan. The aid of the microscope is needed in examining the results of the reaction, and the test is then extremely delicate and characteristic.

Preparation for Homœopathic Use.—The pure sulphate of cinchonia is prepared by trituration, as directed under Class VII.

CINNABARIS.

Proper Name, Mercuric Sulphide.

Synonyms, Hydrargyri Sulphuretum Rubrum. Mercurius Sulphuratus Ruber.

Common Names, Vermilion. Red Sulphide of Mercury. Cinnabar.

Formula, Hg S.

Molecular Weight, 232.

Preparation of Cinnabar.—Mercuric sulphide in the native state is the chief source from which the metal mercury is obtained. It is readily prepared artificially, by subliming an intimate mixture of six parts of mercury and one of sulphur, and reducing the product to very fine powder. It is advised to use a pure commercial article rather than prepare it in the pharmaceutical laboratory.

Properties and Tests.—Mercuric sulphide comes in commerce as a fine powder of a brilliant scarlet-red color, the brilliancy of the tint depending in some degree upon the fineness of the powder. Its specific gravity is 7.75, while that of the native sulphide is 8. It is without odor or taste. Upon heating, it becomes darker in color and finally black, but upon cooling again it recovers its bright hue. Heated out of contact with air to a low red heat, it sublimes unchanged without previous fusion. If heated thus in the air it burns with the flame of burning sulphur, forming sulphurous oxide and liberating metallic mercury, which volatilizes without residue, if the article be pure. It is not decomposed by alkaline solutions, but nitro-muriatic acid dissolves it with the separation of sulphur. The absence of any residue after its volatilization on platinum foil, will show its freedom from iron oxide, red lead and lead chromate, which are used as adulterants. Arsenic and antimony may be detected by treating it with a warm alkaline solution, filtering, and after acidification, testing the filtrate with hydrogen sulphide in the usual way.

Cinnabar was introduced into the Homœopathic Materia Medica by Hahnemann.

Preparation for Homœopathic Use.—The pure cinnabar is prepared by trituration, as directed under Class VII.

CINNAMOMUM.

Synonyms, Cinnamomum Zeylanicum, *Nees.* Laurus Cinnamomum, *Linn.*

Nat. Ord., Lauraceæ.

Common Name, Cinnamon.

C. Zeylanicum is a small evergreen tree with a profuse foliage of beautiful shining leaves, somewhat glaucous beneath. Its flowers are greenish, in panicles, and possess a disagreeable odor. The tree is a native of Ceylon, where it grows at varying elevations in the forests. The bark is used in medicine, and the best varieties come from a strip of country twelve to fifteen miles broad, on the south-west coast of Ceylon, in the region of Colombo.

Description.—Ceylon cinnamon of the finest quality comes in sticks about three feet in length and three-eighths of an inch in thickness. The sticks are made up of tubular pieces of bark, ingeniously arranged one within the other so as to form an even rod of some firmness. The sticks are somewhat flattened-cylindrical in outline. The bark itself is extremely thin, often less than $\frac{1}{100}$ of an inch thick. It has a dull surface of light brown color, and upon it faintly marked waves are noticeable, as well as scars and holes outlining the points of insertion of leaves and twigs. The inner surface of the bark is of a darker hue. Cinnamon has a peculiar and agreeable odor, and an agreeable, sweet, pungent, aromatic taste.

Preparation.—The Ceylon cinnamon bark is coarsely powdered, and covered with five parts by weight of alcohol. Having poured it into a well-stoppered bottle, it is allowed to remain eight days in a dark, cool place, shaking it twice a day. The tincture is then poured off, strained and filtered.

Drug power of tincture, $\frac{1}{10}$.

Dilutions must be prepared as directed under Class IV.

CISTUS.

Synonyms, Cistus Canadense, *Linn.* Helianthemum Canadense, *Michaux.* Heteromeris Canadense.

Nat. Ord., Cistaceæ.

Common Names, Frost Wort. Holly Rose. Rock Rose.

A perennial herbaceous plant, found growing in all parts of the United States. It has a stem at first simple, leaves lanceolate, about an inch long, simple and entire. The primary or earlier flowers are large, yellow, and solitary. The secondary or later ones are small, axillary and nearly sessile, at times without petals. The large flowers and stem, hairy-pubescent. The fruit is a one-celled capsule. The plant gets its popular name from the fact that in late autumn moisture issues from the cracks in the bark near the root and is found congealed into ice-crystals in the early morning.

This remedy was introduced into our Materia Medica by Dr. Hering.

Preparation.—The fresh plant in flower is chopped and pounded to a pulp and weighed. Then two parts by weight of alcohol are taken, the pulp mixed thoroughly with one-sixth part of it and the rest of the alcohol added. After stirring the whole well, and pouring it into a well-stoppered bottle, it is allowed to remain eight days in a dark, cool place. The tincture is then separated by decanting, straining and filtering.

Amount of drug power, $\frac{1}{6}$.

Dilutions must be prepared as directed under Class III.

CLEMATIS.

Synonyms, Clematis Erecta, *Linn.* Flammula Jovis.
Nat. Ord., Ranunculaceæ.
Common Name, Upright Virgin's Bower.

In Central and Southern Europe this plant is to be found on sunny hills, among bushes and on the sides of forests. The stem is three to four feet high, erect, hollow, striped and smooth, has pinnate-cleft leaves, the incisions of which on the base are cordate or ovate, pointed and entire. Flowers, multipartite cymes, the sepals oblong-spatulate, naked, having at the margin on the outer side hair-like down; petals white, four. The fresh plant has a pungent acridity, irritating the nose and blistering the tongue when chewed.

It was first proven by Hahnemann, aided by Stapf and others.

Preparation.—The fresh leaves and stems of the plant just coming into bloom are chopped and pounded to a pulp, enclosed in a piece of new linen and submitted to pressure. The expressed juice is then, by brisk agitation, mingled with an equal part by weight of alcohol. This mixture is allowed to stand eight days in a dark, cool place, and then filtered.

Drug power of tincture, $\frac{1}{2}$.

Dilutions must be prepared as directed under Class I.

CLEMATIS VIRGINIANA, *Linn.*

Synonyms, Clematis Cordata. Clematis Purshii.
Nat. Ord., Ranunculaceæ.
Common Name, Common Virgin's Bower.

This is an indigenous climber, growing on river-banks, climbing over shrubs. Stems are smooth. Leaves with three ovate acute leaflets, which are deeply incised and somewhat cordate at the base; tails of the fruit plumose. The axillary peduncles bear clusters of numerous white flowers; the fertile ones succeeded in autumn by the conspicuous feathery tails of the fruit. Flowers appear in July and August.

Preparation.—The fresh leaves are chopped and pounded to a pulp and weighed. Then two parts by weight of alcohol are taken, the pulp mixed thoroughly with one-sixth part of it, and the rest of the alcohol added. After stirring the whole well, pour it into a well-stoppered bottle and let it stand eight days in a dark, cool place. The tincture is then separated by decanting, straining and filtering.

Drug power of tincture, $\frac{1}{6}$.

Dilutions must be prepared as directed under Class III.

CLEMATIS VITALBA, *Linn.*

Nat. Ord., Ranunculaceæ.
Common Names, Old Man's Beard. Traveller's Joy.

This is a climbing under-shrub growing in hedges and thickets, most common on chalky soil, in Europe, from Holland southward,

Northern Africa and Western Asia. Leaflets two to three inches long, ovate-cordate, entire, toothed or lobed; petioles persistent when twining. Flowers one inch in diameter, odorous, greenish-white. Sepals four, pubescent. Achenia hairy; awns one inch, feathery. Flowers appear in July and August.

Preparation.—The fresh leaves are chopped and pounded to a pulp and weighed. Then two parts by weight of alcohol are taken, the pulp mixed thoroughly with one-sixth part of it, and the rest of the alcohol added. After stirring the whole well, it is poured into a well-stoppered bottle, and allowed to stand eight days in a dark, cool place. The tincture is then separated by decanting, straining and filtering.

Drug power of tincture, $\frac{1}{6}$.

Dilutions must be prepared as directed under Class III.

COBALTUM METALLICUM.

Common Names, Cobalt. Metallic Cobalt.

Symbol, Co.

Atomic Weight, 58.8.

Cobalt is a metal not very abundant in nature; it exists in the free state only in meteorites. It is found in combination in the minerals *cobaltite*, *smaltite* and *erythrite*, all arsenical compounds. It is also found associated with nickel.

Preparation.—Cobalt is a steel-gray metal having a tinge of red. It is hard, granular in fracture and brittle, but at a red heat it becomes malleable; its specific gravity is about 8.8. In masses it tarnishes upon exposure to moist air, and at a red heat it oxidizes. It is dissolved slowly by hydrochloric and sulphuric acids; nitric acid dissolves it readily. For homœopathic use the metal is obtained in the spongy form by reducing the chloride, by passing through its solution a current of pure hydrogen.

Tests.—The precipitated metal is to be dissolved in hydrochloric acid; the solution is of a light red color, and by evaporating it the color changes toward the end of the operation to blue. The metal may be contaminated with nickel or the salts of the metal may contain arsenic. On dissolving the metal in hydrochloric acid and adding potassium cyanide a brownish-white precipitate of cobaltous cyanide occurs, which dissolves easily in an excess of the precipitant, from which solution it cannot be again precipitated by acids. If nickel be present the addition of hydrogen chloride to the solution of the cyanide precipitated as above stated produces the separation of a greenish, nickelous-cobalti-cyanide. Arsenic, if present in a salt of cobalt, may be detected by dissolving, acidifying with HCl and treating with H_2S, when the well known yellow sulphide of arsenic will fall.

Cobalt was introduced into the Homœopathic Materia Medica by Dr. Hering.

Preparation for Homœopathic Use.—The pure metal is prepared by trituration, as directed under Class VII.

COCA.

Synonyms, Erythroxylon Coca, *Lamarck.* Hayo. Ipadu.

Nat. Ord., Lineæ (sub-order, Erythroxyleæ).

Common Name, Coca.

E. Coca is a shrub about four feet in height, indigenous to Peru and Bolivia, where it is cultivated, as it is also in some parts of Brazil and other parts of South America. The leaves are the parts used in medicine; their average length is about two inches, and their greatest breadth is about one inch; they are ovate or obovate, sometimes obtuse, often emarginate, glabrous. The upper surface is dirty-green, the under is paler. The midrib is prominent, and on each side of it, about a quarter of an inch from its central point, is a curved line extending from base to apex. The portion of the leaf between the two curved lines is distinctly darker in color than the rest, as may be seen by examining the leaf by transmitted light but in very young leaves this characteristic is somewhat difficult to recognize. Their odor is weakly aromatic, and their taste is somewhat warm, bitter and aromatic. The leaves are sun-dried for use, but they lose their virtues in great part upon prolonged exposure to the air. After a year's keeping they should be rejected.

It was first proven under Dr. Clotar Müller's direction, in Germany.

Preparation.—The dried leaves, coarsely powdered, are covered with five parts by weight of alcohol, and allowed to remain eight days in a well-stoppered bottle, in a dark, cool place, and shaken twice a day. The tincture is then poured off, strained and filtered.

Drug power of tincture, $\frac{1}{10}$.

Dilutions must be prepared as directed under Class IV.

COCCINELLA.

Synonyms, Chrysomela Septempunctata, *Linn.* Coccinella Septempunctata.

Class, Insecta.

Order, Coleoptera.

Family, Coccinellidæ.

Common Names, Lady-Bird. Lady-Cow. Sun-Chafer.

This is a very well known and widely spread insect, living on vegetables in gardens and fields. Its head and thorax are black, flat, underbody and feet black, wing-shells arched, oval, red or orange-yellow, with black dots, usually seven in number, of unequal size, the wings nearly as long again as the body. When touched with the hand there issues from the joints of the feet a thickish juice, yellow like gamboge.

It was proven by Dr. Claussnitzer, Germany.

Preparation.—The live insects, collected in the month of June, are pounded to a pulp and covered with five parts by weight of alcohol. Having poured the mixture into a well-stoppered bottle, it is allowed to remain eight days in a dark, cool place, and shaken twice a day. The tincture is then poured off, strained and filtered.

Drug power of tincture, $\frac{1}{10}$.

Dilutions must be prepared as directed under Class IV.

COCCULUS.

Synonyms, Anamirta Cocculus, *Wight and Arnott.* Cocculus Indicus. Menispermum Cocculus, *Linn.*

Nat. Ord., Menispermaceæ.

Common Name, India Berries.

A. Cocculus is a strong climbing shrub found in the eastern parts of the Indian Peninsula, in Eastern Bengal and in the Malay Islands. The fruit, a purple drupe, is used in medicine, and when removed from the stalk and dried, has the appearance of a small, round berry. It is about as large as a pea, somewhat oval or nearly reniform, with a blackish, wrinkled, dry pericarp, covering a thin, woody endocarp, within which is a single reniform kernel or seed. The seed is bitter and oily. The drug is preferred when of dark color, free from stalks, fresh and with the seeds evidently well preserved.

The drug was first proved by Hahnemann.

Preparation.—The dried fruit, coarsely powdered, is covered with five parts by weight of alcohol, poured into a well-stoppered bottle, and allowed to remain eight days at a moderate temperature in a dark place, being shaken twice a day. The tincture is then poured off, strained and filtered.

Drug power of tincture, $\frac{1}{10}$.

Dilutions must be prepared as directed under Class IV.

COCCUS CACTI, *Linn.*

Synonym, Coccinella Indica.

Class, Insecta.

Order, Hemiptera.

Family, Coccidæ.

Common Name, Cochineal.

The cochineal insect is a true hemipterous cicada; it is a native of Mexico, but is found in the West and East Indies, as well as in Spain and Java.

The male insect is red, small, gnat-like, more active and less bulky than the female. The female is larger than the male, of oval form with thorax and back convex, without wings, body transversely striated and of a dark red color. The back is covered with a white down. After fecundation the females enlarge greatly, and attach themselves to the cactus plants and die; the eggs mature within the dead parent and the young soon emerge. The latter are allowed to grow till the females are fecundated, when, with the exception of a few left for breeding, they are brushed off the plants, killed by hot water and sun-dried.

It was proven by Dr. Wachtel and other Austrian provers.

Preparation.—The dried insects, previously cleansed by agitation with tepid water, are coarsely powdered, and then covered with five parts by weight of alcohol; having poured the whole into a well-stoppered bottle, it is allowed to remain fourteen days in a dark, cool place, and shaken twice a day. The tincture is then poured off, strained and filtered.

Drug power of tincture, $\frac{1}{10}$.

Dilutions must be prepared as directed under Class IV.

CODEINUM.

Synonyms, Codeia. Codeine. Codein.

Formula, $C_{18}\,H_{21}\,NO_3$.

Codeine is one of the alkaloids existing in opium.

Preparation.—In the process of extracting morphia from opium (see article Morphinum), the hydrochlorates of both morphia and codeine are formed. They are separated by treating their solution with ammonia which precipitates the greater part of the morphia, leaving the codeine in solution. The filtrate is evaporated over the water-bath to expel the excess of ammonia, the morphine salt remaining in the solution being at the same time precipitated; after filtering, the saline solution is concentrated and precipitated by potassium hydrate, and the precipitate of codeine is washed, dried and redissolved in ether whence it is deposited in crystals.

Properties.—Codeine crystallizes from anhydrous ether in small anhydrous rectangular octohedrons, truncated and modified in various ways. It dissolves in water more readily than does morphine, especially if the water be boiling, requiring eighty parts of water at medium temperatures and seventeen at 100° C. (212° F.). When heated with a quantity of water insufficient to dissolve it, it melts to an oily mass which remains at the bottom of the liquid. It dissolves easily in alcohol and hydrated ether, less readily in anhydrous ether. It is insoluble in potash solution. Codeine is a strong base, restoring the blue color to reddened litmus paper, and precipitating the salts of lead, iron, copper, nickel, etc. Its salts are generally crystallizable and of a very bitter taste. From water or hydrated ether it crystallises in large rhombic prisms.

Tests.—It is indifferent to ferric chloride and to iodic acid, and thus is distinguished from morphine. When dissolved in concentrated sulphuric acid it forms a nearly colorless solution, but if a trace of ferric chloride be added a blue or violet coloration occurs. Treated with Frohde's reagent, which is made by dissolving 0.01 gramme of molybdate of sodium in 10 CC. of concentrated sulphuric acid, and prepared freshly when needed, a green color first appears, soon followed by blue, and after some hours changing to yellow. Commercial codeine may contain morphia, and the drug is said to be not infrequently sophisticated with sugar and gum arabic. Morphia or its salts may be detected by their insolubility in ether and their behavior when treated with ferric chloride; the presence of sugar will be known by the greater solubility of the specimen in water and by its smaller solubility in alcohol. Gum arabic may be detected by the brown color of the solution in concentrated sulphuric acid.

It was first proved by Dr. E. E. Marcy, United States.

Preparation.—The pure codeia is prepared by trituration as directed under Class VII.

COFFEA.

Synonyms, Coffea Arabica, *Linn.* Coffea Cruda.
Nat. Ord., Rubiaceæ.
Common Name, Coffee.

This well known, universally spread, and important article of trade requires no particular description. For medicinal use we select the sort sold under the surname Levantic (Mocha beans), consisting of small, more roundish than flat, not very dark, yellowish-gray-green beans, and having a peculiar, strong smell of coffee.

It was proved by Hahnemann.

Preparation.—One part of the best unroasted coffee-beans is coarsely powdered in an iron mortar, moderately heated, and macerated eight days with six parts of strong alcohol, and then filtered. The residuum is then boiled down in a glass retort with forty parts of distilled water, so far that its filtrate and the alcoholic extract mixed together make ten parts by weight.

Drug power of tincture, $\frac{1}{10}$.

Dilutions.—This tincture is potentized according to Class IV, with regard to strength, but the 2x and 3x and 1 dilutions, must be prepared with dilute alcohol.

COLCHICUM.

Synonym, Colchicum Autumnale, *Linn.*
Nat. Ord., Melanthaceæ.
Common Names, Colchicum. Meadow Saffron. Naked Lady.

This perennial plant grows in many districts of Germany, France and the south of Europe, in meadows, where it flowers in autumn and announces the beginning of winter. The root forms a bulb, of the size of a pigeon's egg, round on one side and flat on the other, and furnished with fibrous radicles at its base; naturally it is covered with dark coats, of which the external one is brown, the inner shining and of a clear color; in the fresh state it contains a milky juice of an acrid, bitter taste, and disagreeable odor. The flower rises in autumn immediately from a lateral bulb which the bulb of the preceding year has produced, and which has grown during winter and spring; the flowers are rose-colored, with long tubes, disappearing in a few days, and are followed by leaves only in the following spring; the leaves are large, flat, erect, spear-shaped, about five inches long and one inch broad at the base, and come off with the capsules, which are triangular, sessile, three-pointed; the seeds are round, ovoid, wrinkled, and deep brown.

The first provings were by E. Stapf, Hahnemann, and others in Germany.

Preparation.—The fresh bulb, gathered shortly before coming into bloom, is chopped and pounded to a fine pulp, enclosed in a piece of new linen and subjected to pressure. The expressed juice is then, by brisk agitation, mingled with an equal part by weight of alcohol. This mixture is allowed to stand eight days in a well-stoppered bottle, in a dark, cool place, and then filtered.

Drug power of tincture, $\frac{1}{2}$.

Dilutions must be prepared as directed under Class I.

COLLINSONIA.

Synonym, Collinsonia Canadensis, *Linn.*

Nat. Ord., Labiatæ.

Common Names, Horse-Weed. Knot-Root. Stone-Root.

This is an indigenous plant, found growing in rich, moist woods, from Canada to Florida, and west to Michigan. Root perennial, knotty, depressed, very hard, with many slender fibres; stem smooth, simple, round, straight, one to three feet high; leaves serrate, with broad teeth, pointed, long-petioled, only two or three pairs, these cordate at base, broadly ovate, acuminate, surface smooth, with small veins. Flowers opposite, on long peduncles, with short subulate bracteoles, forming a terminal leafless panicle with branched racemes. Corolla two-thirds of an inch long, yellow, tubular at base, spreading above in two lips, upper lip very short and notched, lower lip fringed. Stamens two, long, protruding, filaments filiform, anther oval, style protruding. Seeds often abortive, only one ripening.

Proved by Dr. Burt, U. S.

Preparation.—The fresh root, collected either in early spring or late autumn, is chopped and pounded to a pulp and weighed. Then two parts by weight of alcohol are taken, the pulp mixed thoroughly with one-sixth part of it, and the rest of the alcohol added. After stirring the whole well, it is poured into a well-stoppered bottle, and allowed to stand eight days in a dark, cool place. The tincture is then separated by decanting, straining and filtering.

Drug power of tincture, $\frac{1}{6}$.

Dilutions must be prepared as directed under Class III.

COLOCYNTHIS.

Synonyms, Citrullus Colocynthis, *Schrader.* Cucumis Colocynthis, *Linn.*

Nat. Ord., Cucurbitaceæ.

Common Names, Bitter Cucumber. Colocynth.

The colocynth plant is slender, scabrous, has a perennial root, and grows in warm and dry regions of the Western Hemisphere. It is found in immense quantities in upper Egypt and Nubia. The fruit is a pepo, of the size and shape of a small orange, having a smooth, marbled-green surface. It is usually peeled with a knife and dried, and is found in commerce as a light, pithy, nearly white ball, consisting of the dried internal pulp of the fruit with the seeds imbedded therein. The pulp is nearly inodorous, but has an intensely bitter taste.

Colocynth was introduced into our Materia Medica by Hahnemann.

Preparation.—The dried fruit, freed from the outer yellow rind and seeds, is reduced to coarse powder and weighed. Then five parts by weight of alcohol are poured upon it, and having been put into a well-stoppered bottle, the mixture is allowed to remain eight days in a dark, cool place, being shaken twice a day. The tincture is then poured off, strained and filtered.

Drug power of tincture, $\frac{1}{10}$.

Dilutions must be prepared as directed under Class IV.

COMOCLADIA DENTATA, *Jacq.*

Synonym, Guao.

Nat. Ord., Anacardiaceæ.

Common Names, Bastard Brazil Wood. Tooth-leaved Maiden-Plum.

This is a very common tree in the island of Cuba, where it is found growing near the coast, luxuriating mostly on barren or stony soils. It is from six to eight feet high, having beautiful dark green leaves, with a brownish border. The flowers are small, bluish-brown, in clusters. The trunk and branches contain a milky fluid that turns black on exposure to sunlight, discoloring the skin, linen, etc. A superstition is entertained that death results from sleeping in its shade.

Preparation.—The fresh bark is chopped and pounded to a pulp and weighed. Then two parts by weight of alcohol are taken, the pulp mixed thoroughly with one-sixth part of it, and the rest of the alcohol added. After stirring the whole well, and pouring it into a well-stoppered bottle, it is allowed to stand eight days in a dark, cool place. The tincture is then separated by decanting, straining and filtering.

Amount of drug power, $\frac{1}{6}$.

Dilutions must be prepared as directed under Class III.

CONDURANGO.

Synonym, Gonolobus Cundurango, *Triana.*

Nat. Ord., Asclepiadaceæ.

Common Name, Condor Plant.

What is known as condurango is the bark of a climbing shrub growing in Ecuador at an altitude of from 3000 to 5000 feet above the sea-level. The bark comes in quills and in half-cylindrical pieces of various lengths, ashy-gray in color, having attached to it different varieties of lichen, forming greenish or dark-colored blotches. Its fracture is fibrous, and the ends are studded with fine yellow points. The taste of the dried bark is aromatic and bitter.

The drug was proved by Dr. J. C. Burnett, England.

Preparation.—The dried bark, coarsely powdered, is covered with five parts by weight of alcohol, and allowed to remain eight days in a well-stoppered bottle, in a dark, cool place, being shaken twice a day. The tincture is then poured off, strained and filtered.

Drug power of tincture, $\frac{1}{10}$.

Dilutions must be prepared as directed under Class IV.

Triturations are prepared from the dried bark finely powdered, as directed under Class VII.

CONIUM.

Synonyms, Conium Maculatum, *Linn.* Coriandrum Cicuta.

Nat. Ord., Umbelliferæ.

Common Name, Spotted Hemlock. Poison Hemlock.

This plant is a native of Europe, but has been naturalized in the eastern portion of the United States, where it is found growing in wet meadows and in waste grounds. The root is biennial, whitish and spindle-shaped. Stem herbaceous, round, hollow and marked with purple-brown splashes or spots. Lower leaves tri-ternate; the upper ones bi-ternate. Leaflets one to three inches long, finely serrate, deep green above, paler beneath. Flowers, small, white in compound terminal umbels, with no involucre, involucels of five or six short bracts. Petals five, obcordate, with inflected points.

Conium was first proven by Hahnemann.

Preparation.—The entire fresh plant, root excepted, gathered about the time the flowers begin to fade, is chopped and pounded to a fine pulp, enclosed in a piece of new linen and subjected to pressure. The expressed juice is then, by brisk agitation, mingled with an equal part by weight of alcohol. This mixture is allowed to stand eight days in a well-stoppered bottle, in a dark, cool place, and then filtered.

Drug power of tincture, $\frac{1}{2}$.

Dilutions must be prepared as directed under Class I.

CONVALLARIA.

Synonym, Convallaria Majalis, *Linn.*

Nat. Ord., Liliaceæ.

Common Name, Lily of the Valley.

A perennial herb, found in shady woods in the United States from Virginia to Georgia, although cultivated farther north. It is found also in Europe. The rhizome is creeping and slender, and from it arises a slender scape bearing a one-sided raceme of small, elegant, white, bell-shaped flowers Leaves radical, two or at times three, smooth and elliptical. Perianth of six united segments which are recurved. The flowers are sweet-scented and appear in May.

Preparation.—The entire fresh plant, gathered when coming into flower, is chopped and pounded to a fine pulp, enclosed in a piece of new linen, and subjected to pressure. The expressed juice is then, by brisk agitation, mingled with an equal part by weight of alcohol.

This mixture is allowed to stand eight days in a well-stoppered bottle, in a dark, cool place, and then filtered.

Drug power of tincture, $\frac{1}{2}$.

Dilutions must be prepared as directed under Class I.

CONVOLVULUS.

Synonyms, Convolvulus Arvensis, *Linn.*

Nat. Ord., Convolvulaceæ.

Common Name, Bindweed.

This perennial is very common in Europe, Asia, Africa, and America, in fields, near the coast. Its low stem is procumbent or twining; leaves ovate-oblong, saggitate, lobes at the base acute; peduncles mostly one-flowered; bracts minute, remote; corolla white or tinged with red, about three-quarters of an inch long; calyx naked at the base; corolla infundibular or campanulate; stamens included; style one; stigmas two, elongated, linear, often revolute. Pod two-celled; the cells two-seeded. Flowers in June.

Preparation.—The fresh blooming plant, allowed to wither a little before manipulation, is chopped and pounded to a pulp and weighed. Then two parts by weight of alcohol are taken, the pulp mixed thoroughly with one-sixth part of it, and the rest of the alcohol added. After having stirred the whole well, pour it into a well-stoppered bottle, and let it stand eight days in a dark, cool place. The tincture is then separated by decanting, straining and filtering.

Drug power of tincture, $\frac{1}{6}$.

Dilutions must be prepared as directed under Class III.

CONVOLVULUS DUARTINUS.

Synonyms, Ipomœa Bona Nox, *Linn.* Calonyetion Speciosum, *De Candolle.*

Nat. Ord., Convolvulaceæ.

Common Name, Morning Glory (not the common Morning Glory which is *I. purpurea, Lam.*).

This is a climbing plant, native of the West Indies, but cultivated in America and Europe. Its leaves are large, entire, cordate, alternate, on long petioles, generally arising from the axils of the flower-bearing branches. Calyx with five unequal folioles, the three outer ones sharp, the two inner ones oval and foliaceous. Corolla white, large, expanding into a large circular limb. Stamens five, adhering by their filaments to the tube of the corolla which is shorter than the stamens. Anthers linear, acuminate. The base of the ovary is surrounded by a glandular disk; style very long, filiform, terminated by a shaggy, bi-lobate stigma; fruit with a coriaceous tegument. There are two or three flowers on the flower-bearing pedicles; they resemble a trumpet in shape, whence their Brazilian name, "herva trombetta."

The drug was proven by Dr. Manoel Duarte Moreira, Brazil.

Preparation.—The fresh flowers are pounded to a pulp and weighed. Then two parts by weight of alcohol are taken, the pulp mixed thoroughly with one-sixth part of it, and the rest of the alcohol added. After stirring the whole well, pour it into a well-stoppered bottle, and let it stand eight days in a dark, cool place. The tincture is then separated by decanting, straining and filtering.

Drug power of tincture, $\frac{1}{6}$.

Dilutions must be prepared as directed under Class III.

COPAIBA OFFICINALIS.

Species' Name, Copaifera Officinalis, *Linn.*

Nat. Ord., Leguminosæ.

Common Name, Balsam of Copaiba.

Balsam of copaiba is the product of trees belonging to the genus *Copaifera,* natives of the warmer countries of South America. The best known is *C. officinalis,* a large tree found in the hot coast-region of New Granada, Venezuela and Trinidad.

In order to collect the oleo-resin, holes are bored into the wood of the tree, whence it soon pours out. The secretion is very abundant, and indeed it is stated on good authority, that occasionally in the untapped trees, the oleo-resin collects in such quantity within the numerous ducts, that the trunk is actually burst asunder.

Description.—Copaiba is a more or less viscid fluid, whose color varies from pale yellow to light golden-brown. It has a peculiar aromatic odor which is not unpleasant, and a persistent, acrid, bitter taste. Its specific gravity is between 0.94 and 0.99. By keeping, it becomes more viscid. When the number of species of copaiba-bearing trees is considered, it will be seen that its composition and even its physical properties must vary; but a specimen may be considered pure if it dissolve in several times its weight of alcohol, specific gravity, 0.830; if, when treated with one-third its own volume of ammonia, it give a mixture perfectly transparent, and if when its volatile oil is evaporated, only a hard resin remain (without any non-volatile oil). It should not possess in any degree the odor of turpentine.

Hahnemann mentions the drug in his Fragmenta, and under Teste, in France, a number of provings were made.

Preparation.—The balsam is dissolved in the proportion of one part by weight, to ninety-nine parts by weight of 95 per cent. alcohol, and designated mother-tincture.

Drug power of tincture, $\frac{1}{100}$.

Dilutions must be prepared as directed under Class VI—β.

COPTIS.

Synonyms, Coptis Trifolia, *Salisbury.* Helleborus Trifolius, *Linn.*

Nat. Ord., Ranunculaceæ.

Common Name, Gold-Thread.

This plant is a small evergreen, indigenous to the northern part of North America, and indeed to the higher latitudes of both hemispheres.

Its root is perennial, creeping, of long, bright yellow fibres, whence the common name of the plant. From it arises a naked, slender, one-flowered scape, three to five inches high. The flowers are small, white, having five to seven petals. Leaves radical, glabrous, ternately divided; leaflets of obovate wedge form, obscurely three-lobed, and sharply dentate. The plant is glabrous, without odor, and has a strongly bitter taste. Flowers appear in May.

Preparation.—The fresh root is chopped and pounded to a pulp and weighed. Then two parts by weight of alcohol are taken, the pulp mixed thoroughly with one-sixth part of it, and the rest of the alcohol added. After stirring the whole well, pour it into a well-stoppered bottle, and let it stand eight days in a dark, cool place. The tincture is then separated by decanting, straining and filtering.

Drug power of tincture, $\frac{1}{6}$.

Dilutions must be prepared as directed under Class III.

CORALLIUM RUBRUM.

Synonyms, Corallium Rubrum, *Lamarck.* Gorgonia Nobilis. Isis Nobilis, *Linn.*

Class, Zoophytes.

Family, Gorgoniadeæ.

Common Name, Red Coral.

Red coral is the skeleton of the coral zoophyte. In most instances it branches into shrub-like forms. The variety we use is pinkish-red in color. The chemical constituents are calcium carbonate, with a trace of magnesium carbonate and a little more than four per cent. of ferric oxide as coloring matter; there is also a small amount of animal matter.

The red coral was first proved by Dr. Attomyr, in Germany.

Preparation.—For homœopathic use the small, branchy, striated pieces, which often have a white calcareous covering, are reduced to a fine powder, and triturated as directed under Class VII.

CORALLORHIZA ODONTORHIZA, *Nuttall.*

Synonym, Corallorhiza Wistariana, *Conrad.*

Nat. Ord., Orchidaceæ.

Common Name, Coral Root.

This plant is a parasite, of a light brown or purplish color, with much branched, toothed, coral-like root-stocks; stem rather slender, bulbous, at the base, and from six to sixteen inches high, bearing from six to twenty flowers; pedicels rather slender; lip entire, or merely denticulate, thin, broadly ovate or obovate, abruptly contracted into a claw-like base, the lamellæ a pair of short projections; the spur represented by a small cavity wholly adnate to the summit of the ovary; pod at first very acute at the base, at length short-oval, about four lines long. Perianth about three lines long. Flowers small, lip whitish or purplish, often mottled with crimson, appear from May to July. The plant is found in rich woods, from New York to Michigan, and especially southward.

Preparation.—The fresh root is chopped and pounded to a pulp and weighed. Then two parts by weight of alcohol are taken, the pulp mixed thoroughly with one-sixth part of it, and the rest of the alcohol added. After having mixed the whole well together, pour it into a well-stoppered bottle, and let it stand eight days in a dark, cool place. The tincture is then separated by decanting, straining and filtering.

Amount of drug power, $\frac{1}{6}$.

Dilutions must be prepared as directed under Class III.

CORNUS CIRCINATA, *L'Heritier.*

Synonyms, Cornus Rugosa. Cornus Tomentulosa.

Nat. Ord., Cornaceæ.

Common Names, Cornel. Green Osier. Round-Leaved Dogwood. Swamp Sassafras.

A shrub six to ten feet high, with green, warty branches, large roundish leaves, pointed, and woolly beneath; flowers white, in flat cymes. The fruit is a light blue drupe. The plant is a native of the United States, extending from Canada to Maryland. It flowers in June.

The first provings were made by Dr. E. E. Marcy, U. S.

Preparation.—The fresh bark is chopped and pounded to a pulp and weighed. Then two parts by weight of alcohol are taken, the pulp mixed thoroughly with one-sixth part of it, and the rest of the alcohol added. After stirring the whole well, pour it into a well-stoppered bottle, and let it stand eight days in a dark, cool place. The tincture is then separated by decanting, straining and filtering.

Drug power of tincture, $\frac{1}{6}$.

Dilutions must be prepared as directed under Class III.

CORNUS FLORIDA, *Linn.*

Nat. Ord., Cornaceæ.

Common Name, American Boxwood. Flowering Dogwood. New England Boxwood.

A small indigenous tree, usually from twelve to thirty feet high. It is of short growth; the stem is compact, and covered with a brownish bark, which is minutely divided by numerous superficial fissures. The leaves are opposite, ovate, pointed, acute at the base, dark green above, glaucous beneath. The flowers are small, aggregated in heads, surrounded by an involucre, corolla-like, of four inversely heart-shaped white leaves, very showy. Fruit a brilliant red drupe.

Preparation.—The fresh bark is chopped and pounded to a pulp and weighed. Then two parts by weight of alcohol are taken, the pulp mixed thoroughly with one-sixth part of it, and the rest of the alcohol added. After stirring the whole well, pour it into a well-stoppered bottle, and let it stand eight days in a dark, cool place. The tincture is then separated by decanting, straining and filtering.

Drug power of tincture, $\frac{1}{6}$.
Dilutions must be prepared as directed under Class III.

CORNUS SERICEA, *L'Heritier.*

Synonyms, Cornus Alba. Cornus Cœrulea. Cornus Cyanocarpus.
Nat. Ord., Cornaceæ.
Common Names, Silky Cornel. Blue-Berried Cornus. Female Dog-wood. Swamp Dogwood.
A shrub, usually three to ten feet in height, with erect stems, which are covered with a shining reddish bark. The young shoots are more or less pubescent. Branches spreading, purplish, leaves narrow, ovate, pointed and silky-downy underneath, often rust-colored. Flowers yellowish-white, in flat close cymes. Fruit a pale blue drupe. It is found in the United States from Canada to Carolina, in moist woods, in swamps, and on the borders of streams. It flowers in June and July.
Preparation.—The fresh bark is chopped and pounded to a pulp and weighed. Then two parts by weight of alcohol are taken, the pulp mixed thoroughly with one-sixth part of it, and the rest of the alcohol added. After having stirred the whole well, pour it into a well-stoppered bottle, and let it stand eight days in a dark, cool place. The tincture is then separated by decanting, straining and filtering.
Drug power of tincture, $\frac{1}{6}$.
Dilutions must be prepared as directed under Class III.

CORYDALIS FORMOSA, *Pursh.*

Synonyms, Dicentra Eximia, *De Candolle.* Dielytra.
Nat. Ord., Fumariaceæ.
Common Names, Fumitory. Squirrel Corn. Stagger Weed. Turkey Pea.
A native plant, growing on rocks in New York and southward to North Carolina. Its rhizome is scaly; leaves radical, numerous, somewhat tri-ternate; flowers nodding, purple, in compound racemes; corolla oblong, with short, obtuse, incurved spurs.
Preparation.—The fresh root is chopped and pounded to a pulp and weighed. Then two parts by weight of alcohol are taken, the pulp mixed thoroughly with one-sixth part of it, and the rest of the alcohol added. Having stirred the whole well, pour it into a well-stoppered bottle, and let it stand eight days in a dark, cool place. The tincture is then separated by decanting, straining and filtering.
Amount of drug power, $\frac{1}{6}$.
Dilutions must be prepared as directed under Class III.

COTYLEDON.

Synonyms, Cotyledon Umbilicus, *Linn.* Umbilicus Pendulinus, *De Candolle.*

Nat. Ord., Crassulaceæ.

Common Names, Kidneywort. Navelwort. Pennywort.

A perennial herbaceous plant, native of Western Europe, growing on rocks, old walls, etc. From its fleshy, tuberous root rises a stem, six inches high, bearing in the form of a spike, numerous, small, greenish-yellow, tubular, bell-shaped flowers. The leaves are fleshy, smooth, peltate, crenate, the upper ones somewhat smaller than the lower.

Cotyledon was proven by Dr. Wm. Craig, England.

Preparation.—The fresh leaves are chopped and pounded to a pulp and weighed. Then two parts by weight of alcohol are taken, the pulp mixed thoroughly with one-sixth part of it, and the rest of the alcohol added. After stirring the whole well, pour it into a well-stoppered bottle, and let it stand eight days in a dark, cool place. The tincture is then separated by decanting, straining and filtering.

Drug power of tincture, $\frac{1}{6}$.

Dilutions must be prepared as directed under Class III.

CROCUS.

Synonyms, Crocus Sativus, *Linn.* Crocus Autumnalis. Crocus Hispanicus.

Nat. Ord., Iridaceæ.

Common Name, Saffron.

Crocus sativus is a small plant having a fleshy, bulb-like corm and grassy leaves. It has a large, elegant, purple-colored flower. The style terminates in three long tubular and filiform stigmas projecting beyond the perianth. The stigmas are orange-red in color and possess a peculiar aromatic smell and pungent taste. The stigmas are the part used in medicine.

The drug was first proven by Stapf, in Germany.

Preparation.—The dried stigmas of the flowers are coarsely pulverized and weighed, and then covered with nine parts by weight of alcohol. After having poured the mixture into a well-stoppered bottle, let it remain eight days in a dark, cool place, shaking twice a day. The tincture is then poured off, strained and filtered.

Drug power of tincture, $\frac{1}{10}$.

Dilutions must be prepared as directed under Class IV.

CROTALUS CASCAVELLA.

Class, Reptilia.

Order, Ophidia.

Family, Crotalidæ.

Common Name, Brazilian Rattlesnake.

This terrible serpent is found in the Province of Ceara. This species generally attains a length of from four to five feet, but the animal from which the poison was taken for the provings, was three feet long. Its oval-triangular head, one half of which is provided with shields, shows a round depression in front of the eyes, which are covered with a large elliptical shield, serving as a lid. The body is big, conical; its movements are sluggish; its upper surface is covered with scales, the dorsal scales being keeled and somewhat lanceolate, the scales of the tail being quadrangular and smaller. The belly is provided with one hundred and seventy large transversal plates; there are twenty-five plates belonging to the tail, the first three of which are divided in shields. The extremity of the tail is furnished with seven or eight capsules of the consistence of parchment, which, when agitated, produce a shrill sound. The color of the crotalus is yellowish-brown, much lighter under the belly, with twenty-six regular long rhomboidal lines on each side of the back. When irritated and during the excessive heat, the crotalus emits a very fetid musk-like odor. The fangs are long and inserted in exceedingly dilatable jaws. The poison of this reptile acts with a frightful intensity, and it was not without great danger that Drs. Mure and Martins succeeded in obtaining a few drops of it.

This drug was introduced into our Materia Medica by Dr. Mure, of Brazil.

Preparation.—The poison, obtained by compressing the secreting gland of the living animal is triturated as directed under Class VIII.

CROTALUS HORRIDUS, *Linn.*

Synonym, Crotalus Durissus.
Order, Ophidia.
Family, Crotalidæ.
Common Name, Rattlesnake.

This poisonous serpent is frequently found in the mountainous and adjacent regions of the Northern and Southern States. It attains a length of from four to six feet, gradually swelling towards the middle, where it is from five to eight inches in circumference; back and sides covered with keeled scales; belly with unkeeled scales, which are always single under the tail. Head broad and triangular, with a large pit on each side below and in front of the eye; fangs one-half to one inch long; the tail has seven or eight capsules of the consistency of parchment, which, when agitated, produce a shrill rattle. Ground color of back varies from yellowish-tawny to brownish-grey. There are a central and two lateral rows of dark spots along the back, confluent on posterior half of body. Tail generally black.

The provings were made from triturations of the venom with sugar of milk and from dilutions prepared from them.

The venom of this deadly snake may be obtained by pressing the poison gland situated between the ear and eye, the serpent being either pinioned or chloroformed, and as the venom drops from the fangs it is received on pulverized sugar of milk, with which it is triturated, in proportion of one to ninety-nine.

Of late the preservation and potentiation of the venom in glycerine has been recommended, but we fail to see any valid reason for departing from Hering's mode of preparing the poison by trituration, especially as the provings were made from such preparations.

The drug was first proven by Dr. Hering.

Preparation.—The poison obtained as explained above is triturated as directed under Class VIII.

CROTON TIGLIUM, *Linn.*

Synonyms, Tiglium Officinale, *Klotsch.* Grana Tiglii.

Nat. Ord., Euphorbiaceæ.

Common Names, Croton Oil. Croton Tree. Purging Nut.

Croton tiglium is a small tree fifteen to twenty feet high, indigenous to India, and cultivated in many parts of the East. The tree has small inconspicuous flowers. The fruit is a brown capsule, three-celled, each cell containing one seed.

Description.—The croton seed is somewhat larger than a coffee bean, ovoid, having two faces, one arched constituting the dorsal, the other and flatter the ventral side. The surface of the seed is covered with a cinnamon-brown epidermis, beneath which is a thin, brittle black testa filled with a whitish, oily kernel. The taste of the seed is at first merely oily, but soon becomes acrid and unpleasant.

Properties.—From the kernels is obtained by expression croton oil, the *Oleum crotonis*, or Oleum tiglii of pharmacy, to the amount of fifty or sixty per cent. The oil is a transparent, sherry-colored, viscid liquid, slightly fluorescent, has a faint rancid smell, and an oleaginous acrid taste.

The attention of the homœopathic profession seems to have been first called to the drug by Dr. Hermann, and subsequent provings were collected by Dr. Buchner, in Germany.

Preparation for Homœopathic Use.—One part by weight of pure croton oil is dissolved in ninety-nine parts by weight of alcohol.

Amount of drug power, $\frac{1}{100}$.

Dilutions must be prepared as directed under Class VI—*β*.

Triturations are prepared as directed under Class VIII.

CUBEBA.

Synonyms, Piper Cubeba, *Linn.* Cubeba Officinalis, *Miquel.*

Nat. Ord., Piperaceæ.

Common Names, Cubeb Pepper. Cubebs.

Piper cubeba is a climbing, woody, diœcious shrub, indigenous to Java, Borneo and Sumatra.

Properties.—The fruit is a globose berry, of which a considerable number are attached by rather long stalks to a common rachis. The berries as found in commerce are spherical, wrinkled, and grayish-brown or blackish in color. Cubebs have a strong aromatic taste, with some bitterness; their odor is aromatic and not unpleasant.

Preparation.—The dried berries are coarsely powdered and covered with five parts by weight of alcohol. After mixing well, pour the whole into a well-stoppered bottle, and let it remain eight days in a dark, cool place, shaking it twice a day. The tincture is then poured off, strained and filtered.

Drug power of tincture, $\frac{1}{10}$.
Dilutions must be prepared as directed under Class IV.

CUCURBITA PEPO, *Linn.*

Nat. Ord., Cucurbitaceæ.
Common Name, Pumpkin.

This plant is an annual, a native of the Levant, but has been long cultivated as a garden vegetable or as food for cattle. The plant is hispid and scabrous, with procumbent stem; leaves large, cordate, palmately five-lobed or angled, denticulate; flowers are axillary, large, yellow, on long peduncles; fruit very large, at times two or three feet in diameter, roundish or oblong, furrowed, smooth, and when mature orange-yellow in color. Flowers in July.

Preparation.—The fresh stems are pounded to a pulp and weighed. Then two parts by weight of alcohol are taken, the pulp mixed thoroughly with one-sixth part of it, and the rest of the alcohol added. After having stirred the whole well, pour it into a well-stoppered bottle, and let it stand eight days in a dark, cool place. The tincture is then separated by decanting, straining and filtering.

Amount of drug power, $\frac{1}{6}$.
Dilutions must be prepared as directed under Class III.

CUPRUM.

Synonym, Cuprum Metallicum.
Common Name, Copper.
Symbol, Cu.
Atomic Weight, 63.5.

Origin.—Copper exists in nature in the free state, and also in combination as oxide, sulphide, carbonate, etc.

Properties.—Copper is a metal of a reddish color, softer than iron, is both malleable and ductile, and has considerable tenacity. It crystallizes in the isometric system. In masses it is unaltered in the air at ordinary temperatures, but when heated to redness it oxidizes superficially. It is dissolved easily by nitric acid, and chlorine and sulphur attack it readily. It is also acted upon by weak acids and alkalies as well as by solutions of many salts. Its specific gravity is 8.95.

Tests.—Copper in a finely divided state may be obtained by boiling a concentrated solution of sulphate of copper, not containing free acid, with distilled zinc. As soon as the liquid loses its color, which it does in a short time, the zinc is removed and the copper powder well boiled with dilute sulphuric acid, then washed uninterruptedly with water till the washings run free from any trace of the acid; it is then pressed between folds of bibulous paper and dried at 75° C. (167° F.). Thus prepared it is a dark red, dull-looking powder, which easily acquires the ordinary lustre of the metal by pressure and rubbing with a burnisher.

It was introduced into our Materia Medica by Hahnemann.

Preparation for Homœopathic Use.—The precipitated metal is prepared by trituration, as directed under Class VII.

CUPRUM ACETICUM.

Synonyms, Cupric Acetate. Cupri Acetas. Ærugo Destillata.
Common Names, Acetate of Copper. Verdigris.
Formula, $Cu\ (C_2\ H_3\ O_2)_2,\ H_2\ O$.
Molecular Weight, 199.5.
Preparation of Acetate of Copper.—Dissolve verdigris (*cupri subacetas*) in dilute acetic acid, evaporate gently, and allow to crystallize.

Properties.—Acetate of copper is in oblique, rhombic, prismatic crystals, which are opaque and have a dark bluish-green color. Upon exposure to the air they become covered with a bright bluish-green powder from superficial efflorescence. They are soluble in five parts of boiling water, in fourteen of water at a medium temperature, and in fifteen of alcohol.

Tests.—The salt when dissolved in strong ammonium carbonate solution in excess should produce a solution of a deep blue color; a turbidity, or precipitate shows the presence of lead oxide, ferrous oxide, or the earthy metals. A portion of the salt brought to a red heat and then treated with water should give no alkaline reaction (absence of the fixed alkalies).

Preparation for Homœopathic Use.—The pure acetate of copper is prepared by trituration, as directed under Class VII.

Tinctura Cupri Acetici Rademacheri.—Rademacher's tincture of acetate of copper is prepared by dissolving one part of crystallized acetate of copper in ten parts of warm water and then adding eight parts of alcohol. Eighteen parts of the tincture with eighty-two parts of dilute alcohol will yield the 2x dilution.

Further dilutions must be prepared as directed under Class V—β.

CUPRUM AMMONIATUM.

Proper Name, Tetrammonio-Cupric Sulphate.
Synonyms, Cuprum Sulphuricum Ammoniatum. Ammonio-Sulphate of Copper.
Common Name, Ammoniated Copper.
Formula, $4\ NH_3,\ Cu\ SO_4,\ H_2O$.
Molecular Weight, 245.5.
Preparation of Ammoniated Copper.—One part of crystalline cupric sulphate dissolved in three parts of ammonium hydrate solution, is filtered if necessary and mixed with six parts of alcohol; the precipitated salt is to be collected and dried without the aid of heat by pressing it between folds of bibulous paper.

Properties.—Ammonio-sulphate of copper is a dark blue crystalline powder having a weak, ammoniacal odor and a disagreeable metallic and ammoniacal taste. Its reaction is alkaline. It is soluble in one and one-half parts of cold water, but by the addition of a large amount of water a salt of paler blue separates out, which contains a less proportion of ammonia. By heating to 250° C. (482° F.), it loses its ammonia and water and there remains only cupric sulphate.

Tests.—The color of the crystals and the rapid and complete solution of the salt in two parts of distilled water will suffice. Upon the addition of a caustic fixed alkali to the solution, ammonia will be evolved. A preparation made with ammonium carbonate instead of the hydrate is not crystalline and effervesces on the addition of an acid.

In his chapter on Cuprum, Hahnemann calls attention to the use of the ammoniated sulphate of copper.

Preparation for Homœopathic Use.—The pure ammoniated copper is prepared by trituration, as directed under Class VII.

CUPRUM ARSENICOSUM.

Synonyms, Arsenious Oxide of Copper. Arsenite of Copper. Cuprum Oxydatum Arsenicosum. Hydric Cupric Arsenite.

Common Name, Scheele's Green.

Formula, $Cu\ H\ As\ O_3$.

Preparation of Arsenite of Copper.—Boil three parts of pulverized white arsenic (arsenious acid) with eight parts of caustic potash in sixteen parts of water, until the arsenic is dissolved. The result is an alkaline liquid containing potassium di-arsenite $(K\ As\ O_2)_2\ As_2\ O_3 + H_2\ O$. On mixing this solution with cupric sulphate till the precipitation is complete, and drying the precipitate at 100° C. (212° F.), the compound so obtained consists of a mixture of $Cu\ H\ As\ O_3$ with arsenious oxide.

The chemically pure cupric hydrogen arsenite may be obtained by precipitation of aqueous arsenious acid with pure ammonio-sulphate of copper. This precipitate when air-dried consists of $Cu\ H\ As\ O_3$, $H_2\ O$, and after drying in a vacuum over concentrated sulphuric acid its constitution is $Cu\ H\ As\ O_3$.

Properties.—Arsenite of copper is a light green powder, which dissolves in excess of ammonia without color, yielding a solution of arsenic acid and cuprous oxide. It is insoluble in water and alcohol.

The first systematic provings were made under the direction of Dr. W. James Blakely, United States.

Preparation for Homœopathic Use.—The pure arsenite of copper is prepared by trituration, as directed under Class VII.

CUPRUM CARBONICUM.

Synonyms, Hydrated-dibasic Cupric Carbonate. Cupri Carbonas.

Common Name, Carbonate of Copper.

Formula, $Cu\ C\ O_3$, $Cu\ O$, $2\ H_2O$.

Preparation of Carbonate of Copper.—This salt exists in nature in the form of blue carbonate (malachite) and anhydrous carbonate. It is also obtained by precipitating a solution of sulphate of copper with a solution of carbonate of soda. The precipitate is collected and washed with cold distilled water. This salt is of a magnificent blue color.

Preparation for Homœopathic Use.—The pure carbonate of copper is prepared by trituration, as directed under Class VII.

CUPRUM SULPHURICUM.

Synonyms, Cupric Sulphate. Cupri Sulphas. Cuprum Vitriolatum.

Common Names, Sulphate of Copper. Blue Vitriol. Blue-stone.

Formula, $Cu\,SO_4$, $5\,H_2\,O$.

Molecular Weight, 249.5.

Preparation of Sulphate of Copper.—Of pure copper foil in clippings, three parts are to be digested with the aid of heat in ten parts of concentrated sulphuric acid. After solution is complete, the crystals may be obtained by evaporation. Cupric sulphate is in transparent, oblique, rhombic crystals of a blue color and a disagreeable, metallic taste. They are soluble in three and a half parts of cold, and in one-third part of boiling water, and are insoluble in alcohol. The watery solution has an acid reaction. By heating to 200° C. (392° F.), the crystals become anhydrous and form then a white powder, which eagerly absorbs water from the air or other media.

Tests.—Dissolve a few crystals of the salt in ten volumes of distilled water with the aid of heat, add then a few drops of chlorine water and of dilute sulphuric acid, precipitate the copper as sulphide by means of hydrogen sulphide, and evaporate some drops of the filtered solution in a watch glass; there should be no residue. If there be a residue, it may contain iron, zinc, potassium, sodium, magnesium or calcium. For further tests of the residue, recourse must be had to appropriate group reagents, followed by individual tests.

Preparation for Homœopathic Use.—The pure sulphate of copper is prepared by trituration, as directed under Class VII.

CURARE.

Synonyms, Urari. Woorari. Wourari. Wourali. Woorara.

Origin.—The arrow-poison of South America is a black paste or extract. Its source is not positively known, but the substance is believed to contain ingredients which are from different species of Strychnos. *Cocculus toxifera*, *Didelphys cancrivora* and *Paullinia Cururu*, are said by different writers to contribute some share in its preparation.

Properties.—Curare is a dry, brownish-black, resinous extract, having a very bitter taste. It is soluble in dilute alcohol, forming a red solution; it is also soluble in water and in absolute alcohol. From it there has been isolated an alkaloid *curarin*, which contains no oxygen.

Preparation for Homœopathic Use.—Curare is prepared by trituration, as directed under Class VII.

CYCLAMEN.

Synonyms, Cyclamen Europæum, *Linn.* Artanita Cyclamen.
Nat. Ord., Primulaceæ.
Common Name, Sow-bread.

C. Europæum is a perennial, herbaceous, stemless plant, indigenous in Southern Europe. Its globular root gives off many branched fibres, is nearly black externally and white internally, and without odor; in the fresh state it has a bitter, acrid, burning taste. The leaves are long-petiolate, roundish, veined, shining dark green, white-spotted above, purple or rosy below. Flowers pendulous, rose-colored (or white), sweet-scented, without stems, on scapes; corolla revolute; berries covered with a capsule.

Preparation.—The fresh root, gathered in autumn, is chopped and pounded to a pulp, enclosed in a piece of new linen and subjected to pressure. The expressed juice is then, by brisk agitation, mingled with an equal part, by weight, of alcohol. This mixture is allowed to stand eight days in a dark, cool place, and then filtered.

It was introduced into the Homœopathic Materia Medica by Hahnemann.

Drug power of tincture, $\frac{1}{2}$.

Dilutions must be prepared as directed under Class I.

CYPRINUS BARBUS.

Synonyms, Barbus Fluviatilis. Ova Barbæ.
Class, Pisces.
Order, Physostomi.
Family, Cyprinoidei.
Common Names, Common Barb or Barbel. Carp.

The fish lives in the clear running waters of Asia and the south of Europe, and is frequently caught in those of France. It is distinguished by the four feelers on the upper jaw, to which it owes its name. The body is commonly covered with a viscous mucus; its flesh is white, tender, and tastes the more agreeably the older the fish is, but is of difficult digestion to weak stomachs. The eggs are considered poisonous, and contain an acrid, bitter substance.

Preparation.—The roe, collected in the month of May, from a large adult barbel, is prepared by trituration, as directed under Class IX.

The fresh roe, obtained in May, from a large adult barbel, is crushed, covered with five parts by weight of alcohol, and allowed to remain eight days in a well-stoppered bottle, in a dark, cool place, being shaken twice a day. This tincture is then poured off, strained and filtered.

Drug power of tincture, $\frac{1}{10}$.

Dilutions from tincture must be prepared as directed under Class IV.

CYPRIPEDIUM.

Synonym, Cypripedium Pubescens, *Willd.*
Nat. Ord., Orchidaceæ.
Common Names, Lady's Slipper. Moccasin Plant.

An indigenous plant, the shape and color of whose flower give it its popular name. Its stem is simple, a foot or two in height. Leaves ovate-lanceolate, acuminate, large and many-veined, alternate, sheathing at the base. The solitary flower irregular, as in all the orchis family, the lip being a large inflated sac; it is yellow in color. Leaves and stems pubescent. The plant is found in bogs and low woods.

Preparation.—The fresh root, gathered in autumn, is chopped and pounded to a fine pulp and weighed. Then two parts by weight of alcohol are taken, and after mixing the pulp thoroughly with one-sixth part of it, the rest of the alcohol is added. After having stirred the whole well, pour it into a well-stoppered bottle, and let it stand eight days in a dark, cool place. The tincture is then separated by decanting, straining and filtering.

Drug power of tincture, $\frac{1}{6}$.

Dilutions must be prepared as directed under Class III.

DAMIANA.

Synonyms, Turnera Microphylla, *De Candolle.* Turnera Aphrodisiaca, *Ward.*
Nat. Ord., Turneraceæ.
Common Name, Damiana.

The Turneraceæ are a small family of (chiefly) tropical American plants. The flowers are small and yellow, sub-sessile, near the ends of the small branches. *T. aphrodisiaca* is found in commerce as broken leaves mixed with fragments of the branches, and sometimes with seed-pods. Leaves less than an inch long, obovate, wedge-shaped, tapering at the base to a short, slender leaf-stalk; they are light green in color, and covered with whitish, short hairs. Their taste is aromatic.

Preparation.—The recently dried leaves, coarsely powdered, are covered with five parts by weight of alcohol. Having poured the mixture into a well-stoppered bottle, let it remain eight days in a dark, cool place, shaking it twice a day. The tincture is then poured off, strained and filtered.

Amount of drug power, $\frac{1}{10}$.

Dilutions must be prepared as directed under Class IV.

DAPHNE.

Synonyms, Daphne Indica, *Linn.* Daphne Lagetta. Daphne Odora. Lagetta Lintearea, *Lamarck.*
Nat. Ord., Thymelaceæ.
Common Name, Sweet-scented Spurge-Laurel.

This moderately-sized branching shrub is a native of the West Indies and China. Leaves are alternate, ovate-cordate, glabrous. Flowers are white, richly scented, in terminal bunches of ten to fifteen almost sessile flowers on a common peduncle, furnished with several bracts at its base.

It was proved by Dr. Bute, United States.

Preparation.—The fresh bark is chopped and pounded to a pulp and weighed. Then two parts by weight of alcohol are taken, the pulp mixed thoroughly with one-sixth part of it, and the rest of the alcohol added. After having stirred the whole well, pour it into a well-stoppered bottle, and let it stand eight days in a dark, cool place. The tincture is then separated by decanting, straining and filtering.

Amount of drug power, $\frac{1}{6}$.

Dilutions must be prepared as directed under Class III.

DATURA ARBOREA, *Linn*

Synonym, Brugmansia Gardneri, *Ruiz et Pav.*

Nat. Ord., Solanaceæ.

Common Name, Tree Stramonium.

This is a native of the Pacific coast, northward from Peru to California. The flowers are long, tubular, bent downward, snowy-white, and of a very sweet odor.

It was introduced to the homœopathic profession by Dr. Poulson, United States.

Preparation.—The fresh flowers are chopped and pounded to a pulp and weighed. Then two parts by weight of alcohol are taken, the pulp mixed thoroughly with one-sixth part of it, and the rest of the alcohol added. After having stirred the whole well, pour it into a well-stoppered bottle, and let it stand two weeks in a dark, cool place. The tincture is then separated by decanting, straining and filtering.

Amount of drug power, $\frac{1}{6}$.

Dilutions must be prepared as directed under Class III.

DELPHINUS AMAZONICUS.

Synonym, Delphinus Geoffroyi.

Class, Mammalia.

Order, Cetacea.

Family, Delphinida.

Common Name, Amazonian Dolphin.

This dolphin is from nine to ten feet long; its body is large and cylindrical, of a brownish-gray color above and pure white below. Its jaws, of equal length, are long, narrow, linear, armed on each side with twenty-six large, conical, somewhat rugose teeth, with wide crowns. Its forehead is bomb-shaped, the eyes a little above the commissure of the lips. The pectoral fins are of considerable size, brownish at their extremities, and placed very low; the dorsal fin is elevated and semilunar. This dolphin, as its name shows, inhabits the mouth of the Amazon. It has a thick and fibrous skin, which we employ in medicine.

Introduced into our Materia Medica by Dr. Mure, Brazil.

Preparation.—The fresh skin is prepared by trituration, as directed under Class IX.

DICTAMNUS.

Synonyms, Dictamnus Albus, *Willd.* D. Fraxinella, *Linn.*
Nat. Ord., Rutaceæ.
Common Names, White or Bastard Dittany. Fraxinella.

This perennial plant grows in the south of Germany, in Italy, France, Russia, in mountain woods, and on stony hills. Root elongated, of the thickness of a finger, branchy, succulent, somewhat spongy; stem upright, from two to three feet high, slightly angular, streaked green, furnished with red, resinous glands, and terminating in a beautiful spike; leaves alternate, shining, pinnated; flowers terminal, in spikes, of a snowy-white or a clear red, with stripes of a deeper color; seeds ovoid, black. When fresh, the whole plant emits a strong, resinous odor, and exhales a quantity of ethereal oil, which, when a lighted candle is brought near in a dry and hot air, inflames without any injury to the plant.

Preparation.—The fresh rootlets and the bark only of the larger roots are chopped and pounded to a pulp and weighed. Then two parts by weight of alcohol are taken, the pulp mixed thoroughly with one-sixth part of it, and the rest of the alcohol added. After having stirred the whole well, pour it into a well-stoppered bottle and let it stand eight days in a dark, cool place. The tincture is then separated by decanting, straining and filtering.

Drug power of tincture, $\frac{1}{6}$.

Dilutions must be prepared as directed under Class III.

DIGITALIS.

Synonyms, Digitalis Purpurea, *Linn.*
Nat. Ord., Scrophulariaceæ.
Common Names, Foxglove. Fairy Fingers. Purple Glove.

D. purpurea is a beautiful plant common throughout Europe, and growing best on siliceous soils, in thickets and bushy ground and waste places. In the warm parts of Europe it is a mountain plant. The root is biennial or perennial, from which in the second year ascends a single, erect, leafy stem, from two to five feet high. The lower leaves are ovate, sometimes a foot or more long, upon winged stalks. The upper ones are sparse and lanceolate. Both have margins crenate, or at least sub-serrate. The segments of the calyx are ovate-oblong; corolla campanulate, obtuse, upper lip entire, purple, internally white, with black spots. The flowers are numerous, in a long simple spike.

The drug was proven by Hahnemann.

Preparation.—The fresh leaves, from the uncultivated plant in its second season, gathered when about to bloom, are chopped and pounded to a pulp, enclosed in a piece of new linen and subjected to pressure.

The expressed juice is then, by brisk agitation, mingled with an equal part by weight of alcohol. This mixture is allowed to stand eight days in a well-stoppered bottle, in a dark, cool place, and then filtered.

Drug power of tincture, ½.

Dilutions must be prepared as directed under Class I.

DIOSCOREA.

Synonyms, Dioscorea Villosa, *Linn.* Dioscorea Quinata. Dioscorea Paniculata. Ubium Quinatum.

Nat. Ord., Dioscoreaceæ.

Common Names, China Root. Colic Root. Devil's Bones. Wild Yam.

This is an indigenous perennial creeper, twining over bushes and fences, in thickets and hedges. Its stems are slender, from knotty and matted root-stocks; leaves mostly alternate, sometimes whorled in fours, downy underneath, heart-shaped, somewhat pointed, nine to eleven-ribbed; flowers pale greenish-yellow, the sterile in panicles, the fertile in simple racemes, both drooping. The flowers are very small. Stamens six, at the base of the divisions of the six-parted perianth. Pods eight to ten lines long, three-celled, three-winged, loculicidally three-valved. Seeds one or two in each cell, flat, with a membranaceous wing. The plant grows from New England to Wisconsin, and is common in Southern States.

The first provings were by Dr. A. M. Cushing, U. S.

Preparation.—The fresh root is chopped and pounded to a pulp and weighed. Then two parts by weight of alcohol are taken, the pulp mixed thoroughly with one-sixth part of it, and the rest of the alcohol added. After having stirred the whole well, pour it into a well-stoppered bottle, and let it stand eight days in a dark, cool place. The tincture is then separated by decanting, straining and filtering.

Drug power of tincture, $\frac{1}{6}$.

Dilutions must be prepared as directed under Class III.

DIPSACUS SYLVESTRIS, *Miller.*

Nat. Ord., Dipsaceæ.

Common Name, Wild Teasel.

This plant is a native of Europe, from Denmark southward, Northern Africa and Western Asia. Its stem is three to four feet high, stout, rigid; ribs prickly. Leaves radical, on the first year's growth only, spreading; cauline six to eight inches long, oblong-lanceolate, entire or crenate; midrib prickly. Heads two to three inches long; bracts linear, rigid, longer than the head; floral bracts very long, rigid, subulate, strict, ciliate; involucre pubescent, four-angled in fruit. Calyx-limb deciduous. Corolla purplish. Flowers appear in July and September.

Preparation.—The fresh plant in flower, is chopped and pounded to a pulp and weighed. Then two parts by weight of alcohol are taken, the pulp mixed thoroughly with one-sixth part of it, and the rest of the alcohol added. After having stirred the whole well, pour it into a well-stoppered bottle, and let it stand eight days in a dark, cool place. The tincture is then separated by decanting, straining and filtering.

Drug power of tincture, $\frac{1}{6}$.

Dilutions must be prepared as directed under Class III.

DIPTERIX ODORATA, *Willdenow.*

Synonyms, Coumarouna Odorata, *Aublet.* Baryosma Tongo.

Nat. Ord., Leguminosæ.

Common Names, Tonka Bean. Tongo or Tonquin Bean.

Tonka beans are the seeds of a tree growing in Guiana. They are enclosed each in a single pod, and are from one and a half to two inches long, and a quarter to a third of an inch wide, covered by a dark brown, nearly black, shining skin. They have a peculiar, agreeable, aromatic odor, resembling in some degree that of new mown hay. Their taste is aromatic and bitter.

Preparation.—The dried seeds, coarsely powdered, are covered with five parts by weight of alcohol. Having poured the mixture into a well-stoppered bottle, let it remain eight days in a dark, cool place, shaking it twice a day. The tincture is then poured off, strained and filtered.

Amount of drug power, $\frac{1}{10}$.

Dilutions must be prepared as directed under Class IV.

DIRCA PALUSTRIS, *Linn.*

Nat. Ord., Thymelaceæ.

Common Names, Leatherwood. Mooswood. Ropebark. Wicopy.

A shrub found growing in rich, damp woods in the United States as far south as Georgia. The nearly sessile leaves are alternate, oval-obovate, with acute ends, and tomentous and pale green beneath. The flowers appear before the leaves, are small, funnel-shaped, clustered in threes. The bark is from the interlacing of its fibres extremely tough; it is smooth, yellowish-brown, or greyish-brown in color.

It was first proved by Dr. E. H. Spooner, U. S.

Preparation.—The fresh inner bark of the twigs is chopped and pounded to a pulp and weighed. Then two parts by weight of alcohol are taken, the pulp mixed thoroughly with one-sixth part of it, and the rest of the alcohol added. After having stirred the whole well, pour it into a well-stoppered bottle, and let it stand eight days in a dark, cool place. The tincture is then separated by decanting, straining and filtering.

Amount of drug power, $\frac{1}{6}$.

Dilutions must be prepared as directed under Class III.

DOLICHOS PRURIENS, *Linn.*

Synonyms, Mucuna Pruriens, *De Candolle.* Carpopogon Pruriens. Stitzolobium Pruriens.

Nat. Ord., Leguminosæ.

Common Names, Cowhage. Cowitch. Kiwach.

The word cowhage is a corruption of the Sanscrit *Kapi-Kachchu,* meaning monkey's itch. The substance is furnished by *D. pruriens,* Linn., a lofty climbing plant with large dark purple papilionaceous flowers, and downy legumes, in size and shape somewhat like those of the sweet pea. The tree is common to the tropical regions of India, Africa and America. The pods are densely covered with rigid, pointed, brown hairs about one-tenth of an inch in length. The hairs are readily removable from the epidermis, but the operator should wear gloves to protect the skin of the hands from the pointed barbs of the hairs.

The drug was proved by Dr. Jacob Jeanes, U. S.

Preparation.—The hair, carefully scraped from the epidermis of the pod, is covered with five parts by weight of alcohol, and allowed to remain eight days in a well-stoppered bottle, in a dark, cool place, being shaken twice a day. The tincture is then poured off, strained and filtered.

Drug power of tincture, $\frac{1}{10}$.

Dilutions must be prepared as directed under Class IV.

DORYPHORA DECEMLINEATA.

Class, Insecta.

Order, Coleoptera.

Family, Chrysomelina.

Common Names, Colorado Beetle. Potato Bug.

This insect makes its home among the foot-hills of the Rocky Mountains, where it feeds upon a species of solanum growing in that locality. It attacks the other solanaceæ (the potato, tomato), and commits widespread devastation.

The drug was first proven by Dr. C. Ruden, U. S.

Preparation.—The live insect is crushed and covered with five parts by weight of alcohol. Having been poured into a well-stoppered bottle, it is allowed to remain eight days in a dark, cool place, being shaken twice a day.

Amount of drug power, $\frac{1}{10}$.

Dilutions must be prepared as directed under Class IV.

DRACONTIUM FŒTIDUM, *Linn.*

Synonyms, Symplocarpus Fœtidus, *Salisbury.* Pothos Fœtidus, *Michaux.* Ictodes Fœtidus, *Bigelow.*

Nat. Ord., Araceæ.

Common Names, Skunk Cabbage. Fœtid Hellebore. Polecat Weed.

D. fœtidum is a horribly ill-smelling perennial plant, found in low moist grounds throughout the United States. The large, abrupt root puts out numerous fleshy fibres two feet or more in length. In the early spring the spathe first appears, purple-spotted, enclosing the spadix, which is oval, the latter being covered with dull purple flowers. The leaves appear after the flowers, are numerous, bright green in color and very large.

Preparation.—The fresh root, gathered in spring, is chopped and pounded to a pulp and weighed. Then two parts by weight of alcohol are taken, the pulp mixed thoroughly with one-sixth part of it, and the rest of the alcohol added. After having stirred the whole well, pour it into a well-stoppered bottle, and let it stand eight days in a dark, cool place. The tincture is then separated by decanting, straining and filtering.

Drug power of tincture, $\frac{1}{6}$.

Dilutions must be prepared as directed under Class III.

DROSERA.

Synonyms, Drosera Rotundifolia, *Linn.* Rorella Rotundifolia. Ros Solis.

Nat. Ord., Droseraceæ.

Common Names, Round-leaved Sundew. Moor-grass. Red Rot. Youth Wort.

This plant grows on turfy ground, thickly covered with short moss, in the north of Europe, Bavaria, Northern Asia and America. The perennial root is thin, of a deep brown color; stem erect, thin, glabrous, rough, from two to eight inches high, and, previous to flowering, rolled upon itself at the summit. The leaves have long peduncles, are circular or transversely oval, disposed in a circle, somewhat juicy and breaking easily, pale green on the lower surface, and on the upper surface covered with many red hairs which are provided, at their extremities, with purple-red follicles, which when exposed to the sun, exude a clear, viscid juice. The flowers are alternate, on short peduncles, white, and open during dry, fine weather for a moment about noon.

It was first proven by Hahnemann.

Preparation.—The entire fresh plant, gathered at the commencement of flowering, is chopped and pounded to a fine pulp, enclosed in a piece of new linen and subjected to pressure. The expressed juice is then, by brisk agitation, mingled with an equal part by weight of alcohol. This mixture is allowed to remain eight days in a well-stoppered bottle, in a dark, cool place, and then filtered.

Drug power of tincture, $\frac{1}{2}$.

Dilutions must be prepared as directed under Class I.

DULCAMARA.

Synonyms, Solanum Dulcamara, *Linn.* Dulcis Amara.

Nat. Ord., Solanaceæ.

Common Names, Bitter-Sweet (not Climbing Bitter-Sweet, or Celastrus). Woody Nightshade (not Deadly Nightshade, or Belladonna).

A climbing, shrubby plant, found growing in moist situations in many parts of the world. Its stem is round, slender and woody, giving off flexuose branches, and is six to ten feet high, but when supported frequently extends to twice that length. Its leaves are alternate, on petioles, ovate, acuminate, the lower ones entire, the upper becoming auriculate or hastate. Flowers drooping, in cyme-like clusters from the side of the stem. Corolla of five reflexed segments, purple, with two green spots at the base of each. The odor of the leaves and stem nauseous and narcotic; their taste is first sweet and then bitter.

It was proven by Hahnemann.

Preparation.—The fresh green stems covered with a gray epidermis, pliant, not ligneous, and the leaves gathered before flowering, are chopped and pounded to a fine pulp, enclosed in a piece of new linen and subjected to pressure. The expressed juice is then, by brisk agitation, mingled with an equal part by weight of alcohol. This mixture is allowed to stand eight days in a well-stoppered bottle, in a dark, cool place and then filtered.

Drug power of tincture, ½.

Dilutions must be prepared as directed under Class I.

ELAPS CORALLINUS.

Class, Reptilia.
Order, Ophidia.
Family, Elapidæ.
Common Name, Coral Viper.

The elaps corallinus is found quite frequently in the woods all along the coast of Brazil, and its bite is much dreaded. Its colors are more brilliant and more agreeably combined than those of any other serpent in Brazil. Its head is small, covered with large polygonal scales; it swells behind and is continuous with the neck, from which it is scarcely distinguished as regards size. It has round and small eyes; the jaws which are little dilatable, are furnished with sharp teeth, accompanied by fangs that rest on the venomous glands. The body is about two feet and a half in length; it is round, rather large in proportion to the head, and terminates in a sharp tail. The upper part is covered with smooth rhomboidal scales; the belly is covered with two hundred transverse shields; the tail has fifty shields, which are arranged in two parallel rows. Its colors are disposed in the shape of rings of a vermillion-red, alternating with black rings, each two rings being separated by circular lines of a greenish-white. The upper part of the head is black, likewise the first colored ring of the neck; the shields of the jaws are white, and are separated from each other by black lines.

The drug was introduced into the Homœopathic Materia Medica by Dr. Mure, Brazil.

Preparation.—The poison, pressed from the jaws of the living animal by means of steel pincers, is triturated as directed under Class VIII.

ELAIS GUINEENSIS, *Jacquin.*

Nat. Ord., Palmæ.

Common Name, Palm Tree.

This species is spread all over South America; it prefers cultivated and sunny regions. Its trunk, which is from twenty-five to thirty feet high, is covered by the persistent bases of the leaves. The top-leaves form a thick tuft; they are large, pinnate, with numerous folioles, ensiform, alternate and sessile, attached to a strong rachis or spike, the petiolar portion of which is garnished with long and sharp prickles. The flowers are monœcious, with a papyraceous perianth having six divisions. The male flowers have six stamens and three internal, erect and converging folioles. They form ramose spathes in fusiform masses, placed between the bases of the leaves. The female flowers are scattered; the ovary is sub-cylindrical, surmounted by a short style with a bilobate stigma. The fruit is oval, oleaginous, reddish-yellow, surrounded by a hard and angular pericarp.

The drug was introduced into our Materia Medica by Dr. Mure, Brazil.

Preparation.—The ripe fruit is prepared by trituration, as directed under Class IX.

ELATERIUM.

Synonyms, Ecbalium Elaterium, *Richard.* Momordica Elaterium, *Linn.* Cucumis Agrestis.

Nat. Ord., Cucurbitaceæ.

Common Names, Elaterium. Squirting Cucumber.

E. elaterium is a coarse, fleshy, decumbent plant, without tendrils. It has a thick, white, perennial root. It is common in the countries bordering on the Mediterranean. The fruit is cucumber-like in appearance, ovoid-oblong, nodding, about one and one-half inches long, covered with numerous, short, fleshy prickles, which terminate in white, lengthened points. It is fleshy and green while young, yellowish when mature. It is three-celled, and contains numerous oblong seeds, in a very bitter, juicy pulp. The fruit when ripe separates suddenly from the stalk, and at the same moment the seeds and juice are forcibly expelled from the aperture left by the detached stem. Hence for medicinal purposes, the fruit must be collected before the period of maturity.

It was first proved by Dr. Caleb B. Matthews, United States.

Preparation.—The fruit, not quite ripe, is pounded to a pulp, enclosed in a piece of new linen and subjected to pressure. The expressed juice is then, by brisk agitation, mingled with an equal part by weight of alcohol, and allowed to stand eight days in a well-stoppered bottle, in a dark, cool place, and then filtered.

Drug power of tincture, $\frac{1}{2}$.

Dilutions must be prepared as directed under Class I.

EPIGÆA REPENS, *Linn.*

Nat. Ord., Ericaceæ.

Common Names, Trailing Arbutus. Ground Laurel.

This indigenous plant grows in sandy woods and rocky soils, generally preferring the sides of hills, with a northern exposure. It is more commonly found eastward. A prostrate or trailing plant, almost shrubby, pubescent, with evergreen, cordate-ovate alternate leaves, on slender petioles, flowers white or rose-colored, in small axillary clusters. Corolla salver-form; the tube villous inside, as long as the green calyx. Stamens ten, filaments slender; anthers oblong, opening lengthwise. Style slender; stigma five-lobed. Capsule five-lobed, five-celled, many-seeded.

Preparation.—The fresh leaves are pounded to a fine pulp and weighed. Then two parts by weight of alcohol are taken, and after thoroughly mixing the pulp with one-sixth part of it, the rest of the alcohol is added. After stirring the whole well, pour it into a well-stoppered bottle, and let it stand eight days in a dark, cool place. The tincture is then separated by decanting, straining and filtering.

Drug power of tincture, $\frac{1}{6}$.

Dilutions must be prepared as directed under Class III.

EQUISETUM ARVENSE, *Linn.*

Nat. Ord., Equisetaceæ.

Common Names, Common Horsetail. Horsetail Rush.

This is a leafless plant, with rush-like, simple, smooth, fertile stem, appearing in March or April, and soon perishing. The barren stems are slender, one or two feet high, green, jointed, about twelve-furrowed, simple or few-branched, bearing at the joints four teeth.

Preparation.—The fresh plant is chopped and pounded to a pulp and weighed. Then two parts by weight of alcohol are taken, the pulp mixed thoroughly with one-sixth part of it, and the rest of the alcohol added. After stirring the whole well, pour it into a well-stoppered bottle and let it stand eight days in a dark, cool place. The tincture is then separated by decanting, straining and filtering.

Drug power of tincture, $\frac{1}{6}$.

Dilutions must be prepared as directed under Class III.

EQUISETUM HYEMALE, *Linn.*

Nat. Ord., Equisetaceæ.

Common Names, Scouring Rush. Shave Grass.

This is a leafless plant of the same genus as the preceding. It has a simple, erect stem, about two feet high, round, rough, the ridges rough by the grooves, sheaths lengthened, and with about twenty narrow linear teeth, with a black girdle at the base and tip at the joints.

The drug was first proven by Dr. Hugh M. Smith, U. S.

Preparation.—The fresh plant is chopped and pounded to a pulp and weighed. Then two parts by weight of alcohol are taken, the pulp mixed thoroughly with one-sixth part of it, and the rest of the alcohol added. After having stirred the whole well, pour it into a well-stoppered bottle and let it stand eight days in a dark, cool place. The tincture is then separated by decanting, straining and filtering.

Drug power of tincture, $\frac{1}{6}$.

Dilutions must be prepared as directed under Class III.

ERECHTHITES HIERACIFOLIA, *Rafinesque.*

Synonym, Senecio Hieracifolius, *Linn.*

Nat. Ord., Compositæ.

Common Name, Fireweed.

This is an indigenous plant, growing in moist woods; common especially northward, springing up where the ground has been burned over, hence the popular name. Its grooved stem is from one to five feet high, frequently hairy. Its leaves are alternate, lanceolate or oblong, acute, sharp-dentate, sessile; the upper auricled and clasping at the base. Flowers whitish, in corymbous heads. The flowers are all tubular and fertile, without rays; involucre cylindrical, scales in a single row, linear, acute. Receptacle naked. Pappus of numerous, fine, capillary bristles. The plant has a very rank odor. Flowers from July to September.

Preparation.—The fresh plant, in flower, is chopped and pounded to a pulp and weighed. Then two parts by weight of alcohol are taken, the pulp mixed thoroughly with one-sixth part of it, and the rest of the alcohol added. After having stirred the whole well, pour it into a well-stoppered bottle and let it stand eight days in a dark, cool place. The tincture is then separated by decanting, straining and filtering.

Drug power of tincture, $\frac{1}{6}$.

Dilutions must be prepared as directed under Class III.

ERIGERON CANADENSE, *Linn.*

Nat. Ord., Compositæ.

Common Names, Canada Fleabane. Horse Weed.

This is an indigenous annual plant, stem two to six feet high, bristly-hairy, and divided into many branches. The leaves linear-lanceolate, entire except those at the root, which are dentate. The flower-heads are very small, numerous, white and panicled. Their oblong calyx and minute rays, help to distinguish this from other Erigerons. It flowers in July and August.

It was proved by Dr. W. H. Burt, United States.

Preparation.—The fresh plant when in bloom is chopped and pounded to a pulp and weighed. Then two parts by weight of alcohol are taken, the pulp mixed thoroughly with one-sixth part of it, and the rest of the alcohol added. After having stirred the whole well, pour it into a well-stoppered bottle and let it stand eight days in a dark, cool place. The tincture is then separated by decanting, straining and filtering.

Drug power of tincture, $\frac{1}{6}$.
Dilutions must be prepared as directed under Class III.

ERIODICTYON CALIFORNICUM, *Bentham.*

Synonyms, Eriodictyon Glutinosum, *Bentham.* Yerba Santa.
Nat. Ord., Hydrophyllaceæ.
Common Names, Mountain Balm. Consumptive's Weed. Bear's Weed.

An evergreen shrub indigenous to California and Northern Mexico, where it inhabits the mountainous regions. Its leaves are used in medicine. They are elliptical, lanceolate, finely serrate or nearly entire, green, the upper surface exuding a varnish-like substance which covers them; white and hirsute underneath. The conspicuous purple-blue flowers are clustered in racemes. The leaves have an aromatic and balsamic taste and odor.

This drug was introduced to the homœopathic profession by provings made under the direction of Dr. G. M. Pease, United States.

Preparation.—The fresh leaves are chopped and pounded to a pulp and weighed. Then two parts by weight of alcohol are taken, the pulp mixed thoroughly with one-sixth part of it, and the rest of the alcohol added. After having stirred the whole well, pour it into a well-stoppered bottle, and let it stand eight days in a dark, cool place. The tincture is then separated by decanting, straining and filtering.

Drug power of tincture, $\frac{1}{6}$.
Dilutions must be prepared as directed under Class III.

ERYNGIUM AQUATICUM, *Linn.*

Synonyms, Eryngium Petiolatum. Eryngium Yuccæfolium, *Michaux.*
Nat. Ord., Umbelliferæ.
Common Names, Button Snakeroot. Water Eryngo.

This is an indigenous perennial herb having a simple stem one to five feet high, with a perennial tuberous root. Leaves a foot or two in length, ensiform below, broadly linear above. Flowers white, inconspicuous, in globose heads. The plant is not aquatic in its habit, but is found growing in dry or damp pine barrens South and West. Flowers in July and August.

It was first proven by Dr. C. H. McClelland, United States.

Preparation.—The fresh root is chopped and pounded to a pulp and weighed. Then two parts by weight of alcohol are taken, the pulp mixed thoroughly with one-sixth part of it, and the rest of the alcohol added. After having stirred the whole well, pour it into a well-stoppered bottle, and let it stand eight days in a dark, cool place. The tincture is then separated by decanting, straining and filtering.

Drug power of tincture, $\frac{1}{6}$.
Dilutions must be prepared as directed under Class III.

ERYNGIUM MARITIMUM.

Nat. Ord., Umbelliferæ.

Common Name, Sea Holly.

This plant is a native of Europe and Northern Africa, growing on sandy shores. Rootstock creeping, stoloniferous. Stems one to two feet high, stout, three-chotomously branched. Radical leaves two to five inches in diameter, suborbicular, three-lobed, spinous, margins cartilaginous; cauline palmate. Heads about three together, half an inch to one inch in diameter, at length ovoid. Primary involucre of three bracts; partial of five to seven ovate spinous-serrate bracts; bracteoles trifid, equalling the flowers. Flowers one-eighth inch in diameter, bluish-white, appearing in July and August.

Proven by E. B. Ivatts, Dublin, Ireland.

Preparation.—The fresh plant is chopped and pounded to a pulp and weighed. Then two parts by weight of alcohol are taken, the pulp mixed thoroughly with one-sixth part of it, and the rest of the alcohol added. After having stirred the whole well, pour it into a well-stoppered bottle, and let it stand eight days in a dark, cool place. The tincture is then separated by decanting, straining and filtering.

Drug power of tincture, $\frac{1}{6}$.

Dilutions must be prepared as directed under Class III.

EUCALYPTUS GLOBULUS, *Labillardière.*

Nat. Ord., Myrtaceæ.

Common Names, Fever-tree. Australian Gum-tree. Blue Gum-tree.

The blue gum-tree is found in Australia, in valleys and in moist regions upon the mountain sides. It reaches a height of 200, and at times of 300 feet; it is a very rapid grower. The leaves are nearly a foot in length, thick, coriaceous, lanceolate or lanceolate-oval, and entire. Their color is yellowish-green and they are studded with numerous oil-glands; the midrib is very prominent and near the margin are two lateral veins. The odor of the leaves is balsamic, and the taste is bitter, aromatic and pungent, followed by a cooling sensation on the tongue.

The drug was introduced into our Materia Medica by Dr. A. Maurin, France.

Preparation.—The fresh leaves are chopped and pounded to a pulp and weighed. Then two parts by weight of alcohol are taken, the pulp thoroughly mixed with one-sixth part of it, and the rest of the alcohol added. After having stirred the whole well, pour it into a well-stoppered bottle, and let it stand eight days in a dark, cool place. The tincture is then separated by decanting, straining and filtering.

Drug power of tincture, $\frac{1}{6}$.

Dilutions must be prepared as directed under Class III.

EUGENIA JAMBOS, *Linn.*

Synonyms, Jambosa Vulgaris, *De Candolle.* Myrtus Jambos.

Nat. Ord., Myrtaceæ.

Common Names, Malabar Plum-tree. Rose-apple.

This beautiful tree is a native of the Indies and the warm countries of America; it is never without flowers or fruit, and attains a height of twenty to forty feet; the bark of the trunk is reddish-brown, that of the branches cracked but smooth; leaves alternate, entire, lancinate veined, and full of points, in length six to eight lines, of a deep green above, pale green below; peduncles terminal, ramose, multifloral; flowers large, of a dull yellow; fruit almost spherical, of the size of a medium pear, of a fine pale yellow, approaching to rose color; seeds monospermous, with four angles, and enveloped in a thin pellicle; the fruit is eaten, but the seeds, and above all the envelope, are considered poisonous; the root of this tree, it is said, contains one of the most violent poisons.

This drug was proven by Dr. Hering.

Preparation.—The fresh seeds are chopped and pounded to a pulp and weighed. Then two parts by weight of alcohol are taken, the pulp mixed thoroughly with one-sixth part of it, and the rest of the alcohol added. After having stirred the whole well, pour it into a well-stoppered bottle, and let it stand eight days in a dark, cool place. The tincture is then separated by decanting, straining and filtering.

Drug power of tincture, $\frac{1}{6}$.

Dilutions must be prepared as directed under Class III.

EUONYMUS ATROPURPUREUS, *Jacquin.*

Synonyms, Euonymus Carolinensis. Euonymus Tristis.

Nat. Ord., Celastraceæ.

Common Names, Wahoo. Spindle-tree. Burning-bush.

This is a shrub (from four to ten feet in height). Leaves opposite, petiolate, elliptic-ovate, pointed, serrate. The small and dark purple flowers are four-parted. The capsule or pod is smooth, crimson, and deeply four-lobed. The plant is indigenous throughout the Northern and Western States.

Preparation.—The fresh bark of the twigs and root of the uncultivated plant, is chopped and pounded to a pulp and weighed. Then two parts by weight of alcohol are taken, the pulp thoroughly mixed with one-sixth part of it, and the rest of the alcohol added. After having stirred the whole well, pour it into a well-stoppered bottle, and let it stand eight days in a dark, cool place. The tincture is then separated by decanting, straining and filtering.

Drug power of tincture, $\frac{1}{6}$.

Dilutions must be prepared as directed under Class III.

EUONYMUS EUROPÆUS, *Linn.*

Nat. Ord., Celastraceæ.

Common Name, Spindle-tree.

The common spindle-tree is a bush occurring everywhere in Europe, in hedges and woods, becoming sometimes as large as a tree. It has lanceolate, at the margin crenate, leaves, and small, pale green raceme four-petaled flowers on forked peduncles. The fleshy seed-capsule, rose-colored when ripe, mostly quadrilocular, contains as many roundish, saffron-yellow seeds, of a disagreeable smell and bitter taste.

Preparation.—The fresh fruit, as soon as it begins to turn red, is pounded to a pulp, enclosed in a piece of new linen and subjected to pressure. The expressed juice is then, by brisk agitation, mingled with an equal part by weight of alcohol, and allowed to stand eight days in a well-stoppered bottle, in a dark, cool place, and then filtered.

Drug power of tincture, ½.

Dilutions must be prepared as directed under Class I.

EUPATORIUM AROMATICUM, *Linn.*

Nat. Ord., Compositæ.

Common Names, Pool Root. White Snake-Root.

This is an indigenous plant, growing in copses, from Massachusetts to Virginia and southward, near the coast. The entire plant is slightly pubescent. The stem is slender, nearly simple, about two feet high. Leaves corymbous at summit, petiolate, opposite, lance-ovate, obtusely serrate, not pointed. The large heads are ten and fifteen flowered, white and aromatic.

Preparation.—The fresh root, gathered in autumn, is chopped and pounded to a pulp and weighed. Then two parts by weight of alcohol are taken, the pulp mixed thoroughly with one-sixth part of it, and the rest of the alcohol added. After having stirred the whole well, pour it into a well-stoppered bottle and let it stand eight days in a dark, cool place. The tincture is then separated by decanting, straining and filtering.

Drug power of tincture, ⅙.

Dilutions must be prepared as directed under Class III.

EUPATORIUM PERFOLIATUM, *Linn.*

Synonym, Eupatorium Salviæfolium.

Nat. Ord., Compositæ.

Common Names, Ague Weed. Boneset. Thoroughwort. Vegetable Antimony.

This is a hairy perennial, found throughout the United States and Canada. The round, erect stem is from two to four feet high, branching near the summit. Leaves opposite, perfoliate-connate, crenate-serrate, pale beneath. Flowers are white, in dense flat-topped corymbs. It flowers from July to September.

The drug was first proven by Drs. W. Williamson and Neidhard, U. S.

Preparation.—The fresh herb, just in bloom, is chopped and pounded to a fine pulp and weighed Then two parts by weight of alcohol are taken, the pulp thoroughly mixed with one-sixth part of it, and the rest of the alcohol added. After having stirred the whole well, pour it into a well-stoppered bottle, and let it stand eight days in a dark, cool place. The tincture is then separated by decanting, straining and filtering.

Drug power of tincture, $\frac{1}{6}$.

Dilutions must be prepared as directed under Class III.

EUPATORIUM PURPUREUM, *Linn.*

Nat. Ord., Compositæ.

Common Names, Gravel-root. Joe Pye Weed. Purple Boneset. Queen of the Meadow. Trumpet Weed.

This is a herbaceous perennial plant, with a green, sometimes purple stem, five or six feet high, leaves ovate, serrate, rugosely veined, petiolate, whorled in fours or fives. The flowers are pale purple, in a lax corymb. It grows in low grounds, from Virginia northward. Flowers in August and September.

The provings were made under direction of Dr. B. L. Dresser, United States.

Preparation.—The fresh root, gathered in autumn, is chopped and pounded to a pulp and weighed. Then two parts by weight of alcohol are taken, the pulp thoroughly mixed with one-sixth part of it, and the rest of the alcohol added. After having stirred the whole well, pour it into a well-stoppered bottle, and let it stand eight days in a dark, cool place. The tincture is then separated by decanting, straining and filtering.

Drug power of tincture, $\frac{1}{6}$.

Dilutions must be prepared as directed under Class III.

EUPHORBIA COROLLATA, *Linn.*

Nat Ord., Euphorbiaceæ.

Common Names, Bowman's Root. Large-flowering Spurge. Milk Weed. Wild Ipecac.

An erect, smooth, perennial plant, growing in various States of the Union, and abundantly in the south and west. The full grown root is one and a half to two feet long, cylindrical and but little branched. Stem simple, two to three feet high. Leaves oblong-ovate, linear, obtuse. Flowers in umbels, dichotomously branched. The large, white calyx resembles a corolla; it is rotate, has five petal-like segments, each having a greenish gland at the base. It flowers in July and August.

It was introduced into our Materia Medica by Dr. E. M. Hale, U. S.

Preparation.—The fresh root is chopped and pounded to a pulp and weighed. Then two parts by weight of alcohol are taken, the pulp mixed thoroughly with one-sixth part of it, and the rest of the alcohol added. After having stirred the whole well, pour it into a well-stoppered bottle, and let it stand eight days in a dark, cool place. The tincture is then separated by decanting, straining and filtering.

Drug power of tincture, $\frac{1}{6}$.

Dilutions must be prepared as directed under Class III.

EUPHORBIA HYPERICIFOLIA, *Linn.*

Nat. Ord., Euphorbiaceæ.

Common Names, Milk Parsley. Spurge.

This plant is indigenous to the United States, where it is very common in open places and cultivated soils. Its stem is smooth or sparsely hirsute, erect, a foot or two high; leaves oblique at the obtuse or slightly cordate base, ovate-oblong or oblong-linear, sometimes falcate, serrate (half an inch to one and a half inch long), often spotted or margined with red; stipules triangular; peduncles longer than the petioles, collected in loose leafy cymes at the ends of the branches; appendages of the involucre entire, larger and white, or smaller and sometimes red; pod glabrous, obtusely angled; seeds ovate, obtusely angled, wrinkled and tubercled, half a line long, blackish.

Preparation.—The fresh plant is chopped and pounded to a pulp and weighed. Then two parts by weight of alcohol are taken, the pulp mixed thoroughly with one-sixth part of it, and the rest of the alcohol added. After having stirred the whole well, pour it into a well-stoppered bottle, and let it stand eight days in a dark, cool place. The tincture is then separated by decanting, straining and filtering.

Amount of drug power, $\frac{1}{6}$.

Dilutions must be prepared as directed under Class III.

EUPHORBIA VILLOSA.

Synonyms, Euphorbia Pilosa, *Linn.* Euphorbia Sylvestris.

Nat. Ord., Euphorbiaceæ.

Common Name, Spurge.

This variety is indigenous to Europe from Southern France and Germany southwards, and Western Siberia, where it is found growing in copses and hedges. Rootstock stout; stems one to three feet high, stout, leafy, much branched above; leaves two to five inches long, obtuse, narrowed at the base, lower obscurely petioled, upper sessile; bracts short, often orbicular; involucre large; glands large, oblong, purple; capsule one-fifth inch long, glands prominent, with pencils of hairs; seeds broad, brown. Flowers appear in May and June.

Preparation.—The fresh root is chopped and pounded to a pulp and weighed. Then two parts by weight of alcohol are taken, the pulp mixed thoroughly with one-sixth part of it, and the rest of the alcohol added. After having stirred the whole well, pour it into a well-stoppered bottle, and let it stand eight days in a dark, cool place. The tincture is then separated by decanting, straining and filtering.

Amount of drug power, $\frac{1}{6}$.

Dilutions must be prepared as directed under Class III.

EUPHORBIUM.

Synonyms, Euphorbia Resinifera, *Berg.* Euphorbium Tenella.

Nat. Ord., Euphorbiaceæ.

Common Name, Euphorbium.

E. resinifera is a leafless, glaucous, perennial plant, native of Morrocco, where it grows on the lower slopes of the Atlas Mountains. Its stems are ascending, fleshy, four-angled and cactaceous. It is without leaves, simple depressions indicating leaf-buds; below each depression instead of stipules are divergent, horizontal, straight spines studding the stem at intervals. At the summits of the branches are pedunculate cymes of three flowers. Upon making incisions in the green fleshy branches of the plant a milky juice exudes, which hardens by exposure to the air as it flows down, and thus encrusts the stems. The gum resin is collected in the latter part of the summer, and the gatherers are obliged to protect mouth and nostrils, by tying a cloth over them, against the acridity of the irritating dust. Euphorbium, as found in commerce, is in irregular pieces, seldom more than one inch in their greatest diameter. It is a waxy-looking, brittle substance of a dull yellow or brown color, with portions of the spiny stem imbedded in it, or if the spines have shrunken and fallen out, their places are represented by holes. The dust arising when powdering the drug excites sneezing, and if it be inhaled is extremely poisonous. Its odor is slightly aromatic and its taste is persistent and acrid.

The drug was introduced into our Materia Medica by Hahnemann.

Preparation.—The powdered gum resin is covered with five parts by weight of alcohol, and allowed to remain eight days in a well-stoppered bottle, in a dark, cool place, being shaken twice a day. The tincture is then poured off, strained and filtered.

Drug power of tincture, $\frac{1}{10}$.

Dilutions must be prepared as directed under Class IV.

EUPHRASIA.

Synonym, Euphrasia Officinalis, *Linn.*

Nat. Ord., Scrophulariaceæ.

Common Name, Eyebright.

This little annual plant grows in the meadows on the borders of forests, all over Europe. The root is very small, hairy; the stem rounded, downy, from five to twelve inches high, ramose at the base, and sometimes simple; leaves alternate, sessile, oval, obtuse, glabrous, thick, sharp-toothed; flowers axillary, in a terminal spike; calyx cylindric, four-leaved; corolla white, labiated, lobed; capsule double, oval, oblong; anthers two-horned, spinous at the base, on one of the lobes.

It was proven by Hahnemann.

Preparation.—The fresh plant, omitting the root, gathered when in flower in July and August, principally from poor-soiled, sunny places, is chopped and pounded to a pulp and weighed. Then take two-thirds by weight of alcohol, and moisten the chopped plant with as much of it as is necessary to make a thick pulp, and stir well; add the rest of the alcohol, mix thoroughly and strain *lege artis* through a piece of new linen. The tincture thus obtained is allowed to stand eight days in a well-stoppered bottle, in a dark, cool place, and then filtered.

Drug power of tincture, $\frac{1}{2}$.
Dilutions must be prepared as directed under Class II.

EUPION.

This is one of the products resulting from the dry distillation of wood. Mention is made of it under the article Kreosotum.

It was proven by Dr. Bertoldi, Italy.

Preparation for Homœopathic Use.—One part by weight of eupion is dissolved in ninety-nine parts by weight of 95 per cent. alcohol.

Drug power of tincture, $\frac{1}{100}$.

Dilutions must be prepared as directed under Class VI—β.

FAGOPYRUM ESCULENTUM, *Mœnch.*

Synonym, Polygonum Fagopyrum, *Linn.*
Nat. Ord., Polygonaceæ.
Common Name, Buckwheat.

This is an annual, indigenous to Central Asia, but is cultivated in most parts of the world. Its stem is smooth, with triangular cordate or hastate leaves, semi-cylindrical sheaths. Flowers white or whitish, in corymbose racemes or panicles. Calyx petal-like, equally five-parted, withering and nearly unchanged in fruit. Interposed between the eight stamens are eight honey-bearing, yellow glands. Styles three, stigma capitate. Achenium three-sided, acute and entire, longer than the calyx.

It was proven by Dr. Dexter Hitchcock, United States.

Preparation.—The fresh, mature plant, is chopped and pounded to a pulp and weighed. Then two parts by weight of alcohol are taken, the pulp mixed thoroughly with one-sixth part of it, and the rest of the alcohol added. After having stirred the whole well, pour it into a well-stoppered bottle, and let it stand eight days in a dark, cool place. The tincture is then separated by decanting, straining and filtering.

Amount of drug power, $\frac{1}{6}$.

Dilutions must be prepared as directed under Class III.

FARFARA.

Synonym, Tussilago Farfara, *Linn.*
Nat. Ord., Compositæ.
Common Name, Coltsfoot.

This perennial herb is found growing in damp heavy soil in Europe and Northern Asia. It has a creeping root-stock a foot or foot and a half long, yellowish or grayish-white in color. The leaves are radical, on long petioles, are nearly six inches in length, roundish-cordate, sharp-serrate; their upper surface is dark green and smooth, the under whitish and tomentous. The flower-heads have yellow ligulate rays, in many rows, the florets of the disk are tubular and number about twenty.

Preparation.—The fresh herb is chopped and pounded to a pulp and weighed. Then two parts by weight of alcohol are taken, the pulp mixed thoroughly with one-sixth part of it, and the rest of the alcohol added. After having stirred the whole well, pour it into a well-stoppered bottle, and let it stand eight days, in a dark, cool place. The tincture is then separated by decanting, straining and filtering.

Drug power of tincture, $\frac{1}{6}$.

Dilutions must be prepared as directed under Class III.

FERRI ET STRYCHNIÆ CITRAS.

Citrate of Iron and Strychnia.

Preparation of Citrate of Iron and Strychnia.— Take of the citrate of iron and ammonium 98 parts; strychnia, citric acid, each one part; distilled water 120 parts. Dissolve the citrate of iron and ammonium in 100 parts, and the strychnia together with the citric acid in 20 parts of the distilled water. Mix the two solutions, evaporate the mixture by means of a water-bath, at a temperature not exceeding 140° F., to the consistence of syrup; and spread it upon plates of glass, so that when dry, the salt may be obtained in scales.

This is a mixture of citrate of strychnia with citrate of iron and ammonium.

Properties.—This compound is in thin transparent scales, garnet-red in color, and deliquescent. They are without odor and have a chalybeate, bitter taste; they dissolve easily in water, but in alcohol they are only slightly soluble.

Tests.—If prepared from materials previously tested and found free from impurities, the compound will be pure. For identification the following tests may be used: Dissolve one part of the double salt in four parts of water, then add one part of liquor potassæ; the whole is to be agitated with two parts of chloroform. The chloroformic layer is to be removed, and after evaporation will leave a residue which can be identified as strychnia by the tests mentioned in the article Strychninum. Ammonia gas will be evolved by heating a watery solution of the double salt with potassium hydrate. Ferric iron will be indicated by adding to a dilute solution of the compound a few drops of potassium ferrocyanide solution, when after acidification with HCl, a blue coloration will appear, the color being destroyed by adding ammonia in excess. When a portion of the citrate is ignited on platinum foil, acid fumes come off, whose odor is similar to that of burnt sugar, but not identical with the odor from an ignited tartrate.

Preparation for Homœopathic Use.—Citrate of iron and strychnia is prepared by trituration, as directed under Class VII.

FERRUM.

Synonyms, Ferrum Metallicum. Ferrum Redactum. Ferrum Reductum. Ferrum Hydrogenio Reductum.

Common Name, Iron.

Preparation of Iron by Hydrogen.—There are three stages in this process. 1. The preparation of a pure ferric hydrate from ferric chloride, drying and powdering the same; 2. Submitting the ferric hydrate at a red heat to the reducing action of a continuous stream of pure hydrogen gas as long as vapor of water comes off; and finally continuing the stream of hydrogen until the reduced iron has cooled. The process is hardly suitable to the pharmaceutical laboratory, and perfectly pure reduced iron is obtainable. It is stated on high authority that preparations of iron by hydrogen, made in France, are more or less impure and not free from ferrous sulphide.

Properties.—Iron reduced by hydrogen is an odorless, tasteless, fine, gray powder (not black), somewhat lighter in weight than powdered iron. It can be readily compacted by strong pressure; when rubbed thus in a mortar it shows metallic streaks, and when a small amount is hammered on an anvil, a brilliant scale of the metal is produced. A lighted match inflames it readily, the powder burning to ferric oxide.

Tests.—Its complete solubility in dilute hydrochloric acid is a real test of its value. One part of reduced iron is treated with twelve parts of the dilute acid, and after hydrogen gas ceases to be evolved, the mixture is heated to boiling; a greenish or greenish-yellow solution should result. When treated with one hundred volumes of a 3 per cent. bromine-water and digested with the aid of a gentle heat, the bromine will, in the course of half an hour, unite with the pure iron; after diluting with an equal quantity of water, the undissolved residue of ferroso-ferric oxide is to be collected on a tared filter, washed with dilute alcohol and weighed; its amount should not exceed 50 per cent. of the weight of the reduced iron originally taken for the test. Ferrous sulphide, if present, will be detected on first dissolving the reduced iron in dilute hydrochloric acid, when the evolved gas will blacken filter paper moistened with a solution of lead acetate

Ferrum was proven by Hahnemann.

Preparation for Homœopathic Use.—Pure reduced iron is prepared by trituration, as directed under Class VII.

FERRUM ACETICUM.

Synonyms, Ferri Acetas. Ferric Acetate. Ferrum Oxydatum Aceticum.

Common Name, Acetate of Iron.

Formula, $Fe_2\ (C_2\ H_3\ O_2)_6$.

Preparation of Acetate of Iron—"Take of solution of persulphate of iron, two and a half fluid ounces; acetate of potash, two ounces (avoird.); rectified spirit, a sufficiency. Dissolve the acetate of potash in ten fluid ounces, and add the persulphate of iron to eight fluid ounces of the spirit; then mix the two solutions in a two-pint bottle, and shake them well together, repeating the agitation several times during an hour."—Br. P. After the precipitate settles, decant the clear liquid and evaporate to dryness at a temperature of about 60° C. (140° F.).

Properties and Tests.—Ferric acetate is a dark brown uncrystallizable mass, having a strongly astringent taste. It should be kept in well-stoppered bottles, as it readily suffers decomposition; it must be protected from light. It is soluble in three or four parts of cold water (boiling water decomposes it). Its alcoholic solution, when precipitated by ammonium hydrate in excess, will give a filtrate which should evaporate without residue.

Ferrum aceticum was used by Hahnemann, and is included in his provings of Ferrum Metallicum.

Preparation for Homœopathic Use.—One part by weight of acetate of iron is dissolved in nine parts by weight of distilled water.

Amount of drug power, $\frac{1}{10}$.

Dilutions must be prepared as directed under Class V—*a*.

The solutions and dilutions do not keep well, and should, therefore, always be freshly prepared.

Triturations are prepared as directed under Class VII.

FERRUM ARSENICICUM.

Synonyms, Ferroso-ferric Arsenate. Ferri Arsenias. Ferrum Arseniatum.

Common Name, Arsenate of Iron.

Formula, $2\ Fe_3\ As_2\ O_8,\ 4\ Fe\ As\ O_4,\ Fe_2\ O_3, 32\ H_2\ O$.

Molecular Weight, 2408.

Preparation of Arsenate of Iron.—"Take of sulphate of iron, nine ounces; arsenate of soda, dried at 300° F., four ounces; acetate of soda, three ounces; boiling distilled water, a sufficiency. Dissolve the arsenate and acetate of soda in two pints, and the sulphate of iron in three pints of the water, mix the two solutions, collect the white precipitate which forms, on a calico filter, and wash until the washings cease to be affected by a dilute solution of chloride of barium. Squeeze the washed precipitate between folds of strong linen in a screw press, and dry it on porous bricks in a warm air-chamber, whose temperature shall not exceed 100° F."—Br. P.

Properties.—Arsenate of iron, as prepared by the above process, is an amorphous powder of a greenish or bluish-green color, and is insoluble in water and alcohol. It dissolves readily in dilute hydrochloric acid, forming a bright yellow solution. The solution, when treated with ferro-cyanide or ferri-cyanide of potassium, gives a blue precipitate, more abundant and of a deeper tint when the latter reagent is used. The acid solution, when treated with hydrogen sulphide, shows a white precipitate at first, of separated sulphur; this is followed by the precipitation of the yellow sulphide of arsenic. The substance resembles phosphate of iron in appearance, but may be differentiated from the phosphate by its behavior when boiled with caustic soda in excess and exactly neutralized by nitric acid, and then treated with silver nitrate solution; a brick-red precipitate occurs. The phosphate of iron under like conditions gives a yellow precipitate.

Preparation for Homœopathic Use.—The pure arsenate of iron is prepared by trituration, as directed under Class VII.

FERRUM BROMATUM.

Synonym, Ferrous Bromide. Ferri Bromidum.
Common Name, Bromide of Iron.
Formula, $Fe Br_2$.
Molecular Weight, 216.

Preparation of Bromide of Iron.—Bromine combines readily with iron. The preparation may be conveniently made by adding to one part of iron filings or iron wire clippings in some water, two parts of bromine; the mixture is to be digested until the liquid assumes a green tint, and then the whole is thrown upon a filter. The filtrate is to be evaporated to dryness on a water-bath.

Properties.—Is a grayish-black amorphous mass; it readily oxidizes on exposure to the air, and then becomes brown in color. Heated to redness in the air it is decomposed into ferric oxide and ferric bromide, the latter volatilizing and condensing in yellow scales. It is a dangerous poison.

Preparation for Homœopathic Use.—The pure bromide of iron is prepared by trituration, as directed under Class VII.

FERRUM CARBONICUM.

Synonyms, Ferrous Carbonate. Ferri Carbonas Saccharata.
Common Name, Saccharated Carbonate of Iron.
Formula, $Fe CO_3, H_2 O$.
Molecular Weight, 134.

Preparation.—Five parts of pure sulphate of iron, dissolved in twenty parts of distilled water, are mixed with four parts of bicarbonate of soda dissolved in fifty parts of distilled water, and for two hours exposed to a temperature of 100° C. (212° F.). The precipitate thoroughly freed from sulphuric acid, collected and as well pressed out as possible, is then mixed with eight parts by weight of sugar and thoroughly dried in a water-bath.

This preparation contains one-fifth of ferrum carb., and when triturated with the same quantity of sugar of milk gives the first decimal trituration.

Further triturations are prepared as directed under Class VII.

FERRUM IODATUM.

Synonyms, Ferrous Iodide. Ferri Iodidum.
Common Name, Iodide of Iron.
Formula, $Fe I_2$.
Molecular Weight, 310.

Preparation of Iodide of Iron.—"Take of fine iron wire, one and a half ounces; iodine, three ounces; distilled water, fifteen fluid ounces. Put the iodine, iron, and twelve ounces of the water into a flask, and having heated the mixture gently for about ten minutes, raise the heat and boil until the froth becomes white. Pass the solution as quickly as possible through a wetted calico filter into a dish of polished iron, washing the filter with the remainder of the water, and boil down until a drop of the solution taken out on the end of an iron wire solidifies on cooling. The liquid should now be poured out on a porcelain dish, and, as soon as it has solidified, should be broken into fragments and inclosed in a well-stoppered bottle."—Br. P.

Properties and Tests.—Ferrous iodide, if anhydrous, is white in color; if prepared as above directed, and protected from the air, it is in green deliquescent crystals containing five molecules of water of crystallization. When the iodide is obtained by heating or triturating iodine with a slight excess of iron filings, it is a brown compound which melts at a red heat, forms a gray laminar mass on cooling, and volatilizes at a stronger heat. It dissolves readily in water, forming a pale green solution, which, by evaporation, yields the green crystals of the officinal process. Both crystals and solution, when exposed to the air, very quickly turn brown from the formation of oxy-iodide and the separation of ferric hydrate and iodine. It cannot be kept unaltered either in the solid state or in solution. Its constituents are readily identified, potassium ferricyanide producing in its solutions a dark blue precipitate (ferrous iron); if chlorine be added to its solution, the latter will color starch mucilage blue (presence of iodine).

It was proven by Dr. Müller, Germany.

Preparation for Homœopathic Use.—The pure and freshly prepared iodide of iron is triturated, as directed under Class VII.

FERRUM LACTICUM.

Synonyms, Ferrous Lactate. Ferri Lactas.

Common Name, Lactate of Iron.

Formula, $Fe(C_3H_5O_3)_2, 3H_2O$.

Molecular Weight, 288.

Preparation of Lactate of Iron.—Ferrous lactate is prepared by boiling dilute lactic acid with iron filings. To a pint of distilled water add one fluid ounce of lactic acid and half an ounce (troy) of iron filings; the whole is to be digested in an iron vessel, and the volume of the mixture is to be kept intact by the addition of distilled water from time to time, to supply the loss by evaporation. When the evolution of gas has wholly ceased, the liquid is to be filtered while hot, and the filtrate set aside in a glass or porcelain vessel to crystallize. At the end of two days the crystals may be removed, washed with alcohol and dried between folds of bibulous paper.

Properties.—Officinal ferrous lactate is a whitish or white with a pale yellowish-green tinge, crystalline powder, whose taste is sweetish and weakly metallic. It is soluble in fifty parts of cold and in ten of boiling water, and is insoluble in alcohol. Its solutions react acid to test paper, and when exposed to the air become brown in color from the formation of the ferric compound.

Tests.—Ferrous lactate should, when treated with fifty parts of cold water, form a greenish-yellow solution; this solution after filtration should, when treated with neutral solution of lead acetate, give only a faint turbidity, a marked turbidity or precipitate showing the presence of ferrous sulphate or tartrate. A solution of ferrous lactate when treated with caustic alkali in excess, the filtered solution warmed and treated with cupric sulphate, should not coagulate (absence of gum), nor should any precipitate occur when boiled (absence of dextrin and milk-sugar).

It was proven by Dr. Müller, Germany.

Preparation for Homœopathic Use.—The pure lactate of iron is prepared by trituration, as directed under Class VII.

FERRUM MAGNETICUM.

Synonyms, Ferroso-ferric Oxide. Ferrum Oxydatum Magneticum. Ferri Oxidum Magneticum.

Common Names, Magnetic Oxide of Iron. Black Oxide of Iron. Loadstone.

Formula, $Fe_3 O_4 = Fe O, Fe_2 O_3$.

Molecular Weight, 232.

Preparation of Magnetic Oxide of Iron.—Take of solution of persulphate of iron, five and one-half fluid ounces; sulphate of iron, two ounces; solution of soda, five pints; distilled water, a sufficiency. Dissolve the sulphate of iron in two and one-half pints of the water, and add to it the solution of persulphate of iron; then mix this with the solution of soda, stirring them well together. Boil the mixture, let it stand for two hours, stirring it occasionally; then put it on a calico filter and wash until the washings cease to give a precipitate with chloride of barium. Lastly, dry the precipitate at a temperature not exceeding 120° F.—Br. P.

Properties and Tests.—It is a tasteless, brownish-black powder, which is strongly attracted by the magnet; it dissolves without effervescence in warm hydrochloric acid diluted with half its volume of water, and this solution gives blue precipitates with ferrocyanide and ferricyanide of potassium. When heated in a test-tube it gives off moisture which condenses in the cool part of the tube, and when the heat is continued in contact with the air, red ferric oxide is left. Its solution in HCl, when treated with H_2S, should only show a white precipitate of separated sulphur. The presence of sulphate from incomplete washing, will be shown by agitating a portion of the powder with distilled water, and then testing the water with barium chloride in the usual way.

Preparation for Homœopathic Use.—The pure magnetic oxide of iron is prepared by trituration, as directed under Class VII.

FERRUM MURIATICUM.

Synonyms, Ferric Chloride. Ferri Chloridum. Ferrum Sesquichloratum.

Common Names, Chloride of Iron. Muriate of Iron. Sesquichloride (Perchloride) of Iron.

15

Formula, $Fe_2 Cl_6, 12H_2 O$.

Molecular Weight, 541.

Preparation of Chloride of Iron.—In a two pint flask place eight fluid ounces of hydrochloric acid, and add to the acid two ounces of iron wire in clippings; heat the mixture till effervescence has ceased and filter. To the filtrate add four more ounces of hydrochloric acid; place the mixture in a large, porcelain capsule and heat nearly to boiling, adding nitric acid in small successive portions, as long as red fumes continue to be evolved, or till a drop of the liquid no longer gives a blue precipitate with potassium ferricyanide. The liquid is now to be evaporated at a gentle heat, till it is reduced to eight troy ounces and three-quarters, when it may be set aside, protected by a cover glass, to crystallize.

Properties.—Ferric chloride, prepared by the above mentioned process, is in pale, orange-yellow, opaque, hemispherical nodules, which are crystalline in structure. It is deliquescent and readily soluble in water, alcohol and ether. The solutions are yellowish-brown in color, acid in reaction, and have a strong chalybeate taste.

Tests.—Ferric chloride solution should give no precipitate with barium chloride (absence of sulphate); and if precipitated by ammonium hydrate in excess, should yield a filtrate that, after evaporation, leaves only ammonium chloride, which volatilizes without residue when heated to redness.

Preparation for Homœopathic Use.—One part by weight of pure chloride of iron is dissolved in nine parts by weight of alcohol.

Amount of drug power, $\frac{1}{10}$.

Dilutions must be prepared as directed under Class VI—*a*.

FERRUM PHOSPHORICUM.

Synonyms, Ferroso-ferric Phosphate. Ferri Phosphas.

Common Name, Phosphate of Iron.

Formula, $Fe_3 2PO_4, Fe PO_4, 12H_2 O$.

Molecular Weight, 725.

Preparation of Phosphate of Iron.—To ten parts of pure crystallized ferrous sulphate dissolved in sixty parts of cold, distilled water, is to be added a cold solution of thirteen parts of crystallized sodium phosphate in fifty of distilled water. The resulting precipitate is to be thrown on a filter and well washed with cold distilled water, then spread upon an unglazed tile or upon bibulous paper, and dried without the aid of artificial heat, when the dried mass is to be rubbed to a fine powder.

Properties and Tests.—The officinal phosphate of iron is a bluish-gray powder without odor or taste. It is soluble in acids, but insoluble in water and alcohol. Its solution in hydrochloric acid has a yellow color, and when treated with barium chloride exhibits only a faint turbidity, and with hydrogen sulphide, shows no change. The powder becomes greenish-gray in color when warmed, and at a higher temperature grayish-brown. The influence of daylight upon the salt is to preserve its color. When treated with hot, distilled water, the latter should evaporate without residue by heating on platinum foil.

It was proven by Dr. J. C. Morgan, United States.

Preparation for Homœopathic Use.—The pure phosphate of iron is prepared by trituration as directed under Class VII.

FERRUM PYROPHOSPHORICUM.

Synonyms, Ferric Pyrophosphate. Ferri Pyrophosphas.

Common Name, Pyrophosphate of Iron.

Preparation of Pyrophosphate of Iron.—Take of phosphate of sodium any quantity; heat it in a porcelain capsule till it melts in its water of crystallization, and finally to complete dryness. It is now to be placed in a shallow iron dish and heated to low redness, without permitting it to fuse. The resulting pyrophosphate of sodium is to be dissolved in about six parts of water, with gentle heating; after filtering and cooling the solution, it may be crystallized.

Next, 100 parts of ferric chloride solution of specific gravity 1.480 to 1.484 is to be diluted with 300 parts of cold distilled water, and with constant stirring is to be mixed with a cold solution of 97 parts of crystallized sodium pyrophosphate (obtained in the preliminary operation described above), in 2000 parts of distilled water and 500 parts of alcohol. The resulting mixture is to be set aside for a day, the precipitate thrown upon a moistened filter and washed with cold distilled water until the washings become turbid. The precipitate is then to be dried between folds of bibulous paper at a moderate temperature and finally reduced to powder.

Properties.—Pyrophosphate of iron, prepared as above directed, is a white, almost tasteless, powder, very slightly soluble in water and almost insoluble in solution of sodium chloride. It dissolves in dilute acids and in caustic ammonia, its solution in the latter being yellow. It contains 35 per cent. of anhydrous ferric oxide. It should be kept in well-closed glass vessels protected from daylight.

Tests.—Boil one part of pyrophosphate of iron and two of crystallized sodium carbonate with twenty parts of water for some minutes and then filter. After acidifying the filtrate with acetic acid and treating it with silver nitrate solution, a white precipitate should occur (a yellow precipitate indicates the presence of orthophosphoric acid). According to the Pharmacopœia Germanica a trace of chlorine in this preparation is allowable.

Preparation for Homœopathic Use.—Pyrophosphate of iron is prepared by trituration, as directed under Class VII.

FERRUM SULPHURICUM.

Synonyms, Ferrous Sulphate. Ferri Sulphas.

Common Name, Sulphate of Iron.

Formula, $Fe\,SO_4, 7H_2\,O$.

Molecular Weight, 278.

Preparation of Sulphate of Iron.—Ferrous sulphate may be obtained pure by dissolving 1 part of iron in 1½ parts of sulphuric acid diluted with 4 parts of water. The solution, if filtered quickly, deposits the salt in beautiful transparent, bluish-green crystals, containing seven equivalents of water.

Properties.—The crystals of ferrous sulphate effloresce slightly in dry air, and if at all moist absorb oxygen and become covered with a reddish-yellow crust of basic ferric sulphate; but if crushed and deprived of hygrometric moisture by strong pressure between folds of bibulous paper they may be preserved in a bottle without change by oxidation. The salt dissolves easily in water, but is insoluble in alcohol and in ether; the watery solution is of a pale greenish-blue color, has an acid reaction, and when exposed to the air for some time absorbs oxygen and deposits a yellowish sediment of basic ferric sulphate. The taste of the salt is styptic.

Tests.—A solution of the salt in water acidulated with sulphuric acid, should, when treated with hydrogen sulphide, give no colored turbidity; at most only a faint, whitish cloudiness from separated sulphur due to some ferric oxide, is permissible. Upon treating a solution of the salt with ammonium sulphide in excess and removing the precipitated sulphide of iron by filtration, there should result a filtrate which, upon evaporation, yields a residue that volatilizes completely upon ignition.

Preparation for Homœopathic Use.—The pure sulphate of iron is prepared by trituration, as directed under Class VII.

FILIX MAS.

Synonyms, Aspidium Filix Mas, *Swartz.* Polypodium Filix Mas, *Linn.*

Nat. Ord., Filices.

Common Name, Male Fern.

The male fern is very widely distributed in temperate regions, and is found in abundance in most countries of the northern hemisphere, except in the Eastern United States, where it grows somewhat sparsely in shady pine woods. Its rhizome is perennial, short, two to three inches in diameter, decumbent or rising only a few inches above the ground, and bearing on its summit a tuft of fronds which are thickly beset in their lower part with brown, chaffy scales. Fronds twice pinnate, large fruit-dot borne in the back near the mid-vein, and usually confined to the lower half of each fertile pinnule.

It was proven by Dr. Berridge, of England.

Preparation.—The fresh main root, gathered in July or August, is chopped and pounded to a pulp and weighed. Then two parts by weight of alcohol are taken, the pulp mixed thoroughly with one-sixth part of it, and the rest of the alcohol added. After having stirred the whole well, pour it into a well-stoppered bottle, and let it stand eight days in a dark, cool place. The tincture is then separated by decanting, straining and filtering.

Drug power of tincture, $\frac{1}{6}$.
Dilutions must be prepared as directed under Class III.

FORMICA RUFA.

Class, Insecta.
Order, Hymenoptera.
Family, Formicariæ.
Common Names, Ant. Wood-ant. Red-ant. Pismire.

The ants are found most frequently in pine forests. Their characters are, a flattened, rust-colored chest; black head; a big, oval abdomen, attached to the corslet by a pediele which bears a small scale or vertical knot; antennæ filiform and broken; antennulæ of unequal size; mandibles strong; tongue truncated, concave, short. There are male, female and neuter ants. The two former, when fully developed, have four long, white, transparent wings; they leave the hills, fly in the air and there couple; the males die shortly after, the females return to the hills. Only a few of them are admitted, which lay eggs and are taken care of by the neuters as among the bees. The females and neuters have, at the extremity of their abdomen, two glands, by means of which they secrete a peculiar liquor, which is acid, and which, on a delicate skin, causes itching and eruptions.

Preparation.—The live insect is crushed, covered with five parts by weight of alcohol, and allowed to remain eight days in a well-stoppered bottle, in a dark, cool place, being shaken twice a day. The tincture is then poured off, strained and filtered.

Drug power of tincture, $\frac{1}{10}$.
Dilutions must be prepared as directed under Class IV.

FRAGARIA VESCA, *Linn.*

Synonyms, Fragulæ. Trifolii Fragiferi.
Nat. Ord., Rosaceæ.
Common Name, Wood-Strawberry.

This perennial plant grows in woods, meadows, fields and hills, over the whole of Europe, and a great portion of America. The root is brown, horizontal, with long, creeping sprouts that take root again; stem erect, round, hairy, of the length of a finger or more; leaves ternate, plicated, petiolated, downy on the upper surface and hairy on the lower; flowers white, inodorous; berry oval, red, of a delicious odor and exquisite taste.

Preparation.—The ripe berries are crushed to a pulp and weighed. Then two parts by weight of alcohol are taken, the pulp mixed thoroughly with one-sixth part of it, and the rest of the alcohol added. After having stirred the whole well, pour it into a well-stoppered bottle, and let it stand eight days in a dark, cool place. The tincture is then separated by decanting, straining and filtering.

Drug power of tincture, $\frac{1}{6}$.
Dilutions must be prepared as directed under Class III.

FRASERA CAROLINENSIS, *Walter.*

Synonyms, Frasera Walteri, *Michaux.* Swertia Difformis.
Nat. Ord., Gentianaceæ.
Common Names, American Colombo. Indian Lettuce.

An indigenous biennial or triennial. Its root is long, fusiform, yellow in color and fleshy. The stem is upright, simple; leaves whorled in fours, oblong-lanceolate, the lowest ones spatulate. Flowers numerous, yellowish-white, in a terminal pyramidal panicle; corolla four-parted, rotate, each division with a glandular and fringed pit on the face, and dotted brown-purple. Filaments awl-shaped, somewhat monadelphous at base, style with two-lobed stigma. Fruit an oval flattened pod, about twelve-seeded. It flowers in the third year from May to July.

Preparation.—The fresh two year old root, gathered in October or November, or the three year old root, gathered in March or April, is chopped and pounded to a pulp and weighed. Then two parts by weight of alcohol are taken, the pulp mixed thoroughly with one-sixth part of it, and the rest of the alcohol added. After having stirred the whole well, pour it into a well-stoppered bottle, and let it stand eight days in a dark, cool place. The tincture is then separated by decanting, straining and filtering.

Drug power of tincture, $\frac{1}{6}$.

Dilutions must be prepared as directed under Class III.

FUCUS VESICULOSUS, *Linn.*

Synonym, Quercus Marina.
Nat. Ord., Algæ.
Common Names, Sea-wrack. Bladder-wrack. Sea-kelp.

This sea-weed is found growing on the rocky shores of Europe and America. Its length is from one to three feet, and its branching flat thallus is from one-half to one inch wide, with entire margins, and when in the fresh state, brownish-green in color. The vesicles are in pairs, one on each side of the mid-rib, spherical or oblong-spherical. The plant becomes shrivelled in drying and its color is then nearly black. It has the usual odor of sea-weeds, and its taste is saline, nauseous and mucilaginous.

Preparation.—The fresh alga, gathered in May or June, is pounded to a pulp and weighed. Then two parts by weight of alcohol are taken, the pulp mixed thoroughly with one-sixth part of it, and the rest of the alcohol added. After stirring the whole well, and pouring it into a well-stoppered bottle, it is allowed to stand eight days in a dark, cool place. The tincture is then separated by decanting, straining and filtering.

Drug power of tincture, $\frac{1}{6}$.

Dilutions must be prepared as directed under Class III.

GALIUM APARINE, *Linn.*

Nat. Ord., Rubiaceæ.

Common Names, Cleavers. Goose-grass. Poor Robin. Savoyan.

This plant is indigenous to Europe, Asia, and North America. The stem is one to five feet long, weak, struggling, often forming matted masses, very rough, bristle-prickly backwards, hairy at the joints; leaves six to eight in a whorl, lanceolate, tapering to the base, mucronate, rough on edges and midrib, from one to two inches long. Cymes usually three-flowered, flowers white; fruit (large) supplied with hooked prickles, purplish, dry or fleshy, globular, twin, separating when ripe into the two seed-like, indehiscent, one-seeded carpels. Flowers appear in June and July.

Preparation.—The fresh herb, in flower, is chopped and pounded to a pulp and weighed. Then two parts by weight of alcohol are taken, the pulp mixed thoroughly with one-sixth part of it, and the rest of the alcohol added. After stirring the whole well, pour it into a well-stoppered bottle, and let it stand eight days in a dark, cool place. The tincture is then separated by decanting, straining and filtering.

Drug power of tincture, $\frac{1}{6}$.

Dilutions must be prepared as directed under Class III.

GAMBOGIA.

Synonyms, Gummi Gutti. Cathartieum Aureum.

Nat. Ord., Guttiferæ.

Common Name, Gamboge.

Gamboge is a gum-resin obtained from *Garcinia Morella* (Desrousseaux) var. *pedicellata.*

A small sized tree, with handsome laurel-like foliage and small yellow flowers, found in Camboja, Siam, and in Cochin China.

The gum-resin is contained in ducts in the middle layer of the bark, and exudes therefrom when the bark is incised. The collectors, in the beginning of the rainy season, make a spiral incision half around the circumference of the tree and collect in a joint of bamboo the gum-resin which slowly exudes for several months.

The drug is in commerce in what are called pipes, *i. e.*, sticks or cylinders one to two and a half inches in diameter, and four to eight inches long, bearing striæ impressed on them from the inside of the bamboo.

A good specimen is brownish-orange in color and with water forms a yellow emulsion. Gamboge is dense, homogeneous, and breaks with a conchoidal fracture. Its taste is disagreeable and acrid; it is without odor, but its powder is irritating to the Schneiderian membrane, producing sneezing.

Gamboge was first proven by Dr. Nenning, Germany.

Preparation.—One part by weight of pure gamboge is dissolved in nine parts by weight of alcohol.

Amount of drug power, $\frac{1}{10}$.

Dilutions must be prepared as directed under Class IV.

GELSEMIUM.

Synonyms, Gelsemium Sempervirens, *Ait.* Gelsemium Nitidum, *Michaux.* Bignonia Sempervirens, *Linn.*

Nat. Ord., Loganiaceæ.

Common Name, Yellow Jessamine.

The true yellow jessamine is a climbing plant, indigenous to the Southern States. It grows to great length, ascending high trees. Stem smooth; leaves opposite, perennial, short-petiolate, entire and lanceolate. Flowers large, yellow, in axillary clusters. Calyx five-parted; corolla infundibuliform, with five-lobed border. Fruit a flattened elliptical pod, two-celled, containing winged seeds. The flowers have a delicious odor.

The first provings of this valuable remedy were by Dr. Henry, for an Inaugural Dissertation, Phila. Hom. Coll., 1852.

Preparation.—Pieces of the fresh root, not thicker than a goose-quill, are chopped and weighed. Then two parts by weight of alcohol are taken, and after thoroughly mixing the mass with one-sixth part of it, the rest of the alcohol is added. After stirring the whole well, put it into a wide-mouthed bottle, and let it stand eight days in a dark, cool place. The tincture is then separated by decanting, straining and filtering.

Drug power of tincture, $\frac{1}{6}$.

Dilutions must be prepared as directed under Class III.

GENTIANA CRUCIATA, *Linn.*

Synonym, Gentiana Minoris.

Nat. Ord., Gentianaceæ.

Common Name, Cross-Wort Gentian.

Stem two to twelve inches high. Leaves oblong-lanceolate, three-nerved at base, connected sheath-like. Flowers in dense corymbs, the topmost sessile, compressed like a bud. Calyx bell-shaped, corolla ovoid tubular, light blue within, and greenish-blue without. Is found on dry hills, and especially on calcareous soil. Flowers in July and September.

It was introduced to the Homœopathic profession by Dr. Watzke's provings, Austria.

Preparation.—The fresh root is chopped and pounded to a pulp and weighed. Then two parts by weight of alcohol are taken, the pulp mixed thoroughly with one-sixth part of it, and the rest of the alcohol added. After having stirred the whole well, pour it into a a well-stoppered bottle, and let it stand eight days in a dark, cool place. The tincture is then separated by decanting, straining and filtering.

Drug power of tincture, $\frac{1}{6}$.

Dilutions must be prepared as directed under Class III.

GENTIANA LUTEA, *Linn.*

Synonyms, Gentiana Majoris. Gentiana Rubra.
Nat. Ord., Gentianaceæ.
Common Names, Bitter-Wort Gentian. Yellow Gentian.

This plant is indigenous to the mountainous regions of Europe. Its root is perennial, thick, long and branching. Stem three to four feet high. Radical leaves, are petiolate, stem leaves opposite, sessile, acute-oval, bright green, glaucous, five-nerved. Flowers large, on peduncles, in axillary whorls; they have a yellow, rotate corolla, in five or six lanceolate segments, with the same number of stamens, shorter than the corolla.

The first provings were made under Dr. Buchner, Germany.

Preparation.—The fresh root is chopped and pounded to a pulp and weighed. Then two parts by weight of alcohol are taken, the pulp mixed thoroughly with one-sixth part of it, and the rest of the alcohol added. After having stirred the whole well, pour it into a well-stoppered bottle, and let it stand eight days in a dark, cool place. The tincture is then separated by decanting, straining and filtering.

Drug power of tincture, $\frac{1}{6}$.

Dilutions must be prepared as directed under Class III.

GERANIUM MACULATUM, *Linn.*

Nat. Ord., Geraniaceæ.
Common Names, Wild Cranesbill. Spotted Geranium.

A perennial herb, whose root is fleshy, horizontal, and has many short fibres. Stem round, erect, hairy, from one to two feet in height. Leaves five-parted, with lobed and incised divisions; as the leaves grow older they become marked with blotches, paler in color than the pale green of the surrounding portions. Radical leaves on long leaf stalks; stem leaves petiolate below, gradually becoming sessile towards the top, opposite and with stipules. Flowers large, light purple, with five entire obovate petals bearded on the claw. Stamens ten, five short, the five longer ones furnished with glands at their base. The plant is indigenous to the United States, growing in low grounds and damp woods. Flowers from May to July.

It was first proven by Dr. E. C. Beckwith, U. S.

Preparation.—The fresh root, gathered in autumn, is chopped and pounded to a pulp and weighed. Then two parts by weight of alcohol are taken, the pulp mixed thoroughly with one-sixth part of it, and the rest of the alcohol added. After having stirred the whole well, pour it into a well-stoppered bottle, and let it stand eight days in a dark, cool place. The tincture is then separated by decanting, straining and filtering.

Drug power of tincture, $\frac{1}{6}$.

Dilutions must be prepared as directed under Class III.

GERANIUM ROBERTIANUM, *Linn.*

Nat. Ord., Geraniaceæ.
Common Name, Herb-Robert.

This plant is indigenous to Europe and North America, growing in moist woods and shaded ravines. It is glabrous or slightly hairy, reddish. Leaves three-divided, or pedately five-divided, the divisions twice pinnatifid; the leaves are from one to three inches broad; petioles half an inch to one inch long; stipules ovate. Flowers half an inch in diameter, sepals awned, shorter than the (red-purple) petals; calyx angular. Claw of petals glabrous. Carpels attached by silky hairs to the axis. Pods wrinkled; seeds smooth. Flowers appear from June to October. The plant is strong-scented.

Preparation.—The fresh plant, in flower, is chopped and pounded to a pulp, enclosed in a piece of new linen and subjected to pressure. The expressed juice is then, by brisk agitation, mingled with an equal part by weight of alcohol. This mixture is allowed to stand eight days in a well-stoppered bottle, in a dark, cool place and then filtered.

Drug power of tincture, $\frac{1}{2}$.

Dilutions must be prepared as directed under Class I.

GINSENG.

Synonyms, Panax Quinquefolium, *Linn.* Aralia Quinquefolia.
Nat. Ord., Araliaceæ.
Common Names, Ginseng. Tartar Root. Five Fingers.

This plant is a native of America, China, etc. It has a fusiform root, whitish, thick and fleshy, aromatic, four to nine inches in length, ending in fibrous prolongations. Stem round, smooth, one foot high, and at the top bears a terminal whorl of three compound, five-foliate leaves, the leaflets being oval, acuminate, serrate and petiolate. Within these is a central pedicel bearing a simple umbel of small, greenish flowers on short pedicels. Fruit, a scarlet reniform berry. The root in the dried state is wrinkled externally, yellowish-white in color, with a soft, whitish bark, surrounding a harder core. Its taste is sweetish and resembles that of liquorice.

It was first proven by Dr. Jouve, Geneva.

Preparation.—The genuine, dried root, coarsely powdered, is covered with five parts by weight of alcohol, and allowed to stand eight days in a well-stoppered bottle, in a dark, cool place, being shaken twice a day. The tincture is then poured off, strained and filtered.

Drug power of tincture, $\frac{1}{10}$.

Dilutions must be prepared as directed under Class IV.

GLONOINUM.

Proper Name, Tri-nitroglycerin.
Synonyms, Nitroglycerinum. Glonoin. Glonoine.
Common Name, Nitroglycerine.
Formula, $C_3 H_5 (NO_2)_3 O_3$.

Molecular Weight, 227.

Preparation of Glonoin.—This remarkable body was discovered by Sobrero in 1847, and was proved by Dr. Hering, who gave it the name by which it is known in pharmacy. The first letters from one of its constituents with the symbols of the other, united by a euphonic o, when completed by the terminal *ine*, give the word glonoine.

Preparation.—One part of glycerine is slowly added, with constant stirring, to a mixture of two parts of concentrated sulphuric acid with one of nitric acid of specific gravity 1.47. The mixing vessel is kept cold, so that the temperature of the contents may not rise above 26.6° C. (80° F.). The solution is then poured in a thin stream into a large quantity of water, and the nitro-glycerine precipitates as a nearly colorless, heavy oil. The latter is repeatedly washed in water rendered alkaline.

Properties.—Nitro-glycerine is a nearly colorless, light yellow, oily liquid, whose specific gravity at 15° C. (59° F.) is 1.6; it is without odor and has a pungent, sweet, aromatic taste. It is slightly soluble in water but readily so in alcohol and in ether. When cooled sufficiently, about 8° C. (46.4° F.), it crystallizes in needles, and at 180° C. (356° F.) it boils, and if the heating be done in closed vessels it explodes with terrible force; its exploding point is about 190° C. (374° F.). Its remarkably disruptive power is readily evoked by a direct blow or by concussion of the surrounding air. When ignited in the air it burns quietly. It decomposes by keeping, and among the products of such change are glyceric and oxalic acids, together with the lower oxides of nitrogen. In the frozen state its transportation is extremely dangerous, from its tendency to explode by the friction of the crystals. To obviate this disadvantage different mixtures of it with inert substances are used, the most notable one, dynamite, being simply infusorial earth saturated to a certain degree with nitro-glycerine. It is almost insoluble in water, but is readily dissolved by ether and alcohol.

Preparation for Homœopathic Use.—One part by weight of pure nitro-glycerine is dissolved in nine parts by weight of 95 per cent. alcohol.

Amount of drug power, $\frac{1}{10}$.

NOTE—If the $\frac{1}{10}$ solution is exposed to a temperature of less than 60° F., part of the Glonoin separates and falls to the bottom.

Dilutions must be prepared as directed under Class VI—*a*.

GLYCERINUM.

Proper Name, Propenyl Alcohol.
Synonyms, Glycerina. Glycerin.
Common Name, Glycerine.
Formula, $C_3 H_8 O_3$.
Molecular Weight, 92.

Origin.—Glycerine is produced from most of the fixed oils and solid fats existing in the bodies of plants and animals. It does not, however, occur in them ready formed, except in a few (palm oil and a few other vegetable oils from which it may be obtained by simple treatment with boiling water), but is formed from them, together with a fatty acid by addition of the elements of water, just as alcohol may be produced from acetate of ethyl. In fact, glycerine is a triatomic alcohol of the propenyl series, and its proper title is propenyl alcohol.

Preparation.—When a fatty body is treated with an alkali or other metallic oxide, in the presence of water, or with water itself at a high temperature, there is formed a metallic salt of a fatty acid, and glycerine; for instance, stearine, one of the constituents of mutton suet, consists of propenyl tristearate $(C_3 H_5)(O C_{18} H_{35} O)_3$. When stearine is boiled with a caustic alkali a stearate of the alkali metal is formed, together with glycerine, as shown by the equation, $(C_3 H_5)(O C_{18} H_{35} O)_3 + 3 HKO = 3 KOC_{18} H_{35} O + (C_3 H_5)(O H)_3$. The metallic salts of the fatty acids thus formed are called soaps, and the process, termed *saponification*, was formerly the chief mode of preparing glycerine. It is also obtained by a somewhat similar method from the residue of the manufacture of stearic acid for candles. Glycerine is now produced in enormous quantity and perfect purity by decomposing fatty substances by means of super-heated steam. Here the reaction is simply the assimilation by one molecule of stearine, of three molecules of water, and the resolution of the resulting compound into stearic acid and glycerine, as shown by the equation, $C_3 H_5 (O C_{18} H_{35} O)_3 + 3 H_2 O = 3 H O C_{18} H_{35} O$ (stearic acid) + $C_3 H_5 (OH)_3$ (glycerine). The process is conducted in a still and condensing apparatus, over-heated steam at a temperature between 287.8° C. (550° F.) and 315.5° C. (600° F.), being caused to penetrate the mass of fat. The fat-acids quickly separate from the glycerine and water when the distillate is allowed to stand for a short time and cool.

Properties.—Chemically pure glycerine is a colorless, transparent, somewhat viscid liquid, without odor and having an intensely sweet taste. It is neutral in reaction, and is extremely hygroscopic. It mixes with water in all proportions, as indeed it does with alcohol, but is insoluble in ether, chloroform, benzin, etc. Heated to 290° C. (554° F.) it boils, and in vacuo at 200° C. (392° F.) it distils over unchanged.

The solvent power of glycerine is very great and extends over a wide range, and it forms soluble compounds of many substances insoluble, or nearly so, in water. It dissolves all deliquescent salts and many others; even aqueous glycerine dissolves oxide of lead. Many alkaloids are soluble in it.

Officinal glycerine has a specific gravity 1.25 at 15° C. (59° F.), and contains from six to ten per cent. of water.

Tests.—Six parts of a mixture of equal volumes of absolute alcohol and ether should dissolve one part of glycerine (in such a mixture glucose and sugar are not soluble), and the solution should not separate into layers. Equal volumes of pure concentrated sulphuric acid and glycerine, when mixed together, should give a colorless fluid and should not give rise to effervescence. A rather faint evolution of gas at the moment of mixing is due to the liberation from the glycerine of absorbed air, which is driven off by the heat produced by the union of the two liquids. Should the peculiar crackling sound of effervescence be heard when the test-tube is brought near the ear, the specimen is too irritating for even external use. When the above mixture is slightly heated, a brown or blackish coloration shows the presence of cane sugar. The indifferent behavior of glycerine to litmus paper suffices to show the absence of free acid or alkali. When treated with hydrogen sulphide or ammonium sulphide, no change should take place in the appearance of glycerine, nor should any precipitate occur with silver nitrate and barium chloride solutions. When diluted with water and then treated with silver nitrate and caustic ammonia, no change should occur even upon standing for half an hour. A blackish precipitate of reduced silver indicates the presence of formic acid, acrolein and similar bodies. When 1 CC. of glycerine is gradually heated upon a platinum dish-cover it evaporates, and there is left a carbonaceous mass which, at a red heat, is completely consumed. A decreased specific gravity is due to the presence of water.

Preparation for Homœopathic Use.—One part by weight of pure glycerin is dissolved in nine parts by weight of distilled water.

Amount of drug power, $\frac{1}{10}$.

Dilutions must be prepared as directed under Class V—*a*.

GNAPHALIUM POLYCEPHALUM, *Michaux.*

Nat. Ord., Compositæ.

Common Names, Common Everlasting. Indian Posey.

This is an indigenous, herbaceous annual plant. It has an erect, whitish, woody, much-branched stem, from one to two feet high. Leaves alternate, sessile, linear-lanceolate, acute, entire, scabrous above and whitish-tomentose beneath. Flowers yellow, tubular, in heads clustered at the summit of panicled corymbous branches. Ray florets subulate; disk florets entire. Receptacle naked, flat; pappus pilose, of distinct bristles.

It was first proven by Dr. William Banks, U. S.

Preparation.—The fresh plant is chopped and pounded to a pulp and weighed. Then two parts by weight of alcohol are taken, the pulp mixed thoroughly with one-sixth part of it, and the rest of the alcohol added. After having stirred the whole well, pour it into a well-stoppered bottle, and let it stand eight days in a dark, cool place. The tincture is then separated by decanting, straining and filtering.

Drug power of tincture, $\frac{1}{6}$.

Dilutions must be prepared as directed under Class III.

GOSSYPIUM HERBACEUM, *Linn.*

Synonym, Lana Gossypii.
Nat. Ord., Malvaceæ.
Common Name, Cotton Plant.

This is a biennial or triennial plant, indigenous to Asia, but largely cultivated in the southern portion of the United States. Its root is fusiform and gives off small radicles. The stem is round, pubescent and about five feet high. Leaves hairy, palmate with sub-lanceolate acute lobes. Flowers yellow, petals five with a purple spot near the base. Style simple, stigmas three or five, involved in cotton, reniform and somewhat plano-convex.

It was proven under the direction of Dr. W. Williamson, U. S.

Preparation.—The fresh inner root-bark is chopped and pounded to a pulp and weighed. Then two parts by weight of alcohol are taken, the pulp mixed thoroughly with one-sixth part of it, and the rest of the alcohol added. After having stirred the whole well, pour it into a well-stoppered bottle, and let it stand eight days in a dark, cool place. The tincture is then separated by decanting, straining and filtering.

Drug power of tincture, $\frac{1}{6}$.

Dilutions must be prepared as directed under Class III.

GRANATUM.

Synonym, Punica Granatum, *Linn.*

Nat. Ord., Granateæ.

Common Name, Pomegranate.

P. Granatum is a shrub or low tree with small deciduous leaves and attractive scarlet flowers, indigenous to Northern India and Persia. It is rarely more than twenty feet high, and its root is woody, heavy and knotty. The bark of the root is grayish or yellowish-gray in color externally, but the inner side is distinctly yellow. The bark of the pomegranate root occurs in commerce in thin quills or fragments, three to four inches in length; their outer surface is marked by wrinkled cross striations; the inner surface is smooth or finely fibrous with an occasional strip of the tough, whitish wood attached. Its fracture is short and granular. The bark has but little odor, its taste is astringent and somewhat bitter, and when chewed it colors the saliva yellow.

The drug was first proven by Dr. J. O. Muller, Germany.

Preparation.—The dried root-bark, coarsely powdered, is covered with two parts by weight of dilute alcohol, and allowed to stand eight days in a well-stoppered bottle, in a dark, cool place, being shaken twice a day, and then pressed out *lege artis* in a piece of new linen and filtered.

Drug power of tincture, $\frac{1}{3}$.

Dilutions must be prepared as directed under Class I., except that three parts of tincture are used to seven parts of dilute alcohol for the 1x dilution, and three parts to ninety-seven parts for the 1 dilution.

GRAPHITES.

Synonyms, Plumbago. Carbo Mineralis. Carburetum Ferri. Cerussa Nigra.

Common Name, Black Lead.

Graphite is a mineral carbon. It is found in the greatest purity in the Borrowdale mine, England; but it also occurs very pure in this country, especially near Bustleton in Pennsylvania. It crystallizes in hexagonal scales, whose specific gravity is between 1.8 and 2.6. It is a blackish-gray substance, of metallic lustre, soft and greasy to the touch, inodorous, and a good conductor of electricity. It was formerly supposed to be a carburet of iron, but it is an allotropic form of the element carbon.

To prepare graphite for medical use, it must be boiled for an hour in a sufficient quantity of distilled water, after which the fluid is to be decanted and the graphite to be digested in a solution of equal parts of sulphuric and hydrochloric acids, diluted with twice their volume of water. After repeatedly stirring the mixture for twenty-four hours, decant the fluid, wash the residue with distilled water and dry it. Because of the extraordinary fineness and flexibility of its scaly crystals it resists even the most continual trituration, which has lasted for hours, and shows permanently not inconsiderable portions of shining points. To obviate this, the best means is to triturate the purified graphite in small portions with coarsely powdered sugar of milk, adding as much water, in a roomy porcelain dish, as is necessary to make the whole into a thick paste. This rubbing is to be continued until the water has evaporated and the mass begins to form little lumps. Boiling hot distilled water is then poured over the whole to dissolve the sugar of milk and to separate the coarser from the finer particles of graphites. This graphite is washed repeatedly and dried.

It was first proven by Hahnemann.

Preparation.—The purified graphite, prepared as described above, is prepared by trituration, as directed under Class VII.

GRATIOLA.

Synonyms, Gratiola Officinalis, *Linn.*
Nat. Ord., Scrophulariaceæ.
Common Name, Hedge Hyssop.

This plant, growing in Central and Southern Europe, near the borders of rivers, lakes and water ditches, also on moist meadows, has a creeping, articulate, on the joints fibrillous root, as thick as a quill and whitish; the stem, one-half to one and a half feet high, is erect, little branched, four-sided above. It has opposite, sessile, lanceolate, finely serrate, three-nerved leaves, and solitary axillary whitish or reddish two-lipped flowers, with yellow hairs in the tube. The whole plant is smooth, pale green, inodorous, and has a very bitter, somewhat acrid, taste.

It was first proven by Nenning, Germany.

Preparation.—The fresh plant, gathered before flowering, is chopped and pounded to a pulp, enclosed in a piece of new linen and subjected to pressure. The expressed juice is then, by brisk agitation, mingled with an equal part by weight of alcohol. This mixture is allowed to stand eight days in a well-stoppered bottle, in a dark, cool place, and then filtered.

Drug power of tincture, $\frac{1}{2}$.
Dilutions must be prepared as directed under Class I.

GRINDELIA ROBUSTA, *Nuttall.*

Nat. Ord., Compositæ.
Common Name, Grindelia.

The Grindelias comprise a genus of herbaceous plants, with some plants woody at the base only. They are found in the western part of North America. They are resinous, possess a balsamic odor and a bitter aromatic taste. The composite heads have yellow ray-florets, ligulate and pistillate; the disk-florets are five-pointed, tubular and perfect. Receptacle flat and with alveolar depressions. Pappus of a few stiff awns. *Grindelia robusta* is a species which produces many varieties. Leaves spatulate or oblong, varying to lanceolate, serrate; apex obtuse. Upper ones cordate at the base and frequently clasping.

Preparation.—The fresh herb, in flower, is chopped and pounded to a pulp and weighed. Then two parts by weight of alcohol are taken, the pulp mixed thoroughly with one-sixth part of it, and the rest of the alcohol added. After having stirred the whole well, pour it into a well-stoppered bottle, and let it stand eight days in a dark, cool place. The tincture is then separated by decanting, straining and filtering.

Drug power of tincture, $\frac{1}{6}$.
Dilutions must be prepared as directed under Class III.

GRINDELIA SQUARROSA, *Dunal.*

Nat. Ord., Compositæ.
Common Name, Grindelia.

This species of grindelia is glabrous from a varnish-like exudation. Leaves punctate, spatulate-lanceolate varying to oblong-lanceolate. Upper leaves sessile, somewhat obtuse, finally dentate. Involucre of reflexed, subulate, pointed, squarrose scales.

It was proved by Dr. J. H. Bundy, United States.

Preparation.—The fresh herb, in flower, is chopped and pounded to a pulp and weighed. Then two parts by weight of alcohol are taken, the pulp mixed thoroughly with one-sixth part of it, and the rest of the alcohol added. After having stirred the whole well, pour it into a well-stoppered bottle, and let it stand eight days in a dark, cool place. The tincture is then separated by decanting, straining and filtering.

Drug power of tincture, $\frac{1}{6}$.
Dilutions must be prepared as directed under Class III.

GUACO.

Synonym, Mikania Guaco, *Humboldt* and *Bonpland.*
Nat. Ord., Corymbiferæ.
Common Name, Mikania Guaco.

This plant is indigenous to tropical America. It is climbing, herbaceous, about twenty feet long. Leaves ovate or ovate-elliptical, subacuminate and scarcely dentate, rough above and tomentous beneath. Flowers in corymbs, opposite and axillary. In the fresh state the leaves have a disagreeable odor and bitter taste; both of these properties together with their medicinal powers are greatly lessened by drying.

It was proven by Dr. Petroz, Spain.

Preparation.—The fresh leaves are chopped and pounded to a pulp and weighed. Then two parts by weight of alcohol are taken, the pulp mixed thoroughly with one-sixth part of it, and the rest of the alcohol added. After having stirred the whole well, pour it into a well-stoppered bottle, and let it stand eight days in a dark, cool place. The tincture is then separated by decanting, straining and filtering.

Drug power of tincture, $\frac{1}{6}$.

Dilutions must be prepared as directed under Class III.

GUAIACUM.

Synonyms, Guaiacum Officinale, *Linn.* Lignum Vitæ. Palus Sanctus.

Nat. Ord., Zygophyllaceæ.

Common Name, Guaiac.

Guaiacum officinale is a low or medium-sized evergreen tree, found growing in the West Indies, particularly in Hayti, and on the northern coast of South America. Its leaves are pari-pinnate with ovate, obtuse leaflets in two, and less frequently, in three pairs. Flowers light blue, on long peduncles, in groups of eight or ten in the axils of the upper leaves.

Resin of guaiac occurs as a natural exudation, or as the result of incisions made into the bark, or by the action of heat upon the wood in the following manner: A log of guaiacum wood is supported in a horizontal position above the ground by two upright bars. Each end of the log is then set on fire, and a large incision having been previously made in the middle, the melted resin runs out therefrom in considerable abundance.

The resin occurs in commerce in spherical tears from one-half to one inch in diameter, but commonly it is in compact masses, containing fragments of the wood and bark. It is brittle and breaks with a clean, glassy fracture. The resin is greenish or reddish-brown in color; thin fragments of it are transparent and are greenish-brown by transmitted light. When freshly powdered it becomes grayish-white in color, but exposure to light and air soon causes the powder to assume a green tint. Its odor is faint and balsamic, and its taste, which is at first very slight, is followed by an irritated sensation in the mouth and throat.

By oxidizing agents it acquires a fine blue color, as will be demonstrated by sprinkling with a dilute solution of ferric chloride a thin layer of the residue left upon evaporating its alcoholic solution.

It was first proven by Hahnemann.

Preparation.—Two parts by weight of the resin are dissolved in nine parts by weight of alcohol and then filtered.

Drug power of tincture, $\frac{1}{10}$.

Dilutions must be prepared as directed under Class VI—*a*.

GUANO AUSTRALIS.

Common Name, Guano.

Origin.—Guano is the accumulated deposit of the excrement of sea birds; it is found upon barren islands off the western coast of South America, those in the latitude of Peru furnishing the largest amount.

Description.—As generally found in commerce it is an amorphous powder, pale brown in color and of a disagreeable ammoniacal odor. Its reaction is generally alkaline, although at times specimens may give in parts an acid reaction. Its specific gravity is 1.64. Its constituents are chiefly uric acid, ammonium urate, with some oxalates, with phosphates of the alkali metals and of magnesium and calcium.

The kind used by Dr. Mure, who introduced it into our Materia Medica, is from Patagonia, and is probably not in any respect different from that obtained from Peru.

Preparation.—The guano, obtained as fresh as possible, is prepared by trituration, as directed under Class VII.

GUARANA.

Synonym, Paullinia Sorbilis, *Martius*.

Nat. Ord., Sapindaceæ.

Common Name, Brazilian Cocoa.

Guarana is a preparation made from a climbing shrub, *Paullinia sorbilis*, indigenous to Northern and Western Brazil. The plant has pinnate leaves, leaflets five, dentate and oval-oblong. Flowers small, in panicles. Fruit a pear-shaped capsule, beaked, containing not more than three dark brown, nearly black, almost globular seeds. The preparation guarana is made from the seeds by powdering them and making a paste with water. The paste is rounded into masses and either fire-dried or sun-dried. The masses of guarana are hard, irregular in surface, reddish-brown in color externally, but lighter within; they break with a vitreous fracture. The taste of guarana is bitter and astringent, and it has a faint odor which is peculiar.

Preparation.—The dried paste made from the seeds, as described above, is covered with five parts by weight of alcohol, and allowed to remain eight days in a well-stoppered bottle, in a dark, cool place, being shaken twice a day. The tincture is then poured off, strained and filtered.

Drug power of tincture, $\frac{1}{10}$.

Dilutions must be prepared as directed under Class IV.

GUAREA TRICHILOIDES, *Linn.*

Nat. Ord., Meliaceæ.

Common Names, Ball-wood. Red-wood.

This medium-sized tree grows in Dominica, St. Vincent and Guadeloupe.

Calyx four-toothed or four-lobed. Petals oblong, two to three inches long, imbricative. Stameneal tube quite entire. Anthers sessile, internally, near its mouth. Ovary four-celled; cells one-ovulate or two-ovulate, with the ovules superimposed. Pericarp woody, at length loculicidal. Leaves abruptly pinnate; the pairs appearing successively along the petiole; panicles simply racemiform, axillary.

It was proven by Dr. Petroz, Spain.

Preparation.—The bark is finely powdered and covered with five parts by weight of alcohol, and then poured into a well-stoppered bottle, and allowed to remain eight days in a dark, cool place, being shaken twice a day. The tincture is then poured off, strained and filtered.

Drug power of tincture, $\frac{1}{10}$.

Dilutions must be prepared as directed under Class IV.

GYMNOCLADUS CANADENSIS, *Lamarck.*

Synonym, Guilandin Dioica.

Nat. Ord., Leguminosæ.

Common Names, American Coffee Tree. Chicot. Kentucky Coffee Tree.

This is a tall, large tree, growing in rich woods, along rivers, from Western New York and Pennsylvania to Illinois and southwestward. It is also cultivated as an ornamental tree. The compound leaves are two to three feet long, with several large partial leafstalks bearing seven to thirteen ovate stalked leaflets, the lowest pair with single leaflets. Flowers are whitish, in terminal racemes. Pod, which is from six to ten inches long and about two inches broad, contains several large flattish seeds.

It was introduced into our Materia Medica by Dr. Hering.

Preparation.—The fresh pulp within the pod surrounding the seeds is crushed and weighed. Then two parts by weight of alcohol are taken, the pulp mixed thoroughly with one-sixth part of it, and the rest of the alcohol added. After stirring the whole well, pour it into a well-stoppered bottle, and let it stand eight days in a dark, cool place. The tincture is then separated by decanting, straining and filtering.

Amount of drug power, $\frac{1}{6}$.

Dilutions must be prepared as directed under Class III.

HÆMATOXYLON.

Synonyms, Hæmatoxylon Campechianum, *Linn.* Lignum Campechianum.

Nat. Ord., Leguminosæ.
Common Names, Logwood. Peachwood.

H. Campechianum is a medium-sized tree, indigenous to the countries about the Gulf of Campeachy, but it is successfully cultivated in other portions of Central America and in the West India Islands. Its numerous, spreading, crooked branches are furnished with alternate leaves made up of obcordate, nearly sessile leaflets in three or four pairs. The flowers are small, yellow, five-parted, in loose racemes. The tree is cut down when about ten years old, and only the red heart-wood is used. In commerce logwood is in logs from three to four feet long, of a blackish-purple color externally, and of a brownish-red within. Its specific gravity is about 1.6; it has a slight, peculiar odor and an agreeable, sweet, slightly astringent taste.

It was introduced into our Materia Medica by Dr. Jouve, Bibl. Hom. de Geneve, I. 47.

Preparation.—The best Campeachy logwood, in fine chips, is covered with five parts by weight of alcohol, and allowed to remain eight days in a well-stoppered bottle, in a dark, cool place, being shaken twice a day. The tincture is then poured off, strained and filtered.

Drug power of tincture, $\frac{1}{10}$.

Dilutions must be prepared as directed under Class IV.

HAMAMELIS.

Synonyms, Hamamelis Virginica, *Linn.* Trilopus Dentata.
Nat. Ord., Hamamelaceæ.
Common Name, Witch-Hazel.

This shrub is indigenous to the United States and Canada, where it grows in damp woods. It reaches a height of from six to ten feet; the stem and branches are crooked. On the younger branches the bark is brown in color and smooth, but that covering the older portions of the wood is brownish-gray and fissured. Leaves alternate, oval, somewhat cordate at the base, wavy-toothed, and when young somewhat downy. Flowers yellowish-green, in axillary clusters. Pod two-celled and two-seeded. It flowers late in autumn, but the seeds do not mature till September of the following year.

It was first proven by Dr. H. C. Preston, United States.

Preparation.—The fresh bark of the twigs and root is chopped and pounded to a pulp and weighed. Then two parts by weight of alcohol are taken, the pulp mixed thoroughly with one-sixth part of it, and the rest of the alcohol added. After having stirred the whole well, pour it into a well-stoppered bottle, and let it stand eight days in a dark, cool place. The tincture is then separated by decanting, straining and filtering.

Drug power of tincture, $\frac{1}{6}$.

Dilutions must be prepared as directed under Class III.

HEKLA LAVA.

Dr. Garth Wilkinson, of London, states in a letter to Dr. Wm. H. Holcombe, of New Orleans:

"Its known pathological effects on the sheep in the vicinity of Hekla are immense exostoses of the jaws.

"The finer ash, which fell on the pastures in distant localities, was particularly deleterious, while the gross ash near the mountain was inert.

"These accounts are from a Danish account of the eruptions of Hekla and their consequences to nature, to man, beast and vegetable. Hekla lava, according to Prof. Morris, of University College, London, has for general constituents, combinations of silica, alumina, lime, magnesia, with some oxide of iron; sometimes it contains anarthite and other minerals." (Vide Tr. Am. Inst., 1870, p. 441.)

Preparation.—For homœopathic use the above-mentioned fine ash is triturated according to Class VII.

HEDEOMA.

Synonyms, Hedeoma Pulegioides, *Persoon.* Cunila Pulegioides, *Linn.* Melissa Pulegioides. Ziziphora Pulegioides.

Nat. Ord., Labiatæ.

Common Names, American Pennyroyal. Squaw Mint. Tickweed.

This is an annual plant, indigenous to the United States and Canada, from nine to fifteen inches high. Its root is small, branching, fibrous, yellowish; stem erect, pubescent and branched. Leaves opposite, oblong, nearly acute, ovate, scarcely serrate, rough or pubescent, glandular-punctate on the under surface. The flowers are small, pale blue, on short peduncles, in axillary cymose whorls upon the branches. Its odor is mint-like and its taste aromatic.

Preparation.—The fresh plant is chopped and pounded to a pulp and weighed. Then two parts by weight of alcohol are taken, the pulp mixed thoroughly with one-sixth part of it, and the rest of the alcohol added. After having been stirred, it is poured into a well-stoppered bottle, and allowed to stand eight days in a dark, cool place. The tincture is then separated by decanting, straining and filtering.

Drug power of tincture, $\frac{1}{6}$.

Dilutions must be prepared as directed under Class III.

HEDYSARUM ILDEFONSIANUM.

Synonym, Carapicho.

Nat. Ord., Leguminosæ.

Common Name, Brazilian Burdock.

This plant is a native of Brazil. The brownish and ligneous stem is about three feet high; it is ramose, pubescent, especially above. Leaves alternate, pinnate, trifoliate; folioles oval and slightly tomentose, on a hairy, bistipulate petiole. The flowers which are small and seated on filiform, unifloral peduncles, form loose, terminal spikes. Fruit oval, hairy, on bent peduncles, attaching itself very intimately to clothes and to the hairy skin of animals, on which account the Brazilians call it "barba de boi."

It was introduced into our Materia Medica by Dr. Mure, Brazil.

Preparation.—The dried leaves are coarsely pulverized and weighed, covered with five parts by weight of alcohol, and allowed to remain eight days in a well-stoppered bottle, at the ordinary temperature, in a dark place, being shaken twice a day. The tincture is then poured off, strained and filtered.

Drug power of tincture, $\frac{1}{10}$.

Dilutions must be prepared as directed under Class IV.

HELIANTHUS.

Synonym, Helianthus Annuus, *Linn.*

Nat. Ord., Compositæ.

Common Name, Sunflower.

The sunflower is a native of tropical America, but is cultivated very generally in the temperate zones. Stem from ten to fifteen feet high, rough. Leaves large, on petioles, alternate, three-ribbed, ovate, the lower ones cordate, serrate, rough. The flower-heads often a foot in diameter; ray flowers bright yellow, ligulate; disk flat; achenia dark purple, four-sided, laterally compressed, at the base embraced by the persistent chaff, and the principal angles surmounted by a pappus of two chaffy scales.

It was proven by Dr. Cessoles, Switzerland (?).

Preparation.—The ripe seeds (achenia), coarsely powdered, are covered with five parts by weight of dilute alcohol, and allowed to remain eight days in a well-stoppered bottle, in a dark, cool place, being shaken twice a day. The tincture is then poured off, strained and filtered.

Drug power of tincture, $\frac{1}{10}$.

Dilutions must be prepared as directed under Class IV, except that the 2x and 3x, and the 1 and 2, require dilute alcohol.

HELLEBORUS.

Synonyms, Helleborus Niger, *Linn.* Melanpodium. Veratrum Nigrum.

Nat. Ord., Ranunculaceæ.

Common Names, Black Hellebore. Christmas Rose.

The black hellebore has a perennial, knotted root, one to three inches long, blackish on the outside, white within, and sends off numerous long, simple rootlets, which are brownish-yellow in the recent state, but when dried, dark brown. The rootlets are very brittle. Upon section, the rhizome shows a rather thick bark, brownish-gray in color, and a whitish pith occupying centrally about one-half the diameter of the section; imbedded in the pith but not reaching its centre, are six to ten wedge-shaped bundles of wood-fibre, which radiate and extend into the substance of the bark. The leaves are pedately divided, dark green in color, on long foot-stalks from the root. Each leaf is seven to nine-lobed, one terminal. The leaflets are ovate-lanceolate, smooth, shining coriaceous and serrated above. The flower-stem rises from the root, and is round, tapering, and reddish towards the base, having one or two large, rose-like flowers. It is indigenous to the mountainous regions of southern and temperate Europe. It flowers from December to March.

It was first proved by Hahnemann.

Preparation.—The root, gathered immediately after the period of flowering, is cautiously dried and powdered, covered with five parts by weight of alcohol, and allowed to remain eight days in a well-stoppered bottle, in a dark, cool place, being shaken twice a day. The tincture is then poured off, strained and filtered.

Drug power of tincture, $\frac{1}{10}$.

Dilutions must be prepared as directed under Class IV.

HELONIAS DIOICA, *Pursh.*

Synonyms, Chamælirium Luteum, *Gray.* Veratrum Luteum, *Linn.* Chamælirium Carolinianum, *Willd.* Helonias Lutea, *Aiton.*

Nat. Ord., Liliaceæ.

Common Names, Blazing Star. Starwort. False Unicorn.

The plant is indigenous to the United States, where it grows in low grounds. The herb is smooth; stem wand-like, from a thick and abrupt tuberous rootstock, and terminated by a long, wand-like, spiked raceme (four to nine inches long) of small, bractless flowers; fertile plant more leafy than the staminate. Leaves are flat, lanceolate, the lowest spatulate, tapering into a petiole. Flowers diœcious. Perianth of six spatulate-linear (white) spreading sepals, withering, persistent. Filaments like threads. Anthers two-celled, yellow, extrorse; fertile flowers with rudimentary stamens. Styles linear-club-shaped, stigmatic along the inner side. Pod ovoid-oblong, not lobed, many-seeded. Flowers in June.

Preparation.—The fresh root, gathered just before flowering, is chopped and pounded to a pulp and weighed. Then two parts by weight of alcohol are taken, the pulp mixed thoroughly with one-sixth part of it, and the rest of the alcohol added. After having stirred the whole well, and poured it into a well-stoppered bottle, it is allowed to stand eight days in a dark, cool place. The tincture is then separated by decanting, straining and filtering.

Drug power of tincture, $\frac{1}{6}$.

Dilutions must be prepared as directed under Class III.

HEPAR SULPHURIS CALCAREUM.

Synonyms, Calcarea Sulphuratum. Calx Sulphurata.

Common Names, Hepar Sulphuris. Impure Calcium Sulphide.

Preparation of Hepar Sulphuris.—This must be prepared according to Hahnemann's direction, viz., by mixing equal parts of finely powdered and calcined oyster-shells and pure well-washed flowers of sulphur, placing them in a clay crucible, covered with a thick layer of moistened powdered chalk, and keeping the mixture at a white heat for at least ten minutes. When cold, open the crucible and preserve the hepar in well-closed bottles protected from the light.

Properties and Tests.—Hepar sulphuris is in white, porous, friable masses, or is a white, amorphous powder, having the odor and taste of sulphuretted hydrogen; it is insoluble in cold water, but dissolves in hot hydrochloric acid with evolution of hydrogen sulphide. The solution gives a white precipitate with oxalate of ammonia.

Preparation for Homœopathic Use.—Hepar sulphuris, prepared as above, is triturated as directed under Class VII.

Though a solution or so-called tincture, made of one part hepar sulphuris, with ninety-nine parts of dilute alcohol, has been recommended, it should not be relied on, as its strength is very uncertain.

HEPAR SULPHURIS KALINUM.

Synonyms, Kalium Sulphuratum. Potassii Sulphuratum.

Common Names, Sulphurated Potash. Liver of Sulphur. Sulphuret of Potassium.

Preparation of Sulphuret of Potassium.—Take of sublimed sulphur, one part; carbonate of potassium, two parts. Dry the carbonate of potassium, then rub it with the sulphur, and gradually heat the mixture in a covered crucible until it ceases to swell and is perfectly fused. Then pour the mass on a marble tile, and when cold break it into pieces. It should be kept in a well-stoppered bottle protected from the light.

Properties.—The sulphide of potassium prepared recently and according to the process given above, is in flattish pieces of a liver-brown color, which, upon exposure to air or by prolonged keeping, become brownish-yellow or greenish-yellow. It is without crystalline structure. Its reaction is alkaline. It forms with water a yellow solution having the odor of hydrogen sulphide, and when an acid is added, that gas is evolved and a precipitation of separated sulphur occurs. It contains, in addition to potassium sulphide, some sulphate of the alkali. It should dissolve completely in water, and almost entirely in alcohol.

Tests.—The presence of sodium is shown by the yellow color of the flame of an alcoholic solution when ignited. Three parts of it dissolved in distilled water and shaken with a solution of four parts of sulphate of copper, should give a filtrate which does not respond to the tests for copper and is not precipitated by hydrogen sulphide.

Preparation for Homœopathic Use.—The pure sulphuret of potassium is triturated, as directed under Class VII.

HEPATICA.

Synonyms, Hepatica Triloba, *Chaix.* Anemone Hepatica, *Linn.*
Nat. Ord., Ranunculaceæ.
Common Name, Liverwort.

This is an indigenous plant, with a perennial fibrous root; leaves radical, three-lobed, cordate at the base, thick, nearly smooth, glaucous, upon hairy footstalks from four to eight inches long, which spring directly from the root. The scapes are several in number, round and hairy, and bear a single white, bluish, or purplish flower. The involucre, at a little distance below the corolla, resembles a calyx. The plant grows upon the sides of hills and mountains. The leaves survive the winter, and the flowers appear in the early spring.

It was proved by Dr. D. G. Kimball, U. S.

Preparation.—The fresh leaves are chopped and pounded to a pulp and weighed. Then two parts by weight of alcohol are taken, the pulp thoroughly mixed with one-sixth part of it, and the rest of the alcohol added. After stirring the whole well, and pouring it into a well-stoppered bottle, it is allowed to stand eight days in a dark, cool place. The tincture is then separated by decanting, straining and filtering.

Drug power of tincture, $\frac{1}{6}$.

Dilutions must be prepared as directed under Class III.

HIPPOMANES.

Hippomanes is the normally white, usually dark olive-green, soft, glutinous, mucous substance, of a urinous odor, which floats in the allantois fluid, or is attached to the allantois membrane of the mare or cow, chiefly during the last months of pregnancy. For the provings, the substance was taken by the veterinary Helffrich from the tongue of a newly-born filly, and when dried was employed.

It was introduced into our Materia Medica by Dr. Hering.

Preparation.—The dried substance is triturated according to Class VII.

HURA BRAZILIENSIS, *Willd.*

Nat. Ord., Rutaceæ.
Common Names (in Brazil), Assacu. Oassacu.

This plant inhabits the equatorial regions of South America, the provinces of Para, Rio Negro, and the neighborhood of the Amazon, where it is very abundant. It resembles the *Hura Crepitans, Linn.*; its leaves are alternate, somewhat cordate, rounded, glabrous, serrate; rolled up and stipulate while young. The petiole is provided at its top with two large glands. Flowers monœcious; the male flowers having a short, urceolate perianth, and covered with a scaly bract; they form elongated, peduncled, terminal husks. The female flowers, which are twice as long as those of the Hura Crepitans, have their perianth resting against the ovary, which is surmounted by a long and infundibuliform style, terminated by a stellate stigma; they are solitary and placed near the male flowers. It is from this tree that the Indians draw the milky juice called Assacu by the Brazilians.

It was introduced into our Materia Medica by Dr. Mure, Brazil.

Preparation.—The fresh sap, obtained by boring the trunk of the tree, is mixed with an equal part by weight of alcohol.

Amount of drug power, $\frac{1}{2}$.

Dilutions must be prepared as directed under Class I.

HYDRASTIS.

Synonyms, Hydrastis Canadensis, *Linn.* Warneria Canadensis.

Nat. Ord., Ranunculaceæ.

Common Names, Golden Seal. Yellow Root. Yellow Puccoon.

This plant is a small, herbaceous perennial, found growing in rich woods in the United States, but especially in the north and west. Its rhizome is knotted, thick, fleshy and yellow in color, and furnished with long rootlets. Stem simple, hairy, nearly a foot high. It has one radical leaf and two from the stem. The leaves are rounded, cordate at the base, five to seven-lobed, doubly serrate; a single greenish-white flower terminates the stem; petals none, calyx colored, corolla-like, caducous. Fruit a red or purple berry, in globular masses.

The first provings were made under the direction of Dr. Lippe, U. S.

Preparation.—The fresh root is chopped and pounded to a pulp and weighed. Then two parts by weight of alcohol are taken, and after thoroughly mixing the pulp with one-sixth part of it, the rest of the alcohol is added. After stirring the whole well, and pouring it into a well-stoppered bottle, it is allowed to stand eight days in a dark, cool place. The tincture is then separated by decanting, straining and filtering.

Drug power of tincture, $\frac{1}{6}$.

Dilutions must be prepared as directed under Class III.

HYDROCOTYLE ASIATICA, *Linn.*

Synonyms, Hydrocotyle Nummularioides. Hydrocotyle Pallida.

Nat. Ord., Umbelliferæ.

Common Names, Indian Pennywort. Water Pennywort.

This perennial creeping plant is indigenous to tropical regions in both continents. Leaves smooth petiolate, grouped on the nodes of the stem, round-kidney shape, dark green in color, an inch broad, with crenate margin. Flowers pinkish, in three-flowered umbels. The fresh bruised leaves have a peculiar odor, and a bitter pungent taste.

It was introduced into the Homœopathic Materia Medica by Dr. Audouit, France.

Preparation.—The carefully dried plant is coarsely powdered, covered with five parts by weight of alcohol, and allowed to remain eight days in a well-stoppered bottle, in a dark, cool place, being shaken twice a day. The tincture is then poured off, strained and filtered.

Drug power of tincture, $\frac{1}{10}$.
Dilutions must be prepared as directed under Class IV.

HYDROPHYLLUM VIRGINICUM, *Linn.*

Nat. Ord., Hydrophyllaceæ.
Common Names, Burr Flower. Waterleaf.
This plant is indigenous, found growing in damp woods. Its stem is smooth, from one to two feet high. The pinnately divided leaves have five to seven divisions, ovate-lanceolate or oblong pointed, sharply dentate, the lowest mostly two-parted, the uppermost confluent; peduncles forked, longer than the petioles of the upper leaves. Calyx-lobes narrowly linear, bristly-ciliate. Corolla campanulate, five-cleft; the tube has five longitudinal linear appendages opposite the lobes, cohering by their middle, with their edges folded inwards, forming a nectariferous groove. Stamens and style mostly exserted; filaments more or less bearded; anthers linear; ovary bristly hairy; spherical pod, ripening one to four seeds. Flowers appear from June to August.
It was introduced into our Materia Medica by Dr. P. B. Hoyt, United States.
Preparation.—The fresh plant, in bloom, is chopped and pounded to a pulp and weighed. Then two parts by weight of alcohol are taken, the pulp thoroughly mixed with one-sixth part of it, and the rest of the alcohol added. After stirring the whole mixture well, pour it into a well-stoppered bottle, and let it stand eight days in a dark, cool place. The tincture is then separated by decanting, straining and filtering.
Drug power of tincture, $\frac{1}{6}$.
Dilutions must be prepared as directed under Class III.

HYDROPIPER.

Synonym, Polygonum Hydropiper, *Linn.*
Nat. Ord., Polygonaceæ.
Common Names, Common Smartweed. Water-Pepper.
This annual, growing from one to two feet high, is a native of Europe and North America, where it is found growing in moist or wet grounds. Stem is smooth; spikes nodding, generally short or interrupted; flowers greenish; stamens six; style two or three-parted; achenium dull, minutely striate, either flat or obtusely triangular. The whole herb is pungent and acrid. Flowers appear late in summer or early in autumn.
Preparation.—The fresh plant is chopped and pounded to a pulp and weighed. Then two parts by weight of alcohol are taken, the pulp mixed thoroughly with one-sixth part of it, and the rest of the alcohol added. After having stirred the whole well, pour it into a well-stoppered bottle, and let it stand eight days in a dark, cool place. The tincture is then separated by decanting, straining and filtering.
Amount of drug power, $\frac{1}{6}$.
Dilutions must be prepared as directed under Class III.

HYOSCYAMUS.

Synonyms, Hyoscyamus Niger, *Linn.* Jusquiami.
Nat. Ord., Solanaceæ.
Common Names, Henbane. Hogbean. Poison Tobacco.

This plant is usually a biennial, with a long, conical, whitish, fleshy, slightly branching root, somewhat like that of parsley, for which it has been mistaken with poisonous results. The stem which rises in the second year, is round, branching, erect and very leafy. Leaves large, oblong, cut sinuously into pointed lobes, clasping at the base. The whole plant is viscid, hairy, sea-green in color, and fetid. Flowers are on one-sided, terminal, depending spikes; calyx tubular, five-cleft; corolla funnel-shaped, five-lobed and unequal, straw-yellow in color, with a network of dark purple veins. Fruit a two-celled pyxis, containing numerous seeds. The plant is a native of Europe, where it grows on roadsides, amid rubbish, etc.

This drug was first proven by Hahnemann.

Preparation.—The fresh blooming plant is chopped and pounded to a pulp, enclosed in a piece of new linen and subjected to pressure. The expressed juice is then, by brisk agitation, mingled with an equal part by weight of alcohol. The mixture is allowed to stand eight days in a well-stoppered bottle, in a dark, cool place, and then filtered.

Drug power of tincture, $\frac{1}{2}$.

Dilutions must be prepared as directed under Class I.

HYPERICUM.

Synonyms, Hypericum Perforatum, *Linn.* Fuga Dæmonum. Herba Solis.
Nat. Ord., Hypericaceæ.
Common Name, St. John's Wort.

This perennial herb is abundant both in Europe and this country, often covering whole fields, and proving extremely annoying to farmers. It is from one to two feet high. The stem is erect, much branched, smooth, two-edged, set with small, opposite, half-clasping, oblong-oval, obtuse, smooth leaves, pellucid-punctate. The flowers in terminal panicles, are on short petioles, are star-shaped, yellow, at the margin black-punctate. Fruit a three-celled pod.

It was proven by Dr Geo. F. Müller, Germany.

Preparation.—The fresh, blooming plant, is chopped and pounded to a pulp and weighed. Then two parts by weight of alcohol are taken, the pulp mixed thoroughly with one-sixth part of it, and the rest of the alcohol added. After having stirred the whole well, pour it into a well-stoppered bottle, and let it stand eight days in a dark, cool place. The tincture is then separated by decanting, straining and filtering.

Drug power of tincture, $\frac{1}{6}$.

Dilutions must be prepared as directed under Class III.

IBERIS AMARA, *Linn.*

Synonym, Lepidium Iberis.
Nat. Ord., Cruciferæ.
Common Name, Bitter Candy-Tuft.

This plant is indigenous to Europe. It is cultivated in gardens on account of its bright, milk-white flowers, and appears occasionally in corn fields in England. It is an herbaceous plant, about a foot in height, with a few erect branches forming a terminal flat corymb. Leaves oblong-lanceolate or broadly linear, with a few coarse teeth, or slightly pinnatifid. Flowers white. Pod nearly orbicular, the long style projecting from the notch at the top.

This drug was proven under the direction of Dr. E. M. Hale, United States.

Preparation.—The ripe seeds are coarsely powdered, covered with five parts by weight of alcohol, and allowed to remain eight days in a well-stoppered bottle, in a dark, cool place, being shaken twice a day. The tincture is then poured off, strained and filtered.

Amount of drug power, $\frac{1}{10}$.

Dilutions must be prepared as directed under Class IV.

IGNATIA.

Synonyms, Strychnos Ignatia, *Lindley.* Faba Ignatii. (Ignatia Amara, *Linn.*)
Nat. Ord., Loganiaceæ.
Common Names, Ignatia. Bean of St. Ignatius.

S. Ignatia is a large shrub or small tree, climbing in habit, found growing in the Phillippine Islands and Cochin China. It has opposite, ovate, entire and glaucous leaves. The flowers are white and fragrant, tubular, nodding, in short axillary racemes. The fruit is oblong or sub-globular in shape, berry-like in character, and within the brittle pericarp is a bitter pulp enclosing from twenty to twenty-four seeds. The seeds are about an inch long, oblong or ovate in shape, obscurely angular, with one convex and one flat side, and having a conspicuous hilum at one end. In the fresh state they are covered with a silky down, beneath which is the brown epidermis. In commerce the seed is found deprived of the pericarp, and it consists simply of the albumen whose surface is granular and gray. The albumen is translucent and difficult to split. The name Ignatia Amara, *Linn.*, is not the title of the plant furnishing the St. Ignatius bean, and should be dropped from such connection.

The drug was proven by Hahnemann.

Preparation.—The powdered seeds are covered with five parts by weight of alcohol, and allowed to remain eight days in a well-stoppered bottle, in a dark, cool place, being shaken twice a day. The tincture is then poured off, strained and filtered.

Drug power of tincture, $\frac{1}{10}$.

Dilutions must be prepared as directed under Class IV.

Triturations are prepared from the powdered seed as directed under Class VII.

ILEX OPACA, *Aiton.*

Synonyms, Ageria Opaca. Ilex Aquifolium
Nat. Ord., Aquifoliaceæ.
Common Name, American Holly.

This tree, from twenty to forty feet in height, grows in moist woodlands, from Maine to Pennsylvania, near the coast, but is commoner from Virginia southward. Leaves oval, flat, margins wavy, sparsely spinous-dentate; flowers in loose clusters along the base of the young branches and in the axils; calyx-teeth acute. Drupe red, its nutlets ribbed, veiny, or one-grooved on the back. Flowers appear in June.

Preparation.—The fresh leaves, gathered in June, are chopped and pounded to a pulp and weighed. Then two parts by weight of alcohol are taken, the pulp mixed thoroughly with one-sixth part of it, and the rest of the alcohol added. After having stirred the whole well, pour it into a well-stoppered bottle, and let it stand eight days in a dark, cool place. The tincture is then separated by decanting, straining and filtering.

Amount of drug power, $\frac{1}{6}$.

Dilutions must be prepared as directed under Class III.

INDIGO.

Synonyms, Color Indicus. Indicum. Pigmentum Indicum.
Nat. Ord., Leguminosæ.
Common Name, Indigo.

A blue dye stuff, the product of several species of indigoferæ, chiefly *Indigofera tinctoria.* The genus indigoferæ is made up of herbaceous plants, or of plants woody only at the base. The juices of the plants contain indican, $C_{26} H_{31} NO_{17}$, which, when boiled with acids or submitted to the action of ferments, absorbs water and splits up into indigo-blue, $C_8 H_5 N O$, and indiglucin, $C_6 H_{10} O_6$, as shown by the equation $C_{26} H_{31} N O_{17} + 2H_2 O = C_8 H_5 N O + 3 (C_6 H_{10} O_6)$. The change was formerly supposed to be due to the oxidation of a substance called indigo-white or chromogen, which was held to be a constituent of the plants, but the researches of Schunk showed that as indigo-white requires free alkali for its solution, it could not exist in the sap of plants, which is always acid. To obtain indigo from the plants which produce it the chopped leaves and twigs are macerated in water for twelve or fifteen hours and allowed to ferment, after which the liquid is poured into shallow vats and repeatedly stirred. The indigo thereby deposited is separated from the brown liquid, boiled with water and dried. Commercial indigo contains from fifty to sixty per cent. of pure indigo-blue, the remainder consisting of indiglucin, indigo-red, indigo-brown and a number of resinous products. It may be purified by different methods. By submitting the commercial article to sublimation between two platinum crucible-lids, kept not more than three-eighths of an inch apart, crystals of pure sublimed indigo may be obtained.

Properties.—The sublimed substance is in purple-red prisms of a metallic lustre. The precipitated indigo is in dark blue masses or cakes. When rubbed with a hard body, the substance becomes distinctly coppery in appearance. It is without odor or taste, is insoluble in ordinary solvents, but is dissolved by nitro-benzol, chloroform, chloral hydrate and fuming sulphuric acid, the solution in the latter being called sulph-indigotic acid.

It was first proven by Drs. Martin and Schüler, Germany.

Preparation for Homœopathic Use.—Indigo is triturated as directed under Class VII.

INDIUM METALLICUM.

Synonyms, Indium. Metallic Indium.
Symbol, In.
Atomic Weight, 74.

Origin.—This metal was discovered by Reich and Richter, in the zinc-blende of Freiberg. Its spectrum is characterized by two indigo-colored lines, one very bright and more refrangible than the blue line of strontium, the other fainter but still more refrangible, approaching the blue line of potassium. It was the production of this peculiar spectrum that lead to the discovery of the metal, and its name is indicative of the color of the lines. The ore, consisting chiefly of blende, galena, and arsenical pyrites, was roasted to expel sulphur and arsenic, then treated with hydrochloric acid, and the solution was evaporated to dryness. The impure zinc chloride thus obtained exhibited, when examined by the spectroscope, the first of the indigo lines above mentioned. The chloride was afterwards obtained in a state of greater purity, and from this the hydrate and the metal itself were prepared. The first line then came out with much greater brilliancy and the second was likewise observed.

Properties.—Indium has hitherto been obtained in such very small quantities that its properties have been but imperfectly studied. It appears, however, to belong to the iron group. The metal itself is of a lead-grey color, soft, very malleable, and its streak is like that of lead. It dissolves easily in hydrochloric acid, forming a deliquescent chloride. From the solution of this salt, it is precipitated by ammonia and potash as a hydrate, insoluble in excess of either reagent. Hydrogen sulphide does not precipitate it from an acid solution. The oxide heated on charcoal with soda, yields a metallic globule, which, when reheated, oxidizes to a yellowish powder. The compounds of indium impart a violet tint to the flame of a Bunsen burner.

It was introduced into our Materia Medica by Dr. J. B. Bell, U. S.

Preparation for Homœopathic Use.—Indium is triturated as directed under Class VII.

INULA.

Synonyms, Inula Helenium, *Linn.* Corvisartia Helenium.
Nat. Ord., Compositæ.

Common Names, Elecampane. Scabwort.

This plant is a native of Europe and of Northern and Central Asia, but has become naturalized in the United States, where it is found growing on road sides, in the Eastern, Middle and Western States. Its root is perennial, from which ascends annually a round, furrowed, branching, downy stem four to six feet high. Radical leaves, large, petiolate, serrate. Stem leaves alternate, ovate, amplexicaul, rugous, downy beneath. Flower-heads large, solitary and terminal. Involucre of ovate scales in rows. Ray flowers numerous, pistillate, spreading, trifid at apex. Disk flowers perfect. The fresh root is branched, the cylindrical divisions having many fibrous rootlets; it has a somewhat camphoraceous smell and a taste at first rancid and soapy, but after chewing the root, becoming bitter and aromatic.

The drug was proven by Dr. Fischer, Germany.

Preparation.—The fresh roots, dug in autumn, and in their second year, are chopped and pounded to a pulp and weighed. Then two parts by weight of dilute alcohol are taken, the pulp mixed thoroughly with one-sixth part of it, and the rest of the alcohol added. After having stirred the whole well, pour it into a well-stoppered bottle and let it stand eight days in a dark, cool place. The tincture is then separated by decanting, straining and filtering.

Drug power of tincture, $\frac{1}{6}$.

Dilutions must be prepared as directed under Class III.

IODIUM.

Synonyms, Iodinium. Iodum. Jodium.

Common Name, Iodine.

Symbol, I.

Atomic Weight, 127.

A non-metallic element.

Origin.—The element iodine exists in nature only in the combined state. It occurs in sea-water and in mineral springs. It is found in certain land-plants, *e. g.*, in tobacco, and a species of *Salsola* growing in the floating gardens on the fresh-water lakes near the city of Mexico. Various marine animals contain it, viz., the common sponge, the horse-sponge, the oyster, etc. It is contained in cod-liver oil to the amount of .03 or .04 per cent. It is found, too, in several minerals, as iodide of potassium, sodium or magnesium, in Chili saltpetre; as iodide of calcium or magnesium in certain dolomites. Sea-water is the great source of it, whence it is appropriated by marine plants and animals, especially by certain algæ, notably *Fucus palmatus*. These plants are collected on the coast of Scotland, Jersey and other places, and burnt to ashes in shallow pits to form kelp or varec. Iodine exists in kelp in the form of iodide of potassium and of sodium, which, being much more soluble than the other constituents, remain in the mother liquor after the carbonates and chlorides have crystallized out.

Preparation.—Iodine is prepared commercially by adding manganese di-oxide and sulphuric acid to the mother liquor, placing the mixture in a retort and distilling and condensing the vapors; the process is similar to that used in the preparation of bromine. Sometimes cyanide of iodine is found in the receivers—in white, needle-shaped crystals, and if the temperature at which the distillation is conducted be much higher than 100° C. (212° F.), the product is contaminated with chloride of iodine. Iodine thus obtained may be purified by washing with a small quantity of water, pressing between folds of bibulous paper, drying and subliming, or by dissolving it in alcohol, filtering and precipitating with water.

Properties.—Re-sublimed iodine crystallizes in rhombic scales or in orthorhombic octohedrons. It is bluish-black in color, has a metallic lustre, and in thin sections is red when viewed by transmitted light. Its odor is somewhat pungent, recalling that of chlorine; its taste is caustic and acrid. It is soft and easily pulverized. Its chemical affinities are those of chlorine and bromine, but much weaker, and it is displaced from most of its combinations by either of these bodies. It destroys coloring matters, but only slowly; upon organic tissues, the skin, paper, etc., it produces a yellow-brown stain, which disappears after a while under the influence of heat, if the contact had not been too prolonged. Its specific gravity is 4.95. In the open air, iodine volatilizes at the ordinary temperature; when heated to 107° C. (224.6° F.) it melts, and at 180° C. (356° F.) it boils, evolving a dense vapor of a magnificent violet-purple tint. This vapor is the heaviest known, being 8.72 times as heavy as air. Iodine is very slightly soluble in water, 7,000 parts of the latter being required to take up one of iodine. It dissolves easily in alcohol, ether, carbon disulphide and chloroform; in the latter two the solutions are of a beautiful purple tint, in the former two of a brown color. It is very soluble in aqueous solutions of iodides.

Tests.—Starch is the most characteristic reagent for free iodine. When to a starch solution is added a drop of a weak iodine solution, a deep blue coloration immediately ensues. On heating the mixture the blue color disappears, but it is restored upon cooling. A number of successive heatings will, however, destroy the color permanently. The test is very delicate, detecting one part of iodine in 400,000 of water. Re-sublimed or officinal iodine is usually very pure. To assure one's self of that fact, heat a small portion in a test-tube; it should volatilize completely and condense in crystals in the cool portion of the tube. If cyanide of iodine be present the crystals already mentioned will appear among those of the iodine. A pure specimen of iodine should dissolve without residue in from ten to fifteen parts of alcohol; if chloride of iodine be present the water will become colored brownish-yellow. Finally, on volatilizing a portion of the iodine in a porcelain capsule there should be no residue.

Iodine was introduced into our Materia Medica by Hahnemann.

Preparation for Homœopathic Use.—One part by weight of resublimed iodine is dissolved in ninety-nine parts by weight of alcohol.

Amount of drug power, $\frac{1}{100}$.

Dilutions must be prepared as directed under Class VI—β.

Triturations are prepared as directed under Class VII.

IODOFORMIUM.

Synonym, Iodoformum.
Common Name, Iodoform.
Formula, $C\,H\,I_3$.
Molecular Weight, 394.

Preparation of Iodoform.—Iodoform may readily be prepared by adding alcoholic solution of potassium hydrate to tincture of iodine, avoiding excess. In a long-necked flask or in a retort with a wide tubulus, are placed 100 parts of iodine, and to it are added 100 parts of potassium bicarbonate, 1200 of distilled water, and 250 of alcohol. After attaching a receiver, the mixture is gradually heated to about 80° C. (176° F.), and when the color of the solution has disappeared, twenty-five parts of iodine are added, and successive additions of twenty, and finally of ten parts of iodine, waiting before each addition until the liquid is decolorized. Should too much iodine have been added (known by the non-discharge of its color), the distillate is to be poured back into the retort or flask, and the whole treated with small, successive portions of caustic potash, until the color finally disappears. The liquid residue is to be poured in a porcelain dish and set aside for twenty-four hours. The crystals are to be collected on a filter, and washed with cold, distilled water, until a drop of the washings when evaporated from platinum foil ceases to leave any residue, and finally, dried at a medium temperature on bibulous paper.

Properties.—Iodoform is in lemon-yellow, glistening, crystalline plates, which have a greasy feel, are saffron-like in odor and have a sweetish taste. The crystals are practically insoluble in water, one part of the salt requiring 14,000 of water at 15° C. (59° F.) for solution. They dissolve in seventy-five parts of 95 per cent. alcohol in the cold, but in ten parts if boiling. They are readily soluble in ether, chloroform, carbon disulphide, and in the ethereal and fatty oils. Heated to 115° C. (239° F.), they melt to a brown liquid, and at a higher temperature are decomposed into vapor of iodine, hydriodic acid and other products, leaving behind a carbonaceous mass. Iodoform is somewhat volatile at ordinary temperatures, and when distilled with boiling water comes over unchanged. A watery solution of caustic alkali does not affect it, but an alcoholic solution decomposes iodoform into formate and iodide of potassium.

Tests.—In addition to the properties above given, the carbonaceous mass left when a portion of iodoform is heated on platinum foil, should at a higher temperature be consumed without leaving a residue.

The drug was first proven by Dr. B. F. Underwood, United States.

Preparation for Homœopathic Use.—Iodoform is triturated as directed under Class VII.

IPECACUANHA.

Synonym, Cephælis Ipecacuanha, *A. Richard.*
Nat. Ord., Rubiaceæ.
Common Name, Ipecac.

This plant is a small shrub abounding in moist, shady woods in Brazil, between the 8th and 20th degrees of south latitude. Its root is from four to six inches long, of the thickness of a goose-quill, wrinkled annularly, often branched. It penetrates the ground obliquely, and at intervals puts out long slender rootlets. The stem begins below the surface of the ground, is often procumbent near the base, so that but little more than one foot of it appears above. The stem is smooth, destitute of leaves below, ashy or brown in color, and gives off rooting shoots. The upper portion is green and hairy. Leaves rarely more than six, are opposite, on petioles, oval, acute, entire, with deciduous stipules clasping the stem. Flowers small, white, in a nearly globular head of about twelve. Fruit, an ovoid, purple-black berry.

It was introduced into our Materia Medica by Hahnemann.

Preparation.—The dried root is coarsely powdered, and covered with five parts by weight of alcohol; having been poured into a well-stoppered bottle, it is allowed to remain eight days in a dark, cool place, being shaken twice a day. The tincture is then poured off, strained and filtered.

Drug power of tincture, $\frac{1}{10}$.

Dilutions must be prepared as directed under Class IV.

IRIDIUM.

Symbol, Ir.

Atomic Weight, 198.

Origin and Preparation of Iridium.—When crude platinum is dissolved in nitro-muriatic acid, a small quantity of a gray, scaly, metallic substance usually remains behind, having altogether resisted the action of the acid; this is a native alloy of iridium and osmium, called *osmiridium* or *iridosmine;* it is reduced to powder, mixed with an equal weight of dry sodium chloride, and heated to redness in a glass tube, through which a stream of moist chlorine gas is transmitted. The farther extremity of the tube is connected with a receiver containing solution of ammonia. The gas, under these circumstances, is rapidly absorbed, iridium chloride and osmium chloride being produced; the former remains in combination with the sodium chloride; the latter, being volatile, is carried forward into the receiver, where it is decomposed by the water into osmic and hydrochloric acids, which combine with the alkali. The contents of the tube when cold are treated with water, by which the iridium and sodium chloride is dissolved out; this is mixed with an excess of ammonium chloride, and the iridium is precipitated as a dark red-brown ammonio-chloride, 2 $(NH_4\ Cl)$, $Ir\ Cl_4$; upon heating this to redness iridium only is left behind.

Properties.—Iridium is a white brittle metal, fusible with great difficulty before the oxy-hydrogen blow-pipe. Deville and Debray, by means of their powerful oxy-hydrogen blast furnace, have fused it completely into a pure white mass, resembling polished steel, brittle in the cold, somewhat malleable at a red heat, and having a density equal to that of platinum, viz., 21.15 (21.8 Hare). By moistening the pulverulent metal with a small quantity of water, pressing it tightly, first between filtering paper, then very forcibly in a press, and calcining it at a white heat in a forge-fire, it may be obtained in the form of a compact, very hard mass, capable of taking a good polish, but still very porous, and of a density not exceeding 16.0. After strong ignition it is insoluble in all acids, but when reduced by hydrogen at low temperatures, it oxidizes slowly at a red heat, and dissolves in nitromuriatic acid. It is usually rendered soluble by fusing it with nitre and caustic potash, or by mixing it with common salt, or better, with a mixture of the chlorides of potassium and sodium, and igniting it in a current of chlorine, as above described.

Preparation for Homœopathic Use.—Iridium is triturated as directed under Class VII.

IRIS VERSICOLOR, *Linn.*

Synonym, Iris Hexagona.

Nat. Ord., Iridaceæ.

Common Names, Blue Flag. Flower-de-luce. Liver Lily.

This is an indigenous species whose root is a perennial, fleshy, horizontal rhizome. Stem two to three feet high, angled and frequently branching. Leaves are sheathed at the base, sword-shaped, and striated. The flowers are two to six in number, blue or purple, but variegated greenish-yellow or white, and purple-veined. Fruit a pod, oblong, three-valved, three-sided, with obtuse angles, containing numerous flat seeds. The plant is found in all parts of the United States, in low wet places, in meadows, and on borders of swamps. Flowers in June.

It was first proved by Dr. J. G. Rowland, Inaugural Thesis, Phila., 1852.

Preparation.—The fresh root, gathered in late autumn or early spring, is chopped and pounded to a pulp and weighed. Then two parts by weight of alcohol are taken, and after thoroughly mixing the pulp with one-sixth part of it, the rest of the alcohol is added. After having stirred the whole well, pour it into a well-stoppered bottle, and let it stand eight days in a dark, cool place. The tincture is then separated by decanting, straining and filtering.

Drug power of tincture, ⅙.

Dilutions must be prepared as directed under Class III.

JABORANDI.

Synonyms, Pilocarpus Pennatifolius, *Lemaire.* Pilocarpus Pinnatus, *Martins.* Pilocarpus Selloanus, *Eng.*

Nat. Ord., Rutaceæ.

Common Name, Jaborandi.

P. pennatifolius is a slightly branched shrub growing in Brazil. The leaves are on long stalks, impari-pennate; leaflets opposite in from two to five pairs, the terminal one being on a large petiole. Leaves entire, ovate-oblong, apex tapering, rounded or emarginate, base tapering or rounded. The leaflets are coriaceous, possess a prominent midrib and have slightly revolute margins. They are punctated with oil glands. The taste of the leaves is bitter and aromatic, followed by a tingling sensation in the mouth and an increased flow of saliva; their odor is not noticeable till they are bruised, when it is perceived to be slightly aromatic.

P. Selloanus occurs in Southern Brazil and Paraguay, and does not differ greatly from the above-described plant.

The first systematic proving of this drug seems to have been by Dr. W. L. Watkins, N. Y., although a number of "physiological experiments" have been made from time to time in 1874–5 by Gubler, Coutinho and Robin in France, and by Ringer and Gould in England.

Preparation.—The dried leaves and stems are coarsely powdered, covered with five parts by weight of alcohol, and allowed to remain eight days in a well-stoppered bottle, in a dark, cool place, being shaken twice a day. The tincture is then poured off, strained and filtered.

Drug power of tincture, $\frac{1}{10}$.

Dilutions must be prepared as directed under Class IV.

JACARANDA CAROBA, *De Candolle.*

Synonyms, Bignonia Caroba. Jacaranda Braziliensis.
Nat. Ord., Bignoniaceæ.
Common Name, Caroba.

The caroba is very common in Brazil, in gardens and on plantations. It is a tree with white wood, the ramose top of which attains a height of from twenty to twenty-eight feet. Leaves pinnate, tri- or quadrijugate, composed of from five to nine opposite, sessile, glabrous and oval folioles. Flowers large, violet-colored, on pedicels that are expanded at their extremities, and forming ramose terminal panicles. Calyx tubulous, with five teeth; corolla tubulous, slightly pubescent externally, and expanding at its summit into a limb with five obtuse divisions. Stamens five, one of which is rudimentary; ovary ovoid, surmounted by a simple style terminating in a bilamellary stigma. The husks are linear and flat. Blossoms appear in September.

It was introduced into the Homœopathic Materia Medica by Dr. Mure, Brazil.

Preparation.—The fresh flowers are pounded to a pulp and weighed. Then two parts by weight of alcohol are taken, and, having mixed the pulp thoroughly with one-sixth part of it, the rest of the alcohol is added. After having stirred the whole well, pour it into a well-stoppered bottle and let it stand eight days in a dark, cool place. The tincture is then separated by decanting, straining and filtering.

Amount of drug power, $\frac{1}{6}$.

Dilutions must be prepared as directed under Class III.

JALAPA.

Synonyms, Ipomœa Purga, *Hayne.* Exogonium Purga, *Bentham.* Convolvulus Purga, *Wenderoth.* Mechoacanna Nigra.

Nat. Ord., Convolvulaceæ.

Common Name, Jalap.

This is a tuberous-rooted plant, having a twining, herbaceous stem, furnished with cordate, entire, pointed, smooth leaves on long stalks. Its flowers are deep pink in color, salver-shaped and stand two or three on long peduncles. The plant is a native of Mexico, deriving its name from Xalapa, in the State of Vera Cruz. The Jalap of commerce consists of irregular, ovoid roots, whose sizes vary from that of a hazelnut to that of an egg, but at times specimens are found as large as a man's fist. They are of a dark brown hue, with numerous transverse light-colored scars. The large roots are gashed longitudinally to permit of more ready drying, or are halved or quartered; the smaller specimens are usually found entire. A good specimen of jalap is heavy, hard, tough and often horny; it becomes brittle when kept long and breaks with a resinous, non-fibrous fracture. Its color internally is dirty white or pale dull brown. Its odor is smoky, from the mode in which it is dried, and its taste acrid and disagreeable.

It was introduced into our Materia Medica by Noack and Trinks.

Preparation.—The heavy, resinous root, carefully dried and coarsely pulverized, is covered with five parts by weight of alcohol, and allowed to remain eight days in a well-stoppered bottle, in a dark, cool place, being shaken twice a day. The tincture is then poured off, strained and filtered.

Drug power of tincture, $\frac{1}{10}$.

Dilutions must be prepared as directed under Class IV.

JANIPHA MANIHOT, *Kunth.*

Synonyms, Jatropha Manihot, *Linn.* Manihot Utilissima, *Pohl.* Manioca Mandi.

Nat. Ord., Euphorbiaceæ.

Common Names, Tapioca Plant. Manioca. Cassava.

The cassava plant is probably a native of Brazil, where it has long been cultivated for its nutritious root. It is bushy in habit, with a ramose stem, growing three feet or more in height. Its leaves are sea-green in color, petiolate, alternate, palmately divided, having five to seven lanceolate, smooth, entire lobes. The flowers are in panicles, terminal or axillary; the perianth is bell-shaped, five-parted, light yellow, changing to brown at the end. The roots are white, fleshy, tuberous, and often weigh over twenty-five pounds each. They abound in a milky juice, which is poisonous, but which is removable by pressure and drying. The residue is starchy in character and is a food-staple.

It was proved by Dr. J. Vincente Martins, Brazil.

Preparation.—The milky juice of the fresh root is triturated as directed under Class VIII.

JATROPHA CURCAS, *Linn.*

Synonyms, Curcus Purgans, *Adanson.* Ficus Infernalis. Ricinus Majoris.

Nat. Ord., Euphorbiaceæ.

Common Names, Physic Nut. Purging Nut.

This plant is a shrub, indigenous to tropical regions, and found growing in the West Indies and South America. Its leaves are heart-shaped, smooth, entire; flowers campanulate, greenish-yellow, in paniculate cymes. The fruit is a three-celled capsule, each cell one-seeded; seeds are blackish, oblong-ovoid, nearly an inch long, convex on one side, flat on the other, with a whitish hilum at one end. Within the envelope is the kernel, whose taste is somewhat sweet but followed by an acrid, burning sensation.

It was introduced into our Materia Medica by Dr. Hering.

Preparation.—The ripe seeds are coarsely powdered and covered with five parts by weight of alcohol, and allowed to remain eight days in a well-stoppered bottle, in a dark, cool place, being shaken twice a day. The tincture is then poured off, strained and filtered.

Drug power of tincture, $\frac{1}{10}$.

Dilutions must be prepared as directed under Class IV.

JUGLANS CINEREA, *Linn.*

Synonym, Juglans Cathartica.

Nat. Ord., Juglandaceæ.

Common Names, Butternut. Oil Nut. White Walnut.

This is a well-known indigenous forest tree, often forty to fifty feet high, with a thick but short trunk. The young branches are smooth and of a grayish color. Leaves alternate, twelve to twenty inches long, pinnate; leaflets fifteen to seventeen in pairs, with one terminal, lanceolate, serrate, rounded at base, pointed, soft pubescent beneath. Barren flowers in long aments, fertile ones in short spikes. Fruit drupaceous, with a spongy epicarp, within which is an oblong pointed nut, dark in color, rugous and irregularly furrowed.

The drug was first proven by Dr. J. P. Paine, Inaugural Thesis, Phila., 1852.

Preparation.—The fresh, young, inner bark (especially of the root), collected in May or June, is chopped and pounded to a pulp and weighed. Then two parts by weight of alcohol are taken, the pulp mixed thoroughly with one-sixth part of it, and the rest of the alcohol added. After having stirred the whole well, pour it into a well-stoppered bottle and let it stand eight days in a dark, cool place. The tincture is then separated by decanting, straining and filtering.

Drug power of tincture, $\frac{1}{6}$.

Dilutions must be prepared as directed under Class III.

JUGLANS REGIA, *Linn.*

Synonym, Nux Juglans.

Nat. Ord., Juglandaceæ.

Common Name, Common European Walnut.

This is a beautiful tree cultivated from Southern Europe to Central Germany, and has large, unequally pinnate, long-petiolate leaves, with smooth, entire, petiolate, sweet-scented leaflets.

The drug was first proven by Dr. Clotar Müller, Germany.

Preparation.—In June and July, from the unripe, smooth, green fruit, the hulls are taken and, with an equal part of green leaves, are chopped and pounded to a pulp and weighed. Then two parts by weight of alcohol are taken, the pulp mixed thoroughly with one-sixth part of it and the rest of the alcohol added. After stirring the whole well, pour it into a well-stoppered bottle, and let it stand eight days in a dark, cool place. The tincture is then separated by decanting, straining and filtering.

Drug power of tincture, ⅙.

Dilutions must be prepared as directed under Class III.

JUNCUS EFFUSUS, *Linn.*

Nat. Ord., Junceaceæ.

Common Names, Bulrush. Common or Soft Rush.

This perennial rush, growing in marshy grounds in Europe, Asia and America, rises from matted running rootstocks, to the height of from two to four feet. The scape is soft and pliant; with short leafless or rarely leaf-bearing sheaths at the base; leaves, if any, terete, knotless and similar to the scape; inner sheaths awned; panicle diffusely much-branched, many-flowered; flowers numerous, small, greenish; sepals lanceolate, very acute, as long as the triangular-obovate retuse and pointless greenish-brown pod; anthers and filaments of equal length; style very short; seeds small. Flowers in spring.

It was proven by Dr. Wahle, Germany.

Preparation.—The fresh root, gathered in spring, is chopped and pounded to a pulp and weighed. Then two parts by weight of alcohol are taken, the pulp mixed thoroughly with one-sixth part of it, and the rest of the alcohol added. After stirring the whole well, pour it into a well-stoppered bottle, and let it stand eight days, in a dark, cool place. The tincture is then separated by decanting, straining and filtering.

Drug power of tincture, ⅙.

Dilutions must be prepared as directed under Class III.

JUNCUS PILOSUS.

Synonym, Luzula Pilosa, *Willd.*

Nat. Ord., Junceaceæ.

Common Name, Wood-Rush.

This is a perennial found growing usually in dry ground in shady places in Europe, Asia, Africa and North America. Its stem is slender, cyme lax, branches few, reflexed in fruit, flowers subsolitary, perianth-segments acuminate, shorter than the very broadly ovoid obtuse capsule, crest of seeds long curved terminal. Rootstock short, tufted; stolons slender. Stems many, one-half to one foot high. Leaves about half as long as the stem, one-sixth to one-quarter inch broad, soft, sparingly hairy. Cyme with capillary branches and pedicles. Flowers one-sixth to one-fifth inch, chestnut-brown, rarely in pairs; bractlets broad, short. Capsule very broad below, suddenly contracted to a conical top above the middle. Flowers appear in April and May.

Preparation.—The fresh root, gathered in spring, is chopped and pounded to a pulp and weighed. Then two parts by weight of alcohol are taken, the pulp mixed thoroughly with one-sixth part of it, and the rest of the alcohol added. After stirring the whole well, pour it into a well-stoppered bottle, and let it stand eight days in a dark, cool place. The tincture is then separated by decanting, straining and filtering.

Drug power of tincture, $\frac{1}{6}$.

Dilutions must be prepared as directed under Class III.

JUNIPERUS COMMUNIS, *Linn.*

Nat. Ord., Coniferæ.

Common Names, Common Juniper. Juniper.

J. communis is an evergreen shrub found growing throughout Europe and in the greater part of Asia. It is also distributed over the northern portion of North America. In northern regions, such as Norway and Sweden, it is a small tree, attaining a height of from thirty to thirty-six feet, while throughout Europe generally, it does not rise above six feet. In high mountainous regions it becomes decumbent (*J. nana*, Willd), and rises only a few inches above the soil. Its branches are numerous, prostrate, the shrub becoming often pyramidal in outline. Leaves in whorls of three, five to eight lines long, acerose-lanceolate, bristly-pointed, mid-vein channelled above, keeled below. Barren flowers are in small, axillary aments; fertile ones, on a different plant, are small, sessile, axillary. The fruit is a galbulus or pseudo-berry, ovate and green during its first year, ripening only in autumn of its second year. In the ripe state it is spherical, from three-tenths to four-tenths of an inch in diameter, and is of a deep purplish tint, covered with a bluish-gray bloom. The thin epicarp encloses a loose, yellowish-brown sarcocarp, imbedded in which, and lying closely together, are three hard, triangular seeds, whose top is sharp-edged, and whose surface is supplied each with several oil sacs. In commerce, juniper berries are about the size of a pea, and shriveled more or less, marked with three furrows at the top and tubercled at the base, from the persistent calyx.

Preparation.—The fresh, ripe berries, are pounded to a pulp and weighed. Then two parts by weight of alcohol are taken, the pulp mixed thoroughly with one-sixth part of it, and the rest of the alcohol added. After having stirred the whole well, pour it into a well-stoppered bottle, and let it stand eight days in a dark, cool place The tincture is then separated by decanting, straining and filtering.

Drug power of tincture, $\frac{1}{6}$.
Dilutions must be prepared as directed under Class III.

KALI ACETICUM.

Synonyms, Potassium Acetate. Acetas Kalicus. Kali Acetas. Potassii Acetas.
Common Name, Acetate of Potash.
Formula, $K\ C_2\ H_3\ O_2$.
Molecular Weight, 98.
Preparation of Acetate of Potassium.—By neutralizing pure officinal acetic acid with bicarbonate of potassium added gradually. After filtering, the solution is to be evaporated carefully on a sand-bath to dryness. The salt should be kept in a well-stoppered bottle.
Properties.—Potassium acetate is a snowy, glistening mass of crystalline powder, which is neutral in reaction or only weakly alkaline; it must not be acid; it has a pungent saline taste. It is soluble in less than its own weight of water at medium temperatures, and in three to four parts of alcohol. Heated to about 280° C. (536° F.) it melts, and at 360° C. (710° F.) it is decomposed, with the production of acetic acid and potassium carbonate. Officinal potassium acetate contains from four to five per cent. of water.
Tests.—In addition to the properties already mentioned, potassium acetate, in dilute solution, should undergo no change when treated with barium chloride and hydrogen sulphide; with silver nitrate an opalescent turbidity, due to the presence of a trace of chloride, is admissible in the German Pharmacopœia.
The first proving was by Vogt, in Germany.
Preparation for Homœopathic Use.—One part by weight of acetate of potassium is dissolved in nine parts by weight of distilled water.
Amount of drug power, $\frac{1}{10}$.
Dilutions must be prepared as directed under Class V—*a*.

KALI ARSENICOSUM.

Synonyms, Potassium Arsenite.
Formula, $H\ K_2\ As\ O_3$.
Take of arsenious acid, one part, of pure and dry carbonate of potash, one part, and of distilled water, one part; boil in a test-tube until a clear liquid results, then add about forty parts of distilled water, and after the liquid has cooled, add enough distilled water to bring the whole to one hundred parts.
This solution will contain one part of kali arsenicosum to one hundred of water, and should be marked 2x.
Prepare further dilutions according to Class V.

KALI BICHROMICUM.

Synonyms, Potassium Dichromate. Potassæ Bichromas. Potassii Bichromas.

Common Name, Bichromate of Potash.

Formula, $K_2\ Cr_2\ O_7$.

Molecular Weight, 295.

Preparation.—Potassium dichromate or anhydrochromate, is prepared by adding to the neutral yellow chromate of potassium in solution, a moderate quantity of one of the stronger acids. As a result, one-half the base is abstracted by the new acid, and the formula of the salt may be expressed, $K_2\ CrO_4,\ CrO_3$. The salt is crystallized by slow evaporation in beautiful red, tabular crystals, derived from a triclinic prism.

Properties.—Potassium dichromate is permanent in the air, reddens litmus paper and has a cooling, bitter and metallic taste. It is soluble in ten parts of water at 15° C. (59° F.), and more abundantly in boiling water; it is insoluble in alcohol. At a little below a red heat it melts to a transparent red liquid, out of which, on slow cooling, may be obtained fine, large crystals, but they crumble to powder at a lower temperature. It is a powerful oxidizer.

Tests.—Potassium dichromate is readily obtainable in a state of purity. Calcium might possibly be present, as it is used in the manufacture of the yellow chromate; if present, the addition of an alkaline carbonate to a solution of the salt will cause a turbidity. A solution of the dichromate acidulated with nitric acid, should show no change when treated with barium chloride (absence of sulphuric acid or sulphate).

The drug was first proved by Dr. Drysdale, England.

Preparation for Homœopathic Use.—One part by weight of bichromate of potassium is dissolved in ninety-nine parts by weight of distilled water.

Amount of drug power, $\frac{1}{100}$.

Dilutions must be prepared as directed under Class V—β, except that distilled water is used for dilutions to the 4x and 2 inclusive.

Triturations of bichromate of potassium are prepared as directed under Class VII.

KALI BROMATUM.

Synonyms, Potassium Bromide. Bromuretum Kalicum. Kalium Bromatum. Potassii Bromidum.

Common Name, Bromide of Potassium.

Formula, $K\ Br$.

Molecular Weight, 119.

Preparation.—Potassium bromide may be produced by treating a solution of bromide of iron with a solution of potassium carbonate as long as any precipitate occurs. The whole is to be thrown upon a filter and the precipitate washed with boiling distilled water, the washings added to the filtrate and the solution evaporated till crystallization is completed. The crystals are to be collected and dried on bibulous paper and kept in a well-stoppered bottle. As prepared by the above process, the bromide has a slight alkaline reaction, but by the

German Pharmacopœia, the compound is required to behave indifferently to both red and blue litmus paper.

Properties.—Potassium bromide is in tolerably large, white, glistening, cubical crystals, which are permanent in the air. They have a pungent, saline taste; their specific gravity is 2.4. They are soluble in two parts of water at 0° C. (32° F.), in one and a half parts at 20° C. (68° F.), in one of boiling water and in 180 parts of 90 per cent. alcohol. When heated, the crystals decrepitate, and at a low red heat melt without decomposition; at a bright red heat they gradually sublime.

Properties.—A solution of potassium bromide, when treated with dilute sulphuric acid, should remain colorless, a reddish or reddish-yellow color indicating the presence of bromine from decomposed bromate. If silver nitrate be added to a solution of the salt, the resulting precipitate should be completely soluble in dilute ammonia or nearly so. A faint opalescent turbidity due to silver bromide is permissible. Should a milky turbidity or a real precipitate occur, it may be due to excess of silver bromide or to silver iodide, or to both; by treating it with caustic ammonia, all the silver bromide will be dissolved, and any residue then is due to silver iodide. The presence of iodide may be also determined by adding to a solution of potassium bromide a drop of chlorine water, when, upon adding starch solution, the well-known blue color of the so-called iodide of starch will be perceived.

Preparation for Homœopathic Use.—One part by weight of pure bromide of potassium is dissolved in ninety-nine parts by weight of distilled water.

Amount of drug power, $\frac{1}{100}$.

Dilutions must be prepared as directed under Class V—β.

Triturations of the pure bromide of potassium are prepared as directed under Class VII.

KALI CARBONICUM.

Synonyms, Potassium Carbonate. Carbonas Kalicus. Potassii Carbonas. Sal Tartari.

Common Names, Carbonate of Potassium. Salt of Tartar.

Formula, $K_2 CO_3$.

Molecular Weight, 138.

Preparation of Pure Carbonate of Potassium.—By placing potassium bicarbonate in a roomy iron crucible, gradually heating the salt to redness and keeping it at that degree of heat for half an hour, the excess of CO_2 is driven off. The potassium carbonate so obtained is to be dissolved in distilled water and evaporated over a slow fire till there results a thick granular mass, which is to be kept in a well-stoppered bottle.

Properties.—Officinal pure potassium carbonate is a dry, white, coarsely granular mass, or a white crystalline powder; it is without odor, has an alkaline taste and reaction. It contains usually about 4 per cent. of hygroscopic moisture. When exposed to the air it deliquesces and ultimately forms a slightly yellowish liquid. It is soluble in its own weight of water at medium temperatures, is insoluble in alcohol, and when treated with acids, evolves CO_2, forming a salt with the acid used.

Tests.—Its solution in water should be perfectly clear, an undissolved residue being due to a not insignificant proportion of potassium bicarbonate. When treated with nitric acid in excess and the result evaporated, the residue should dissolve completely in water, and this solution should give no precipitate with barium chloride or silver nitrate; the *Pharmacopœia Germanica* allows a faint turbidity when the solution acidified with nitric acid is treated with silver nitrate, as the commercially pure salt is seldom entirely free from potassium chloride.

This drug was first proven by Hahnemann.

Preparation for Homœopathic Use.—One part by weight of pure carbonate of potassium is dissolved in nine parts by weight of distilled water.

Amount of drug power, $\frac{1}{10}$.

Dilutions must be prepared as directed under Class V—*a*.

Triturations of the pure carbonate of potassium are prepared as directed under Class VII, but owing to the deliquescence of the salt the 1x will not keep.

KALI CAUSTICUM.

Synonyms, Potassium Hydrate. Lapis Causticus. Potassa Caustica. Potassæ (Potassii) Hydras.

Common Name, Caustic Potash.

Formula, KHO.

Molecular Weight, 56.

Preparation of Caustic Potassa.—The officinal solution of potassa is prepared by adding to a solution of 15 troy ounces of potassium bicarbonate, a mixture of 9 troy ounces of fresh burnt lime in 4 pints of distilled water; each must be brought to the boiling point before mixing and then boiled for ten minutes. The whole is to be strained through muslin and distilled water is added through the strainer until the strained liquid measures 7 pints. Of the solution of potash, any quantity may be taken and boiled down rapidly in a clean silver or iron vessel until a drop of the liquid, when removed on a warm glass-rod, solidifies on cooling. It is then to be poured into moulds, and while still warm placed in well-stoppered bottles. Officinal caustic potash is not pure, and contains appreciable proportions of potassium sulphate, sodium hydrate and alumina. To obtain the substance in the pure state, the officinal preparation is to be dissolved in 2 volumes of water, the solution mixed with 4 volumes of alcohol, filtered and evaporated rapidly to dryness in a silver vessel.

Properties.—Caustic potash is in white, dry, cylindrical pieces, which break with a crystalline fracture. It is extremely deliquescent, and has a strong affinity for carbonic oxide, with which it combines even in the solid state; it is, of course, easily soluble in water, and unlike most of the potassium compounds, is freely soluble in alcohol. When heated strongly it melts to a colorless, oily liquid, and at a full red heat it volatilizes in white vapors without change.

Tests.—As stated above, its solubility in alcohol serves to distinguish it from other potassium compounds, and when dissolved in 2 volumes of water and then mixed with 4 volumes of alcohol, only a slight precipitate or an insignificant watery layer should separate out (absence of other potassium salts, sulphate, chloride or carbonate). When treated with acids, a solution of caustic potash should give no, or at most but very slight, effervescence, and when heated with sulphuric acid in excess, the solution should not discharge the color of indigo solution (absence of nitrate).

Preparation for Homœopathic Use.—One part by weight of pure caustic potassa is dissolved in nine parts by weight of distilled water.

Amount of drug power, $\frac{1}{10}$.

Dilutions must be prepared as directed under Class V—*a*.

KALI CHLORICUM.

Synonyms, Potassium Chlorate. Potassæ Chloras. Potassii Chloras.

Common Name, Chlorate of Potash.

Formula, $K\,Cl\,O_3$.

Molecular Weight, 122.5.

Preparation of Chlorate of Potassium.—"Take of carbonate of potash, twenty ounces; slaked lime, fifty-three ounces; distilled water, a sufficiency; black oxide of manganese, eighty ounces; hydrochloric acid, twenty-four pints. Mix the lime with the carbonate of potash, and triturate them with a few ounces of the water so as to make the mixture slightly moist. Place the oxide of manganese in a large retort or flask, and having poured upon it the hydrochloric acid, diluted with six pints of water, apply a gentle sand heat and conduct the chlorine as it comes over, first through a bottle containing six ounces of water, and then into a large carboy containing the mixture of carbonate of potash and slaked lime. When the whole of the chlorine has come over, remove the contents of the carboy, and boil them for twenty minutes with seven pints of the water; filter and evaporate till a film forms on the surface, and set aside to cool and crystallize. The crystals thus obtained are to be purified by dissolving them in three times their weight of boiling distilled water, and again allowing the solution to crystallize."—Br. P.

Properties.—Pure potassium chlorate forms neutral, permanent, colorless, rhomboidal crystalline plates, which possess a cooling saline taste, are soluble in 16½ parts of water at 15° C. (59° F.) and in less than two parts of boiling water. The salt melts when heated below a red heat, and at a higher temperature parts with one-third of its oxygen, becoming converted thereby into potassium chloride and perchlorate, but with a stronger heat all its oxygen is driven off and the salt is changed into chloride. When rubbed in a mortar with substances that are easily oxidized, *e. g.*, sulphur, carbon, powdered resin, starch, sugar, tannin and metallic sulphides, it decomposes with explosive violence.

Tests.—Pure potassium chlorate, when heated on platinum foil to redness, yields a residue which is neutral in reaction; an alkaline reaction is due to the presence of potassium nitrate. A dilute watery solution of the salt should give no precipitate with barium chloride (sulphate) or with silver nitrate (chloride).

The salt was proven under the direction of Dr. E. Martin, Germany.

Preparation for Homœopathic Use.—One part by weight of pure chlorate of potassium is dissolved in ninety-nine parts by weight of distilled water.

Amount of drug power, $\frac{1}{100}$.

Dilutions must be prepared as directed under Class V—β.

Triturations of pure chlorate of potassium are prepared as directed under Class VII.

KALI CYANATUM.

Synonyms, Potassium Cyanide. Kali Cyanuretum. Kalium Cyanatum. Potassii Cyanidum. Potassii Cyanuretum.

Common Names, Cyanide of Potassium. Cyanuret of Potassium.

Formula, K Cy or K C N.

Molecular Weight, 65.

Preparation of Cyanide of Potassium.—An intimate mixture of eight parts of anhydrous potassium ferrocyanide and three parts of potassium carbonate is introduced by small portions into a cast-iron crucible previously heated to low redness. After all the material has been added the crucible is kept in the fire till a sample of the melted mass appears white and has the aspect of porcelain on cooling; it is then taken out, left at rest until the metallic iron produced by the decomposition has settled down, when the fused mass is poured out. The mass is to be broken up while yet warm and the pieces transferred to a well-stoppered bottle.

Properties.—Potassium cyanide crystallizes from its watery solutions in cubes or in forms derived therefrom; they are transparent and colorless, possess a bitter acrid taste and the odor, to some extent, of bitter almonds. The salt is very fusible, melting at a dull red heat to a transparent liquid which, on cooling, becomes a white, dull, opaque, porcelain-like mass; at a white heat it volatilizes without decomposition. Its reaction is alkaline. Potassium cyanide is deliquescent, is easily soluble in water, dissolves in dilute alcohol, but in absolute alcohol is almost insoluble. The aqueous solution is decomposed by boiling, formate and carbonate of potassium being produced, together with ammonia. Potassium cyanide is intensely poisonous.

Test.—The salt is considered sufficiently pure when its concentrated solution exhibits, upon treatment with hydrochloric acid, no, or at most only very slight, effervescence.

The first provings were by Lembke, Germany.

Preparation for Homœopathic Use.—The pure cyanide of potassium is prepared by trituration as directed under Class VII.

KALI FERROCYANATUM.

Synonyms, Potassium Ferrocyanide. Ferrocyanuret of Potassium. Kalium Borussicum. Kalium Ferrocyanatum. Potassii Ferrocyanidum.

Common Names, Ferrocyanide of Potassium. Yellow Prussiate of Potash.

Formula, $K_4\ Fe\ Cy_6,\ 3H_2\ O$.

Molecular Weight, 422.

Preparation.—Ferrocyanide of potassium is prepared commercially by adding animal matters such as horn, feathers, dried blood, leather clippings, etc., mixed with iron filings, to fused carbonate of potassium, lixiviating the fused mass with water, filtering, and crystallizing by evaporation. The animal matter contains nitrogen and carbon, the latter in larger proportion than is required to form cyanogen with the nitrogen; hence when these substances are fused with carbonate of potassium, the excess of carbon reduces potassium from the carbonate, and the potassium thus set free unites with the cyanogen formed, producing cyanide of potassium, the latter being converted into ferrocyanide in the subsequent lixiviation. The product is afterward purified by recrystallization.

Properties.—Pure potassium ferrocyanide crystallizes with three molecules of water in truncated pyramids, belonging to the dimetric or quadratic system. The crystals are often reduced to the tabular form by the predominance of the lateral faces. They are somewhat soft, permanent in the air, transparent, yellow in color and possess a sweetish saline taste. The salt dissolves with a pale yellow color in four parts of cold and in two of boiling water; it is insoluble in alcohol. Heated to 100° C. (212° F.) the salt parts with its water of crystallization and falls in a white powder; at a red heat it melts, and at a higher temperature decomposes into a mixture of potassium cyanide and carbide of iron. A solution of potassium ferrocyanide gives with solutions of ferric salts a deep blue precipitate of Prussian blue and with ferrous salts a whitish precipitate which gradually becomes blue upon exposure to the air; with cupric salts the precipitate is a dark reddish-brown, but with cuprous salts the color of the precipitate is whitish, becoming reddish-brown upon exposure to the air. Alkalies do not precipitate the iron from the combination in the salt, but on heating the salt with potassium carbonate potassium cyanide is formed with the separation of metallic iron.

Potassium ferrocyanide is usually found in commerce beautifully crystallized, but occasionally there are present with it small crystals of potassium carbonate colored yellow by some admixture of the ferrocyanide. For testing, therefore, the small crystals should be selected. By treating the crystals with dilute sulphuric acid the absence of effervescence will show freedom from carbonate. A solution of the salt in water acidified with hydrochloric acid should not give a white precipitate with barium chloride (absence of sulphate).

In order to detect the presence of chloride a portion of the ferrocyanide should be decomposed by fusion with potassium or ammonium nitrate; the residue is to be dissolved in distilled water, acidified with nitric acid and treated with silver nitrate in the usual way, when, if chloride be present, a white curdy precipitate will appear.

The first provings were made under the direction of Dr. J. B. Bell, United States.

Preparation for Homœopathic Use.—The pure ferrocyanide of potassium is prepared by trituration, as directed under Class VII.

KALI HYPOPHOSPHOROSUM.

Synonyms, Potassium Hypophosphite. Hypophosphis Kalicus. Potassii Hypophosphis. Hypophosphis Potassicus.

Common Name, Hypophosphite of Potash.

Formula, $K\,H_2\,P\,O_2$.

Molecular Weight, 104.

Preparation of Hypophosphite of Potassium.—By boiling an aqueous or alcoholic solution of potassium hydrate with pure phosphorus as long as phosphoretted hydrogen continues to escape, then decanting the solution from the undissolved phosphorus and mixing it with acid potassium carbonate in order to convert the remaining potassium hydrate into carbonate. The solution is then to be evaporated and the residue treated with hot strong alcohol which dissolves the hypophosphite and leaves the carbonate. The solution is to be filtered while hot and set aside to crystallize.

Properties and Tests.—Hypophosphite of potassium usually forms an opaque, indistinctly crystalline mass, sometimes, however, exhibiting six-sided plates. It is very deliquescent, more so even than calcium chloride, is readily soluble in water and dilute alcohol, less soluble in absolute alcohol and insoluble in ether. It may be heated to 100° C. (212° F.) without undergoing any change, but at a red heat out of contact with air it gives off phosphoretted hydrogen. This, like other hypophosphites, acts as a powerful reducing agent. With silver nitrate it forms a white precipitate which quickly turns brown and is converted into metallic silver; with mercuric chloride it acts similarly, the black precipitate being in this case metallic mercury.

Preparation for Homœopathic Use.—One part by weight of pure hypophosphite of potassium is dissolved in nine parts by weight of distilled water.

Amount of drug power, $\frac{1}{10}$.

Dilutions must be prepared as directed under Class V—*a*.

Triturations of pure hypophosphite of potassium are prepared as directed under Class VII, but owing to the deliquescence of the salt, the 1x will not keep.

KALI JODATUM.

Synonyms, Potassium Iodide. Ioduretum Kalicum. Kali hydriodicum. Kalium Iodatum. Potassii Iodidum.

Common Name, Iodide of Potassium.

Formula, K I.

Molecular Weight, 166.

Preparation of Iodide of Potassium.—To a solution of potassium hydrate in boiling distilled water, add iodine in fine powder, in successive portions. After each addition of iodine the mixture is to be stirred until its color disappears, and this procedure is to be repeated till the iodine is in small excess, which will be known by the slight color of the solution. The solution is now to be evaporated, and there is to be intimately mixed with it, by stirring towards the end of the evaporation, powdered charcoal, until its amount equals one-third of the potassium hydrate used. The mixture is then to be reduced to powder, placed in an iron crucible and heated to low redness, and kept so for a quarter of an hour. After cooling, the mass is to be treated with distilled water and the mixture filtered, evaporated and set aside, until the potassium iodide has crystallized out.

Properties.—Pure potassium iodide forms colorless, transparent, glistening, cubical crystals. In commerce it is generally found in crystals, which are white, opaque or porcelain-like in appearance, and which have an alkaline reaction. Both these differences are due to the presence of a minute amount of potassium carbonate. Potassium iodide has a sharp, saline, somewhat bitter taste, and if its reaction be neutral, is only slightly hygroscopic. Four parts of the compound require three parts of water at medium temperatures, or two parts at 100° C. (212° F.) for solution. It is also soluble in ten or eleven parts of ninety per cent. alcohol and in forty of absolute alcohol. Its solutions dissolve iodine freely.

Tests.—Aqueous solution of potassium iodide should give no precipitate when agitated with lime water (absence of potassium carbonate), and when treated with silver nitrate, the resulting precipitate washed, agitated with ammonia and filtered, the filtrate should not give any turbidity when treated with nitric acid in excess. The aqueous solution, when treated with hydrochloric acid, should exhibit no change of coloration; a yellow color is due to the presence of potassium iodate. Its solution mixed with starch solution gives a blue color on the addition of a drop or two of chlorine water (iodine), and a crystalline precipitate occurs with tartaric acid (potassium).

It was introduced into our Materia Medica by Hartlaub and Trinks, Germany.

Preparation for Homœopathic Use.—One part by weight of pure iodide of potassium is dissolved in ninety-nine parts by weight of alcohol.

Amount of drug power, $\frac{1}{100}$.

Dilutions must be prepared as directed under Class V—β.

Triturations of pure iodide of potassium are prepared as directed under Class VII, but the 1x will not keep well.

KALI MURIATICUM.

Synonyms, Potassium Chloride. Kali Chloratum. Kali Chloridum. Potassii Chloridum.

Common Names, Chloride of Potash. Chloride of Potassium.

Formula, K Cl.

Molecular Weight, 74.5.

Preparation of Chloride of Potassium. Potassium chloride is a constituent of the mineral *carnallite*—a double chloride of potassium and magnesium found in large quantity at Stassfurth near Magdeburg, in Germany. The deposit is worked for the extraction of the chloride, by dissolving the double chloride in water and leaving the solution to cool. The greater part of the potassium chloride separates out, while magnesium chloride remains in solution.

Potassium chloride may be prepared by neutralizing pure aqueous hydrochloric acid with pure potassium carbonate or hydrate. The solution is to be evaporated to crystallization.

Properties.—Potassium chloride crystallizes in cubes, often prismatically elongated, and occasionally in octohedrons. The crystals are colorless or white, are permanent in the air, decrepitate when heated, melt at a low red heat, and at a higher temperature volatilize without decomposition. The substance tastes like common or table salt. It is soluble in three parts of cold, and in two of boiling water, and is insoluble in strong alcohol.

Tests.—According to German pharmaceutical authority, the presence of sodium chloride to an amount not exceeding two per cent., is permissible in potassium chloride for internal use. To determine the presence of a greater proportion of the sodium compound, a handful of the crystals of potassium chloride is to be reduced to powder and quickly dried. Of this dry powder 0.2 gram, together with 0.49 gram of pure silver nitrate are placed in a test-tube with water, and dilute nitric acid added. The mixture is to be warmed, thoroughly shaken, and after cooling, filtered. The filtrate when treated with silver nitrate solution, should not exhibit the least turbidity, otherwise the proportion of the sodium compound is in excess of the limit prescribed.

Preparation for Homœopathic Use.—The pure chloride of potassium is prepared by trituration, as directed under Class VII.

KALI NITRICUM.

Synonyms, Potassium Nitrate. Nitras Kalicus. Nitrate of Potassium. Nitrum. Potassæ Nitras. Potassii Nitras.

Common Names, Nitrate of Potash. Nitre. Saltpetre.

Formula, KNO_3.

Molecular Weight, 101.

Origin and Preparation of Nitrate of Potassium.—Potassium nitrate is widely diffused in nature, although in small proportion, as a constituent of vegetable soil and in spring and river water. It is never found in large beds as is nitrate of sodium; it occurs in veins in sandstone in Pennsylvania and in calcareous soil in other parts of the world. In South America and in some districts of India, Arabia, Persia, Spain and Hungary, nitrates are found widely disseminated through the soil, but never at a depth lower than can be easily penetrated by the air. The formation of nitric acid in these localities is in all probability dependent on the oxidation of ammonia, for the production of saltpetre is always found to take place most abundantly where there is a large quantity of vegetable or animal matter in a state of putrefaction, or where the air contains a considerable amount of ammonia resulting from such decomposition. The luxuriant vegetation of the tropics supplies by its decay a never failing source of ammonia, and the high temperature and moisture of the air facilitate its oxidation, so that in the tropics the amount of naturally produced saltpetre is vastly in excess of that formed in Europe. An indispensable condition for the formation of nitrates in large quantity, is the presence of alkaline or earthy bases to fix the nitric acid as soon as formed. Nitrate of calcium is formed artificially in several countries in Europe, by mixing decomposing vegetable and animal matters with cinders, chalk, marl, etc., moistening the mass repeatedly with urine, exposing it freely to the air for two or three years, and then lixiviating. Nitrates are found in the juices of plants, particularly those with fleshy, tuberous roots, and are probably acquired from the soil by direct imbibition. The commercially pure salt has to be further purified before it is used in pharmacy, but this is done by the manufacturing chemist.

Properties.—Chemically pure potassium nitrate forms either a dry, snow-white, crystalline mass, or colorless, permanent, large six-sided, striated, rhombic prisms. They dissolve in four parts of water at medium temperatures, in less than half their weight of boiling water, and are insoluble in alcohol. The solutions are neutral in reaction. The crystals contain longitudinal cavities filled with the mother liquor, so that when triturated a damp powder is produced, but through the spontaneous and slow evaporation of a saturated solution, solid crystals are readily obtainable. The taste of the salt is saline, cooling and slightly bitter. The salt melts below a red heat without decomposition to a colorless liquid, and on cooling solidifies to a white, opaque, radiate-crystalline mass. At a higher temperature it is decomposed with the evolution of oxygen and nitrogen, and the formation of nitrite of potassium. When thrown upon glowing coal, it deflagrates and leaves a residue which is alkaline in reaction.

Tests.—A portion of the salt dissolved in 50 times its volume of distilled water should give no turbidity with silver nitrate (absence of chloride), nor with barium chloride (absence of sulphate), nor with sodium carbonate (absence of earthy metals), nor with hydrogen sulphide (absence of heavy metals); its solution treated with ammonium hydrate and carbonate and then with sodium phosphate, will give a white precipitate of ammonio-magnesium phosphate if magnesium be present. The presence of sodium may be detected by dissolving a portion of the salt in aqueous alcohol and igniting the latter, a yellow-colored flame indicating the presence of sodium.

The first provings were made under Jörg, in Germany.

Preparation for Homœopathic Use.—One part by weight of pure nitrate of potassium is dissolved in nine parts by weight of distilled water.

Amount of drug power, $\frac{1}{10}$.

Dilutions must be prepared as directed under Class V—*a*.

Triturations of pure nitrate of potassium are prepared as directed under Class VII.

KALI PERMANGANICUM.

Synonyms, Potassium Permanganate. Kali Hypermanganicum Crystallizatum. Potassæ Permanganas. Potassii Permanganas.

Common Name, Permanganate of Potash.

Formula, $K_2\ Mn_2\ O_8$.

Molecular Weight, 316.

Preparation of Permanganate of Potassium.—"Take of caustic potash, five ounces; black oxide of manganese in fine powder, four ounces; chlorate of potash, three and a half ounces; diluted sulphuric acid, a sufficiency; distilled water, two and a half pints. Reduce the chlorate of potash to fine powder, and mix it with the oxide of manganese; put the mixture into a porcelain basin, and add to it the caustic potash, previously dissolved in four ounces of water. Evaporate to dryness on a sand-bath, stirring diligently to prevent spurting. Pulverize the mass, put it into a covered Hessian or Cornish crucible, and expose it to a dull red heat for an hour, or till it has assumed the condition of a semi-fused mass. Let it cool, pulverize it, and boil with a pint and a half of the water. Let the insoluble matter subside, decant the fluid, boil again with half a pint of the water, again decant, neutralize the united liquors accurately with the diluted sulphuric acid, and evaporate till a pellicle forms. Set aside to cool and crystallize. Drain the crystalline mass, boil it in six ounces of the water and strain through a funnel, the throat of which is lightly obstructed by a little asbestos. Let the fluid cool and crystallize, drain the crystals, and dry them by placing them under a bell-jar over a vessel containing sulphuric acid."—Br. P.

Properties.—Potassium permanganate is in tolerably permanent, neutral, very dark purple, prismatic crystals having a metallic lustre; they are without odor, possess a sweetish astringent taste, and are soluble in 16 parts of cold, and in 2 of boiling water. The solutions are of a deep purple color, and even when quite dilute, show a decided purple tint, and when brought in contact with oxidizable matters, whether organic or inorganic, the color rapidly disappears from loss of oxygen and consequent formation of manganic hydrate; mineral acids discharge the color with the formation of manganous salts.

Test.—Five grains dissolved in water require, for complete decoloration, a solution of 44 grains of granulated ferrous sulphate, acidulated with 2 fluid drachms of dilute sulphuric acid.

The first provings were by Dr. H. C. Allen, U. S.

Preparation for Homœopathic Use.—One part by weight of pure permanganate of potassium is dissolved in ninety-nine parts by weight of distilled water.

Amount of drug power, $\frac{1}{100}$.

Dilutions must be prepared as directed under Class V—β, except that they must be freshly prepared as required.

Owing to its decomposition with organic matter, permanganate of potassium should not be prepared by trituration.

KALI PHOSPHORICUM.

Synonyms, Potassium Phosphate. Potassii Phosphas.

Common Name, Phosphate of Potash.

Formula, $K_2 H P O_4$.

Molecular Weight, 174.

Preparation of Phosphate of Potassium.—This salt is produced by mixing aqueous phosphoric acid with a sufficient quantity of potassium hydrate or carbonate until the reaction is slightly alkaline, and evaporating.

Properties.—The salt crystallizes with difficulty in irregular forms (Berzelius). It is generally obtained as a white amorphous mass, is very deliquescent, is freely soluble in water, and is insoluble in alcohol. By ignition it is converted into pyrophosphate.

Tests.—When prepared as directed above, it is not likely to be contaminated. For identification, it may be dissolved in water and then treated with silver nitrate solution, when a yellow precipitate will be thrown down, showing the presence of orthophosphoric acid, and when treated with tartaric acid, a white crystalline precipitate is evidence of the presence of potassium.

Preparation for Homœopathic Use.—Phosphate of potassium is prepared by trituration, as directed under Class VII.

KALI SULPHURICUM.

Synonyms, Potassium Sulphate. Kali Sulphas. Potassæ Sulphas. Potassii Sulphas.

Common Name, Sulphate of Potash.

Formula, $K_2 S O_4$.

Molecular Weight, 174.

Preparation of Sulphate of Potassium.—This salt occurs native in delicate needle-shaped crystals, or as a crust on many of the Vesuvian lavas, and is designated mineralogically as *Glaserite, Arcanite, Aphthalose* or *Vesuvian salt.* It is obtained as a by-product in several manufacturing processes, as in the preparation of nitric acid from nitrate of potassium, the acid sulphate usually obtained as a residue of this operation being converted into neutral sulphate by addition of potassium carbonate. It likewise crystallizes out from the mother-liquors of sea-water and salt springs, and from the liquors obtained by lixiviating kelp and varec.

Properties.—Potassium sulphate crystallizes in short, permanent, colorless, four and six-sided prisms, and by slow crystallization from a large quantity of its solution in double six-sided pyramids. It is soluble in 10 parts of cold, and in 3 of boiling water, and is insoluble in alcohol. It has a sharp, bitter, saline taste; its specific gravity is 2.66. The crystals decrepitate strongly when heated.

Tests.—A solution of potassium sulphate should be unaffected by treatment with hydrogen sulphide or ammonium sulphide (absence of heavy metals), by potassium carbonate (absence of earths), by antimonate of potassium (sodium), and by silver nitrate (chloride).

Preparation for Homœopathic Use.—The pure sulphate of potassium is prepared by trituration, as directed under Class VII.

KALMIA.

Synonym, Kalmia Latifolia, *Linn.*

Nat. Ord., Ericaceæ.

Common Names, Laurel. Mountain Laurel.

This is an evergreen shrub found growing on rocky hills and damp soil, from Maine to Ohio and Kentucky, four to eight feet high; in the mountains from Pennsylvania southward, it often grows to the height of from 10 to 20 feet. Leaves mostly alternate, bright green both sides, ovate-lanceolate or elliptical, tapering to each end, petioled; corymbs terminal, many flowered, clammy-pubescent; pod depressed, glandular. The flowers appear in May and June, are profuse, large and very showy, varying in color from deep rose to nearly white.

It was first proved by Dr. Buchner, in Germany.

Preparation.—The fresh leaves, collected when flowering, are chopped and pounded to a pulp and weighed. Then two parts by weight of alcohol are taken, the pulp mixed thoroughly with one-sixth part of it, and the rest of the alcohol added. After having stirred the whole well, pour it into a well-stoppered bottle, and let it stand eight days in a dark, cool place. The tincture is then separated by decanting, straining and filtering.

Drug power of tincture, $\frac{1}{6}$.

Dilutions must be prepared as directed under Class III.

KAMALA.

Synonyms, Mallotus Philippinensis, *Müll.* Rottlera Tinctoria, *Roxburgh.* Croton Coccineus.

Nat. Ord., Euphorbiaceæ.

Common Name, Kameela.

This is a large shrub or small tree from 20 to 45 feet in height, growing throughout the Indian peninsulas, in many of the East India Islands, and in China and Australia. The fruit is a roundish three-celled capsule, about the size of a cherry, and is covered with stellate hairs, together with small glands. The berries are collected in large quantities and thrown into large baskets, in which they are rolled about so as to divest them of the glands and hairs. The powder so obtained forms the kamala of commerce, and is light, finely granular and very mobile, consisting of crimson granules, whose bright color is dulled by the admixture of gray stellate hairs and fragments of leaves. It is without odor, but its alcoholic solution poured into water emits a melon-like odor; it is almost without taste, but it feels gritty between the teeth. It yields to alcohol, ether, chloroform or benzol a splendid red resin; from a concentrated ethereal solution allowed to stand a few days, minute, platy, yellow crystals, of a satiny lustre, can be isolated; when decomposed with caustic potash, they yield paraoxybenzoic acid.

Preparation.—The kamecla powder is covered with five parts by weight of alcohol, and having poured the mixture into a well-stoppered bottle, it is allowed to remain eight days in a dark, cool place, being shaken twice a day. It is then poured off, strained and filtered.

Drug power of tincture, $\frac{1}{10}$.

Dilutions must be prepared as directed under Class IV.

Triturations are prepared as directed under Class VII.

KAOLINUM.

Synonyms, Kaolin. Alumina Silicata.

Common Names, Porcelain or China Clay.

This is a mixture of aluminous and silicious earth, or more properly is decomposed felspar, Al K Si_3O_8, found in nature in layers filling hollows between granite and other rocks, and distinguishing itself from other aluminous earths by its being free from iron, and quite white or only pale-colored. The most excellent occurs in the mountains near Misnia in Saxony, near Passau in Bavaria, and near Karlsbad in Bohemia.

Preparation.—Kaolin, first reduced to powder by pounding, is carefully washed with distilled water, and then triturated, as directed under Class VII.

KINO.

Synonyms, Butea Frondosa, *Roxb.* Erythrina Monosperma. Pterocarpus Marsupium, *De Candolle.* Eucalyptus Rostrata, *Schlect,* (Nat. Ord., Myrtaceæ.)

Nat. Ord., Leguminosæ.

Common Names, Buja. Dhak Tree. Australian Red Gum.

Pterocarpus Marsupium is a handsome tree, 40 to 80 feet high, growing in Central and Southern India, and in Ceylon.

Butea frondosa or Dhak tree, grows in India and Burmah, and is conspicuous for its large orange, papilionaceous flowers.

Pterocarpus erinaceus is a native of tropical Western Africa.

The kino, originally used in medicine in the last century, came from the river Gambia, in West Africa, and was the product of P. erinaceus. At the beginning of the present century, East Indian kino, from the Malabar coast, whose botanical origin is P. Marsupium, replaced the African drug, as the latter no longer appeared in commerce. The

Butea kino is used in India in place of the Malabar or East Indian kino. The true East Indian kino is very scarce, the whole amount collected probably not exceeding a ton or two per annum. For some years the drug market has been largely supplied with considerable quantities of kino obtained from Australia; this is the product of numerous species of *Eucalyptus*. It is believed that the better varieties of Eucalyptus kino, such as that from *E. rostrata*, possess the properties of Pterocarpus kino.

The provings were made with kino from E. rostrata.

Properties.—Kino is the juice which exudes from incisions made in the tree, and dried without artificial heat. As it oozes out it has the appearance of red currant jelly, but hardens in a few hours' exposure to the air. Malabar or East India kino is in dark blackish-red, angular fragments, rarely larger than a pea, and when in thin sections is transparent and of a bright garnet hue. The fragments sink in water and upon agitation partially dissolve; they are completely soluble in alcohol. Kino is without odor and has an extremely astringent and sweetish taste.

It was proven by Dr. Blundell, *Month. Hom. Rev.*, 7, 199.

Preparation.—The inspissated juice, obtained from incisions made in the trunk, is powdered, covered with five parts by weight of alcohol, and allowed to remain eight days in a well-stoppered bottle, in a dark, cool place, being shaken twice a day. The tincture is then poured off, strained and filtered.

Drug power of tincture, $\frac{1}{10}$.

Dilutions must be prepared as directed under Class IV.

KRAMERIA.

Synonym, Krameria Triandra, *Ruiz et Pavon.*

Nat. Ord., Polygalaceæ.

Common Names, Mapato. Pumacuchu. Ratanhia. Rhatany.

The rhatany plant is a small, woody shrub with an upright stem about a foot in height, growing in Bolivia and Peru at an elevation of from 3000 to 8000 feet above the sea level. The root is dark reddish-brown and consists of a short, thick crown, sometimes as large as a man's fist, and knotted. The root throws out an abundance of branching woody rootlets, one-quarter to one-half inch thick and several feet long. The woody portion of the root is brownish-yellow and dense; the valuable qualities of the drug are contained in the bark of the root, and hence the superior value of the long rootlets or "long" rhatany in which the woody portion is very small.

It was introduced into the Homœopathic Materia Medica by Hartlaub and Trinks, Germany.

Preparation.—The dried root, coarsely powdered, is covered with five parts by weight of alcohol, and allowed to remain eight days in a well-stoppered bottle, in a dark, cool place, being shaken twice a day. The tincture is then poured off, strained and filtered.

Drug power of tincture, $\frac{1}{10}$.

Dilutions must be prepared as directed under Class IV.

KREOSOTUM.

Synonym, Creosotum.

Common Names, Creasote. Kreosote.

Origin and Preparation.—The substance found in commerce under the name of kreosote is often merely hydrate of phenyl, more or less impure, but the true kreosote extracted by Reichenbach from wood-tar is a perfectly distinct body. In the dry distillation of wood a tar is left, and when it is in its turn distilled the residue acquires the consistence of a pitchy mass, and the liquid contained in the receiver is found to consist of several distinct layers, the lowest of which contains the kreosote. The latter layer is saturated with sodium carbonate, left at rest and after some time a yellowish oil rises to the surface. The oil is decanted, rectified in a glass retort, the lighter portion of the distillate rejected and the heavier portion collected and treated with potash solution of specific gravity 1.12. The kreosote dissolves in the alkaline liquid and the hydrocarbons, including Eupion (*vide infra*), with which it is mixed, remain undissolved. After decanting and boiling, the potash solution is treated with sulphuric acid to set free the kreosote, but the latter is further purified by successive distillations with alkaline water, re-solution in potash and re-separation by sulphuric acid.

Eupion, as shown above, is obtained from wood-tar, and is procured in greater proportion from coal-tar, from rectified bone-oil and from the oil obtained by the dry distillation of hemp-seed and rape-seed. To prepare eupion from rectified bone-oil the latter is mixed with quarter its weight of sulphuric acid; the lighter and clearer liquid which rises to the surface is taken off and distilled with an equal weight of sulphuric acid and a small quantity of nitre; the distillate is again distilled with sulphuric acid, then washed with aqueous potash and with water, rectified, dried under the air-pump and treated with potassium as long as the metal shows signs of oxidation.

Properties of Kreosote.—It is a colorless or faintly yellow, strongly refracting liquid. Its specific gravity is 1.071, as required by the British Pharmacopœia, or 1.046 by United States Pharmacopœia. Its specific gravity varies between 1.040 and 1.090, and its boiling point from 200° to 210° C. (392–410° F.). Its odor is disagreeable, smoky and penetrating and its taste is burning and caustic; it is soluble in eighty parts of cold and in twenty-four of hot water, and in all proportions in alcohol, ether, carbon disulphide and acetic acid. When ignited it burns with a white but very sooty flame. It precipitates gum and albumen from their solutions, but forms a clear mixture with collodion. When kept for some time it gradually becomes brownish in color.

Eupion is a colorless, transparent, extremely mobile liquid, having a low refractive power on light; it is tasteless, but has an odor like that of flowers. Its specific gravity is 0.65 at 20° C. (68° F.); it is very volatile, evaporating perceptibly at common temperatures. Eupion is insoluble in water, dissolves sparingly in aqueous alcohol, but mixes readily with absolute alcohol, ether and the volatile and fixed oils. It is a very stable substance; it is not altered by light; acids and alkalies have no influence upon it, and it is said that potassium permanganate is not reduced by it, while with chlorine, bromine and iodine it unites without undergoing decomposition.

Tests.—The liability of kreosote to contain carbolic acid as a falsification, will call for special tests for presence of the latter. Liquid carbolic acid is soluble in three volumes of a mixture of one part of water with three of glycerine; kreosote is almost insoluble in the same. In ten volumes of strong liquor ammonia kreosote scarcely dissolves; by heating to the boiling point a partial solution takes place, and on cooling, the kreosote separates at the bottom of the vessel as a yellow or brownish layer, and if the whole be allowed to stand for a day, the ammoniacal solution will be found to be colored yellowish or yellowish-brown. Carbolic acid on the other hand, dissolves at once in the caustic ammonia, and when boiled and placed aside for a day, the liquid becomes blue or violet-blue in color. When ten drops of kreosote are thoroughly shaken with ten CC. of water, and then a drop of ferric chloride solution added, a yellowish or greenish or green turbidity occurs, which changes after some time to greenish-brown or brownish. Under similar conditions carbolic acid produces a clear blue fluid and the color is permanent. When equal volumes of kreosote and collodion are mixed together, there results a clear viscid mass. With carbolic acid the collodion gelatinizes, will not flow, and is more or less turbid. A specimen of kreosote is to be considered adulterated when it does not sink upon being dropped into water (with cautious shaking), or if it does not evidence its transparency when lying at the bottom of the water, or if, when treated with ten volumes of strong solution of ammonia and shaken, it dissolves completely or suffers a diminution of its volume; or when mixed with an equal volume of collodion the latter gelatinizes. Kreosote adulterated with carbolic acid does not fail to gelatinize collodion.

The first provings were by Dr. Syrbius, in Germany.

Eupion was proven by Dr. Bertoldi, Italy.

Preparation for Homœopathic Use.—One part by weight of pure beechwood-tar kreosote is dissolved in ninety-nine parts by weight of alcohol.

Amount of drug power, $\frac{1}{100}$.

Dilutions must be prepared as directed under Class VI—β.

LACERTA AGILIS, *L.*

Synonym, Lacerta Stirpium.
Class, Reptilia.
Order, Sauria.
Family, Lacertina.
Common Name, Green European Lizard.

The green lizard is frequently met with in Southern Europe, in some parts of Africa and in Sweden. It is not poisonous; it will bite, but the wounds are not dangerous. It was reputed of old to be an antidote against all poisons, and is yet used occasionally as a popular remedy.

There seems to be some doubt as to the proper preparation; while some prepare a tincture from the fresh pounded lizard, others recommend a trituration from the dried animal.

Preparation.—The entire dried animal is prepared by trituration, as directed under Class VII.

LACHESIS.

Synonym, Trigonocephalus Lachesis, *L.*
Class, Reptilia.
Order, Ophidia.
Family, Crotalidæ.
Common Name, Surukuke or Churukuku.

The lachesis or trigonocephalus inhabits the hot countries of South America; it attains a length of upwards of seven feet, and its poison-fangs are nearly one inch long; the skin is reddish-brown, marked along the back with large rhomboidal spots of a blackish-brown color, each of which encloses two spots of the color of the body. The poison resembles saliva, is less viscous, limpid, inodorous, without any marked taste, in color somewhat greenish; at the extremity of the fang, it easily forms into drops, and falls without threading; exposed to the air, it soon concentrates into a dry, yellow mass, which for an indefinite time preserves its poisonous qualities. This poison introduced into a wound, or injected into a vein, produces the most dreadful symptoms, and generally, death. The virus of this serpent has been more carefully proved than that of any other. The specimen used by Dr. Hering in his experiments was obtained from the living snake, which was stunned with a blow; the poison was then collected on sugar by pressing the poison-fang upwards against the bag, and the three first attenuations prepared by trituration.

Preparation.—The virus is triturated as directed under Class VIII.

LACHNANTHES.

Synonym, Lachnanthes Tinctoria, *Elliott.*
Nat. Ord., Hæmodoraceæ.
Common Names, Red Root. Spirit Weed.

This herb grows in sandy swamps, from Rhode Island and New Jersey southward, near the coast. Its root is red, fibrous and perennial. Leaves ensiform, equitant, clustered at the base and scattered on the stem, which is hairy at the top, and terminated by a dense compound cyme of dingy yellow and loosely woolly flowers. Perianth woolly outside, six-parted down to the adherent ovary Stamens three, opposite the three larger or inner divisions; filaments long, exserted; anthers linear, fixed by the middle. Style thread-like, exserted, declined. Pod globular; seeds few on each fleshy placenta, flat and rounded, fixed by the middle. Flowers appear from July to September.

It was proved under the direction of Dr. Lippe, United States.

Preparation.—The fresh plant in flower is chopped and pounded to a pulp and weighed. Then two parts by weight of alcohol are taken, the pulp mixed with one-sixth part of it, and the rest of the alcohol added. After having stirred the whole well, pour it into a well-stoppered bottle, and let it stand eight days in a dark, cool place. The tincture is then separated by decanting, straining and filtering.

Amount of drug power, ⅙.

Dilutions must be prepared as directed under Class III.

LACTUCA SATIVA, *Linn.*

Synonyms, Lactuca Crispa. Lactuca Sylvestris.

Nat. Ord., Compositæ.

Common Name, Garden Lettuce.

This is an annual plant, cultivated as a salad vegetable. The stem, about two feet high, is erect, round, simple below, and branching above. The lower leaves are sub-orbicular; the upper are cordate and toothed; both are shining, and yellowish-green in color. The flowers are numerous, small, with yellowish corollas. The plant contains a milky, narcotic juice, which is abundant during the period of inflorescence. The plant is widely cultivated in both hot and temperate climates.

Preparation.—The fresh, perfectly developed plant, grown in the garden, is chopped and pounded to a pulp, enclosed in a piece of new linen and subjected to pressure. The expressed juice is then, by brisk agitation, mingled with an equal part by weight of alcohol. This mixture is allowed to stand eight days in a well-stoppered bottle, in a dark, cool place, and then filtered.

Drug power of tincture, ½.

Dilutions must be prepared as directed under Class I.

LACTUCA VIROSA, *Linn.*

Synonyms, Intybus Augustus. Lactuca Fœtida.

Nat. Ord., Compositæ.

Common Name, Acrid or Strong-scented Lettuce.

This plant is a native of Europe. It is a biennial herb, stem three to four feet high, cylindrical, prickly near the base, pale green in color, and often marked with purple spots. Radical leaves are large, petiolate, oblong-ovate, obtuse, prickly on under side along the midrib, margins wavy. The stem leaves are smaller, alternate, sessile, horizontal, with a saggitate and clasping base, and with spinous apex. Flowers in terminal panicles, pale yellow; akenes are oval, flattened, black, with a whitish beak. The plant exudes a milky juice, has a disagreeable, narcotic odor and a bitter, acrid taste.

It was first proven by Dr. Seidel, Germany.

Preparation.—The fresh plant is chopped and pounded to a pulp, enclosed in a piece of new linen and subjected to pressure. The expressed juice is then, by brisk agitation, mingled with an equal part by weight of alcohol. This mixture is allowed to stand eight days in a well-stoppered bottle, in a dark, cool place, and then filtered.

Drug power of tincture, ½.

Dilutions must be prepared as directed under Class I.

LACTUCARIUM.

This substance is the concrete juice of *Lactuca virosa*, *L. sativa*, *L. Scariola* and *L. altissima*. The drug market is supplied with lactucarium from Germany and England, from plants specially grown for this purpose.

Preparation of Lactucarium.—Just before the time of flowering, the stem is cut off about a foot below the top, after which a transverse slice is taken off daily until September. The juice is pure white at first but readily becomes brown on the surface, is collected from the wounded top by the finger and is transferred to earthen cups, from which it is turned out after hardening. German lactucarium comes in commerce in fragments moulded by the collecting cups, externally of a dull reddish-brown color, and internally opaque and wax-like. It has a strong opium-like odor, and a very bitter taste.

Preparation for Homœopathic Use.—The dried milk-juice is triturated, as directed under Class VII.

LAMIUM ALBUM, *Linn.*

Synonyms, Gallopsidis Maculata. Lamium Lævigatum.

Nat. Ord., Labiatæ.

Common Names, Dead Nettle. White Archangel.

This plant grows in Europe, on highways, beside ditches, hedges, etc. Root cylindrical, ramose, hairy; stem straight, quadrangular, downy, simple. Leaves ovate-cordate, serrate, pointed, downy. Flowers white, in axillary clusters; calyx-teeth slender and hairy at base.

This drug was first proven by Hahnemann and Stapf.

Preparation.—Two parts of fresh leaves and one part of fresh blossoms are chopped and pounded to pulp, enclosed in a piece of new linen and subjected to pressure. The expressed juice is then, by brisk agitation, mingled with an equal part by weight of alcohol. This mixture is allowed to stand eight days in a well-stoppered bottle, in a dark, cool place, and then filtered.

Amount of drug power, ½.

Dilutions must be prepared as directed under Class I.

LAPATHUM ACUTUM.

Synonym, Rumex Obtusifolius, *Linn.*

Nat. Ord., Polygonaceæ.

Common Name, Bitter Dock.

This plant is a native of Europe, but has been introduced into America, where it is found growing in fields, etc. Stem somewhat rough; lower leaves ovate-cordate, obtuse, downy on the veins beneath, wavy-margined; the upper lance-oblong, acuminate; whorls distant; valves ovate-hastate, and with some sharp subulate teeth at the base, strongly reticulated, one grain-bearing.

Proven by Dr. Widenhorn, Archiv. de la Med. Hom., 2, 305.

Preparation.—The fresh root, gathered in autumn, is chopped and pounded to a pulp and weighed. Then two parts by weight of alcohol are taken, the pulp mixed thoroughly with one-sixth part of it, and the rest of the alcohol added. After having stirred the whole well, pour it into a well-stoppered bottle, and let it stand eight days in a dark, cool place. The tincture is then separated by decanting, straining and filtering.

Amount of drug power, $\frac{1}{6}$.

Dilutions must be prepared as directed under Class III.

LAPIS ALBUS.

Synonym, Silico-Fluoride of Calcium.

This name, Lapis Albus, is given by Dr. v. Grauvogl, to an unnamed species of *gneiss,* which he first found held in suspension in the waters of the mineral springs of Gastein, Germany. These springs start from the foot of the Tauern Mountains, and flow downward into the valley of the Achen, over formations of gneiss.

The substance proved was a trituration of the solid gneiss rock. Dr. v. Grauvogl calls it a white, primitive, calcium gneiss. Until a careful scientific analysis of the rock used by v. Grauvogl is made, we must only consider as officinal, triturations of the gneiss from the springs of Gastein, Germany.

Preparation.—Genuine Lapis Albus is triturated, as directed under Class VII.

LAUROCERASUS.

Synonyms, Prunus Laurocerasus, *Linn.* Padus Laurocerasus.
Nat. Ord., Rosaceæ.
Common Name, Cherry Laurel.

This is a handsome evergreen shrub growing to a height of eighteen feet or more, and is a native of the Caucasus, of North Western Asia Minor, and of Northern Persia. It has been introduced as an ornamental plant in many parts of Europe. The leaves are alternate, simple, coriaceous, with shining upper surface; they are five to six inches long and nearly two inches wide, oblong or obovate, on thick petioles; margin recurved, sharp-serrate, glandular-dentate. They are paler on lower side, and dull, and marked by eight to ten lateral veins. Flowers small, white, in simple racemes. Fruit an oval, dark red, almost black, drupe. The fresh leaves are inodorous until bruised, when they at once emit the odor of hydrocyanic acid. When chewed, their taste is rough, aromatic and bitter.

It was first proven under Dr. Jörg, Germany.

Preparation.—The mature fresh leaves, gathered in the summer months, are chopped and pounded to a pulp and weighed. Take two-thirds by weight of alcohol, and add it to the pulp, stirring and mixing well together; then enclose in a piece of new linen and subject to pressure. The tincture thus obtained is allowed to stand eight days in a well-stoppered bottle, in a dark, cool place, and then filtered.

Drug power of tincture, $\frac{1}{2}$.

Dilutions must be prepared as directed under Class II.

LEDUM.

Synonyms, Ledum Palustre, *Linn.* Anthos Sylvestris. Rosmarinum Sylvestre.

Nat. Ord., Ericaceæ.

Common Names, Marsh Tea. Wild Rosemary.

This is an evergreen shrub, from two to three feet high. Stem erect, slender, much branched, young branches covered with close rust-colored down. Leaves scattered, horizontal or reflexed, on short petioles, linear or ligulate, entire, with revolute margins, channeled, smooth; upper surface dark green, under surface paler, and the midrib covered with rust-colored down. Flowers numerous, in dense, simple, terminal, bracteated corymbs. Stamens uniformly ten. Pods oval. The whole plant, when bruised, has a strong, oppressive, aromatic odor, and a bitter, astringent, nauseous taste. It grows in moist, swampy grounds in north of Europe, France, Asia and British America.

It was first proven by Hahnemann.

Preparation.—The fresh herb is pounded to a pulp and weighed. Then two parts by weight of alcohol are taken, the pulp mixed thoroughly with one-sixth part of it, and the rest of the alcohol added. After having stirred the whole well, pour it into a well-stoppered bottle, and let it stand eight days in a dark, cool place. The tincture is then separated by decanting, straining and filtering.

Drug power of tincture, $\frac{1}{6}$.

Dilutions must be prepared as directed under Class III.

LEPIDIUM BONARIENSE, *De Candolle.*

Synonym, Lepidium Mastruco.

Nat. Ord., Cruciferæ.

Common Names, Buenos Ayres Pepperwort. Mastruco.

This plant is very common in the neighborhood of Rio, where it is found along the roads and in stony places. It is herbaceous, with numerous glabrous, erect stems, attaining a height of from twenty to thirty inches; the radical leaves are petiolate, finely indented; the superior leaves are alternate, sessile and almost linear. The flowers are in terminal spikes, supported by filiform pedicles; calyx with four folioles; corolla small, cruciform, with four hypogynous petals, six tetradynamous stamens, short style, small, subelliptical pod, which is somewhat crenated at the top; root fibrous, simple, erect.

It blossoms in September.

It was introduced into our Materia Medica by Dr. Mure, Brazil.

Preparation.—The fresh leaves are chopped and pounded to a pulp and weighed. Then two parts by weight of alcohol are taken, the pulp mixed thoroughly with one-sixth part of it, and the rest of the alcohol added. After stirring the whole well, and pouring it into a well-stoppered bottle, it is allowed to stand eight days in a dark, cool place. The tincture is then separated by decanting, straining and filtering.

Drug power of tincture, $\frac{1}{6}$.

Dilutions must be prepared as directed under Class III.

LEPTANDRA.

Synonyms, Leptandra Virginica, *Nutall.* Veronica Virginica, *Linn.* Callistachya Virginica. Eustachya Alba.

Nat. Ord., Scrophulariaceæ.

Common Names, Black Root. Culver's Root. Tall Speedwell. Tall Veronica.

This is a perennial herbaceous plant, with a smooth or slightly downy erect stem, two to six feet high, growing throughout the United States east of the Mississippi. Leaves in whorls of four to seven, on short petioles, lanceolate, pointed and finely serrate. Calyx five-parted. Corolla nearly white, wheel-shaped, tube larger than the limb, segments unequal. Stamens much exserted. Lower part of filaments and corolla pubescent. Fruit a pod, ovate, acuminate, opening at the apex, two celled, many seeded. Flowers in July and August.

It was proven by Dr. W. H. Burt, United States.

Preparation.—The fresh root, of the second year, is chopped and pounded to a pulp. Then two parts by weight of alcohol are taken, the pulp mixed thoroughly with one-sixth part of it, and the rest of the alcohol added. After having stirred the whole well, pour it into a well-stoppered bottle, and allow it to stand eight days in a dark, cool place. The tincture is then separated by decanting, straining and filtering.

Drug power of tincture, $\frac{1}{6}$.

Dilutions must be prepared as directed under Class III.

LILIUM TIGRINUM, *H. K.*

Nat. Ord., Liliaceæ.

Common Name, Tiger Lily.

This plant is a native of China and Japan, but is widely cultivated as a garden plant. Stem from four to six feet high, unbranched, woolly. Leaves scattered, sessile, three-veined, the upper cordate-ovate, the axils bulbiferous. Flowers large, in a pyramid at the summit of the stem, dark orange-colored, with black or very deep crimson, somewhat raised spots, which give the flower the appearance of the skin of the tiger, and from which circumstance it has derived its name; perianth revolute and papillose within. Flowers appear [illegible] August.

It was introduced into our Materia Medica by Dr. W. E. Payne, United States.

Preparation.—The fresh plant, in flower, is chopped and pounded to a pulp and weighed. Then two parts by weight of alcohol are taken, the pulp mixed thoroughly with one-sixth part of it, and the rest of the alcohol added. After having stirred the whole and poured it into a well-stoppered bottle, it is allowed to stand eight days in a dark, cool place. The tincture is then separated by decanting, straining and filtering.

Drug power of tincture, $\frac{1}{6}$.

Dilutions must be prepared as directed under Class III.

LITHIUM BROMATUM.

Synonyms, Lithium Bromide. Lithium Bromatum. Lithium Hydrobromicum. Lithii Bromidum.

Common Name, Bromide of Lithium.

Formula, Li Br.

Molecular Weight, 87.

Preparation and Properties of Bromide of Lithium.—One part of lithium sulphate is to be dried by heating on a water-bath and then digested for an hour with three parts of crystallized barium bromide and three parts of hot distilled water. After cooling, there are to be added four parts of alcohol, and after some hours the whole is to be thrown on a filter; the residue is to be washed on the filter with dilute alcohol, the alcohol distilled off and the rest of the filtrate evaporated to dryness.

Properties.—Lithium bromide is a colorless hygroscopic salt which may be obtained in crystals by slowly evaporating its solution over sulphuric acid. It is readily soluble in water and alcohol.

Preparation for Homœopathic Use.—Bromide of lithium is prepared by trituration, as directed under Class VII.

LITHIUM CARBONICUM.

Synonyms, Lithium Carbonate. Carbonas Lithicus. Lithii Carbonas.

Common Name, Carbonate of Lithium.

Formula, $Li_2\ CO_3$.

Molecular Weight, 74.

Preparation of Carbonate of Lithium.—Carbonate of lithium exists in the waters of Carlsbad, Franzensbad and of other springs. It is prepared by dissolving an excess of ammonium carbonate in a concentrated solution of lithium chloride and washing the resulting precipitate with alcohol.

Properties.—Lithium carbonate is a white light powder, not unlike magnesia in appearance, and has an alkaline taste. It effervesces with acids and when moistened with hydrochloric acid and placed in a loop of platinum wire and held in the flame of an alcohol lamp it colors the flame a carmine-red. It is soluble in about 135 parts of water at medium temperatures, and the solution has an alkaline reaction; in alcohol it is almost insoluble. Heated to redness it fuses, and on cooling solidifies to a crystalline mass; at a white heat it loses four-fifths of its carbonic acid. The lithium carbonate of commerce is frequently a sesquicarbonate, and is soluble in about 100 parts of water; absolutely pure monocarbonate requires 150 parts of cold water for its solution.

Tests.—The solution of lithium carbonate in dilute hydrochloric acid gives, when evaporated, a residue which is soluble in a mixture of equal volumes of ninety per cent. alcohol and ether; the chlorides of potassium and sodium are insoluble, or nearly so in this mixture. The above-mentioned residue after evaporation, when dissolved in 200 volumes of water, should give no turbidity with ammonium oxalate (calcium) nor with sodium carbonate (magnesia). A solution of lithium carbonate in dilute nitric acid should give no precipitate with silver nitrate or barium chloride, nor with hydrogen sulphide or ammonium sulphide.

It was first proven by Dr. Hering.

Preparation for Homœopathic Use.—Pure carbonate of lithium is prepared by trituration, as directed under Class VII.

LOBELIA.

Synonyms, Lobelia Inflata, *Linn.* Rapuntium Inflatum.

Nat. Ord., Lobeliaceæ.

Common Names, Indian Tobacco. Lobelia. Asthma Root. Bugle Weed. Emetic Herb. Puke Root.

This is an indigenous annual plant found growing on roadsides and in neglected fields. Root fibrous, stem erect, angled, from nine to eighteen inches high, pubescent, much branched. Leaves sessile, ovate or oblong, serrate, diminishing into leaf-like bracts. Flowers numerous, short-pedicelled, small, in spike-like racemes. Corolla pale blue, tubular, somewhat two-lipped, the upper lip bifid, the lower trifid. Fruit a two-celled pod, with numerous small, brown seeds. Flowers from July to September.

It was introduced into the Homœopathic Materia Medica by Dr. Jeanes, United States.

Preparation.—The fresh plant is pounded to a pulp and weighed. Then two parts by weight of alcohol are taken, and after thoroughly mixing the pulp with one-sixth part of it, the rest of the alcohol is added. After having stirred the whole well, pour it into a well-stoppered bottle and let it stand eight days in a dark, cool place. The tincture is then separated by decanting, straining and filtering.

Drug power of tincture, $\frac{1}{6}$.

Dilutions must be prepared as directed under Class III.

LOBELIA CARDINALIS, *Linn.*

Nat. Ord., Lobeliaceæ.

Common Names, Cardinal Flower. Red Lobelia.

This species of lobelia is tall, two to four feet high, stem simple, smoothish; leaves oblong-lanceolate, slightly toothed, acute at each end, sessile. Flowers in a terminal branched raceme, on short pedicels. Corolla deep scarlet and large. The plant is common from Canada to the Carolinas, and westward to Illinois.

Preparation.—The fresh plant is chopped and pounded to a pulp and weighed. Then two parts by weight of alcohol are taken, the pulp mixed thoroughly with one-sixth part of it, and the rest of the alcohol added. After stirring the whole well and pouring it into a well-stoppered bottle, it is allowed to remain eight days in a dark, cool place. The tincture is then separated by decanting, straining and filtering.

Drug power of tincture, $\frac{1}{6}$.

Dilutions must be prepared as directed under Class III.

LOBELIA SYPHILITICA, *Linn.*

Synonyms, Lobelia Cœrulea. Lobelia Glandulosa.

Nat. Ord., Lobeliaceæ.

Common Names, Blue Lobelia. Great Lobelia.

An indigenous plant often found in the Western States in wet meadows and along streams. Stem erect, simple, two to four feet high, angular. Leaves oblong-lanceolate, acute at both ends, irregularly serrate. Flowers in a dense raceme or crowded spike. Corolla pale blue, an inch long, showy. Calyx with reflexed sinuses. Flowers in July.

It was first proven by Dr. W. Williamson, United States.

Preparation.—The fresh plant is chopped and pounded to a pulp and weighed. Then two parts by weight of alcohol are taken, the pulp mixed thoroughly with one-sixth part of it, and the rest of the alcohol added. After having stirred the whole well and poured it into a well-stoppered bottle, it is allowed to stand eight days in a dark, cool place. The tincture is then separated by decanting and filtering.

Drug power of tincture, $\frac{1}{6}$.

Dilutions must be prepared as directed under Class III.

LOLIUM TEMULENTUM, *Linn.*

Synonyms, Lolium Arvense. Lolium Robustum.

Nat. Ord., Gramineæ.

Common Name, Bearded Darnel. Darnel. Tare.

This grass is an annual, about two feet high, indigenous to Europe and Western Asia, but found in this country from New England to Pennsylvania. Leaves lance-linear, large and showy, rough-edged. Spikelets five to seven-flowered, much compressed, not longer than the glume. Seeds oblong-ovoid, about one quarter of an inch in length, inner surface grooved, outer convex, smooth, light brown.

It was first proven by Dr. Cordier, France.

Preparation.—The ripe seeds are coarsely powdered, and covered with five parts by weight of alcohol, and allowed to remain eight days in a well-stoppered bottle, in a dark, cool place, being shaken twice a day. The tincture is then poured off, strained and filtered.

Drug power of tincture, $\frac{1}{10}$.

Dilutions must be prepared as directed under Class IV.

LUPULINA.

Common Name, Lupulin.

This is a yellow glandular powder detached from the strobiles of Humulus Lupulus. See Lupulus.

When dry hops are handled, the glandular powder becomes separated and is freed from other matters by sifting; about 10 per cent. of the weight of the hops may be thus procured. Lupulin, when recent, is a yellow, afterwards brown, granular, resinous powder, which has the odor and taste of hops.

Preparation.—The lupulin is triturated, as directed under Class VII

LUPULUS.

Synonym, Humulus Lupulus, *Linn.*

Nat. Ord., Urticaceæ.

Common Names, Hops. Hop Vine.

The hop vine is found growing wild, especially in thickets, on the banks of rivers throughout Europe, and extends to the Caucasus and Central Asia. It has been cultivated for centuries in Europe, and is found in both North and South America. It is a perennial, diœcious plant, producing annually long turning stems, which climb freely over trees and bushes. Leaves opposite, on long petioles, mostly three to five-lobed, serrate, deep green on upper surface, prickly, rough. The male flowers are in a long panicle, the female flowers are in a less conspicuous stalked catkin, made up of a short, central, irregular stalk bearing overlapping, rudimentary leaflets, ultimately forming an ovoid cone or strobile. The leaflets bear at the base the fruit or seeds, and both leaflets (at the base) and seeds are beset with numerous yellow glands, which, when separated, appear in mass as powder.

It was first proven by Dr. Bethmann, in Germany.

Preparation.—The fresh hop-strobiles are chopped and pounded to a pulp and weighed. Then two parts by weight of alcohol are taken, the pulp thoroughly mixed with one-sixth part of it, and the rest of the alcohol added. After having stirred the whole well and poured it into a well-stoppered bottle, it is allowed to stand eight days in a dark, cool place. The tincture is then separated by decanting, straining and filtering.

Drug power of tincture, $\frac{1}{6}$.
Dilutions must be prepared as directed under Class III.

LYCOPERSICUM.

Synonyms, Solanum Lycopersicum, *Linn.* Lycopersicum Esculentum, *Mill.* Poma Amoris.

Nat. Ord., Solanaceæ.

Common Names, Love Apple. Tomato.

This plant is a native of tropical America, but its fruit has come into such high repute that it is cultivated very extensively elsewhere. The tomato plant resembles the potato plant in general aspect. It is hairy; stems herbaceous, weak, growing three to four feet high; leaves unequally pinnatifid, segments cut, glaucous beneath; flowers greenish-yellow, of an unpleasant odor; fruit is large and abundant, torulose, furrowed, smooth, at first green, becoming when ripe a beautiful red; it has an agreeable acid taste.

Introduced by Dr. Gross, Germany.

Preparation.—The fresh herb beginning to flower, is chopped and pounded to a pulp and weighed. Then two parts by weight of alcohol are taken, the pulp mixed thoroughly with one-sixth part of it, and the rest of the alcohol added. After stirring the whole well and pouring the mixture into a well-stoppered bottle, it is allowed to stand eight days in a dark, cool place. The tincture is then separated by decanting, straining and filtering.

Amount of drug power, $\frac{1}{6}$.

Dilutions must be prepared as directed under Class III.

LYCOPODIUM.

Synonyms, Lycopodium Clavatum, *Linn.* Muscus Clavatus. Pes Leoninus. Pes Ursinus.

Nat. Ord., Lycopodiaceæ.

Common Names, Club-Moss. Stag's Horn. Witch Meal. Wolf's Claw.

The common *club-moss* is widely distributed through the greater part of the world, but more especially in northern countries. Its stem is creeping, two to four feet long, with ascending branches. Leaves linear-awl-shaped, incurved. Fertile branches end in slender peduncles supporting two to three linear spikes, with ovate acuminate, erosely dentate bracts. Sporangia in the axils of the bracts. The spikes are gathered just before maturity, and the sporules shaken out and separated from other parts of the plant by means of a fine sieve.

Lycopodium in mass, is a pale yellow powder, so very mobile that its behavior is like that of a liquid when the vessel holding it is inclined from side to side. Under microscopic examination, each sporule is seen to be a roundish or nearly globular body, having three well defined facets on one side forming a short, three-sided pyramid. The surface presents a honey-combed appearance, and the angular edges of the pyramid are furnished with small projections. Bucholz found the constituents of Lycopodium sporules to be in 100 parts as follows: fixed oil 6, sugar 3, mucilage 1.5, and 89.5 of what he designated as pollenin, meaning the residue left after extracting the mass with water, alcohol, ether and cold alkaline solution, and which does not seem to be cellulose. Flückiger and Hanbury find that the fixed oil amounts to 47 per cent., and they were enabled to recover this large amount by first finely dividing the sporules by prolonged trituration with sand, and then exhausting the triturated mass with ether. The oil is bland and does not solidify at even —15° C. (5° F.). By subjecting Lycopodium or its extract to distillation, Stenhouse succeeded in obtaining several volatile bases, although in extremely small proportion. Beneath the net-work already described, is a thin, coherent and dense membrane, yellow in color, which resists the action of such solvents as boiling water and strong potash solution. Sulphuric acid does not affect it in the cold, even after prolonged contact. It affects, however, the membrane in a manner analagous to its action in producing parchment paper, for the pollen grains become transparent; at the same time numerous oil drops quickly exude. Trituration of the sporules alone results in a darkening of the color and increased consistency with evident greasiness of the mass. The toughness of the membrane (and probably the elasticity of the reticulations) render the pollen very difficult to triturate perfectly, but long trituration with such an amount of sugar of milk as will just suffice to isolate each sporule from its neighbors, offers the best means of obtaining as complete rupture and comminution of the pollen grains as can be attained. A method of triturating Lycopodium, and which may give the proper proportions of sugar of milk to sporules, was published in New York *Medical Times*, Vol. X—6.

The drug was first proven by Hahnemann.

Preparation.—To obtain an efficacious tincture of Lycopodium, a previous trituration for hours, first dry, and then with the addition of as much alcohol as is necessary to form a thick paste, will be found of great advantage; after this is done, sufficient strong alcohol is added to make five parts by weight of alcohol to each part by weight of Lycopodium used. This preparation is allowed to remain eight days in a well-stoppered bottle, in a dark, cool place, being shaken twice a day. The tincture is then poured off, strained and filtered.

Drug power of tincture, $\frac{1}{10}$.

Dilutions must be prepared as directed under Class IV.

Triturations of Lycopodium are prepared as directed under Class VII, but the first trituration should be prepared from 1x, made by using one part of Lycopodium to nine of granulated saccharum lactis, and then triturating powerfully for several hours. From this 1x trituration the higher numbers can be made on both scales in the usual way.

LYCOPUS.

Synonym, Lycopus Virginicus, *Linn.*
Nat. Ord., Labiatæ.

Common Names, Bugle-weed. Paul's Betony. Virginia Hoarhound.

This is an indigenous perennial herb found in bogs and wet soils. Stem erect, obtusely four-angled, from twelve to eighteen inches high, generally simple. Leaves opposite, sessile, on petioles, broad-lanceolate, serrate in the middle, entire at both ends, glandular-punctate beneath. The whole plant often takes on a purple tint. Flowers minute, purplish, in small whorls. Corolla four-cleft, nearly regular, upper segment broadest; tube as long as the calyx. Achenia four, truncated obliquely at apex.

It was first proven by Dr. G. E. Chandler, United States.

Preparation.—The fresh plant, in flower, is chopped and pounded to a pulp and weighed. Then two parts by weight of alcohol are taken, and after thoroughly mixing the pulp with one-sixth part of it, the rest of the alcohol is added. After stirring the whole well, and pouring it into a well-stoppered bottle, it is allowed to stand eight days in a dark, cool place. The tincture is then separated by decanting, straining and filtering.

Drug power of tincture, $\frac{1}{6}$.

Dilutions must be prepared as directed under Class III.

LYSSIN.

Synonym, Hydrophobinum.

The virus of the rabid dog.

Preparation.—The virus is prepared by trituration, as directed under Class VIII.

MADAR.

Synonyms, Calotropis Gigantea, *Brown.* Asclepias Gigantea, *Linn.* Mudar.

Nat. Ord., Asclepiadaceæ.

This plant is a native of the East Indies, but has been introduced into the West India Islands. The bark is used as a remedy in East India under the name of *Madar* or *Mudar.* The bark is whitish, is without epidermis, has very little, if any odor, and its taste is nauseous and bitter.

It was proved by E. B. Ivatts, Dublin.

Preparation.—The recently-dried bark, coarsely pulverized, is triturated as directed under Class VII.

MAGNESIA CARBONICA.

Synonyms, Magnesium Carbonate. Carbonas Magnesicus. Magnesii Carbonas. Salis Amari.

Common Name, Carbonate of Magnesia.

Formula, $(Mg\,CO_3)_4,\ Mg\,(H\,O)_2,\ 5H_2\,O$.

Molecular Weight, 484

Preparation of Carbonate of Magnesium.—"Take of sulphate of magnesia, ten ounces; carbonate of soda, twelve ounces; boiling distilled water, a sufficiency. Dissolve the sulphate of magnesia and the carbonate of soda each in a pint of water, mix the two solutions, and evaporate the whole to perfect dryness by means of a sand-bath. Digest the residue for half an hour with two pints of water, and having collected the insoluble matter on a calico filter, wash it repeatedly with distilled water until the washings cease to give a precipitate with chloride of barium. Finally, dry the product at a temperature not exceeding 212° F."—Br. P.

Officinal carbonate of magnesia is a porous, loose coherent mass of dazzling white color, without odor, and having a slightly earthy taste. It is nearly insoluble in water, one part requiring 2500 parts of cold and 9000 of boiling water for its solution. The substance has a weakly alkaline reaction. At a low red heat it loses its CO_2 and water, and magnesia is left.

Tests.—It effervesces on the addition of acids and gives the ordinary reactions of magnesium. It is apt to be contaminated with traces of lime, soda and of sulphuric and hydrochloric acids. When dissolved in dilute nitric acid the solution should give no precipitate with barium nitrate (sulphate) nor with silver nitrate (chloride), and when the solution is neutralized with ammonia no precipitate should occur upon the addition of ammonium oxalate (calcium). The precipitate formed upon adding ammonia in excess to the solution, should redissolve in ammonium chloride (undissolved residue indicating the presence of alumina), and the ammoniacal solution, when treated with hydrogen sulphide, should not give a white precipitate (zinc).

It was first proven by Hahnemann.

Preparation for Homœopathic Use.—The pure carbonate of magnesia is triturated as directed under Class VII.

MAGNESIUM METALLICUM.

Synonym, Magnesium.

Symbol, Mg.

Atomic Weight, 24.

Origin.—The metal magnesium occurs abundantly in nature, but never in the free state. It is found as hydrate in the mineral *brucite*, as carbonate in *magnesite*, as sulphate in *epsomite*, as fluo-phosphate in *wagnerite*. Its silicates are well known,—*meerschaum*, *mica*, *serpentine*, etc.; magnesian limestone is a double carbonate of magnesium and calcium, and magnesium chloride exists in many natural waters, especially in sea-water.

Preparation.—The metal is prepared on the large scale by heating to full redness a mixture of six parts of magnesium chloride, one of sodium chloride, one of calcium fluoride and one of sodium, out of contact with air. The magnesium is obtained then in metallic globules, which are further purified by distillation in an atmosphere of hydrogen.

Properties.—The metal is silver-white in color, very brilliant in lustre and has a specific gravity of 1.75. It is malleable and ductile, fuses at a red heat and at a higher temperature volatilizes. When heated to redness in a strong alcohol flame it takes fire, burning with a dazzling white light which is very rich in actinic rays and by means of which photographs can be taken in otherwise darkened chambers. It is permanent in dry air, and is attacked readily by acids.

Preparation for Homœopathic Use.—The metal magnesium is triturated as directed under Class VII.

MAGNESIA MURIATICA.

Synonyms, Magnesium Chloride. Chloras Magnesicus. Magnesii Chloridum.

Formula, $Mg\ Cl_2$.

Molecular Weight, 95.

Common Name, Muriate of Magnesia.

Preparation of Muriate of Magnesia.—Divide a quantity of pure hydrochloric acid into two parts; neutralize one part with magnesia and the other with ammonium hydrate or carbonate. The solutions are to be mixed and evaporated to dryness and then heated to redness in a loosely covered porcelain crucible. Ammonium chloride is driven off and fused magnesium chloride remains behind. The latter is to be poured out on a clean stone and when cold transferred to a well-stoppered bottle.

Properties.—Magnesium chloride is a white mass, crystalline in structure. It is very deliquescent and extremely soluble in water. It cannot be recovered by evaporation from its watery solution, because the last portions of the water are retained with such obstinacy that the latter's decomposition ensues as a result of the affinity of chlorine for hydrogen and of magnesia for oxygen, the hydrochloric acid formed being then expelled, and magnesia only, remaining. Anhydrous chloride of magnesia is in flexible crystalline plates, having a pearly lustre and a sharp bitter taste. The hydrated chloride (with six molecules of water) is deposited from a hot concentrated solution on cooling, in needles and prisms. The crystals are highly deliquescent, dissolve in two-thirds their weight of cold and in one-fifth their weight of hot water; they are soluble in two parts of alcohol of specific gravity 0.817.

Tests.—Its solution should, when acidified with HCl, give no precipitate with barium chloride, and after adding ammonia in excess and then ammonium oxalate, no precipitate should occur.

It was first proven by Hahnemann.

Preparation for Homœopathic Use.—Muriate of magnesia is triturated, as directed under Class VII.

MAGNESIA PHOSPHORICA.

Formula, $Mg\ HPO_4,\ 7H_2\ O$.

Two parts of sulphate of magnesia are to be dissolved in thirty-two parts of distilled water, mixed with a solution of three parts of phosphate of soda in thirty-two parts of distilled water and set aside to crystallize. The salt separates in the course of twenty-four hours in tufts of prisms or needles.

Properties.—Crystallized magnesium phosphate forms small six-sided needles, having a cooling, sweetish taste. It is sparingly soluble in water, 322 parts of water taking up one of the salt after long standing. By boiling the solution, the salt becomes decomposed through a partial separation of trimagnesian salt. Magnesium phosphate dissolves easily in dilute acids; its crystals effloresce in warm air, and when heated to 100° C. (212° F.) give off more than half of their water, and at 170° C. (248° F.) the remaining portion. At a red heat the basic hydrogen is driven off and magnesium pyrophosphate is left. It may be tested for impurities in the way mentioned under the two previous articles, *mutatis mutandis.*

Preparation for Homœopathic Use.—The salt is triturated according to Class VII.

MAGNESIA SULPHURICA.

Synonyms, Magnesium Sulphate. Magnesii Sulphas.
Common Names, Epsom Salt. Sulphate of Magnesia.
Formula, $Mg\ SO_4 . 7H_2\ O$.
Molecular Weight, 246.

Origin and Preparation.—Sulphate of magnesium occurs native in the mineral *epsomite* and it is found in the waters of certain bitter saline springs, as those of Epsom in England, whence the popular name applied to this salt. The salt is made in large amount by acting on magnesian limestone with dilute sulphuric acid and separating the resulting magnesium sulphate from the greater part of the slightly soluble calcium sulphate by filtration. It is purified by re-solution and rapid crystallization.

Properties.—Pure magnesium sulphate, when crystallized slowly from its solutions, forms large, colorless, right-angled prisms. But in commerce it is in small rhombic prisms. The salt is neutral, is without odor, and has a saline, bitter taste. At ordinary temperatures it is soluble in two parts of cold water, but boiling water takes up more than its own weight of the salt. By heat, the salt melts, gradually gives up six molecules of its water, and between 200° and 230° C. (392° to 446° F.) it yields the remaining molecule. The anhydrous salt is a white powder, which melts at a full red heat to an enamel-like mass, without decomposition. It is soluble in dilute and slightly so in absolute alcohol.

Tests.—Caustic alkalies precipitate magnesium sulphate from its solutions. Its solutions should be neutral in reaction, and when diluted should not be affected when treated with silver nitrate (chloride), with ammonium carbonate (calcium and zinc compounds), with potassium ferrocyanide (zinc and other metallic salts), nor with ammonium sulphide (iron manganese and other metals). The presence of ammonium compounds may be recognized by treating the solution of the salt with caustic alkali and holding near the mouth of the test-tube a glass rod moistened with hydrochloric acid; the occurrence of white fumes will show the presence of ammonia. When one part of magnesium sulphate is rubbed in a mortar with two and a half parts of barium carbonate, and the mixture boiled with 20 CC. of distilled water for some minutes, and after cooling filtered, the filtrate should, when treated with barium chloride solution, give no turbidity, otherwise potassium or sodium sulphate is present in more than mere traces.

It was proven by Nenning, in Germany.

Preparation for Homœopathic Use.—Pure sulphate of magnesium is triturated, as directed under Class VII.

MAGNESIA USTA.

Synonyms, Magnesium Oxide. Magnesia Calcinata. Calcined Magnesia.

Common Name, Magnesia.

Formula, $Mg\,O$.

Molecular Weight, 40.

Preparation.—Calcined magnesia is prepared by exposing magnesium carbonate in an earthen vessel, to a red heat for two hours or until all the CO_2 is driven off; during the process, the mass is to be constantly stirred with an iron spoon.

Properties.—Officinal magnesia is a white, odorless powder having an earthy taste. It has a weakly alkaline reaction, and is almost insoluble in water. At a red heat it is unchanged, becoming only more dense; it dissolves in dilute acids without effervescence. Its specific gravity is between 2.75 and 3.25. When exposed to the air it absorbs moisture and CO_2, and becomes in part altered to carbonate. When mixed with water it forms a hydrate.

Tests.—Even when kept in well-stoppered bottles, it absorbs some moisture and a small amount of CO_2. When a pinch of it is shaken up with a few CC. of water, it should not effervesce so as to be appreciated by the sense of sight, although when the ear is placed to the test-tube, a minute crepitation then observable may be considered as not worth notice. Its behavior with reagents should be that described under the article Magnesium Carbonicum.

Preparation for Homœopathic Use.—Pure calcined magnesia is triturated as directed under Class VII.

MAGNOLIA.

Synonym, Magnolia Glauca, *Linn.*

Nat. Ord., Magnoliaceæ.

Common Names, Laurel Magnolia. White Laurel. White Bay. Sweet Bay.

This shrub or small tree is indigenous to the Middle and Southern States, and is found growing in marshy grounds near the coast. In favorable situations in the South it reaches a height of twenty feet. Leaves oval-obtuse, shining above, glaucous-white beneath. Flowers two inches broad, cup-shaped; calyx of three white or greenish sepals; petals concave, fragrant. Carpels one to two-seeded, aggregated into a cone-like fruit; upon their opening at maturity the seeds are suspended by a funicle.

Preparation.—The fresh flowers are chopped and pounded to a pulp and weighed. Then two parts by weight of alcohol are taken, the pulp mixed thoroughly with one-sixth part of it, and the rest of the alcohol added. After stirring the whole well, and pouring it into a well-stoppered bottle, it is allowed to stand eight days in a dark, cool place. The tincture is then separated by decanting, straining and filtering.

Amount of drug power, $\frac{1}{6}$.

Dilutions must be prepared as directed under Class III.

MAJORANA.

Synonyms, Origanum Majorana, *Linn.* Majorana Hortensis, *Mœnch.*

Nat. Ord., Labiatæ.

Common Name, Sweet Marjoram.

This annual is frequently cultivated as a pot-herb. It is indigenous to Western Asia and Southeastern Europe. Leaves entire, oval or spatulate, grayish-green in color, downy and pellucid-punctate. Flowers small, white, in heads. The odor of the plant is peculiar, but agreeable and aromatic.

Preparation.—The fresh plant, in flower, is chopped and pounded to a pulp and weighed. Then two parts by weight of alcohol are taken, the pulp mixed thoroughly with one-sixth part of it, and the rest of the alcohol added. After stirring the whole well and pouring it into a well-stoppered bottle, it is allowed to stand eight days in a dark, cool place. The tincture is then separated by decanting, straining and filtering.

Amount of drug power, $\frac{1}{6}$.

Dilutions must be prepared as directed under Class III.

MANCINELLA.

Synonym, Hippomane Mancinella, *Linn.*

Nat. Ord., Euphorbiaceæ.

Common Name, Manchineel.

Although the toxic properties of the mancinella have been greatly exaggerated, it is nevertheless a very poisonous tree, which is becoming more and more rare, owing to its being rooted up with great care wherever it shows itself. It is a native of the West Indies, is from twelve to fifteen feet high, with a trunk having a white and soft wood, covered with a grayish bark. Its leaves are alternate, oval-acute, somewhat cordate at the base, with fine indentations, and a red gland at the apex. They are attached to long petioles; stipulate while young. Flowers monœcious, forming long terminal spikes, the male flowers being above, the female below or at the axils of the leaves. The male flowers have a bifid perianth whence emanate the stamens, the united filaments of which form a column that supports the anthers. The female flowers have a perianth with two or three divisions and a rudimentary foliole; the ovary is round and superior; style straight, terminating in six or seven red, radiating, reflexed stigmata. The fruit is round, pulpy, from five to six inches in diameter, umbilicate at the top, and enclosing a woody kernel with seven monospermous compartments.

It was introduced into our Materia Medica by Dr. Mure, Brazil.

Preparation.—Equal parts of the fresh leaves, bark and fruit are chopped and pounded to a pulp and weighed. Then two parts by weight of alcohol are taken, the pulp mixed thoroughly with one-sixth part of it, and the rest of the alcohol added. After stirring the whole well and pouring it into a well-stoppered bottle, it is allowed to stand eight days in a dark, cool place. The tincture is then separated by decanting, straining and filtering.

Amount of drug power, ⅙.

Dilutions must be prepared as directed under Class III.

MANGANUM ACETICUM.

Synonyms, Manganous Acetate. Acetas Manganosus. Manganesii Acetas.

Common Name, Acetate of Manganese.

Preparation of Acetate of Manganum.—By saturating pure acetic acid with Manganese Carbonate and crystallizing.

Properties.—The salt crystallizes in colorless or pale reddish, shining, rhomboidal prisms, which are persistent in the air and easily soluble in water. Their taste is metallic and astringent. Their solution undergoes no change with silver nitrate, and when acidified with HCl is not affected by hydrogen sulphide.

It was introduced into our Materia Medica by Hahnemann.

Preparation for Homœopathic Use.—Acetate of manganese is triturated as directed under Class VII.

MANGANUM CARBONICUM.

Synonyms, Manganous Carbonate. Carbonas Manganosus. Manganesii Carbonas.

Common Name, Carbonate of Manganese.

Preparation of Carbonate of Manganum.—Ten parts of distilled water are deprived of atmospheric air by boiling, and one part of crystallized manganous sulphate is dissolved therein, and this solution is mixed, with constant stirring, with a filtered solution of one part of sodium bicarbonate in fifteen parts of distilled water. After a day or two the precipitate is collected, spread upon filter paper and dried in the sun or in a warm place.

Properties.—Manganous carbonate is a fine, whitish or reddish-white powder. It is without taste or odor and is almost insoluble in water. It dissolves in solutions of CO_2, and when treated with dilute sulphuric acid evolves CO_2, a pale, reddish, clear solution resulting.

Tests.—Manganous carbonate when shaken with distilled water, does not dissolve therein, and in dilute hydrochloric acid is easily soluble without the slightest turbidity. This solution should be divided and tested in parts. With hydrogen sulphide no change should occur, or at most, a faint, white turbidity due to the presence of manganic oxide (a colored turbidity or precipitate shows the presence of other metals). The portion already saturated with hydrogen sulphide should not give, after the abundant addition of sodium acetate solution, any white turbidity (absence of zinc). The solution in dilute hydrochloric acid, when treated with tincture of galls, should not become violet or dark-colored (absence of iron); or when treated with a plentiful addition of ammonium chloride and then with caustic ammonia, should remain clear (absence of alumina), as it also should upon the addition of ammonium oxalate (absence of calcium).

It was introduced into our Materia Medica by Hahnemann.

Preparation for Homœopathic Use.—Carbonate of manganese is triturated, as directed under Class VII.

MANGANUM METALLICUM.

Synonym, Metallic Manganese.

Symbol, Mn.

Molecular Weight, 27.7.

Preparation and Properties of Metallic Manganese.—Manganese was discovered by Scheele and Bergmann in 1774, in the mineral *Braunstein.* As this mineral had been confounded with magnetic iron, it received the Latin name of that substance, magnesia nigra, and hence the name given at first to the new metal was magnesium. In order to distinguish this metal from the real magnesium the name was afterward altered into manganesium. Manganese is found in a number of minerals.

Preparation and Properties.—The metal is obtained by reducing its oxide by heating it to redness with charcoal. It is hard, grayish-white in color, looks like cast-iron, and is very brittle. Its specific gravity is about 8. When exposed to the air it oxidizes readily, and it is easily attacked by acids.

Preparation for Homœopathic Use.—Metallic manganese is triturated, as directed under Class VII.

MATICO.

Synonyms, Piper Angustifolium, *Ruiz et Pavon.* Artanthe Elongata, *Miquel.* Steffensia Elongata, *Kunth.*

Nat. Ord., Piperaceæ.

Common Names, Soldier's Herb. Narrow-leaved Piper.

This is a shrub growing in moist woods in Bolivia, Peru and other portions of South America. It has nearly sessile leaves, lance-oval, acuminate, in length from two to six inches and in breadth about one or one and a half inches, bright green above, paler and downy beneath. The leaves are rather thick and their whole upper surface is traversed by minute sunk veins producing a tesselated appearance; on the under side are corresponding depressions. The leaves have an aromatic odor and a similar taste with some bitterness.

Preparation.—The dried leaves are coarsely powdered and covered with five parts by weight of alcohol; having been poured into a well-stoppered bottle, the mixture is allowed to remain eight days in a dark, cool place, being shaken twice a day. The tincture is then poured off, strained and filtered.

Drug power of tincture, $\frac{1}{10}$.

Dilutions must be prepared as directed under Class IV.

MELASTOMA ACKERMANNI.

Synonym, Melastoma Tapixirica.
Nat. Ord., Melastomaceæ.
Common Name, Tapixirica.

This is a bush with round branches, triangular at their extremities, and covered with a brownish bark. The leaves are opposite, supported by short and hairy petioles; their limb is oval, reticulate, covered with stiff hairs, and traversed on the lower surface by five thick, almost parallel, nerves, running from the base to the summit of the leaf. The flowers are sessile, supported by terminal axes. This bush is a native of tropical America.

Introduced into our Materia Medica by Dr. Mure, Brazil.

Preparation.—The fresh leaves are chopped to a pulp and weighed. Then two parts by weight of alcohol are taken, the pulp mixed with one-sixth part of it, and the rest of the alcohol added. After stirring the whole well and pouring it into a well-stoppered bottle, it is allowed to stand eight days in a dark, cool place. The tincture is then separated by decanting, straining and filtering.

Drug power of tincture, $\frac{1}{6}$.

Dilutions must be prepared as directed under Class III.

MELILOTUS.

Synonym, Melilotus Alba, *Lamarck.*
Nat. Ord., Leguminosæ.
Common Names, White Melilot. Sweet Clover.

This plant is indigenous to Europe, where it is found along roadsides and in cultivated fields; it has been partly naturalized in the United States. It is three to six feet high, leaves trifoliate, with smooth, entire, awl-shaped stipules; the leaflets truncate, the upper ones lanceolate. The flowers are in one-sided racemes, white and very fragrant.

Preparation.—The fresh flowers are pounded to a pulp and weighed. Then two parts by weight of alcohol are taken, the pulp mixed thoroughly with one-sixth part of it, and the rest of the alcohol added. After stirring the whole well, and pouring it into a well-stoppered bottle, it is allowed to stand eight days in a dark, cool place. The tincture is then separated by decanting, straining and filtering.

Amount of drug power, $\frac{1}{6}$.

Dilutions must be prepared as directed under Class III.

MELILOTUS OFFICINALIS, *Willd.*

Synonym, Trifolium Officinale.

Nat. Ord., Leguminosæ.

Common Names, Yellow Melilot. Sweet Clover.

This plant is indigenous to Europe, but is naturalized in the United States Stem upright, two to four feet high, leaves trifoliate; leaflets obovate-oblong, obtuse, dentate. Corolla yellow and very fragrant.

Preparation.—The fresh flowers are pounded to a pulp and weighed. Then two parts by weight of alcohol are taken, the pulp mixed thoroughly with one-sixth part of it, and the rest of the alcohol added. After having stirred the whole well, and poured it into a well-stoppered bottle, allow it to stand eight days in a dark, cool place. The tincture is then separated by decanting, straining and filtering.

Amount of drug power, $\frac{1}{6}$.

Dilutions must be prepared as directed under Class III.

MELOË MAJALIS.

Synonym, Meloë Proscarabæus.

Class, Insecta.

Order, Coleoptera.

Family, Vesicantia.

Common Name, Oil-Beetle. (This must not be confounded with the common May-beetle, Scarabæus Melolantha.)

The meloë proscarabæus is without wings, an inch or an inch and a half long, and about as big as a finger. It is soft, with the head bent downwards as is that of the cantharis; antennæ moniliform, of twelve joints, corslet almost rounded and flexible, punctated elytræ which cover scarcely one-half of the oval abdomen. The color of the head, feet and abdomen verges on reddish. The fore feet have five, the hind feet four joints.

The meloë majalis is the smaller of the two; its body is coppery-red, or bronze-black; the elytræ are black-green, and the back is furnished with red incisions.

The two kinds have a disagreeable odor, and emit, when seized, an acrid, yellowish humour, staining the fingers, and smelling something like the violet, of a sweetish taste at first, then acrid and caustic, and causing an itching and blister-like eruption on the skin.

These insects are found all over Europe in the spring, on the grass, low plants, on dry meadows and sunny hills. They have to be gathered with great care, so that the juice which they emit will not get lost, and they should at once be placed in the vessel in which they are to be kept.

Preparation.—The living insect carefully put into the glass used for the pharmaceutical preparation, so as not to lose any of the juice, is drenched with five parts by weight of alcohol, and macerated eight days, being shaken twice a day. The tincture is then poured off, strained and filtered.

Amount of drug power, $\frac{1}{10}$.

Dilutions must be prepared as directed under Class IV.

MENISPERMUM CANADENSE, *Linn.*

Synonym, Cissampelos Smilacina.

Nat. Ord., Menispermaceæ.

Common Names, Yellow Parilla. Canadian Moonseed. Vine Maple.

This is a climbing indigenous plant, growing on the banks of streams. The root or rhizome is long, and has a bitter taste. Leaves peltate near the edge, three to seven angles or lobes. Flowers whitish or greenish-yellow, in axillary panicles, appear in June and July. Sepals four to eight. Petals six to eight, short. Stamens twelve to twenty in the sterile flowers, as long as the sepals; anthers four-celled. Pistils two to four in the fertile flowers, raised on a short common receptacle; stigma broad and flat. Drupe globular, having the mark of the stigma near the base, with a laterally flattened stone (putamen), crescentic or ring-shaped. Drupes ripen in September, looking like frost grapes.

Preparation.—The fresh root is chopped and pounded to a pulp and weighed Then two parts by weight of alcohol are taken, and the pulp mixed thoroughly with one-sixth part of it, and the rest of the alcohol added. After stirring the whole well and pouring it into a well-stoppered bottle, it is allowed to stand eight days in a dark, cool place. The tincture is then separated by decanting, straining and filtering.

Drug power of tincture, $\frac{1}{6}$.

Dilutions must be prepared as directed under Class III.

MENTHA PIPERITA, *Hudson.*

Synonyms, Mentha Hercina. Mentha Viridi Aquatica.

Nat. Ord., Labiatæ.

Common Name, Peppermint.

This plant is found growing in wet places in Europe and North America, and is also cultivated. It is perennial, and increases by throwing out runners. Stem purplish, four-angled, about three feet high. Leaves dark green, opposite, on long petioles, sharply serrate, ovate-lanceolate. Flowers pale purplish-red, in spikes, oblong or cylindrical and obtuse; appear in August and September. Fruit four separable achenia.

It was proven by Dr. Demeures, France.

Preparation.—The fresh plant, in flower, is chopped and pounded to a pulp and weighed. Then two parts by weight of alcohol are taken, the pulp mixed thoroughly with one-sixth part of it, and the rest of the alcohol added. After having stirred the whole well, and having poured it into a well-stoppered bottle, it is allowed to stand eight days in a dark, cool place. The tincture is then separated by decanting, straining and filtering.

Amount of drug power, ⅙.

Dilutions must be prepared as directed under Class III.

MENYANTHES.

Synonyms, Menyanthes Trifoliata, *Linn.* Trifolium Amarum.

Nat. Ord., Gentianaceæ.

Common Names, Buckbean. Marsh Trefoil. Water Shamrock.

This is a perennial plant, growing in North America, Europe and Asia, in swamps, on margins of ponds, etc. It has a fleshy rootstock about as thick as a finger, black and descending deep into the earth. Stem eight to twelve inches high. Leaves on long footstalks, trifoliate; leaflets sessile, obovate. Flowers in a terminal pyramidal raceme, on a long, naked peduncle. Corolla rotate, flesh-colored, bearded in the tube.

The drug was first proven by Hahnemann.

Preparation.—The fresh plant, just coming into bloom, is chopped and pounded to a pulp, enclosed in a piece of new linen and subjected to pressure. The expressed juice is then, by brisk agitation, mingled with an equal part by weight of alcohol. This mixture is allowed to stand eight days in a well-stoppered bottle, in a dark, cool place, and then filtered.

Drug power of tincture, ½.

Dilutions must be prepared as directed under Class I.

MEPHITIS.

Synonyms, Mephitis Putorius. Viverra Putorius.

Class, Mammalia.

Order, Carnivora.

Family, Mustelidæ.

Common Names, Skunk. Polecat.

The polecat is a quadruped of the family of martins, inhabiting the United States; it is of the size of a martin; has a round head; snout elongated, three-rowed moustaches on the upper jaw, a dry nose and the neck a little marked. Its coat is black, but has a white streak along the back to the tail, and two other streaks on each side parallel to the first; the posterior part of its body is larger than that of the martin; its tail is as if cropped, and furnished with long hairs, nearly all white; the under part of the body is whitish; the fore part of the feet elongated and fortified with five strong nails; near the anus there is, as in all the genus viverra, a pouch where follicular glands deposit an unctuous matter of such pungent and insupportable odor, that at the approach of the animal, at the moment when he squirts this liquor, a person inhaling its vapor is almost stifled. The liquor is nearly puriform, of a deep yellow color, and has an alliaceous odor.

Preparation.—One part by weight of the liquid obtained from the anal glands of the animal is dissolved in ninety-nine parts by weight of alcohol.

Amount of drug power, $\frac{1}{100}$.

Dilutions must be prepared as directed under Class VI—β.

MERCURIALIS PERENNIS, *Linn.*

Synonyms, Cynocrambes. Mercurialis Montana.

Nat. Ord., Euphorbiaceæ.

Common Name, Dog Mercury.

This plant is indigenous to Europe, where it occurs in shaded, mountainous forests, on stony or moist ground. It is distinguished from *mercurialis annua* (to which it is nearly related, and which occurs more frequently) by its creeping, knotty, articulate root, which is verticillately fibred on the joints; by its single, low, below leafless stem and the short-petiolate, serrated and short-haired, elliptic-lanceolate leaves. Flowers appear in early spring.

Preparation.—The fresh plant, in flower, is chopped and pounded to a pulp and weighed. Then two-thirds of that weight of alcohol is taken, and having mixed it thoroughly with the pulp, the mixture is pressed out *lege artis* in a piece of new linen, and filtered.

Amount of drug power, $\frac{1}{2}$.

Dilutions must be prepared as directed under Class II.

MERCURIUS ACETICUS.

Synonyms, Mercurous Acetate. Hydrargyrum Aceticum.

Common Name, Acetate of Mercury.

Preparation of Acetate of Mercury.—A solution of the nitrate of mercury, as is mentioned under the head *Mercurius solubilis*, is prepared and decomposed by pure carbonate of soda, dissolved in twice its weight of distilled water. The carbonate of mercury obtained in this way is well washed, heated in a porcelain dish with eight parts of distilled water to 100° C. (212° F.), and then acetic acid added gradually till all is dissolved. The hot filtered liquid yields after cooling scale-like, crystalline laminæ, nacreous in appearance, and greasy to the touch; they are removed from the mother-liquor, washed rapidly with diluted alcohol, dried between bibulous paper, and kept in bottles well protected from light.

Preparation for Homœopathic Use.—Pure acetate of mercury is triturated as directed under Class VII.

MERCURIUS AURATUS.

Preparation of Mercurius Auratus.—Mercury is capable of uniting with most other metals, forming compounds called *amalgams*, some of which are liquid while others are solid. The liquid amalgams may be regarded as solutions of definite compounds in an excess of mercury, for when they are subjected to pressure between chamois leather, mercury containing but a small amount of the other metal passes through, leaving behind a solid amalgam, which has very frequently a definite atomic constitution. A native amalgam of gold is found in small yellowish crystals, in the native mercury of Mariposa, in California. It contains from 39 to 41.6 per cent. of gold; its sp. gr. is 15.47.

An amalgam, which has been prescribed in Germany, may be prepared by adding two parts of mercury to one of gold leaf, in a closed vessel with agitation; heat may be used to facilitate the amalgamation, but it should not in any case be higher than 300° C., the boiling point of mercury being about 350° C. (662° F.). The agitation is to be kept up until the vessel has completely cooled, when the mass is to be gently pressed through chamois leather and the residue transferred to a well-stoppered bottle.

Preparation for Homœopathic Use.—Mercurius auratus, as prepared above, is triturated as directed under Class VII.

MERCURIUS CYANATUS.

Synonyms, Mercuric Cyanide. Hydrargyri Cyanidum. Cyanuretum Hydrargyricum.

Common Names, Cyanide of Mercury. Cyanuret of Mercury.

Formula, $Hg\ Cy_2$ or $Hg\ (CN)_2$.

Molecular Weight, 252.

Preparation of Cyanide of Mercury.—Dissolve five troy ounces of ferrocyanide of potassium in twenty fluid ounces of water, and add the solution to four troy ounces of sulphuric acid diluted with ten fluid ounces of water, previously placed in a glass retort. The retort is to be connected with a receiver containing ten fluid ounces of water and three troy ounces of red oxide of mercury. The mixture in the retort is to be distilled nearly to dryness. Two fluid ounces of the liquid in the receiver after the operation, are to be set aside, and to the remainder more red oxide of mercury is to be added gradually until the odor of hydrocyanic acid disappears. After filtering the solution, the two ounces of the reserved liquid are to be added to the filtrate and the whole evaporated in a dark place, that mercuric cyanide may crystallize out. The crystals are to be dried and placed in a well-stoppered bottle protected from light, otherwise they decompose and become black.

Properties.—Mercuric cyanide is in white, more or less transparent, quadratic prisms and pyramids; the crystals are without odor, and have a sharp, nauseating, metallic, disagreeable taste. The salt is soluble in ten parts of cold, in two of hot water, and in twenty of alcohol at ordinary temperatures. The solutions do not affect litmus paper. It is not decomposed by sulphuric or nitric acid, nor by alkaline hydrates or carbonates. Hydrochloric acid decomposes it with the formation of mercuric chloride and hydrocyanic acid; similarly a solution of the salt when treated with hydrogen sulphide, gives a precipitate of mercuric sulphide (the black modification) and hydrocyanic acid. The solution, when treated with a solution of potassium iodide, gives a yellow precipitate, which quickly changes to bright red, and is readily soluble in excess of either reagent. By careful heating, the salt may be decomposed into its constituents, the cyanogen readily igniting and burning with a pinkish-purple flame; when rapidly heated, the liberated cyanogen is changed into paracyanogen, a carbonaceous body which remains behind.

Tests.—In addition to the above described properties, the salt, when heated upon platinum foil, should be dissipated without residue. Mercuric cyanate, if present, is only slightly soluble in water, and its solution has an alkaline reaction with turmeric paper; it can be transformed into the cyanide by dissolving in boiling water, neutralizing with hydrocyanic acid and recrystallizing.

Preparation for Homœopathic Use.—One part by weight of pure cyanide of mercury is dissolved in ninety-nine parts by weight of distilled water.

Amount of drug power, $\frac{1}{100}$.

Dilutions must be prepared as directed under Class V—β.

Triturations of pure cyanide of mercury are prepared as directed under Class VII.

MERCURIUS DULCIS.

Synonyms, Mercurous Chloride. Hydrargyri Chloridum Mite. Hydrargyri Subchloridum. Hydrargyrum Chloratum Mite. Calomelas. Mild Chloride of Mercury. Subchloride of Mercury. Submuriate of Mercury.

Common Name, Calomel.

Formula, Hg_2Cl_2.

Molecular Weight, 471.

Preparation of Calomel.—Take of mercury 48 parts, of sulphuric acid 36 parts, and of sodium chloride 18 parts. Boil half of the mercury with the sulphuric acid on a sand-bath until a white, dry mass is left. Add to this, when cold, the remainder of the mercury, in an earthenware mortar, and rub together until they are intimately mixed. The sodium chloride is now to be added and all the ingredients rubbed together till globules of mercury are no longer visible, when the mixture is to be sublimed into a roomy receptacle in order that the sublimate may settle as a powder. The sublimate is to be washed with boiling distilled water as long as the washings give a precipitate with ammonium hydrate, and the precipitate is then to be dried.

Properties.—Calomel is an odorless, tasteless substance, having no influence on test paper. When prepared by sublimation, it is in microscopic prismatic crystals, generally aggregated in masses. Its specific gravity is from 7.2 to 7.25. By exposure to sunlight, it suffers partial decomposition into metallic mercury and mercuric chloride, and it acquires thereby a grayish tinge; when boiled with water, the same change takes place slowly, and even a mixture of calomel with sugar contains, after some time, an appreciable amount of the higher chloride. When heated, it sublimes in white vapors without undergoing change. It is insoluble in water, alcohol and the simple solvents.

Tests.—Calomel should volatilize completely (a residue shows fixed impurities). A portion of calomel well shaken with ten volumes of distilled water and thrown upon a double filter previously moistened, should yield a filtrate which is not changed in appearance by treatment with hydrogen sulphide or silver nitrate (absence of mercuric chloride), and the filtrate, when agitated with dilute acetic acid, should undergo no change when tested with hydrogen sulphide or silver nitrate (absence of ammonia compounds of mercury).

Although this drug has been in the Homœopathic Materia Medica since Hahnemann's time, the first provings seem to have been made by Dr. D. S. Kimball, U. S.

Preparation for Homœopathic Use.—Pure calomel is triturated as directed under Class VII.

MERCURIUS IODATUS FLAVUS.

Synonyms, Mercurous Iodide. Hydrargyrum Iodatum. Protoiodide of Mercury. Hydrargyrum Iodidum. Hydrargyrum Iodatum Flavum. Hydrargyri Iodidum Viride. Yellow Iodide of Mercury. Green Iodide of Mercury.

Common Name, Yellow Iodide of Mercury.

Formula, $Hg_2 I_2$.

Molecular Weight, 654.

Preparation of Yellow Iodide of Mercury.—Take 48 parts of mercury and 30 parts of resublimed iodine, mix the ingredients in a mortar, and, with the addition of a small amount of stronger alcohol, triturate till the materials are thoroughly incorporated. After occasional stirrings for two hours triturate again, and forcibly, until the mass is almost dry. The mass is then to be rubbed up with sufficient stronger alcohol, added gradually, until a uniform thin paste is produced; this is to be thrown on a filter and washed with stronger alcohol until the washings, when dropped into a large quantity of water, no longer produce a permanent cloudiness. The residue is to be dried in the dark with the aid of a gentle heat, preserved in a well-stoppered bottle and protected from light.

Properties and Tests.—Mercurous iodide is a greenish-yellow, odorless, tasteless powder, insoluble in water and alcohol in the cold, and is completely dissipated by heating. Under the influence of light it is decomposed with tolerable rapidity, mercuric iodide and metallic mercury being produced, the color in such cases becoming dark green and finally black. By slow heating it is decomposed in the same manner, but by a stronger and more rapid heating, it fuses to a brown fluid and is finally dissipated. A portion of mercurous iodide, when agitated with alcohol and thrown upon a moistened filter, should yield a filtrate which is scarcely changed by treatment with hydrogen sulphide, and with silver nitrate should produce only a faint opalescence. A minute amount of mercuric iodide is admissible, as the best washed preparations show, after two weeks' keeping, distinct traces of the higher iodide.

It was first proven by Dr. I. S. P. Lord, U. S.

Preparation for Homœopathic Use.—Pure yellow iodide of mercury is triturated as directed under Class VII, care being taken to protect from light.

MERCURIUS IODATUS RUBER.

Synonyms, Mercuric Iodide. Biniodide of Mercury. Hydrargyrum Bijodatum Rubrum. Hydrargyri Iodium Rubrum. Deutoioduretum (Biniodidum) Hydrargyri.

Common Name, Red Iodide of Mercury.

Formula, $Hg\ I_2$.

Molecular Weight, 454.

Preparation of Red Iodide of Mercury.—A cold filtered solution of twenty parts of mercuric chloride in 400 parts of distilled water is to be mixed with a cold filtered solution of twenty-five parts of potassium iodide in 100 of distilled water. The resulting precipitate is to be thrown upon a filter, washed with cold distilled water and dried at a gentle heat. The product is to be kept in a well-stoppered bottle.

Properties.—Mercuric iodide is a fine, heavy, crystalline powder of a vivid scarlet-red color, becoming yellow on heating and red again when cooled. It is almost insoluble in water, but it dissolves in 130 parts of cold and in fifteen of hot 90 per cent. alcohol. It is somewhat soluble in ether and readily in the fixed oils and chloroform. It is extremely soluble in solution of potassium iodide. Four parts of mercuric iodide are soluble in one part of a hot concentrated solution of potassium iodide, and when the double solution is allowed to cool, a portion of the mercuric iodide separates out in small, red octohedrons; from the remaining fluid can be obtained by crystallization, potassio-mercuric iodide, $2KI,\ HgI_2,\ 3H_2O$, in long, yellow prisms. The latter are soluble in alcohol and ether. Water decomposes them, about half the mercuric iodide separating out, and the liquid then yields by evaporation a saline mass, regarded by Boullay as $2KI,\ Hg\ I_2$. In addition to the above described properties, mercuric iodide should show no residue after being sublimed from platinum foil (absence of red lead and other fixed compounds), and it should dissolve completely in hot alcohol (absence of vermillion).

Provings of this drug were made by the American Provers' Union, 1856.

Preparation for Homœopathic Use.—Pure red iodide of mercury is triturated, as directed under Class VII.

MERCURIUS NITROSUS.

Synonyms, Mercurous Nitrate (nearly neutral). Hydrargyrum Nitricum Oxydulatum. Protonitrate of Mercury.

Common Name, Nitrate of Mercury.

Preparation of Nitrate of Mercury.—To twenty parts of pure mercury, add, in a very flat porcelain dish, a mixture of nine parts of concentrated nitric acid, of 1.2 specific gravity, and twenty-seven parts of distilled water; cover the mixture lightly, and let it stand in a dark, cool place until the formation of the white octohedral crystals, the salt required, has ceased. From time to time they are taken off the mercury upon whose surface they are floating, after which wash them speedily with a little alcohol, and then dry them between layers of bibulous paper; this done, they are preserved in a well-stoppered bottle. The crystals are permanent in the air, and are perfectly soluble in water that has been acidulated with a few drops of nitric acid.

Preparation for Homœopathic Use.—Pure nitrate of mercury is triturated, as directed under Class VII.

MERCURIUS PRÆCIPITATUS ALBUS.

Synonyms, Dimercuroso-Ammonium Chloride. Hydrargyrum Ammoniatum. Hydrargyri Ammonio-Chloridum. Hydrargyrum Præcipitatum Album.

Common Names, Ammoniated Mercury. White Precipitate.

Formula, NH_2 Hg Cl.

Molecular Weight, 251.5.

Preparation of White Precipitate.—To a solution of one part of mercuric chloride in twenty parts of hot distilled water, are to be added after cooling, with constant stirring, one and one-half parts of a 10 per cent. ammonium hydrate solution. The precipitate is to be thrown on a filter, and after all the fluid has passed through, washed twice with a mixture of ninety parts of distilled water with one of the ammonia. The precipitate is to be dried at a gentle heat in a dark room.

Properties and Tests.—Dimercur-ammonium chloride is a white, loose powder, or is in friable masses. It is insoluble in water, alcohol and ether. By prolonged washing with cold water or by contact with hot water, it turns yellow and is converted into hydrated trimercur-ammonium chloride. It is readily dissolved by acids. When treated with potassium or sodium hydrate, it turns yellow and evolves free ammonia. By heating, it sublimes without decomposition (absence of fixed salts).

Preparation for Homœopathic Use.—Pure ammoniated mercury is triturated, as directed under Class VII.

MERCURIUS PRÆCIPITATUS RUBER.

Synonyms, Mercuric Oxide. Hydrargyrum Oxydatum Rubrum. Hydrargyri Oxidum Rubrum. Hydrargyri Nitrico-Oxidum. Oxydum Hydrargyricum. Red Oxide of Mercury. Peroxide of Mercury.

Common Name, Red Precipitate.

Formula, HgO.

Molecular Weight, 216.

Preparation of Red Oxide of Mercury.—Six parts of nitric acid are to be diluted with eight parts of water, and nine parts of mercury are to be dissolved in the diluted acid, with the aid of a gentle heat. After the solution is complete, the whole is to be evaporated to dryness. The resulting dry mass is to be rubbed to powder and heated in a shallow, porcelain dish until acid vapors cease to come off. It is to be kept in well-stoppered bottles protected from light.

Properties.—When made as above directed, mercuric oxide is a yellowish-red powder, but as found in commerce it is the product of large establishments and is in bright red, lustrous, crystalline scales, which on powdering become orange-red in color, the tint being lighter as the powder is finer. When heated, this oxide becomes darker in color and finally black, but upon cooling it resumes its original appearance. At less than a red heat it suffers decomposition with separation of mercury and evolution of free oxygen. Light acts upon it in a similar manner, but only superficially. It is nearly insoluble in water, and the resulting solution is weakly alkaline in reaction, has a metallic taste, and when treated with hydrogen sulphide turns brownish in color.

Tests.—Mercuric oxide should sublime without residue when heated in a test-tube (absence of fixed salts), and should not give off red fumes (absence of nitrate), and when dissolved in nitric acid there should be no residue; a red, undissolved portion indicates vermillion or other adulteration, a brown one being probably due to plumbic peroxide, in which case the nitric acid solution will be precipitated white by sulphuric acid.

It was first proven by Hahnemann.

Preparation for Homœopathic Use.—Pure red oxide of mercury is triturated, as directed under Class VII.

MERCURIUS SOLUBILIS HAHNEMANNI.

Synonyms, Ammonio-Nitrate of Mercury. Hydrargyrum Oxydulatum Nigrum. Hydrargyrum Oxydulatum Nitricum Ammoniatum.

This preparation is, according to Kane, dimercuroso-ammonium nitrate, $(Hg)_2 H_4 N_2 (NO_3), H_2O$, or according to Mitscherlich, trimercuroso-ammonium nitrate, $(Hg_2)_3 H_2 N_2 (NO_3)_2, 2H_2O$. It is not an oxide, although the black mercurous oxide is formed when a mercurous salt is decomposed by potassium or sodium hydrate in excess. With ammonia, however, the resulting precipitate is that whose formula is given above. Hahnemann abandoned this preparation, preferring to it, *in all cases*, that of metallic mercury, mentioned as *Mercurius vivus*.

Nevertheless, as there are many who believe that metallic mercury is not so efficacious as the uncertain ammonio-nitrate, we give the method recommended by Hahnemann to obtain it.

Preparation of Mercurius Solubilis Hahnemanni.—Having purified the mercury, as described under mercurius vivus, it is dissolved, cold, in strong nitric acid, which requires many days; the salt which results is dried on blotting-paper, and triturated in a glass mortar for half an hour, adding one-fourth of its weight of the best alcohol. The alcohol which has been converted into ether is thrown aside, and the trituration of the mercurial is continued with fresh alcohol for half an hour each time, until this fluid no longer has the smell of ether. That being done, the alcohol is decanted and the salt dried on blotting-paper, which is renewed from time to time. Afterwards it is triturated for a quarter of an hour, in a glass mortar, with twice its weight of distilled water; the clear fluid is decanted, the salt is again washed by a second trituration with a fresh quantity of water, the clear fluid is united to the preceding, and thus we have the aqueous solution of all that the saline mass contained of mercurial nitrate really saturated. The residuum is composed of other mercurial salts, of chloride and sulphate. Finally, this aqueous solution precipitates, by caustic ammonia, the so-called *black oxide of mercury.*

Properties.—The soluble mercury of Hahnemann is a velvet black powder, has a slight metallic taste and is volatilized by heat, with decomposition; it contains no metallic globules.

Preparation for Homœopathic Use.—Mercurius solubilis Hahnemanni, prepared according to above formula, is triturated as directed under Class VII.

MERCURIUS SUBLIMATUS CORROSIVUS.

Synonyms, Mercuric Chloride. Hydrargyri Chloridum Corrosivum. Hydrargyri Perchloridum. Hydrargyrum Bichloratum Corrosivum. Corrosive Chloride of Mercury. Perchloride of Mercury. Bichloride of Mercury.

Common Name, Corrosive Sublimate.

Formula, $Hg\ Cl_2$.

Molecular Weight, 271.

Preparation of Bichloride of Mercury.—Boil four parts of mercury with six parts of sulphuric acid, over a sand-bath, unto dryness. The white residue is to be rubbed when cold with three parts of sodium chloride in an earthenware mortar, and the mixture is then to be sublimed by the aid of a gradually increasing heat.

Properties.—Corrosive sublimate when prepared by rapid sublimation, forms white, transparent radio-crystalline masses; by slow sublimation it may be obtained in small, white, glistening, rhombic crystals. It is without odor, has a disagreeable, sharp, metallic taste, and is a powerful irritant poison. It dissolves in twelve parts of water at 20° C. (68° F.), in four parts at 80° C. (176° F.) and in two of boiling water; it is more soluble in alcohol, requiring only two and one-half parts in the cold and one and one-fourth parts at 100° C. (212° F.), and it dissolves almost as readily in ether. When its solutions are evaporated small portions of the compound are carried off with the vapor of the solvent. Its watery solutions are weakly acid in reaction, but such reaction is neutralized when chlorides of the alkalies are present. The solid substance is not affected by light, but the solutions are decomposed with the liberation of hydrochloric acid and calomel. Organic substances such as sugar, gum, extracts, resin, etc., slowly decompose it. Its specific gravity is 5.4. The aqueous solution when treated with lime-water, or potassium or sodium hydrate, gives a yellow precipitate of mercuric oxide, and with silver nitrate a white precipitate of silver chloride; with ammonia it yields the well-known white precipitate of ammoniated mercury. Stannous chloride and other reducing agents produce a separation of calomel, and if in excess, with the aid of heat, liberate mercury in the metallic state. The oxygen acids in general do not act upon the salt, and nitric and hydrochloric acids dissolve a considerable amount of it.

Tests.—Mercuric chloride should volatilize completely by heat (a residue shows fixed impurities); in six parts of alcohol or ether it should dissolve completely and clearly (a residue is probably calomel). Arsenic, if present, may be detected by adding potassium hydrate in excess, then some fragments of pure zinc, and loosely closing the test-tube with a cork into whose inner face is inserted a strip of filtering paper moistened with silver nitrate solution; upon heating the test-tube the appearance of a black spot upon the paper indicates arsenic.

It was introduced into our Materia Medica by Hahnemann.

Preparation for Homœopathic Use.—One part by weight of pure corrosive sublimate is dissolved in ninety-nine parts by weight of alcohol.

Amount of drug power, $\frac{1}{100}$.

Dilutions must be prepared as directed under Class VI—β.

Triturations are prepared, as directed under Class VII.

The alcoholic solution is to be preferred on account of its stability.

MERCURIUS SULPHURETUM NIGRUM.

Synonyms, Black Sulphuret of Mercury. Æthiops Mineralis. Hydrargyrum Sulphuretum Nigrum.

A mixture of black amorphous sulphide of mercury, Hg S, with sulphur in large excess.

Preparation of Æthiops Mineralis.—Equal parts of pure metallic mercury and pure sublimed sulphur are to be triturated together with repeated sprinkling with alcohol to prevent the rising of dust, until with a lens no metallic globules are observable.

Properties.—Æthiops mineral is a fine, heavy, black, odorless and tasteless powder, and is not soluble in water or hydrochloric acid. When heated in the air it ignites, exhibiting the blue flame of burning sulphur and with sublimation of metallic mercury; when heated in a test-tube mercuric sulphide (red) sublimes and condenses in the cold part of the tube. When boiled with hydrochloric acid the acid liquid should give no precipitate when thrown into water (absence of antimony).

Preparation for Homœopathic Use.—The pure black sulphide of mercury is triturated as directed under Class VII.

MERCURIUS SULPHURICUS.

Synonyms, Mercuric Sulphate. Hydrargyri Sulphas. Hydrargyrum Sulphuricum.

Common Names, Sulphate of Mercury. Persulphate of Mercury.

Formula, Hg SO_4.

Molecular Weight, 296.

Preparation of Sulphate of Mercury.—Take of mercury by weight, twenty ounces; sulphuric acid, twelve fluid ounces. Heat the mercury with the sulphuric acid in a porcelain vessel, stirring constantly until the metal disappears, then continue the heat until a dry white salt remains.—Br. P.

Properties and Tests.—Mercuric sulphate is a white crystalline powder, which bears an incipient red heat without alteration, but melts at a higher temperature to a brown liquid, and is volatilized completely with decomposition. When treated with a large amount of water it is resolved into a soluble acid salt and an insoluble basic one; with a small quantity of water it forms a hydrate which crystallizes with one molecule of water in colorless quadratic prisms.

It was first proven under Dr. Neidhard's direction, United States.

Preparation for Homœopathic Use.—Pure sulphate of mercury is triturated as directed under Class VII.

MERCURIUS VIVUS.

Synonyms, Hydrargyrum. Argentum Vivum. Mercury.

Common Name, Quicksilver.

Symbol, Hg.

Atomic Weight, 200.

Origin.—Mercury occurs in nature in the free state in very small quantity; its chief ore is *cinnabar*, a sulphide of the metal which is found in Almaden in Spain, in Idria in Austria, in Peru, in China and in New Almaden in California.

Preparation.—By roasting the ore the sulphide sublimes and the vapor being ignited by flame let into the chamber, the mercury is set free and is volatilized; by special arrangements varying in different countries, the vaporized mercury is condensed and collected in the liquid state. The ore is also distilled with lime or with blacksmiths' scales, in closed vessels.

Metallic mercury comes in commerce in iron bottles or flasks, each holding about seventy-five pounds, and is contaminated with small amounts of other metals; it has to be purified by redistillation or by prolonged digestion with a mixture of equal parts of nitric acid and distilled water. The contaminating metals are thus oxidized and dissolved, and the mercury is separated from the acid solution, well washed with water, and dried by means of bibulous paper.

Properties.—Mercury is a brilliant silver-white metal, which is liquid at ordinary temperatures, but when cooled to — 40° C. (— 40° F.) solidifies to a tin-like mass, which is easily cut and hammered; it is then crystalline in structure, the crystals being regular octohedrons. In the pure state it does not adhere to glass, but when contaminated with other metals it drags upon glass or "tails." It is slightly volatile at ordinary temperatures, and when heated to 350° C. (662° F.) it boils, yielding a colorless vapor. It is unalterable in the air, the film often seen upon specimens of the metal being due to the presence of an amalgam with other metals; it readily unites with other metals, such alloys being called *amalgams.* Heated to its boiling point in the air, it slowly oxidizes, forming the red or mercuric oxide. Mercury is not attacked by hydrochloric or dilute sulphuric acid, but is dissolved readily by boiling strong sulphuric acid and by dilute nitric acid. It combines with chlorine, bromine, iodine and sulphur.

The purity of the metal may be in general assured by its possessing the characteristics above given. When a portion of the metal is agitated with a solution of ferric chloride free from ferrous chloride, and the metal then separated from the chloride, the latter, on the addition of potassium ferrocyanide, should not give a blue precipitate; such change, if present, is dependent upon the presence in the mercury of a foreign metal, which has reduced the ferric compound to the ferrous state.

It was introduced into our Materia Medica by Hahnemann.

Preparation for Homœopathic Use.—Pure mercury is triturated, as directed under Class VII.

MEZEREUM.

Synonyms, Daphne Mezereum, *Linn.* Chamædaphne. Chamælia Germanica. Coccus Chamelacus.

Nat. Ord., Thymelaceæ.

Common Names, Mezereon. Spurge Olive.

This is a small shrub, three or four feet high, native of Northern and Central Europe. Its leaves are deciduous, without petioles, obovate-lanceolate; light green, nearly glaucous beneath. Flowers rose red in color, fragrant, in small clusters. The bark, which is the part used in medicine, comes in long strips, about half an inch wide and less than a line in thickness. These strips are folded and arranged in bundles, or rolled in flat masses, with the inner surface of the bark presenting externally. The outer surface is yellowish-brown or paler, and has a shining coppery appearance. It is dotted with many small, black, wart-like elevations. The pale green outer bark is readily separable from the corky layer. The inner surface is hairy in appearance, silky and whitish in color. In the dry state it is without odor, and possesses an acrid, burning taste.

It was first proven by Hahnemann.

Preparation.—The fresh bark, gathered in early spring before the flowers appear, is chopped and pounded to a pulp and weighed. Then two-thirds by weight of alcohol are taken, the pulp well mixed with it, and then strained *lege artis* through a piece of new linen. This tincture is then poured into a well-stoppered bottle, and allowed to stand eight days in a dark, cool place and filtered.

Drug power of tincture, $\frac{1}{2}$.

Dilutions must be prepared as directed under Class II.

MILLEFOLIUM.

Synonyms, Achillea Millefolium, *Linn.* Achillea Myriophylli.

Nat. Ord., Compositæ.

Common Names, Yarrow. Milfoil. Nose-bleed.

This common perennial herb is found growing in old fields, on the borders of woods, etc., in both North America and Europe. It is about a foot high, stem furrowed. Leaves bi-pinnatifid; segments linear, dentate, mucronate. Flowers white, in a dense, flat-topped corymb at the summit of the stem; they have an agreeable pungent taste and smell. Flowers from June to September.

The drug was proven by Nenning, Germany.

Preparation.—The fresh plant, gathered when flowering begins and before the stems are ligneous, is chopped and pounded to a pulp and then pressed out *lege artis* in a piece of new linen. The expressed juice is by brisk agitation mingled with an equal part by weight of alcohol. This mixture is allowed to stand eight days in a well-stoppered bottle, in a dark, cool place, and then filtered.

Drug power of tincture, $\frac{1}{2}$.

Dilutions must be prepared as directed under Class I.

MIMOSA HUMILIS, *Linn.*

Nat. Ord., Leguminosæ.

This species, which is one of the smallest of the genus mimosa, is found in the prairies around Rio Janeiro. Its stem is feeble, rather woody, ramose, pubescent above and covered with very sharp prickles. The leaves are bipinnate, the pinnæ being three or four-paired, with small, linear folioles, which close at the least contact; there are from six to twelve on each side of the spike. The flowers are small, sessile, forming pretty silky tufts of a violet color. The fruit is somewhat triangular, flattened, covered with long and stiff hairs, and surrounded by a persistent pericarp, divided in two capsules, each of which contains one seed.

It was introduced into our Materia Medica by Dr. Mure, Brazil.

Preparation.—The fresh leaves are chopped and pounded to a pulp and weighed. Then two parts by weight of alcohol are taken, the pulp mixed with one-sixth part of it, and the rest of the alcohol added. After having stirred the whole well, pour it into a well-stoppered bottle, and let it stand eight days in a dark, cool place. The tincture is then separated by decanting, straining and filtering.

Drug power of tincture, $\frac{1}{6}$.

Dilutions must be prepared as directed under Class III.

MITCHELLA REPENS, *Linn.*

Nat. Ord., Rubiaceæ.

Common Names, Checker Berry. Partridge Berry. Squaw Vine.

This plant must not be confounded, on account of its popular name, with the *Gaultheria procumbens.* It is a small evergreen indigenous plant, with a creeping stem. Leaves round, ovate, petiolate, shining, dark green and furnished with minute stipules. Flowers in pairs on the double ovary. Corolla funnel-shaped, generally four-lobed, hairy within, white or tinged with red, very fragrant. Fruit a drupe composed of the united ovaries. Flowers in June and July.

It was first proven by Dr. T. C. Duncan, United States.

Preparation.—The fresh plant is chopped and pounded to a pulp and weighed. Then two parts by weight of alcohol are taken, the pulp mixed thoroughly with one-sixth part of it, and the rest of the alcohol added. After having stirred the whole well, pour it into a well-stoppered bottle and let it stand eight days in a dark, cool place. The tincture is then separated by decanting, straining and filtering.

Drug power of tincture, $\frac{1}{6}$.

Dilutions must be prepared as directed under Class III.

MOMORDICA BALSAMINA, *Linn.*

Synonym, Balsamina.

Nat. Ord., Cucurbitaceæ.

Common Name, Balsam Apple.

This plant is a native of the East Indies, but is sometimes cultivated in this country. It is an annual, and is climbing in its habit. The fruit somewhat resembles a cucumber, is ovate, narrowed at each end, obscurely ridged, with wart-like elevations, is orange-colored or orange-red, and separates by lateral division. The seeds are numerous, flat, oval, brownish and wrinkled, enclosed in the fleshy red arillus.

It was proven under the direction of Dr. A. Mercier, United States.

Preparation.—The ripe fruit is chopped and pounded to a pulp and pressed out *lege artis* in a piece of new linen. The expressed juice is then, by brisk agitation, mingled with an equal part by weight of alcohol. This mixture is allowed to stand eight days in a well-stoppered bottle, in a dark, cool place and then filtered.

Amount of drug power, $\frac{1}{2}$.

Dilutions must be prepared as directed under Class I.

MONOBROMATUM CAMPHORÆ.

Synonym, Camphora Monobromata.

Common Names, Monobromated Camphor. Bromated Camphor.

Formula, $C_{10}\ H_{15}$ Br O.

Molecular Weight, 231.

Preparation of Monobromated Camphor.—Into a large tubulated retort, whose neck has been closed, place 13 ounces of camphor, broken into small pieces, and then bring the neck into a somewhat erect position; by using a funnel-tube passing through the tubulure, four ounces of bromine are to be introduced into the retort, the last portion of the bromine being washed down with about half a drachm of alcohol. A marked reaction will begin in fifteen or a few more minutes, and after its subsidence and the complete cooling of the retort, four successive additions of an ounce each of bromine are to be made; a fresh addition is not to be made until the reaction from the previous one has ended. When the last addition of bromine has been made, and the resulting reaction has subsided, the retort is to be gradually and cautiously heated to 130° C. (266° F.) and then the contents, after being partially cooled, are to be dissolved in warm petroleum-benzine and the solution set aside to crystallize. The crystals are to be collected in a funnel and purified by re-solution and crystallization in the benzine.

Monobrom-camphor is in colorless transparent prisms, having a camphor-like odor and taste. They are easily soluble in alcohol, ether and chloroform and in less than their own volume of hot petroleum-ether; they are somewhat soluble in glycerine, and not at all in water. The crystals fuse at 65° C. (149° F.) and at 270° C. (518° F.) they boil, but suffer partial decomposition.

Preparation for Homœopathic Use.—Monobromated camphor is triturated as directed under Class VII.

MONOTROPA UNIFLORA, *Linn.*

Synonym, Monotropa Morisoniana.

Nat. Ord., Ericaceæ.

Common Names, Indian Pipe. Bird's Nest. Corpse Plant. Ice plant.

This is a low and fleshy herb, found in dark and rich woods from Maine to Carolina and westward to Missouri. The clustered stems spring from a ball of matted fibrous rootlets, furnished with scale-like bracts in place of leaves; the flowering summit at first nodding, in fruit erect. The plant is smooth, dirty white (turning black in drying), inodorous, with a single sessile, nodding, five-petaled flower at the summit; the calyx of two to four irregular scales or bracts; anthers transverse, opening by two chinks; style short and thick; stigma naked. It flowers from June to September.

Preparation.—The whole plant in flower is chopped and pounded to a pulp and weighed. Then two parts by weight of alcohol are taken, the pulp mixed thoroughly with one-sixth part of it, and the rest of the alcohol added. After having stirred the whole well, pour it into a well-stoppered bottle, and let it stand eight days in a dark, cool place. The tincture is then separated by decanting, straining and filtering.

Amount of drug power, $\frac{1}{6}$.

Dilutions must be prepared as directed under Class III.

MORPHIUM.

Synonyms, Morphium Purum. Morphia.
Common Name, Morphine.
Formula, $C_{17}\ H_{19}\ NO_3,\ H_2\ O$.
Molecular Weight, 303.

Preparation of Morphia.—Ten parts of opium are to be digested with three volumes of boiling water for half an hour; the liquid is then strained, and the residue, after being expressed, is again twice treated with water in the same way. The united liquids are to be boiled down to half their bulk and then stirred into a boiling milk of lime made from caustic lime whose weight is equal to one-fourth the amount of opium taken. The mixture is to be boiled for a quarter of an hour and then strained and the calcareous residue again twice boiled in twenty-five parts of water. The whole of the lime-bearing liquors are now to be boiled down to twenty parts and mixed at the boiling temperature with one part of ammonium chloride; the heat is kept up for an hour, or as long as ammonia is given off, the liquid is then allowed to cool, and after eight days the morphia, which separates in the form of brown granules, is to be collected. The mother liquor yields another crop if further boiled down and left to itself. The product is purified by washing in cold water, solution in hydrochloric acid, repeated boiling with excess of milk of lime and precipitation with ammonium chloride.

Properties.—Morphia is in short, colorless, transparent, or white glistening prisms, whose taste is tolerably bitter and whose reaction is alkaline. They are soluble in 1200 parts of cold and in 500 of hot water, in from forty-five to fifty of cold and thirty of hot 90 per cent. alcohol. They are almost insoluble in ether, benzol, petroleum-ether, and the fixed oils, and 150 parts of chloroform are required to take up one of morphia. It neutralizes acids completely and forms thereby crystallizable salts. Morphia is readily soluble in the fixed alkalies and in lime-water, less so in ammonium hydrate or carbonate. When heated, morphia melts with the loss of its water of crystallization, and on cooling solidifies to a radio-crystalline mass. By stronger heating it carbonizes and finally burns without residue. Dry morphia has a very slight taste, but its solutions are bitter. Its salts are soluble in water and in alcohol, but not in ether.

Tests.—The impurities that may be present in morphia are narcotin, lime, and magnesium and ammonium compounds; and as adulterations, other alkaloids, salicin, sugar of different kinds and salts of ammonium. When a small portion of the alkaloid is burned on platinum foil there should remain no ash (absence of lime and magnesia). When to 0.1 gram in a test-tube are added 1.5 to 2 grams of caustic alkaline hydrate solution, there should result a clear, colorless or almost colorless solution (a brown coloration indicates the presence of glucose, and incomplete solubility some foreign alkaloid, especially narcotin). From the alkaline solution ammonia gas should not be evolved (absence of salts of ammonium). In a test-tube is to be placed 0.1

gram of morphia, and there are to be poured upon it about 3 CC. of concentrated sulphuric acid and the mixture slightly agitated. The resulting solution should be colorless, and only after long standing should the color become tinged with red (narcein, thebain, give with concentrated sulphuric acid a red solution, pseudomorphine a green one, and cane-sugar and milk-sugar cause the solution to become blackish). Finally, the solution in sulphuric acid is to be tested by Husemann's method; the solution is heated to about 150° C. (302° F.), and the addition of a little nitric acid causes the color to become violet-blue, changing quickly to blood-red, and after some time to deep orange.

Preparation for Homœopathic Use.—Pure morphia is triturated, as directed under Class VII.

MORPHIUM ACETICUM.

Synonyms, Morphiæ Acetas. Morphinum Aceticum.
Common Name, Acetate of Morphia.
Formula, $C_{17} H_{19} NO_3, C_2 H_4 O_2, H_2 O$.
Molecular Weight, 363.

Preparation of Acetate of Morphia.—Pure morphia is to be dissolved in dilute acetic acid with the aid of a gentle heat, the solution placed in a flat dish set aside in a warm place and evaporated till a friable mass is produced.

Properties and Tests.—Acetate of morphia is a white powder. It has a bitter taste, a weak acetous odor and its reaction is barely alkaline. It is soluble in twenty-five parts of cold and in two of boiling water, in forty-five of cold and in two of boiling alcohol; it is insoluble in ether. Upon keeping, it slowly loses acetic acid and thereby it becomes more alkaline in reaction and less soluble in water, and its color darkens till finally it is brownish. It should then be redissolved in dilute acetic acid and re-evaporated. Its watery solutions also undergo this change, becoming gradually yellow and at last brown in color. It should leave no residue when heated on platinum foil. It may be tested in the way described under the article Morphinum. It is to be noted, however, that a specimen of the acetate kept for some time will not give a colorless solution with sulphuric acid, the color being yellowish.

Preparation for Homœopathic Use.—Pure acetate of morphia is triturated, as directed under Class VII.

MORPHIUM MURIATICUM.

Synonyms, Hydrochlorate of Morphia. Morphiæ Murias. Morphiæ Hydrochloras.
Common Name, Muriate of Morphia.
Formula, $C_{17} H_{19} N O_3, HCl, 3H_2O$.
Molecular Weight, 375.5.

Preparation of Muriate of Morphia.—This salt is readily prepared by neutralizing dilute hydrochloric acid with pure morphia, and crystallizing by evaporating the solution.

Properties and Tests.—The hydrochlorate of morphia forms fine, white, silky, acicular crystals which are without odor and have a very bitter taste. They are soluble in twenty parts of water at medium temperatures, in their own volume of boiling water, in from sixty to seventy of cold and in ten or twelve of boiling alcohol, and in twenty of glycerine. The crystals are permanent in the air; by heat they lose their water of crystallization, and at a high temperature are consumed without leaving a residue. The tests described for morphia will apply to this salt. Its solutions when precipitated by tannin should redissolve on the addition of HCl, any undissolved turbidity being probably due to narcotin.

Preparation for Homœopathic Use.—Pure muriate of morphia is triturated, as directed under Class VII.

MORPHIUM SULPHURICUM.

Synonyms, Morphiæ Sulphas. Morphinum Sulphuricum.

Common Name, Sulphate of Morphia.

Formula, $(C_{17}\ H_{19}\ N\ O_3)_2,\ H_2\ S\ O_4,\ 5H_2O$.

Molecular Weight, 758.

Preparation of Sulphate of Morphia.—This salt may be prepared by neutralizing pure dilute sulphuric acid with pure morphia, partly evaporating the solution in a warm place or over a water-bath and then setting it aside to crystallize.

Properties and Tests.—Sulphate of morphia crystallizes in tufts of colorless prisms having a silky lustre. They are soluble in two parts of water, less readily in alcohol. When heated to 130° C. (266° F.) they give off all their water of crystallization; the solutions are neutral in reaction. The usual tests for morphia apply to this salt.

Preparation for Homœopathic Use.—Pure sulphate of morphia is triturated, as directed under Class VII.

MOSCHUS.

Synonyms, Moschus Orientalis. Moschus Tibetanus. Moschus Tunquinensis.

Class, Mammalia.

Order, Ruminantia.

Family, Moschina.

Common Name, Musk.

A dried preputial secretion from *Moschus moschiferus, Linn.*

Origin.—The musk deer is found in mountainous regions and elevated plateaus in Asia, from India to Siberia. The musk-sac is situated on the abdomen of the male animal between the umbilicus and the preputial orifice, and directly in front of the latter. The bag or sac is oval, about two inches long and somewhat less in width, and about half an inch thick. The bag is made up of two coats, the external one cuticular and hairy except on the upper surface; the lower surface has an aperture about its middle, and toward this the stiff, appressed hairs are directed. The inner coat, composed of muscular and fibrous layers, is thin, somewhat transparent and more or less veined, and in the recent state is bright brown in color; its lining has numerous depressions containing the secreting glands. Musk is in small, irregular grains or crumbs, dark reddish-brown in color, and when near the orifice often mixed with hairs. The grains have a somewhat unctuous lustre, and when fresh are easily crushed. The odor of musk is peculiar, very persistent, and is not agreeable except when quite faint; it is slight in the dry substance, but by moisture is greatly increased. The best variety of musk is the Tonquin, from China and Thibet. It comes in small packages or boxes lined with sheet-lead, each containing about twenty-five sacs, separately wrapped in paper. When this variety of musk is brought into commerce *via* Russia, it is called Russian or Siberian musk, and a variety coming from Siberia, called Cabardine musk, is found in flatter, more oval sacs, less covered with hair and having a less musk-like odor. Only Chinese musk should be used in medicine, and it should not be purchased except in the sacs; the bags should be carefully examined for evidences of the substitution of an artificial sac, made of a portion of the hide of the animal sewn to a membrane. Here the absence of the central aperture and of the circularly arranged hairs surrounding it, will at once expose the fraud. Sometimes genuine sacs are cut open, a portion of their contents removed and other substances substituted; the stitches which hold the edges of the slit in apposition, are evidence of the fact mentioned, but when foreign bodies have been introduced through the natural opening there is no means of detecting this fraud before opening the bag.

Properties.—Good musk contains from 40 to 50 per cent. of constituents soluble in water, and 8 to 10 per cent. of matters soluble in 90 per cent. alcohol. It contains also fatty, waxy, gelatinous and albuminous substances, various salts of the alkalies and of the alkaline earths, with traces of ammonia, and a volatile oil.

The drug was proven by Hahnemann.

Preparation for Homœopathic Use.—A tincture is made, according to Altschul, of the whole bag, with dilute alcohol in the proportion of one to twenty, the dilutions from which must be prepared as directed under Class IV, except that dilute alcohol, in the proportion of twenty to eighty, is used for the 1 and 2x dilutions.

Triturations are prepared as directed under Class VII.

MUREX PURPUREA.

Synonyms, Murex Brandaris, *Buchner.* Purpurea Patula.
Class, Mollusca.
Order, Gasteropoda.
Family, Muricidæ.

This sea-snail is found in large quantities on the coasts of the Adriatic and Mediterranean Seas. The coloring juice is lodged in a bag between the heart and liver, and does not always possess the fine red color, when taken out, but appears as a tough, viscid, colorless or greenish liquid, gradually reddening when exposed to the air.

Preparation.—The fresh juice is triturated, as directed under Class VIII.

A solution of the third trituration in water still shows a fine rose-red color.

MURURE LEITE.

Resin obtained from Yichetea Officinalis.

Preparation.—The resin is triturated, as directed under Class VII.

Introduced into our Materia Medica by Dr. Mure, Brazil.

MYGALE LASIODORA.

Synonym, Mygale Lasiodora Cubana.

A large black Cuban Spider.

It was proven under direction of Dr. John G. Houard, United States.

Preparation.—The live insect is crushed and covered with five parts by weight of alcohol, and allowed to remain eight days in a well-stoppered bottle, in a dark, cool place, being shaken twice a day. The tincture is then poured off, strained and filtered.

Amount of drug power, $\frac{1}{10}$.

Dilutions must be prepared as directed under Class IV.

MYRICA CERIFERA, *Linn.*

Nat. Ord., Myricaceæ.

Common Names, Bayberry. Candle Berry. Sweet Gale. Wax-myrtle.

This is an indigenous shrub four to eight feet high, growing in great abundance along the sea-shore, and also near Lake Erie. Leaves alternate, glabrous, cuneate-oblong, undulate-dentate towards the apex, resinous-punctate, and emitting fragrance when bruised. Flowers diœcious, the sterile ones in cylindrical catkins, the fertile ones in shorter ovoid heads. Fruit a drupe which is covered with a white waxy coating. The bark is externally whitish, somewhat wrinkled, the outer layer separating in small fragments. The inner layer is dark reddish-brown, almost smooth. It has a granular, pale reddish fracture.

This drug was proven by members of the Massachusetts Homœopathic Medical Society (Transactions, 1864).

Preparation.—The fresh bark of the root is chopped and pounded to a pulp and weighed. Then two parts by weight of alcohol are taken, the pulp mixed with one-sixth part of it, and the rest of the alcohol added. After having stirred the whole well, pour it into a well-stoppered bottle, and let it stand eight days in a dark, cool place. The tincture is then separated by decanting, straining and filtering.

Drug power of tincture, $\frac{1}{6}$.
Dilutions must be prepared as directed under Class III.

MYRISTICA SEBIFERA, *Swartz.*

Synonym, Virola Sebifera, *Aublet.*
Nat. Ord., Myristicaceæ.
Common Name, Brazilian Ucuuba.

This tree is found in the provinces of Para and Rio Negro. The tree is of some height, and the trunk and branches are covered with a thick, brownish and reticulate bark. Leaves alternate, oblong, cordate, rather tomentose on their lower surface, and supported by short petioles. Flowers in tufted panicles, ramose, arising from the axils of the leaves or the extremities of the branches; they are diœcious, with a simple, urceolate perigone having three divisions. Male flowers with six stamens, the filaments of which are attached to each other, and are inserted in a glandular disk. The female flowers are smaller, one unilocular ovary, style wanting, stigma bilobed. Capsular berry, with two valves, containing an oleaginous seed, surrounded by an aril crenated above.

It was introduced into our Materia Medica by Dr. Mure, Brazil.

Preparation.—The fresh, red juice, obtained by puncturing the bark, is triturated according to Class VIII.

MYRTUS COMMUNIS, *Linn.*

Nat. Ord., Myrtaceæ.
Common Name, Myrtle.

This shrub is a native of Southern Europe. Leaves opposite, oblong-ovate, shining, smooth, from one to two inches long, on short petioles and pellucid-punctate. Flowers white, solitary, axillary, many stamened. Fruit a two-celled, bluish-black berry, with four or five seeds in each cell. Leaves, flowers and fruit are fragrant.

Preparation.—The fresh, flowering shoots and leaves are chopped and pounded to a pulp and weighed. Then two parts by weight of alcohol are taken, the pulp mixed thoroughly with one-sixth part of it, and the rest of the alcohol added. After having stirred the whole well, pour it into a well-stoppered bottle and let it stand eight days in a dark, cool place. The tincture is then separated by decanting, straining and filtering.

Drug power of tincture, $\frac{1}{6}$.
Dilutions must be prepared as directed under Class III.

NABALUS ALBUS, Var. Serpentarius, *Gray.*

Synonyms, Nabalus Serpentaria, *Hooker.* Prenanthes Alba, *Linn.*
Nat. Ord., Compositæ.
Common Names, Rattlesnake-Root. White Lettuce. Lion's Foot.

This indigenous perennial grows in rich soil on the borders of woods. The stem, two to four feet high, purplish and often deeply so in spots, arises from a spindle-shaped tuberous root. Radical leaves, angular-hastate, more or less deeply lobed. Stem leaves, round-ovate, sinuate-toothed. The lobes or leaves are obtuse. Flower-heads in corymbous panicles at the summit of the stem. Eight to twelve flowered, pappus deep cinnamon-colored. Var. Serpentaria has radical leaves, palmate-sinuate, stem leaves on long petioles, middle segment three-parted.

It was proved by Dr. M. E. Lazarus, United States.

Preparation.—The fresh plant is chopped and pounded to a pulp and weighed. Then two parts by weight of alcohol are taken, the pulp mixed thoroughly with one-sixth part of it, and the rest of the alcohol added. After having stirred the whole well, pour it into a well-stoppered bottle, and let it stand eight days in a dark, cool place. The tincture is then separated by decanting, straining and filtering.

Drug power of tincture, $\frac{1}{6}$.

Dilutions must be prepared as directed under Class III.

NAJA.

Synonyms, Naja Tripudians. Coluber Naja.
Class, Reptilia.
Order, Squamata.
Family, Elapidæ.
Common Names, Cobra di Capello. Hooded Snake.

This species of snake is commonly found in Hindostan. It varies in length from two to four feet. The neck can be dilated so as to give the appearance of a hood covering the head. It is the snake usually employed by the snake-charmers. The fangs are canaliculated, and are in front of the superior maxilla, with smaller solid teeth behind them. The sixth upper labial scale is small, forming a suture with a very large temporal scale; there is generally a spectacle-like mark on the neck.

It was first proved by Dr. Stokes, England.

Preparation.—The poison, obtained by compressing the gland (of the live animal) which secretes it, is triturated as directed under Class VIII.

NAPHTHALINUM.

Synonyms, Naphthalin. Naphthalene.
Formula, $C_{10}H_8$.
Molecular Weight, 128.

Origin.—Naphthalin is generally produced when organic bodies are distilled alone. It may be procured from coal; alcohol, ether vapor and even olefiant gas yield more or less naphthalin when passed through red hot tubes. Petroleum and most essential oils when treated in the latter way also afford it, and camphor vapor when passed over red hot quicklime gives rise to it; from the above considerations it is not remarkable that naphthalin should be found in soot and lamp-black.

Preparation.—Coal-tar from which the lighter oils have been removed by preliminary distillation is distilled in large iron retorts; the distillate is received in puncheons and the process carried on until the liquid is heavier than water. The first two parts out of a charge of seventy contain but little naphthalin, the rest of the distillate abounds in it. To extract the naphthalin from the oily distillate small quantities of sulphuric acid are shaken with it and then after settling for some time, are run off. The supernatant oil on cooling to 0° C. (32° F.), deposits large quantities of the naphthalin. The crude greasy naphthalin is drained and pressed in strong bags to remove the oil and then redistilled, the receiver being changed when the product comes over colorless. To obtain it in large crystals it may be melted over the sand-bath, in basins with covers of paper pasted over them; the basins should be not more than half full. When the contents are melted and begin to sublime, the whole may be allowed to cool, and when quite cold a large quantity of colorless crystals will be found between the cake of naphthalin and the paper cover, and may be removed with a feather.

Properties.—Naphthalin when purified by sublimation is in transparent, colorless, glistening scales; when crystallized from its ethereal solution it forms rhombic tables or prisms. It has a peculiar, somewhat tar-like odor and a rather pungent taste. It is but slightly soluble in water and cold alcohol, but readily dissolves in boiling alcohol as well as in ether, carbon disulphide, the volatile oils, acetic acid and dilute oxalic acid. It is insoluble in watery solutions of the alkalies. It is somewhat volatile at ordinary temperatures, and when ignited burns with a dense smoky flame. When heated to 80° C. (176° F.) it melts, and at 218° C. (424.4° F.) it boils. Its specific gravity is 1.15.

Tests.—Perfectly pure naphthalin volatilizes completely when heated; and with concentrated sulphuric acid it forms a colorless solution. The commercial article usually gives a brownish solution. For its identification Vohl's reaction may be used, as follows: when naphthalin is brought in contact with the strongest nitric acid, a large quantity of water added and the resulting precipitate, after washing with dilute alcohol, mixed with a little hydrate and sulphide of potassium, the residue dissolves in alcohol with a violet-red color. Naphthalin when fused into sticks, like sulphur, has the appearance of alabaster, cracks when held in the warm hand and when rubbed becomes negatively electric.

Preparation for Homœopathic Use.—Pure naphthalin is triturated, as directed under Class VII.

NARCOTINUM.

Synonyms, Narcotina. Narcotin. Narcotia.
Formula, $C_{44}\ H_{23}\ NO_{14}$.

Molecular Weight, 413.

Preparation of Narcotina.—Narcotin exists in opium to the amount of six or eight per cent.; it was the first base extracted from that drug. During the process for obtaining morphia from opium narcotin is also obtained; it may be separated from the morphia by the use of ether, which does not dissolve the latter. The ethereal solution is to be slowly evaporated. It may be obtained directly from opium by treating that substance with ether and evaporating the solution as in the previous method.

Properties.—Narcotin crystallizes in right rhombic prisms, or in needles grouped in bundles, flattened, colorless, transparent and lustrous; it is without odor or taste, and is indifferent to litmus paper. It is almost insoluble in cold water, and of boiling water it requires about 7,000 parts for solution; it dissolves in thirty-five parts of ether, in three of chloroform and in twenty-five of benzol. The alcoholic and ethereal solutions have a bitter taste. Its salts are very unstable.

Tests.—Narcotin is a weaker base than opium, and does not decompose ammonium chloride even at 100° C. (212° F.). With concentrated sulphuric acid it forms at first a colorless solution, but after some minutes the color changes to yellow, and in the course of a day or two it becomes raspberry-red. The caustic alkalies and their carbonates precipitate narcotin from its solutions as a white crystalline powder insoluble in excess of the reagent. Caustic ammonia dissolves it in slight amount. To ferric chloride and iodic acid it is indifferent. Its absence of taste, its neutral reaction, its precipitation by alkalies, its solubility in ether and its not being affected by iron salts and iodic acid, all serve to distinguish it from morphia.

Preparation for Homœopathic Use.—Pure narcotina is triturated as directed under Class VII.

NATRUM ARSENICICUM.

Synonyms, Sodium Arsenate. Arsenias Natricus. Arsenias Sodicus. Natri Arsenias. Sodæ Arsenias. Sodii Arsenias.

Formula, $Na_2\ H\ As\ O_4,\ 7\ H_2O$.

Molecular Weight, 312.

Common Name, Arsenate of Soda.

Preparation of Arsenate of Soda.—960 grains of pure arsenious oxide, finely powdered, and 816 grains of sodium nitrate, finely powdered, and 528 grains of dried sodium carbonate, finely powdered, are to be intimately mixed and placed in a large, covered, clay crucible and exposed to a full red heat until effervescence ceases and the mass is completely fused. The fused product is to be poured on a porcelain tile and as soon as solidification has taken place and before cooling, it is to be put into half a pint of boiling distilled water and the mixture stirred until the salt is dissolved. Then the solution is to be filtered and set aside that crystals may form. The crystals are to be collected, drained, dried rapidly on bibulous paper and transferred to a well-stoppered bottle.

Properties.—Arsenate of soda prepared as above directed is in colorless, transparent, monoclinic prisms, containing seven molecules of water; when crystallized below 18° C. (64.4° F.), it forms large efflorescent crystals isomorphous with ordinary phosphate of sodium, and containing twelve molecules of water; a salt containing twenty-six molecules of water separates from a solution cooled to 0° C. (32° F.). The crystals are slightly efflorescent in dry air, and in moist air they deliquesce somewhat. They dissolve in two or three parts of water, forming an alkaline solution.

Tests.—The usual arsenical reactions are given by this salt after its reduction to the arsenious state, by means of sulphurous acid, or sodium sulphite with some hydrochloric acid.

The drug was proven by Dr. Imbert Gourbeyre, France.

Preparation for Homœopathic Use.—Pure arsenate of sodium is triturated as directed under Class VII.

NATRUM CARBONICUM.

Synonyms, Sodium Carbonate. Carbonas Sodicus. Disodic Carbonate. Sodæ Carbonas. Sal Soda.

Common Name, Washing Soda.

Formula, $Na_2\,C\,O_3,\ 10H_2O$.

Molecular Weight, 286.

Origin and Preparation of Carbonate of Sodium.—Sodium carbonate exists in the soda lakes of Egypt and Hungary, in the volcanic springs of Iceland, etc; it is largely used in the arts, and was formerly obtained from *barilla*, the ash of *Salsola soda* and other plants growing on the sea-shore, and from the ash of sea-weed, called *kelp;* but at present nearly all the soda of commerce is obtained from common salt by first converting the chloride of sodium into sulphate by heating it with sulphuric acid, and then converting the sulphate into carbonate by heating it in a reverberatory furnace with chalk or limestone and coal. The crude soda obtained by this process is dark gray in color and appears partially vitrified; it is purified by lixiviating, and mixing the residue left after evaporation, with sawdust and heating in a reverberatory furnace, at a low red heat, for some hours. To obtain crystallized carbonate, the purified salt is dissolved in water, and the liquid, when clarified, is boiled down till a pellicle forms on the surface. The solution is then run into shallow crystallizing vessels, and after standing for a week the mother liquor is drawn off and the crystals drained and broken up for the market. The crystals thus obtained contain ten molecules of water.

Properties and Tests.—Sodium carbonate is in large, colorless, rhombic crystals or in irregular masses of the same, having an alkaline taste and reaction. They effloresce in the air, and are soluble in two parts of cold and in a quarter of a part of boiling water, and are insoluble in alcohol and ether. Commercially pure carbonate of sodium is generally contaminated with small amounts of chloride and sulphate, and its solutions, when acidified with nitric acid, give some turbidity or precipitate with silver nitrate and with barium nitrate. When the salt is prepared from *cryolite* alumina is likely to be present; it may be detected by acidifying a solution of the carbonate with HCl, boiling and adding ammonia in excess, when aluminium hydrate will separate out in a gelatinous mass. Chemically pure sodium carbonate should not suffer any change when tested in the foregoing methods, and its solution, when acidulated with HCl, should show no change upon treatment with hydrogen and ammonium sulphides (absence of metals).

It was proven by Hahnemann.

Preparation for Homœopathic Use.—Pure carbonate of sodium is triturated as directed under Class VII.

NATRUM BROMATUM.

Synonyms, Sodium Bromide. Bromurctum Sodicum. Sodii Bromidum.

Common Name, Bromide of Sodium.

Formula, Na Br.

Molecular Weight, 103.

Preparation of Bromide of Sodium.—The directions for preparing potassium bromide, as given in the article Kali Bromatum, will, by the substitution of sodium carbonate for the corresponding potassium compound, result in the formation of sodium bromide.

Properties and Tests.—Bromide of sodium, when crystallized out from its solutions at temperatures above 30° C. (86° F.), forms anhydrous cubes which have a slightly alkaline taste and neutral reaction; they are easily soluble in water and alcohol. When crystallized below 30° C. it forms hydrated, oblique rhombic prisms containing two molecules of water.

The solutions of the compound in water should be neutral or at most but very faintly alkaline, and when treated with a large addition of dilute sulphuric acid, should not show a yellow or reddish coloration.

Preparation for Homœopathic Use.—Pure bromide of sodium is triturated as directed under Class VII.

NATRUM HYPOPHOSPHOROSUM.

Synonyms, Sodium Hypophosphite. Sodii Hypophosphis.

Common Name, Hypophosphite of Soda.

Formula, $Na\ H_2\ PO_2,\ H_2O$.

Molecular Weight, 106.

Preparation of Hypophosphite of Sodium.—By decomposing calcium hypophosphite with sodium carbonate (avoiding excess of either), filtering and evaporating. The product contains some calcium carbonate from which it may be freed by re-solution in alcohol, filtering and recrystallizing, the evaporation being at a temperature below 100° C. (212° F.). The directions given for preparing potassium hypophosphite (see article Kalium Hypophosphorosum) will serve equally well for the production of the sodium compound by the substitution of the word "sodium" for "potassium" wherever the latter occurs in the article.

Properties.—Sodium hypophosphite crystallizes in pearly, rectangular tables somewhat less deliquescent than the corresponding potassium salt. It usually is seen as a white powder. It is easily soluble in alcohol and water, but does not dissolve in ether. At a high temperature it decomposes with the evolution of phosphoretted hydrogen and leaves a residue of pyrophosphate and metaphosphate of sodium.

Preparation for Homœopathic Use.—Pure hypophosphite of sodium is triturated as directed under Class VII.

NATRUM MURIATICUM.

Synonyms, Sodium Chloride. Chloruretum Sodicum. Natrium Chloratum Purum. Sodii Chloridum. Chloride of Sodium.

Common Names, Common Salt. Table Salt.

Formula, Na Cl.

Molecular Weight, 58.5.

Origin and Preparation of Chloride of Sodium.—Sodium chloride occurs very abundantly in nature, both in the solid state as rock salt, forming extensive beds in rocks of various ages, and in solution in sea-water, salt lakes and salt springs. The salt is mined from the solid deposits or taken from open cuts, while from saline waters it is obtained by evaporation or by first freezing; the latter mode is followed in Northern countries of Europe, since salt water separates on freezing, into ice containing no salt, and a strong saline lye. After the crystallizing out of sodium chloride the mother liquors containing potassium, sodium, calcium and magnesium sulphates, chlorides and bromides are utilized for the extraction of these compounds and their derivatives.

Properties.—Pure sodium chloride crystallizes from aqueous solutions at ordinary temperatures or higher, in colorless, transparent, anhydrous cubes, but an aqueous solution exposed to a temperature of —10° C. (14° F.) yields hexagonal plates containing two molecules of water; when the temperature rises the water of crystallization is expelled and the crystals are changed into a heap of minute cubes. Ordinarily, sodium chloride is found as a white powder made up of small, glistening, hard cubes, without reaction to test-paper, without odor and possessing a pure saline taste. The crystals are anhydrous, have a specific gravity of 2.16, decrepitate when thrown on red hot coal or when heated upon platinum foil; in a very damp atmosphere they become moist. Salt is soluble in less than three parts of water in the cold, and is scarcely more soluble in boiling water, but the admixture of other salts increases its solubility. It is not taken up by absolute alcohol, and 100 parts of 90 per cent. alcohol dissolve only two parts of it. At a red heat it melts, and on cooling solidifies to a crystalline mass; at a white heat it volatilizes. Its watery solutions have the property of dissolving several bodies insoluble in water, *e. g.*, calcium phosphate, calcium sulphate and silver chloride.

Tests.—The aqueous solution of sodium chloride should be perfectly neutral (absence of carbonate and of free hydrochloric acid); it should not be precipitated by hydrogen sulphide nor by ammonium sulphide (absence of metals), nor by ammonium oxalate (absence of calcium), nor by barium chloride (absence of sulphate), nor by sodium carbonate (absence of the earths, especially magnesia).

This drug was introduced into our Materia Medica by Hahnemann.

Preparation for Homœopathic Use.—One part by weight of pure chloride of sodium is dissolved in nine parts by weight of distilled water.

Amount of drug power, $\frac{1}{10}$.

Dilutions must be prepared as directed under Class V—*a*.

Triturations are prepared as directed under Class VII.

NATRUM NITRICUM.

Synonyms, Sodium Nitrate. Nitras (Azotas) Sodicus. Nitrum Cubicum. Sodii Nitras.

Common Names, Nitrate of Soda. Cubic Nitre. Chili Saltpetre.

Formula, $Na\ NO_3$.

Molecular Weight, 85.

Origin and Preparation.—Nitrate of sodium occurs abundantly as a natural mineral in South America; in the northern part of Peru the dry elevated plains, 3,000 feet above the sea-level, are covered with beds of it several feet in thickness, associated with gypsum, common salt, sulphate of sodium and the shelly residue of an ancient sea. The crude nitre called *caliche* is refined by solution and crystallization, but the great solubility of sodium nitrate renders it difficult to purify the latter from common salt; on a small scale this can be done by heating the powdered salt with nitric acid, by which means the chlorides are destroyed, and then by solution and recrystallization the nitrate is obtained perfectly pure.

Properties.—Pure sodium nitrate crystallizes in obtuse rhombohedrons, which, at a hasty glance, may be mistaken for cubes, whence the name cubic saltpetre. The crystals are colorless, transparent and permanent in the air, but when the salt is contaminated with sodium chloride, they become moist upon exposure, without, however, deliquescing. The salt has a saline, cooling, slightly bitter taste, is soluble in one and a quarter parts of water at ordinary temperatures, and in about half its weight of boiling water, and in 100 parts of 90 per cent. alcohol; the solutions are neutral in reaction. Upon dissolving the salt in water, a considerable fall in temperature is produced. When heated the salt deflagrates, and when mixed with inflammable bodies, it detonates, less strongly, however, than does the corresponding potassium compound; at 310° C. (590° F.) it fuses, and on cooling solidifies to a white mass; at a red heat it is decomposed, giving off oxygen and the lower oxides of nitrogen.

Tests.—Solutions of sodium nitrate should give no turbidity or precipitate with hydrogen sulphide (absence of metals), nor with sodium carbonate (magnesia and calcium compounds), nor with barium nitrate (sulphate), nor with silver nitrate (chloride), or with the latter a faint opalescence is permissible. When a few drops of chlorine water are added to a solution of the salt, and the mixture well agitated with carbon disulphide, the color of the reagent should undergo no change (a violet coloration of the bisulphide indicates the presence of iodine); if the test prove negative, sulphuric acid may be added to the mixture, and if a violet coloration then appear in the layer of carbon disulphide, an iodate is present.

Introduced into the Homœopathic Materia Medica by Dr. Gross, Germany.

Preparation for Homœopathic Use.—Pure nitrate of sodium is triturated as directed under Class VII.

NATRUM PHOSPHORICUM.

Synonyms, Sodium Phosphate. Natri Phosphas. Phosphas Natricus. Sodæ Phosphas. Sodii Phosphas.

Common Name, Phosphate of Soda.

Formula, $Na_2H\,P\,O_4$, $12\,H_2O$.

Molecular Weight, 358.

Preparation of Phosphate of Sodium.—To 10 parts of bone, calcined to whiteness and in fine powder, add 6 parts of sulphuric acid in an earthen vessel and thoroughly mix the ingredients; 22 fluid ounces of water are to be added to the mixture, and the whole thoroughly stirred. The mixture is to be set aside to digest for three days, and during that time is to be frequently stirred and enough water added from time to time to replace that lost by evaporation. At the end of the time, 22 fluid ounces of boiling water are to be added, and the whole thrown upon a muslin strainer, and repeatedly washed by boiling water in small amounts till the liquid comes through tasteless. The strained liquid is then to be set aside to permit the newly formed precipitates to settle; when the precipitation is complete, the clear liquid is decanted off and boiled down to 22 ounces. This concentrated liquid is to be decanted from any fresh precipitate and heated in a vessel of iron, and there is gradually added to it a hot solution of sodium carbonate as long as effervescence ensues, and until the liberated phosphoric acid is entirely neutralized; the liquid is now to be filtered and set aside in a cool place to crystallize. The first crop of crystals is the purest, but a subsequent crop may be obtained by adding sodium carbonate to the liquid as long as crystals are formed; the crystals of the secondary crop must be repurified by solution and recrystallization.

The salt should be kept in a well-stoppered bottle.

Properties.—Officinal sodium phosphate crystallizes in oblique rhombic prisms and tables, which are transparent and colorless, and have a mild, cooling, saline taste. They are soluble in two parts of hot water, and in four or five of water at medium temperatures; they are insoluble in alcohol. The solutions are slightly alkaline in reaction.

Heated to 35° C. (95° F.) they melt in their water of crystallization, and solidify to a crystalline mass on cooling; at 100° C. (212° F.) they give up their water of crystallization, and above 300° C. (572° F.) the salt is converted into pyrophosphate. The aqueous solution of the salt, when treated with silver nitrate solution, precipitates yellow orthophosphate of silver, and the filtered fluid has an acid reaction; the aqueous solution, upon the addition of barium chloride, gives a white precipitate of barium phosphate; both these precipitates are soluble in nitric acid. The solution of the salt after acidulation with HCl should not be changed in any way by hydrogen sulphide (absence of metals, and especially arsenic). The neutral solution should not effervesce upon the addition of an acid (absence of carbonate), and should give no precipitate or turbidity when treated with ammonia (absence of magnesium), or with ammonium oxalate (calcium).

Preparation for Homœopathic Use.—Pure phosphate of sodium is triturated as directed under Class VII.

NATRUM SALICYLICUM.

Synonyms, Sodium Salicylate. Salicylate of Sodium.

Formula, $2\,(Na\,C_7\,H_5\,O_3) + H_2O$.

Molecular Weight, 338.

Preparation.—Six parts of powdered, perfectly pure, sodium carbonate are to be thoroughly mixed with 10 parts of pure salicylic acid, and the mixture gradually added, with constant stirring, to 100 parts of dilute alcohol; the solution is to be dried at a gentle heat over a water-bath.

Properties.—Pure sodium salicylate is in very white and small crystalline plates, or is a crystalline powder; it is almost without odor, has a sweetish, saline and somewhat alkaline taste, and when kept in tightly closed vessels, undergoes no change in color, odor or taste. It is soluble in one part of water and in five or six parts of alcohol, the solutions being colorless and weakly alkaline. Treated with ferric chloride, it gives a dark violet coloration; and with pure concentrated sulphuric acid, it forms a solution which remains colorless for ten or fifteen minutes.

Tests.—Sodium salicylate may be considered pure when it is white in color, dissolves in one and one-half times its volume of distilled water and in six parts of alcohol, forming solutions which are colorless or very nearly so, and when shaken with fifteen volumes of pure concentrated sulphuric acid, it neither colors the acid nor effervesces. When it is heated to redness on platinum foil, an alkaline residue is left, whose weight should be not less than 30 nor more than 32 per cent. of the amount of the salt taken. The residue should give the reactions of pure sodium carbonate. A solution of the salt acidulated with nitric acid should give no turbidity when treated with silver nitrate or barium chloride.

Preparation for Homœopathic Use.—Pure salicylate of sodium is triturated as directed under Class VII.

NATRUM SELENICUM.

Synonyms, Sodium Selenate. Selenate of Soda.
Formula, $Na_2\ Se\ O_4$, 10 H_2O.
Molecular Weight, 369.
Preparation and Properties.—By fusing selenium or selenite of sodium, or selenide of lead with sodium nitrate, dissolving the fused mass in hot water and leaving the concentrated solution to cool and crystallize. The excess of nitrate crystallizes out first, and afterwards the selenate in crystals containing ten molecules of water, exactly resembling those of the normal sulphate (Glauber's salt), and exhibiting like the latter a maximum solubility at about 33° C. (91.4° F.). When crystallization is conducted at a temperature above 40° C. (104° F.), the crystals obtained are anhydrous.
Tests.—The salt, when prepared from pure materials, is not likely to be contaminated. If in doubt, it may be tested, as directed in the article Natrum Sulphuricum. For identification of the constituent selenium, the salt may be heated with charcoal or sodium carbonate in the reducing flame with the blow-pipe; a selenide is produced, recognized by the peculiar odor of decomposing horse-radish.
Preparation for Homœopathic Use.—One part by weight of selenate of soda is dissolved in nine parts by weight of distilled water.
Amount of drug power, $\frac{1}{10}$.
Dilutions must be prepared as directed under Class V—*a*.

NATRUM SULPHO-CARBOLICUM.

Synonyms, Sodii Sulpho-carbolas. Sodium Sulpho-carbolate.
Common Names, Sulphocarbolate of Sodium. Sulphophenate (Phenolsulphonate) of Sodium.
Formula, $Na\ C_6\ H_5\ S\ O_4$, 2 H_2 O.
Molecular Weight, 232.
Origin.—Phenol (carbolic acid) dissolves easily in strong sulphuric acid, forming at ordinary temperatures ortho-phenyl sulphuric acid, but by heating, the result is para-phenyl sulphuric acid. The two acids may be separated by fractional crystallization of their potassium or sodium salts, the para-salt separating out first in elongated hexagonal tables, which are anhydrous; the mother-liquor yields the ortho-salt in long colorless spicules containing two molecules of water. The two acids are not known in the free state. The sodium salt of the para-acid, when heated with manganese dioxide, and sulphuric acid yields *quinone;* the two potassium salts, when fused with excess of potash, yield different results, the ortho-salt giving *pyrocatechin,* and the para-salt *resorcin.*
Preparation.—By treating phenol with excess of strong sulphuric acid, and after about twenty-four hours diluting with water, then saturating the solution with barium carbonate, filtering and evaporating; the crystallized salt thus obtained is to be purified by crystallization from alcohol. The sulphocarbolate of barium is to be redissolved, treated with sodium carbonate or sulphate as long as a precipitate of the insoluble

22

barium sulphate or carbonate is produced, the precipitate filtered off and the filtrate evaporated.

Properties and Tests.—Sodium sulphocarbolate forms a white crystalline powder, or is in transparent, rhombic prisms. As the amount of water of crystallization varies according to the temperature at which the solution is evaporated and the degree of concentration, the anhydrous salt is to be used; this can be obtained by heating the crystals until their water is expelled and a dry white powder is left. Sulpho-carbolate of sodium is easily soluble in water and aqueous alcohol. The salt has a sharp taste and little or no odor.

A very dilute solution of the sulpho-carbolate is colored violet by treatment with ferric chloride (the salicylate gives a similar reaction).

Preparation for Homœopathic Use.—Pure sulphocarbolate of sodium is triturated as directed under Class VII.

NATRUM SULPHURICUM.

Synonyms, Sodium Sulphate. Sodæ Sulphas. Sodii Sulphas.

Common Names, Glauber's Salt. Sulphate of Soda.

Formula, $Na_2 S O_4, 10H_2O$.

Molecular Weight, 322.

Origin and Preparation of Sulphate of Sodium.—This salt occurs rather abundantly in nature, either anhydrous as *Thenardite*, crystallized in right rhombic prisms, or with ten molecules of water as Glauber's salt, in monoclinic prisms. It occurs more abundantly in combination with calcium sulphate as *Glauberite*; it is also found in sea-water, in the waters of most saline springs, and it exists in large quantity in many salt lakes in Russia. Sodium sulphate is prepared in enormous amount by the action of sulphuric acid on common salt, as a preliminary step in the manufacture of sodium carbonate and as a secondary product in many other chemical processes. It is purified by recrystallization.

Properties.—Pure sodium sulphate forms large, colorless, transparent, glistening, oblique rhombic or irregularly six-sided prisms, whose specific gravity is 1.35. They possess a cooling, bitter, saline taste, and in the air, especially in a warm place, they effloresce, becoming a white powder. At 30° C. (86° F.) they melt in their own water of crystallization, and at a higher temperature are rendered anhydrous by the loss of that water. Their behavior to solvents is remarkable. With increase of temperature their solubility increases in water to a certain limit, and decreases again if heated beyond that. The point of greatest solubility is 33° C. (91.4° F.), so that a saturated solution at this temperature will, if either further warmed or cooled, deposit some of the salt as crystals; at this maximum solubility one part of water will take up more than three of the salt.

Tests.—Pure sodium sulphate should be free from other salts, and its solution should undergo no change when treated with hydrogen or ammonium sulphide. In German pharmacy a trace of chloride is permissible, but the precipitate in watery solutions with silver nitrate should not be more than a mere opalescence. The solutions of the salt must be neutral to test-paper, and 100 grains of it dissolved in distilled water and acidulated with hydrochloric acid should give, by the addition of chloride of barium a white precipitate which, when washed and dried, weighs 72.2 grains.

Preparation for Homœopathic Use.—Pure sulphate of sodium is triturated as directed under Class VII.

NEPETA CATARIA, *Linn.*

Synonym, Cataria Vulgaris, *Mœnch.*

Nat. Ord., Labiatæ.

Common Names, Catnep. Catmint.

A perennial herb indigenous to Europe and Asia, but found widely spread in the United States as a common weed. Stem downy, erect, branched, square. Leaves opposite, on petioles, cordate, oblong, deeply crenate, from one to three inches long, whitish-downy beneath. Flowers in cymose clusters, many flowered, forming interrupted spikes or racemes. Corolla whitish, purple-dotted, hairy externally, lower lip crenately three-toothed; upper erect, concave, two-cleft. Stamens four, ascending under the upper lip, the lower pair shorter. The plant has a mint-like odor, but not so agreeable. Flowers from July to September.

Preparation.—The fresh leaves and flowering tops, gathered in June or July, are chopped and pounded to a pulp and weighed. Then two parts by weight of alcohol are taken, the pulp mixed thoroughly with one-sixth part of it, and the rest of the alcohol added. After having stirred the whole well, pour it into a well-stoppered bottle, and let it stand eight days in a dark, cool place. The tincture is then separated by decanting, straining and filtering.

Amount of drug power, $\frac{1}{6}$.

Dilutions must be prepared as directed under Class III.

NICCOLUM CARBONICUM.

Synonyms, Carbonate of Nickel. Nickel Carbonate.

Formula, $Ni\ CO_3$.

Preparation of Carbonate of Nickel.—Ten parts of nickel (commercial) are to be treated with eighty parts of pure nitric acid, specific gravity 1.185, so that a small portion of the metal remains undissolved. The solution after being filtered, is evaporated to dryness, heated to about 150° C. (302° F.), and the saline residue is to be dissolved in 120 parts of distilled water, filtered, and precipitated by a boiling solution of fifty parts of crystallized sodium carbonate. The precipitate is thrown upon a filter, well washed with warm water and treated with hydrochloric acid in considerable excess. The solution is now saturated with hydrogen sulphide, set aside for several hours, then filtered if necessary, and heated to boiling; then two parts of barium carbonate are to be added, the mixture repeatedly agitated and set aside for a day. It is then to be saturated with chlorine gas, filtered, and the filtrate treated with dilute sulphuric acid as long as any precipitate continues to fall. The fluid is again to be filtered and decomposed with a solution of about fifty parts of crystallized sodium carbonate, or as much as may be required to make the reaction of the liquid alkaline. The precipitate is collected on a filter, washed with hot water, and dried at a moderate temperature, and is to be preserved in a well-stoppered bottle. It is a pale, grayish-green, impalpable, nearly insipid powder.

Preparation for Homœopathic Use.—Carbonate of nickel is triturated as directed under Class VII.

NICCOLUM.

Synonyms, Niccolum Metallicum. Metallic Nickel.

Common Name, Nickel.

Symbol, Ni.

Atomic Weight, 58.8.

Origin and Preparation of Nickel.—Nickel is found in tolerable abundance in some of the metal-bearing veins of the Saxon mountains, in Westphalia, Hesse, Hungary and Sweden, chiefly as arsenide. the *kupfernickle* of mineralogists, so-called from its yellowish-red color. The word *nickle* is a term of detraction, having been applied by the old German miners to what was looked upon as a kind of false copper ore.

Nickel is easily prepared by exposing the oxalate to a high white heat, in a crucible lined with charcoal, or by reducing one of the oxides by means of hydrogen at a high temperature. It is a white, malleable metal, having a density of 8.8, a high melting point, and a less degree of oxidability than iron, since it is but little attacked by dilute acids. Nickel is strongly magnetic, but loses this property when heated to 350° F.

The metal was proven by Nenning, Germany.

Preparation for Homœopathic Use.—Nickel is triturated, as directed under Class VII.

NICCOLUM SULPHURICUM.

Synonyms, Nickel Sulphate. Niccoli Sulphas.

Common Name, Sulphate of Nickel.

Formula, $NiSO_4, 7H_2O$.

Preparation of Sulphate of Nickel.—This salt is formed by dissolving carbonate of nickel in dilute sulphuric acid, concentrating the solution and setting it aside to crystallize.

Properties and Tests.—The salt is in emerald-green, prismatic crystals, efflorescent in the air, soluble in three parts of cold water, but insoluble in alcohol and ether. It has a sweet, astringent taste. The solution gives a black precipitate with yellow sulphide of ammonium, slightly soluble in excess, forming a dark brown solution, and with caustic potash a pale green, bulky precipitate.

Preparation for Homœopathic Use.—Sulphate of nickel is triturated, as directed under Class VII.

NICOTINUM.

Synonyms, Nicotia. Nicotina. Nicotylia. Nicotin.
Common Name, Nicotine.
Formula, $C_{10}H_{14}N_2$.
Molecular Weight, 162.
Preparation.—Nicotine is a volatile alkaloid existing in the seeds and leaves of various kinds of tobacco, and of which it is the chief poisonous principle. It may be readily obtained by extraction of the leaves with dilute sulphuric acid and distilling the concentrated extract with potassium hydrate in excess. The distillate which contains the nicotine must be shaken up with ether, and the ether, after decantation, is to be distilled off. The residue of the distillation is odorless, limpid, and contains besides nicotine, water, ether and ammonia; a temperature of 140° C. (284° F.) maintained for twelve hours and assisted by a current of dry hydrogen suffices to expel these three bodies, so that when the temperature is raised subsequently to 180° C. (356° F.), the nicotine passes over pure and colorless.
Properties.—Nicotine is a colorless or slightly yellow, oily liquid, which completely volatilizes by heat. It is weakly hygroscopic, strongly alkaline, and has an odor which is disagreeable and tobacco-like, and its inhalation produces some stupefaction; its taste is sharp and burning. Its specific gravity at 15° C. (59° F.) is 1.027. When cooled to —10° C. (14° F.) it does not solidify, between 150° and 200° C. (302° to 392° F.) it distils over unchanged, and at 240° C. (464° F.) it boils and suffers partial decomposition. It is readily soluble in water, alcohol and ether, and with difficulty in chloroform and carbon disulphide. When exposed to the air it becomes gradually brownish in color and viscid.
Preparation for Homœopathic Use.—One part by weight of pure nicotin is dissolved in ninety-nine parts by weight of alcohol.
Amount of drug power, $\frac{1}{100}$.
Dilutions must be prepared as directed under Class VI—β.

NIGELLA DAMASCENA, *Linn.*

Nat. Ord., Ranunculaceæ.
Common Names, Fennel Flower. Ragged Lady.
This is an annual plant found growing in Southern Europe and Eastern countries bordering on the Mediterranean. Leaves twice and and thrice pinnatifid, resembling those of fennel. Fruit a capsule, five follicled; seeds numerous. The seeds are dull black externally, one-tenth of an inch in length, wrinkled and ovate-triangular. When bruised the seeds emit the odor of strawberries.
Preparation.—The ripe seeds are coarsely powdered, covered with five parts by weight of alcohol, and allowed to remain eight days in

a well-stoppered bottle, in a dark, cool place, being shaken twice a day. The tincture is then poured off, strained and filtered.

Amount of drug power, $\frac{1}{10}$.

Dilutions must be prepared as directed under Class IV.

NITRI SPIRITUS DULCIS.

Synonyms, Spiritus Ætheris Nitrosi. Naphtha Nitri.

Common Name, Sweet Spirits of Nitre.

Preparation.—The officinal (German) spiritus ætheris nitrosi of the pharmacopœia may be prepared by placing in a roomy glass retort 100 parts of 90 per cent. alcohol, adding thereto 25 parts of pure nitric acid, specific gravity 1.185, and distilling the mixture on a water-bath, raising the temperature gradually until 84 parts have come over.

The distillate is to be well shaken with magnesia in order to neutralize any free acid, set aside for a day and is then to be decanted and rectified on a water-bath.

Properties.—Sweet spirit of nitre is a transparent, perfectly volatile, colorless or faintly yellow, inflammable fluid, whose reaction is neutral or slightly acid. It has an agreeable, ethereal, apple-like odor and a sweetish, warm, ethereal taste. Its specific gravity is from 0.840 to 0.850. Exposed to the atmosphere and light, and in contact with water, it decomposes with the production of acetic acid, free nitric acid and the lower oxides of nitrogen. The preparation of the Pharmacopœia Germanica contains more aldehyde than that made after the formula of the United States Pharmacopœia.

It was first proven by Lembke, Germany.

Preparation for Homœopathic Use.—One part by weight of the spirits of nitrous ether is dissolved in nine parts by weight of alcohol.

Amount of drug power, $\frac{1}{10}$.

Dilutions must be prepared as directed under Class VI—*a*.

NUCIS VOMICÆ CORTEX.

Bark of Strychnos Nux Vomica, *Linn.*

Preparation.—The dried bark, coarsely powdered, is covered with five parts by weight of alcohol, and allowed to remain eight days in a well-stoppered bottle, in a dark, cool place, being shaken twice a day. The tincture is then poured off, strained and filtered.

Amount of drug power, $\frac{1}{10}$.

Dilutions must be prepared as directed under Class IV.

NUPHAR LUTEUM, *Smith.*

Synonym, Nymphæa Lutea, *Linn.*

Nat. Ord., Nymphæaceæ.

Common Name, Small Yellow Pond Lily.

This species is a native of Europe, and is also found at Manayunk, a suburb of Philadelphia. The earlier and submersed leaves are very thin and roundish, the floating ones oval, generally with a narrow or closed sinus. Sepals five, nearly equal; petals longer than the sepals and dilated upwards; stigma twelve to sixteen-rayed; fruit globular, with a short narrow neck. The expanded flower measures about two inches across.

It was first proven by Dr. Pitet, France.

Preparation.—The fresh root is chopped and pounded to a pulp and weighed. Then two parts by weight of alcohol are taken, the pulp mixed thoroughly with one-sixth part of it, and the rest of the alcohol added. After having stirred the whole well, it is put into a well-stoppered bottle, and allowed to stand eight days, in a dark, cool place. The tincture is then separated by decanting, straining and filtering.

Drug power of tincture, ½.

Dilutions must be prepared as directed under Class III.

NUX MOSCHATA.

Synonyms, Myristica Moschata, *Thunberg.* Nuces Aromaticæ. Nux Myristica.

Nat. Ord., Myristicaceæ.

Common Name, Nutmeg.

The nutmeg tree is a native of the Molucca Isles, and is now cultivated in the Eastern Archipelago, as well as in India, the West Indies and South America. The tree is much branched, has alternate short-petiolate leaves, which are oval-oblong, pointed, smooth and entire. The flowers are diœcious, small and yellow, the male ones in axillary peduncled clusters, the female solitary, its ovary ripening into a roundish-oval, one-seeded berry. The pericarp and aril are removed and the nut-like seed is carefully dried either by the sun or over a slow fire. After drying, the investing shell is removed and the kernel or nutmeg is fit for export. The nutmeg is so well known that it does not require description.

The drug was first proven by Dr. Helbig, Germany.

Preparation.—The dried nutmeg is coarsely powdered, covered with five parts by weight of alcohol, and the whole poured into a well-stoppered bottle, where it is allowed to remain eight days in a dark, cool place, being shaken twice a day. The tincture is then poured off, strained and filtered.

Drug power of tincture, $\frac{1}{10}$.

Dilutions must be prepared as directed under Class IV.

NUX VOMICA.

Synonym, Strychnos Nux Vomica, *Linn.*

Nat. Ord., Loganiaceæ.

Common Names, Poison Nut. Quaker Buttons.

The tree is of moderate size, indigenous to most of India, and is also found in Burmah, Siam, Cochin China and Northern Australia.

Its trunk is short, thick and at times crooked. Leaves opposite, ovate, shining, from three to five-veined. Flowers whitish, infundibuliform, in terminal, small, paniculate cymes. The fruit is an indehiscent berry, in size and shape like a small orange; it is filled with a white gelatinous, bitter pulp, in which from one to five seeds are placed vertically in an irregular manner. The pulp and probably all parts of the plant contain strychnia. Nux vomica is the seed removed from its thin, somewhat hard, shell or epicarp. It is disk-like, irregularly circular, a little less than an inch in diameter, about a quarter of an inch thick, concave on the dorsal side, flat or convex on the other, and its margin is often broadened and thickened so that the central portion appears depressed. The outside edge is generally ridged or keeled. The seeds are of a light gray color, and have a satiny lustre from their being thickly covered with fine, radiating, appressed hairs. Beneath the hairy covering is a thin brown testa enclosing a yellowish-gray, translucent, horn-like and hard albumen, which, upon softening with water, splits into two parts by a fissure in which lies the embryo. The latter is about three-tenths of an inch long, with two delicate heart-shaped cotyledons and a club-shaped radicle.

It was first proven by Hahnemann.

Preparation.—One part of finely-pulverized seed of nux vomica is covered with five parts by weight of alcohol, and allowed to remain eight days in a well-stoppered bottle, in a dark, cool place, being shaken twice a day. The tincture is then poured off, strained and filtered.

Amount of drug power, $\frac{1}{10}$.

Dilutions must be prepared as directed under Class IV.

Triturations are prepared as directed under Class VII.

NYMPHÆA ODORATA *Aiton.*

Synonyms, Castalia Pudica. Nymphæa Alba.

Nat. Ord., Nymphæaceæ.

Common Names, Sweet-scented Water-Lily. Water Nymph. White Pond Lily.

This plant, found growing in ponds and in still or sluggish waters, is common eastward and southward in the United States. Leaves five to nine inches wide, orbicular, deeply cordate at the base, entire; stipules nearly reniform, notched at the apex, appressed to the rootstock; flowers white, very fragrant (often five and one-half inches in diameter when fully expanded, opening early in the morning, closing in the afternoon); petals obtuse; aril much longer than the stipitate oblong seeds. Sepals four, green outside, nearly free. Petals numerous, in many rows, the innermost gradually transformed into stamens, imbricately inserted all over the surface of the ovary. Stamens indefinite, inserted on the ovary, the outer with dilated filaments. Ovary eighteen to thirty-celled, the summit tipped with a globular projection at the centre, around which are the radiate stigmas. Fruit depressed-globular, covered with the bases of the decayed petals, maturing under water.

It was first proven by Dr. Edwin Cowles, U. S.

Preparation.—The fresh root is chopped and pounded to a pulp and weighed. Then two parts by weight of alcohol are taken, the pulp mixed thoroughly with one-sixth part of it, and the rest of the alcohol added. After having stirred the whole well, and having poured it into a well-stoppered bottle, it is allowed to stand eight days in a dark, cool place. The tincture is then separated by decanting, straining and filtering.

Drug power of tincture, $\frac{1}{6}$.

Dilutions must be prepared as directed under Class III.

OCIMUM CANUM, *DeCandolle.*

Synonym, (in Brazil) Alfavaca.

Nat. Ord., Labiatæ.

Common Name, Hoary Basil.

This is an herbaceous plant, having an aromatic odor, with an erect and ramose stem about sixteen or twenty inches high; it is pubescent, quadrangular, and grooved towards the upper branches. Leaves opposite, oval, finely indented, on petioles of the same length as the limbs of the leaves. Flowers whorled, forming terminal spikes; each whorl is provided with two foliaceous bracts. Calyx with five divisions, the upper being oval, large and entire; the other four are sharp and inferior. Corolla tubular, inverted, with a bilabiate limb; the upper lip divided into four lobes; the lower lip composed of a single lobe, which is longer. Stamens four, with free and outward-bent filaments, and two other stamens, which are shorter and somewhat geniculate at their base; style filiform and bifid. Root vertical, fibrous, rather ramose. This plant is a native of Brazil.

It was introduced into our Materia Medica by Dr. Mure, Brazil.

Preparation.—The fresh leaves are chopped and pounded to a pulp and weighed. Then two parts by weight of alcohol are taken, the pulp thoroughly mixed with one-sixth part of it, and the rest of the alcohol added. After having stirred the whole well, it is poured into a well-stoppered bottle, and allowed to stand eight days in a dark, cool place. The tincture is then separated by decanting, straining and filtering.

Drug power of tincture, $\frac{1}{6}$.

Dilutions must be prepared as directed under Class III.

ŒNANTHE.

Synonyms, Œnanthe Crocata, *Linn.* Œnanthe Apiifolia.

Nat. Ord., Umbelliferæ.

Common Names, Water-Hemlock. Water-Dropwort. Water Lovage. Dead Tongue.

This plant is indigenous to England, Sweden, France and Spain, growing in moist places and swamps. It is a stout, branched species, attaining three to five feet, the root-fibres forming thick, elongated tubers close to the stock; the juice, both of the stem and roots becoming yellow when exposed to the air. Leaves twice or thrice pinnate, the segments always above half an inch long, broadly crenate or rounded, and deeply cut into three or five lobes. Umbels on long terminal peduncles, with fifteen to twenty rays, two inches long or more; the bracts of the involucres small and linear, several in the partial ones, few or none under the general umbel. The pedicellate flowers at the circumference of the partial umbels are mostly, but not always barren, the central fertile ones almost sessile. Fruit somewhat corky, the ribs broad and scarcely prominent.

Preparation.—The fresh root, gathered at the time of blooming, is chopped and pounded to a pulp and weighed. Then two parts by weight of alcohol are taken, and having thoroughly mixed the pulp with one-sixth part of it, the rest of the alcohol is added. After having stirred the whole well, it is poured into a well-stoppered bottle and allowed to stand eight days in a dark, cool place. The tincture is then separated by decanting, straining and filtering.

Drug power of tincture, $\frac{1}{6}$.

Dilutions must be prepared as directed under Class III.

ŒNOTHERA BIENNIS, *Linn.*

Synonyms, Œnothera Gauroides. Œnothera Parviflora. Onagra Biennis. Onosuris Acuminata.

Nat. Ord., Onagraceæ.

Common Names, Evening Primrose. Scabish. Tree Primrose.

This indigenous plant of which there are several varieties, is commonly found in fields and waste places. It has an erect, hairy, simple stem, two to five feet high and often purplish in color. Leaves ovate-lanceolate, nearly entire, sessile on the stem, the radical ones being petiolate, all roughly pubescent. Flowers in a terminal, leafy spike, calyx tubular, adherent to the ovary; petals four, obcordate, yellow. Fruit a four-celled capsule containing numerous seeds.

Preparation.—The fresh plant, gathered when coming into flower, is chopped and pounded to a pulp and weighed. Then two parts by weight of alcohol are taken, the pulp mixed thoroughly with one-sixth part of it, and the rest of the alcohol added. After having stirred the whole well, pour it into a well-stoppered bottle, and let it stand eight days in a dark, cool place. The tincture is then separated by decanting, straining and filtering.

Drug power of tincture, $\frac{1}{6}$.

Dilutions must be prepared as directed under Class III.

OLEANDER.

Synonyms, Nerium Oleander, *Linn.* Nerium Album. Nerium Variegatum.

Nat. Ord., Apocynaceæ.

Common Names, Oleander. Rose-bay. Rose-laurel.

This shrub is common in Southern Europe, Arabia and Northern Africa. It is cultivated elsewhere as an ornamental plant. It grows to a height of ten or fifteen feet. Stem and branches covered with a nearly smooth, grayish bark. Leaves lanceolate, acute at each end, whorled in threes, short-petiolate, smooth, entire, coriaceous, fine-pointed at apex, with prominent transverse veins beneath. Flowers large, rose-colored, in terminal corymbs.

The drug was first proven by Hahnemann.

Preparation.—The fresh leaves, gathered when the plant is coming into bloom, are chopped and pounded to a pulp and weighed. Then take two-thirds by weight of alcohol, add it to the pulp, stir and mix well together, and strain *lege artis* through a piece of new linen. The tincture thus obtained is allowed to stand eight days in a well-stoppered bottle, in a dark, cool place and then filtered.

Drug power of tincture, $\frac{1}{2}$.

Dilutions must be prepared as directed under Class II.

OLEUM ANIMALE ÆTHEREUM.

Synonyms, Oleum Animale Dippelii. Oleum Cornu Cervi.

Common Names, Animal Oil. Dippel's Animal Oil.

Preparation of Animal Oil.—This oil is obtained in large quantity in the preparation of bone-black. Similar products are obtained by the dry distillation of other animal substances. The original Dippel's oil known in pharmacy was produced from stag's horn. Dippel, an apothecary of the seventeenth century, prepared the oil bearing his name from crude fetid animal oil, *ol. cornu cervi fœtidum*, by submitting the latter to repeated rectification alone, until it no longer left any black residue. The oil thus obtained is colorless, highly refractive, has a not unpleasant odor, somewhat like that of cinnamon, and a burning taste with a sweetish after-taste like a mixture of pepper and cinnamon; its specific gravity is 0.865. When kept for some time it turns yellow, especially if exposed to light.

Nearly all the animal oil of commerce is now obtained by the destructive distillation of bones in the manufacture of lamp-black, and the crude product is generally purified by rectifying it with the addition of sand, lime or water. That which is rectified with water is very mobile, has a pungent, disagreeable, smoky, ethereal odor and an acrid, pungent taste, followed by a cool and bitter one. Its specific gravity is about 0.75. It is soluble in eighty parts of water, easily in alcohol and in the fatty and ethereal oils. On submitting it to fractional distillation a number of bases are obtained from it, among which are *pyridine, picoline, lutidine* and *collidine*, together with amines of methyl, propyl, butyl, etc.

It was first proven by Nenning, Germany.

Preparation for Homœopathic Use.—Animal oil is triturated as directed under Class VIII. Or, one part by weight of animal oil is dissolved in nine parts by weight of alcohol.

Amount of drug power, $\frac{1}{10}$.

Dilutions must be prepared as directed under Class VI—*a*.

OLEUM CAJUPUTI.

Synonym, Cajuputum.
Nat. Ord., Myrtaceæ.
Common Names, Oil of Cajuput. Oil of Cajeput. Kayu-puti (white wood).

This is a volatile oil obtained from the leaves of Melaleuca Cajuputi, *Roxburgh* (seu M. Minor, *Smith*).

Origin.—The tree is, according to Bentham, a variety of *M. Leucadendron, Linn.*, widely spread and abundant in the Indian Archipelago and the Malayan Peninsula, and also in Australia.. The tree is small, with entire lance-shaped leaves, and small, white flowers in terminal spikes.

Preparation.—The leaves are submitted to distillation with water, the process being conducted in a very primitive manner.

Properties.—Oil of cajeput is a transparent, mobile fluid, of a clear green color. Its odor is fragrant and camphor-like, and the taste bitterish, aromatic and somewhat camphoraceous; both odor and taste are similar to the flavor of cardamon and rosemary. Its specific gravity is from 0.91 to 0.94. It can be cooled to —13° C. (8.6° F.) without solidifying. It dissolves iodine, at times with the production of reddish vapor. When treated with sulphuric acid it becomes brown in color, the tint changing afterwards to purplish-brown. As the green tint of the oil is due to copper, the color may be discharged by treating the oil with dilute HCl.

It was proved by Dr. C. Ruden, U. S.

Preparation for Homœopathic Use.—One part by weight of oil of cajeput is dissolved in ninety-nine parts by weight of strong (95 per cent.) alcohol.

Amount of drug power, $\frac{1}{100}$.

Dilutions must be prepared as directed under Class VI—β.

OLEUM JECORIS ASELLI.

Synonyms, Oleum Morrhuæ. Oleum Hepatis Morrhuæ.
Class, Pisces.
Order, Teleostia.
Family, Gadida.
Common Names, Cod-Liver Oil. Cod Oil.

This is a fatty oil obtained from the liver of *Gadus Morrhua, L.* and of allied species.

The well-known cod-fish, G. Morrhua, is an inhabitant of the North Atlantic on the banks of Newfoundland, and in their neighborhood. In the same waters are found the *hake* and *haddock*, both species of Gadus, whose livers also furnish the oil. On the coast of Norway the species chiefly used for the purpose is G. Callarius, called *dorse*, but the *coal-fish*, G. Carbonarius, is another source of the oil. The mode of preparation varies in different localities.

On the North American coast, the livers are subjected to gradually increasing heat, which causes the oil to exude from the tissues, and by mechanical separation and filtering, the oil is obtained very pure. In Norway and the neighboring islands the process is conducted in a more primitive and less cleanly manner. The livers are placed in barrels or baskets and kept in a sunny locality, the oil slowly separating out. Sometimes steam is used or the livers are boiled with water, and the oil is removed by skimming.

Properties.—The best cod-liver oil is of a pale yellow color, almost without taste, the fishy flavor being in this kind at its minimum. When prepared at too high a temperature, or when decomposition has set up in the livers, the color is darker, until in some specimens it is a reddish-brown. In the latter case the fishy taste and smell are well marked, and the oil has a decidedly acid reaction; in the pale oil the acid reaction is faint. The specific gravity is nearly alike in the two kinds, the lowest (pale), being about 0.92, the highest (brown), 0.93. Alcohol in the cold will take up about 6 per cent. of the dark brown variety, while it will not dissolve out more than 2.5 per cent. of the pale. Owing to the presence of biliary matters, the addition of sulphuric acid causes a violet coloration, soon changing to brownish-red.

It was first proven by Dr. C. Neidhard, U. S.

Preparation for Homœopathic Use.—Cod-liver oil is triturated, as directed under Class VIII.

OLEUM LIGNI SANTALI.

Synonyms, Oleum Santalum Album. Oleum Santalum Citrinum.

Nat. Ord., Santalaceæ.

Common Name, Oil of Sandal-Wood.

An oil obtained from the wood of Santalum Album, *Linn.*

Origin.—The sandal tree is indigenous to mountainous parts of the Indian Peninsula, and is also found in the islands of the Eastern Archipelago. It grows in dry and open situations, not in forests. The tree attains a height of from twenty to thirty feet, and its trunk is from a foot and a half to three feet in circumference. The tree is felled and the trunk allowed to lie on the ground for several months, in which time most of the inodorous sap-wood is eaten away by ants. The heart-wood only is used, and when distilled yields, even with very rude and imperfect apparatus, from two to five per cent. of the essential oil.

Properties.—The oil is a light yellow, thick liquid, having a characteristic agreeable and aromatic odor and a bitter somewhat acrid taste. Its specific gravity is 0.96; it begins to boil at about 214° C. (417.2° F.).

Preparation for Homœopathic Use.—One part by weight of oil of sandal-wood is dissolved in ninety-nine parts by weight of alcohol.

Amount of drug power, $\frac{1}{100}$.

Dilutions must be prepared as directed under Class VI—β.

Triturations are prepared as directed under Class VIII.

OLEUM RICINI.

Synonyms, Oleum Palmæ Christi. Ricinus Communis. Ricinus Lævis. Ricinus Virdis.

Nad. Ord., Euphorbiaceæ

Common Name, Castor Oil.

A fixed oil from the seeds of Ricinus Communis, *Linn.*

The castor oil plant is a native of India, but is largely cultivated throughout the world. In the United States all or nearly all the castor oil used in the country is the product of home cultivation. In its native habitat it is a tree, but in the Northern States of America it is an annual herbaceous plant, in the Southern a good-sized shrub. The fruit is a tri-coccous capsule, containing one seed in each of its three cells.

Preparation.—The oil is obtained from the seeds by subjecting them to great pressure after the integuments have been removed. When the marc is again pressed with the aid of heat, a second yield of the oil is obtained but it is of inferior quality. The cold-pressed oil is nearly transparent and of a pale yellow tint. It has a faint, mawkish taste and odor and is somewhat viscid. Its specific gravity is about 0.96. It does not solidify until cooled to —18° C. (about 0° F.). When exposed in thin layers it dries up to a varnish-like film. It is distinguished by its property of mixing in all proportions with glacial acetic acid or absolute alcohol. It begins to boil at about 265° C. (509° F.).

Preparation for Homœopathic Use.—One part by weight of castor oil is dissolved in ninety-nine parts by weight of alcohol.

Amount of drug power, $\frac{1}{100}$.

Dilutions must be prepared as directed under Class VI—β.

ONISCUS ASELLUS

Class, Insecta.

Order, Crustacea.

Family, Oniscidæ Isopoda.

Common Names, Common Wood-louse. Sow-Bug.

This little animal is from three to six lines long; it has fourteen feet, four antennæ, of which two are short and almost entirely concealed; the others setaceous, bent, having five or six joints; its body is oval, covered with many crustaceous pieces, transverse, sub-imbricated, and provided at the extremity with two short and very simple appendages. The color is gray, more or less deep, verging on blue or brown, with yellowish streaks or spots. The oniscus is found in cellars, under stones, in humid places, and seems to shun the light; when touched it rolls up in a ball; the taste is sweetish, nauseous; the odor disagreeable, ammoniacal. The *Oniscus asellus* should not be confounded with the *Oniscus armadillo, Linn.*, which has several feet and no bifid tail.

It was first proven by Dr. Hering.

Preparation.—The live animals are crushed and covered with five parts by weight of alcohol, and the mixture allowed to remain eight days in a well-stoppered bottle, in a dark, cool place, being shaken twice a day. The tincture is then poured off, strained and filtered.

Drug power of tincture, $\frac{1}{10}$.

Dilutions must be prepared as directed under Class IV

OLIBANUM.

Nat. Ord., Burseraceæ.

Common Names, Gum Olibanum. Frankincense.

From several species of Boswellia.

Origin.—The different species of Boswellia, from whose stems olibanum is obtained, are not well known. Those furnishing the drug inhabit the hot, dry regions of Eastern Africa. Frankincense has been known since the earliest times, and was held by the ancients to be of great value. The fragrant gum resin is distributed through the leaves and bark of the tree, and, it is said, even exudes as milky juice from the flowers.

Collection.—Longitudinal incisions are made in the bark at the season when the intumescence of the parts beneath is evidenced by the glistening of the cuticle. The gum pours forth at first white as milk, and as it hardens by exposure to the air is suffered to accumulate below the incision or on the ground, to be collected afterwards by the gatherers.

Properties.—The olibanum of commerce varies very much in quality and appearance. It may, however, be described as a dry gum-resin consisting of detached tears of all sizes up to an inch in length, and roundish, oblong or irregular in shape. The color varies from pale yellow to reddish. Their fracture is waxy. The gum-resin softens in the mouth, has a taste resembling somewhat that of turpentine with slight bitterness added; its odor is terebinthinate and balsamic. When heated it softens, burns, and diffuses an agreeable aromatic odor. When rubbed up in a mortar with water it gives a white emulsion. It dissolves almost completely in alcohol.

Preparation for Homœopathic Use.—Pure olibanum is triturated as directed under Class VII.

ONONIS SPINOSA, *Linn.*

Synonyms, Remora Alopecuroides. Remora Aratum. Remora Urinaria. Resta Bovis.

Nat. Ord., Leguminosæ.

Common Name, Common Rest-harrow.

This perennial vegetable is found all over Europe, where it grows in uncultivated fields, dry pasturages, along roads, hedges, etc. The root is as thick as the finger, branchy, descending into the ground two feet or more, reddish-brown externally, whitish internally, of a sweetish-slimy and somewhat acrid-bitter taste; stem recumbent below, erect above, round, ligneous, branchy, spiny; leaves petiolate, sparse, ovoid, serrate, hairy on both sides, the lower ternate, the upper undivided; flowers solitary, axillary, with short peduncles, of a pale purplish color or with rosy veins.

Preparation.—The fresh plant, gathered when beginning to flower, is chopped and pounded to a pulp and weighed. Then two parts by weight of alcohol are taken, the pulp mixed thoroughly with one-sixth part of it, and the rest of the alcohol added. After having stirred the whole well, pour it into a well-stoppered bottle, and let it stand eight days in a dark, cool place. The tincture is then separated by decanting, straining and filtering.

Drug power of tincture, $\frac{1}{6}$.

Dilutions must be prepared as directed under Class III.

OPIUM.

Synonym, Papaver Somniferum, *Linn.*

Nat. Ord., Papaveraceæ.

Common Names, Opium. White Poppy. Succus Thebaicus.

This widely known and extensively cultivated plant is believed to be a native of Asia. It was cultivated by the ancients, and in the present day its product is largely exported from the Levant, India, Persia and other Asiatic countries.

The white poppy is an annual herbaceous plant, often reaching a height of three feet and sometimes more. Its stem is glabrous, glaucous, leaves large, clasping, cut-dentate and alternate; flowers brilliantly white, large and terminal; capsule globose, two to four inches in diameter, containing numerous white seeds. The whole plant abounds in a milky juice, which exudes when any part of the plant is wounded but is most abundant in the capsules. The plant flowers, in Asia Minor, between May and July, according to the elevation of the land. A few days after the fall of the petals, the capsule, then about an inch and a half in diameter, is ready for incision, which is made with a knife, transversely about half way up, extending about two-thirds of the circumference and not deep enough to penetrate the parieties of the capsule. The incisions are done in the afternoon, as a rule, and the next morning are found covered with exuded juice. This is scraped off with a knife and transferred to a poppy leaf, which the gatherer holds in his left hand. Each poppy head is cut only once, but as the plant produces several heads, all of which are not of the proper age at the same time, the operation of incising and gathering has to be repeated two or three times in the same field. As soon as a sufficient quantity of the half-dried juice has been collected to form a cake or lump, it is wrapped in poppy leaves and put for a short time to dry in the shade.

Opium comes in commerce in brown cakes of a somewhat shining appearance externally; the interior is moist and coarsely granular, and varies in tint from light chestnut to blackish-brown. Its odor is peculiar, and is commonly described as narcotic and unpleasant; its taste is bitter.

The black opium from Smyrna is the strongest, and is the kind used for homœopathic preparations.

This drug was first proven by Hahnemann.

Preparation.—The gum opium, dried and powdered, is covered with five parts by weight of dilute alcohol, and allowed to remain eight days in a well-stoppered bottle, in a dark, cool place, being shaken twice a day. The tincture is then poured off, strained and filtered.

Drug power of tincture, $\frac{1}{10}$.

Dilutions must be prepared as directed under Class IV, except that dilute alcohol must be used for the 2x and 1 dilutions.

Triturations are prepared according to Class VII.

OPOPANAX.

Synonyms, Opopanax Chironium, *Koch.* Pastinaca Opopanax, *Linn.*

Nat. Ord., Umbelliferæ.

Common Name, Rough Parsnip.

This is a perennial plant indigenous to the eastern countries bordering on the Mediterranean, and now growing wild in Southern Europe. It has a long, thick, fleshy root, a tall branching stem, pinnatifid leaves with oblong, serrate leaflets, and small yellow flowers in terminal umbels. When the stem is wounded, a yellowish-milky juice exudes, which, upon being dried in the sun, is known in commerce as Opopanax.

Description.—Opopanax is in irregularly angular or sometimes almost globular masses, varying in size from that of a pea to that of a walnut; their color is, in general, yellowish-brown, white-speckled externally, and when broken they exhibit a waxy fracture. The odor is peculiar, strong and disagreeable, the taste bitter and acrid, and when heated the substance softens and emits a garlicky odor.

Preparation.—The gum-resin is powdered and covered with five parts by weight of alcohol, and allowed to remain eight days in a well-stoppered bottle, in a dark, cool place, being shaken twice a day. The tincture is then poured off, strained and filtered.

Drug power of tincture, $\frac{1}{10}$.

Dilutions must be prepared as directed under Class IV.

OPUNTIA VULGARIS, *Miller.*

Synonyms, Cactus Opuntia, *Linn.* Opuntia Humifusa.

Nat. Ord., Cactaceæ.

Common Names, Prickly Pear. Indian Fig.

This is a low, prostrate or creeping plant, pale, with flat ovate joints; the minute leaves ovate-subulate and appressed; the axils bristly, often with a few small spines; flowers large, sulphur-yellow, opening in sunshine for more than a day; berry nearly smooth, crimson, pulpy, eatable. It is found growing in sandy fields and rocky places, from Nantucket, Massachusetts, southward, usually near the coast. Its flowers appear in June.

The drug was introduced into our Materia Medica by Dr. S. P. Burdick, U. S.

Preparation.—The fresh twigs and flowers are chopped and pounded to a pulp and weighed. Then two parts by weight of alcohol are taken, the pulp mixed thoroughly with one-sixth part of it, and the rest of the alcohol added. After having stirred the whole well, pour it into a well-stoppered bottle, and let it stand eight days in a dark, cool place. The tincture is then separated by decanting, straining and filtering.

Drug power of tincture, $\frac{1}{6}$.

Dilutions must be prepared as directed under Class III.

OREOSELINUM.

Synonyms, Athamanta Oreoselinum, *Linn.* Peucedanum Oreoselinum. Apium Montanum.

Nat. Ord., Umbelliferæ.

Common Names, Mountain-Parsley. Speedwell. Galbanum.

This plant, occurring on loose meadows, hills and slopes nearly over all Europe, has a perennial root, almost simple, yellowish-gray, furnished with a cluster of brown fibres. Stem erect, with fine furrows, glabrous, not very branchy, from one to two feet high. Radical leaves petioled, large, tripinnate; leaflets oval, deeply indented, glabrous; the teeth terminate in white points. Corymbs terminal. Involucre consists of a number of lanceolate, revolute leaflets. Petals white. The ripe fruit is almost round, flat, with a broad, pale yellow border. The whole plant has an agreeable aromatic smell and taste, like common parsley.

Preparation.—The fresh plant, gathered shortly before it begins to flower, is chopped and pounded to a pulp and pressed out *lege artis* in a piece of new linen. The expressed juice is then, by brisk agitation, mingled with an equal part by weight of alcohol. The mixture is allowed to stand eight days in a well-stoppered bottle, in a dark, cool place and then filtered.

Drug power of tincture, $\frac{1}{2}$.

Dilutions must be prepared as directed under Class I.

ORIGANUM VULGARE, *Linn.*

Nat. Ord., Labiatæ.

Common Names, Common Marjoram. Mountain Mint. Organg.

This indigenous perennial plant is found growing in poor soils along roadsides and in fields. Its stem is erect, square, purplish and downy, twelve to eighteen inches high, and branching above. Leaves ovate, entire, on petioles, and hairy. Flowers nearly regular, purplish-white, spiked in paniculate corymbs. Corolla funnel-shaped, upper lip erect, lower with three nearly equal segments; stamens four, ascending. The plant has an agreeable aromatic odor and taste. Flowers from June to October.

This drug was proven by Dr. Cessoles, Rev. Hom. du Midi.

Preparation.—The fresh herb, in flower, is chopped and pounded to a pulp and weighed. Then two parts by weight of alcohol are taken, the pulp thoroughly mixed with one-sixth part of it, and the rest of the alcohol added. After having stirred the whole well, pour it into a well-stoppered bottle, and let it stand eight days in a dark, cool place. The tincture is then separated by decanting, straining and filtering.

Drug power of tincture, $\frac{1}{6}$.

Dilutions must be prepared as directed under Class III.

OROBANCHE VIRGINIANA, *Linn.*

Synonym, Epiphegus Americanus, *Nuttall.*

Nat. Ord., Orobancheæ.

Common Names, Beech-drop. Broom Rape. Cancer Root. Squaw Root.

This is a parasitic plant found growing in all parts of North America on the roots of the beech tree. From a ball of rigid, short, brittle rootlets arises a stem one foot high, entirely leafless, glabrous, dull red in color, branching, and flower-bearing in its whole length. The flowers are subsessile, alternate, and brownish-white in color. The plant has a nauseating, bitter, astringent taste.

Preparation.—The fresh plant is chopped and pounded to a pulp and weighed. Then two parts by weight of alcohol are taken, the pulp mixed thoroughly with one-sixth part of it, and the rest of the alcohol added. After having stirred the whole well, pour it into a well-stoppored bottle, and let it stand eight days in a dark, cool place. The tincture is then separated by decanting, straining and filtering.

Drug power of tincture, $\frac{1}{6}$.

Dilutions must be prepared as directed under Class III.

OSMIUM.

Symbol, Os.

Atomic Weight, 199.

Origin and Preparation of Osmium.—The separation of this metal from iridium, ruthenium, and the other metals with which it is associated in native osmiridium, and in platinum residues, depends chiefly on its ready oxidation by nitric or nitro-muriatic acid or by ignition in air or oxygen, and the volatility of the oxide thus produced. To prepare metallic osmium, the solution obtained by condensing the vapor of osmium tetroxide in potash is mixed with excess of hydrochloric acid, and digested with mercury in a well-closed bottle at 40° C. (104° F.). The osmium is then reduced by the mercury, and an amalgam is formed, which, when distilled in a stream of hydrogen till all the mercury and calomel are expelled, leaves metallic osmium in the form of a black powder (Berzelius). The metal may also be obtained by igniting ammonium chloro-osmite with sal-ammoniac.

Properties.—The properties of osmium vary according to its mode of preparation. In the pulverulent state it is black, destitute of metallic lustre, which, however, it acquires by burnishing; in the compact state, as obtained by Berzelius' method above described, it exhibits metallic lustre, and has a density of 10. Deville and Debray, by igniting precipitated osmium sulphide in a crucible of gas-coke, at the melting heat of nickel, obtained it in bluish-black, easily divisible lumps. When heated to the melting point of rhodium, it becomes more compact, and acquires a density of 21.3 to 21.4. At a still higher temperature, capable of melting ruthenium and iridium, and volatilizing platinum, osmium likewise volatilizes, but still does not melt; in fact, it is the most refractory of all metals.

Osmium in the finely divided state is highly combustible, continuing to burn when set on fire, till it is all volatilized as tetroxide. In this state also it is easily oxidized by nitric or nitro-muriatic acid, being converted into tetroxide. But after exposure to red heat, it becomes less combustible, and is not oxidized by nitric or nitro-muriatic acid. Osmium which has been heated to the melting point of rhodium, does not give off any vapor of tetroxide when heated in the air to the melting point of zinc, but takes fire at higher temperatures.

Osmium was introduced into our Materia Medica by Dr. Bojanus, Russia.

Preparation for Homœopathic Use.—Osmium is triturated as directed under Class VII.

OSTRYA VIRGINICA, *Willd.*

Nat. Ord., Cupuliferæ.

Common Names, Hop-Hornbeam. Iron Wood. Lever Wood.

This small tree is spread throughout the United States. It is from 25 to 30 feet high; the bark is brownish, and finely furrowed longitudinally. Leaves oblong-ovate, tapering, twice serrate, downy beneath; buds rather acute. Fertile aments oblong, pendulous. Fruit similar in appearance to hops, consisting of membranous imbricated sacs. The wood is very white and hard, and because of its strength, is much used for making levers, etc.

It was first proven by Dr. W. H. Burt, U. S.

Preparation.—The heart-wood, in coarse powder, is covered with five parts by weight of alcohol, and allowed to remain eight days in a well-stoppered bottle, in a dark, cool place, being shaken twice a day. The tincture is then poured off, strained and filtered.

Drug power of tincture, $\frac{1}{10}$.

Dilutions must be prepared as directed under Class IV.

OXYDENDRUM.

Synonyms, Oxydendrum Arboreum, *DC.* Andromeda Arborea, *Linn.*

Common Names, Sorrel Tree. Sour-Wood.

This tree is found growing in the Middle States and southward along the Alleghanies, and often reaches a height of forty feet. Leaves like those of the peach in size and shape, four to five inches long, deciduous, oblong-lanceolate, acuminate, villous when young, on petioles.

Flowers white, panicled in slender spicate racemes. Calyx of five nearly distinct sepals; corolla urn-shaped, ovate, five toothed. Fruit an oblong pyramidal pod, five-celled and five-valved, many seeded. The foliage is acid to the taste.

Preparation.—The fresh leaves are chopped and pounded to a pulp and weighed. Then two parts by weight of alcohol are taken, and after thoroughly mixing the pulp with one-sixth part of it, the rest of the alcohol is added. After having stirred the whole well, and poured it into a well-stoppered bottle, it is allowed to stand eight days in a dark, cool place. The tincture is then separated by decanting, straining and filtering.

Drug power of tincture, $\frac{1}{6}$.

Dilutions must be prepared as directed under Class III.

PÆONIA OFFICINALIS, *Linn.*

Synonym, Rosa Benedicta.

Nat. Ord., Ranunculaceæ.

Common Name, Peony.

This perennial ornamental plant is said to be a native of Europe. It has a fasciculate, many headed root-stock, which is dark brown externally, and white and granular within. The stem is branched, two feet high, leaves bi-and tri-pinnately divided, green, smooth and shining; leaflets ovate-lanceolate, variously incised. Flowers large, terminal; sepals five; petals five to eight; stamens numerous; ovaries two to five. Petals are obovate, either entire or crenate. Flowers are purple-red, although there are varieties white, pink or flesh-colored.

It was first proven by Dr. Geyer, Germany.

Preparation.—The fresh root, gathered in spring, is chopped and pounded to a pulp, and pressed out *lege artis* in a piece of new linen. The expressed juice is then, by brisk agitation, mingled with an equal part by weight of alcohol. This mixture is allowed to stand eight days in a well-stoppered bottle, in a dark, cool place, and filtered.

Amount of drug power, $\frac{1}{2}$.

Dilutions must be prepared as directed under Class I.

PALLADIUM.

Symbol, Pd.

Atomic Weight, 106.

Preparation of Palladium.—When the solution of crude platinum, from which the greater part of that metal has been precipitated by sal-ammoniac, is neutralized by sodium carbonate, and mixed with a solution of mercuric cyanide, palladium cyanide separates as a whitish, insoluble substance, which, on being washed, dried and heated to redness, yields metallic palladium in a spongy state. The palladium may then be welded into a mass, in the same manner as platinum.

Properties.—Palladium closely resembles platinum in color and appearance; it is also very malleable and ductile. Its density, however, differs very much from that of platinum, being only 11.8, and it is more oxidizable. When heated to redness in the air, especially in the state of sponge, it acquires a blue or purple superficial film of oxide, which is again reduced at a white heat. This metal is slowly attacked by nitric acid; its best solvent is nitro-muriatic acid.

Palladium was proven by Dr. Hering.

Preparation for Homœopathic Use.—Palladium is triturated as directed under Class VII.

PANACEA ARVENSIS.

Common Name, Poorman's Mercury.

This is a tree exceedingly common in Brazil, where it is known as *azougue dos pobres* (mercury of the poor), *cabedula* and *erva carnevra.*

Introduced into our Materia Medica by Dr. Mure, Brazil.

Preparation.—The fresh leaves are chopped and pounded to a pulp and weighed. Then two parts by weight of alcohol are taken, the pulp mixed thoroughly with one-sixth part of it, and the rest of the alcohol added. After having stirred the whole well, pour it into a well-stoppered bottle, and let it stand eight days in a dark, cool place. The tincture is then separated by decanting, straining and filtering.

Amount of drug power, $\frac{1}{6}$.

Dilutions must be prepared as directed under Class III.

PANCREATINUM.

Synonym, Pancreatin.

The pancreas is a large gland, situated deep within the abdominal cavity, and whose function consists in the elaboration of a secretion known as the pancreatic juice. The pancreatic juice has the triple property of acting on starch, whether in the raw or boiled state, with great energy, rapidly converting it into grape sugar; of exercising a solvent action upon proteids similar to the action of the gastric juice upon the same bodies, in so far that by it proteids are converted into peptones; and on fats it has a two-fold action in emulsifying them and splitting up neutral fats into their respective acids and glycerine. The active principle is a nitrogenous ferment called *pancreatin.*

Preparation.—Prof. Scheffer's method, as given in 1875, is as follows: Fresh and finely chopped beef pancreas is macerated for a day in water acidulated with a little hydrochloric acid; the maceration is repeated with water, the strained liquids filtered, neutralized with calcium carbonate, again filtered, and mixed with an equal volume of 95 per cent. alcohol; the precipitate is washed with dilute alcohol, pressed between bibulous paper, and dried at the ordinary temperature.

Properties.—Pancreatin prepared after Scheffer's formula is a yellow transparent mass, which is quite brittle, and looks like albumen dried after solution. It dissolves slowly in water, but not quite completely, and gives a pale yellow solution which is transparent, and neutral to test-paper. It is precipitated by alcohol and by heating, and also by hydrochloric acid; it remains clear when treated with a saturated solution of sodium chloride.

Preparation.—Pure pancreatin is triturated, as directed under Class VII.

PARAFFIN.

Synonym, Paraffinum.

Origin.—The colorless, crystalline, fatty substance known by the name of paraffin is the solid portion of the mixture of oily hydrocarbons, produced together with other substances when various organic bodies are destructively distilled at temperatures not exceeding a low red heat. It also exists as a constituent of many varieties of petroleum, associated with liquid hydrocarbons similar to, if not identical with, those contained in the tar produced by destructive distillation of bituminous and other coals. Native paraffin occurs in the solid state in coal deposits and other bituminous strata in various parts of the world and constitutes the minerals called *fossil wax*, *ozokerite*, etc.

Properties.—Paraffin does not possess any individuality chemically; it is probably a mixture of several hydrocarbons just as the liquid petroleum oil is. The paraffin of commerce, when pure, is a solid, colorless, translucent substance, without odor or taste, and somewhat resembles spermaceti. Its density is about 0.870; it melts between 45° and 65° C. (113–149° F.), forming a colorless oil which on cooling solidifies to a lamino-crystalline mass. It boils at about 370° C. (698° F.). It is insoluble in water, dissolves in 2.85 parts of boiling alcohol, but on cooling is deposited from that solution in snow-white needles, which are soft, friable and greasy to the touch. It is more soluble in ether and oils. It is but slowly attacked by strong sulphuric acid, even in the warmth, and not at all by dilute nitric acid; heated with strong nitric acid for some time, it is said to yield succinic and butyric acids.

Preparation for Homœopathic Use.—Paraffin is triturated, as directed under Class VII.

PAREIRA BRAVA.

Synonyms, Chondodendron Tomentosum, *Ruiz et Pav.* Cocculus Chondodendron, *DC.*

Nat. Ord., Menispermaceæ.

Common Name, Pareira Brava.

Pareira brava is a name meaning in the Portugese language *wild vine;* in medicine it is applied to the roots of a plant which is properly *Chonodendron tomentosum*, Ruiz et Pav., and not *Cissampelos*, a species of which was founded by Linnæus and called by him *C. pareira*, as he erroneously believed the latter to be the source of the medicinal root. Chondodendron tomentosum is a tall climbing shrub with large, simple, long-petioled leaves often a foot in length, generally ovate or ovate at the base. The flowers are minute, unisexual and racemose. The fruit is a one-seeded drupe in bunches resembling grapes in appearance. Pareira brava is a long, branching, woody root, at times two inches or more in diameter, but usually much smaller, giving off rootlets of the thickness of a quill or less, sometimes indeed being scarcely larger than horse hair. The root is very tortuous, transversely ridged and constricted and having long longitudinal wrinkles. The bark is dark brown, or even black, internally it is light yellowish-brown or at times a dull greenish-brown. The root breaks with a coarse fibrous fracture having a somewhat waxy lustre. Beneath the bark are seen on transverse section two or more concentric zones separated by irregular circles of a wax-like tissue; the zones are rayed. Parcira brava is almost without odor, and is bitter in taste.

Preparation.—The carefully dried root, coarsely powdered, is covered with five parts by weight of alcohol, and allowed to stand eight days in a well-stoppered bottle, in a dark, cool place, being shaken twice a day. The tincture is then poured off, strained and filtered.

Drug power of tincture, $\frac{1}{10}$.

Dilutions must be prepared as directed under Class IV.

PARIS QUADRIFOLIA, *Linn.*

Synonyms, Aconitum Pardalianches. Herba Paris. Solanum Quadrifolium Bacciferum. Uva Lupulina.

Nat. Ord., Liliaceæ.

Common Names, Fox Grape. Herb Paris. True Love.

This plant grows all over Europe, in wet woods, thickets, in plains as well as on mountains. The root is perennial, vertical, rampant, rounded, jointed, fleshy, whitish. Stem erect, single, round, uniflorał, a foot high, herbaceous; leaves at the top of the stem, with short peduncles, broad-elliptical or oval, pointed, entire, glabrous, disposed as a cross, shining beneath, veined, with sharp edges and three or four nerves; calyx four-leaved, greenish-yellow; peduncles from one to two inches long, and furrowed; flower yellowish-green; berry dark blue, shining, slightly quadrangular. The fresh leaves and berries have a disagreeable and narcotic odor; the root has a pungent odor and a nauseous taste.

It was first proven by Hahnemann.

Preparation.—The entire fresh plant, gathered at the time of ripening of the berries, is chopped and pounded to a pulp and pressed out *lege artis* in a piece of new linen. The expressed juice is then, by brisk agitation, mingled with an equal part by weight of alcohol. This mixture is allowed to stand eight days in a well-stoppered bottle, in a dark, cool place, and then filtered.

Drug power of tincture, $\frac{1}{2}$.

Dilutions must be prepared as directed under Class I.

PASSIFLORA INCARNATA, *Linn.*

Nat. Ord., Passifloraceæ.

Common Names, May Pop. Passion-Flower.

This is a climbing indigenous plant found in the Southern States as far north as Maryland. Its stem is smooth, often climbing 20 to 30 feet. Leaves deeply three-cleft, the lobes oblong, acute, serrate; petioles furnished with two glands. Flowers large, showy, nearly white, with a triple crown, purple and flesh-colored. Involucre of three obovate glandular bractlets. Calyx of five sepals, cup-shaped, deeply five-parted. Petals five. Stamens five, connate with the stipe of the ovary. Fruit a large, pulpy, pale yellow berry, oval and eatable, called *May Pop*.

Preparation.—The fresh leaves, gathered in May, are chopped and pounded to a pulp and weighed. Then two parts by weight of alcohol are taken, the pulp mixed thoroughly with one-sixth part of it, and the rest of the alcohol added. After having stirred the whole well, pour it into a well-stoppered bottle, and let it stand eight days in a dark, cool place. The tincture is then separated by decanting, straining and filtering.

Drug power of tincture, $\frac{1}{6}$.

Dilutions must be prepared as directed under Class III.

PAULLINIA PINNATA.

Synonym, Paullinia Timbo.

Nat. Ord., Sapindaceæ.

Common Names, (in Brazil) Guaratimbo. Timbo-Sipo.

This beautiful liana is commonly found in the woods of Brazil; its stem, of a flexible and tenacious wood, furnishes slender, slightly pubescent branches with deep parallel furrows. The leaves are alternate, with winged petioles; they are composed of five folioles which are almost sessile, oval-lanceolate, crenulate, irregularly bijugate. The flowers are small, in spikes, situated on axes that are accompanied by leaflets arising from the axils of the leaves. Calyx with five folioles, corolla with four petals, alternating with the folioles of the calyx; eight stamens; ovary with three uni-ovulate chambers. Capsule pear-shaped and sharp, divided at its superior part in three tubercles. Root with long fasciculate branches, which are a little hairy at their extremity.

It was introduced into our Materia Medica by Dr. Mure, Brazil.

Preparation.—The fresh root is chopped and pounded to a pulp and weighed. Then two parts by weight of alcohol are taken, the pulp mixed thoroughly with one-sixth part of it, and the rest of the alcohol added. After having stirred the whole well, pour it into a well-stoppered bottle, and let it stand eight days in a dark, cool place. The tincture is then separated by decanting, straining and filtering.

Amount of drug power, $\frac{1}{6}$.

Dilutions must be prepared as directed under Class III.

PENTHORUM SEDOIDES, *Linn.*

Nat. Ord., Crassulaceæ.

Common Name, Virginia Stone-Crop.

This is a hardy little plant, found growing in open wet situations in Canada and the United States. Stem from ten to sixteen inches high, branches few, short; leaves alternate, scattered, two to three inches long, by one-half to one inch broad, smooth, sharply and unequally serrate, lanceolate, acute; flowers arranged on the upper side of the branches of the cyme, pale yellowish-green; petals generally wanting. Flowers appear from July to September.

It was first proven by Dr. D. B. Morrow, U. S.

Preparation.—The fresh plant is chopped and pounded to a pulp and weighed. Then two parts by weight of alcohol are taken, the pulp mixed thoroughly with one-sixth part of it, and the rest of the alcohol added. After having stirred the whole well, pour it into a well-stoppered bottle, and let it stand eight days in a dark, cool place. The tincture is then separated by decanting, straining and filtering.

Amount of drug power, $\frac{1}{6}$.

Dilutions must be prepared as directed under Class III.

PEPSIN.

All the investigations into the process of stomach digestion tend to prove that the influence of the gastric juice upon proteids, is a ferment-action due to the presence of a ferment-body in the gastric juice. This ferment-body which, as yet, has only been approximately isolated, is called *Pepsin.*

The preparations used in medicine under this name are more or less impure from the presence of various salts, peptones, etc., thus reducing the peptic action of the extract. A good quality of commercial pepsin is made by Prof. Scheffer's process as follows: The well-cleaned fresh stomach of the hog is deprived of its mucous membrane by dissection, and the membrane is finely chopped and allowed to macerate in water which has been acidulated with hydrochloric acid. After standing for several days, the liquid is to be strained, the strained portion allowed to rest and finally decanted from the settlings; it is then to be mixed with its own volume of a saturated solution of sodium chloride, when the pepsin will separate out and float upon the surface of the heavier liquid. The pepsin is then to be thrown upon a muslin strainer and pressed to remove any adhering salt solution; it should not be suffered to dry in this state or it will become leathery and tough. It is to be again dissolved in water and filtered to remove mucus and calcium phosphate, with which it is still contaminated; the filtrate is to be precipitated by sodium chloride solution and again pressed, and on drying, the sodium chloride which still remains attached to it will appear upon its surface as a white efflorescence, and can be removed by a short immersion in water. It is then Scheffer's purified pepsin, which is dissolved readily by water acidulated with hydrochloric acid, forming a clear colorless solution.

Properties.—Purified pepsin is a light powder, yellowish-brown in color, having a faint, peculiar odor which is not repugnant, and a somewhat salty taste without the slightest putridity. It is slightly soluble in water or alcohol. According to Scheffer, one part of his purified pepsin dissolves more than 3,000 parts of coagulated albumen in a few days.

Preparation for Homœopathic Use.—Purified pepsin is triturated as directed under Class VII.

PETIVERIA TETRANDRA, *Gom.*

Synonym, Petiveria Mappa Graveolens.

Nat. Ord., Phytolacaceæ.

Common Name, (in Brazil) Pipi. Erva de Pipi.

This bush is common in the fields around Rio Janeiro, where it blossoms the whole year. Its branches are erect, somewhat sarmentous, slightly pubescent at their extremities, with alternate, glabrous, somewhat undulate leaves. Flowers small, scattered over long axillary or terminal spikes; perianth persistent, herbaceous, with four linear divisions. Stamens four, alternate with the divisions of the perianth, and a little taller. A single ovary, surmounted by a style, divided into ten reflexed stigmata. Capsule flattened, containing a single seed. The roots are branching and very fibrous; they smell strongly of garlic.

It was proven by Dr. Manuel Duarte Moreira, Brazil.

Preparation.—The recently dried root is powdered and covered with five parts by weight of alcohol. Having poured the mixture into a well-stoppered bottle, it is allowed to remain eight days at a moderate temperature in a dark place, being shaken twice a day. The tincture is then poured off, strained and filtered.

Drug power of tincture, $\frac{1}{10}$.

Dilutions must be prepared as directed under Class **IV.**

PETROLATUM.

Common Names, Vaseline. Cosmoline. Geoline.

Under the names, Vaseline, Cosmoline and Geoline, has been introduced a proprietary substance which, from its extreme blandness and from its favorable consistence, has gained general favor as an application in inflammations of the skin.

It is a dense, neutral, concentrated, oleaginous body, obtained by subjecting crude petroleum to distillation for the purpose of expelling the light hydro-carbons. The residue is purified without the use of chemicals, and is deodorized by animal charcoal. It consists essentially of paraffin and some of the heavy coal oils.

Preparation for Internal Use.—Petrolatum is prepared by trituration, as directed under Class IX.

PETROLEUM.

Synonyms, Oleum Petræ. Oleum Terræ. Bitumen Liquidum. Naphtha Montana.

Common Names, Coal Oil. Rock Oil.

The name petroleum is employed so loosely to designate numerous liquid hydrocarbons, that it is important to insure the use of the same substance which Hahnemann employed in his proving. This is made by agitating the liquid portion of commercial petroleum with sulphuric acid, and then rectifying the portion which this acid does not act upon. Its chemical constitution is very complex.

Properties and Tests.—It is a light oily fluid, colorless, or of a pale straw-color and strong characteristic naphthalic smell. When agitated with a mixture of equal volumes of sulphuric acid and water, no change takes place beyond its imparting to the acid any yellow tint it may possess and itself becoming colorless. Dropped on white paper, it evaporates completely, leaving no greasy stain. To secure its freedom from other volatile oils, agitate with twice its bulk of rectified spirit, and filter through bibulous paper previously moistened with rectified spirit; or it may be separated from the spirit by means of a burette. It must be preserved in well-stoppered bottles.

Hahnemann proved the crude Rangoon Rock Oil, a thin light yellow variety.

Preparation for Homœopathic Use.—One part by weight of crude petroleum is dissolved in ninety-nine parts by weight of alcohol.

Amount of drug power, $\frac{1}{100}$.

Dilutions must be prepared as directed under Class VI—β.

PETROSELINUM.

Synonyms, Petroselinum Sativum, *Hoffmann.* Apium Petroselinum, *Linn.* Apium Hortensis. Carum Petroselinum.

Nat. Ord., Umbelliferæ.

Common Name, Parsley.

This well known plant, cultivated everywhere as a pot-herb, is a native of Southern Europe. From its biennial root arises annually a round, erect, branching stem from two to four feet high. Leaves are decompound; segments of the lower ones cuneate-ovate; terminal ones trifid, all incised. Stem leaves have lance-linear sub-entire segments. The flowers are pale yellow, small, in umbels with involucels of three to five awl-shaped bracts. The seeds are small, ovate, five-ribbed, dark green, and have the odor of turpentine.

It was proven by Dr. Bethmann, Germany.

Preparation.—The fresh plant, gathered when coming into bloom, is chopped and pounded to a pulp, and pressed out *lege artis* in a piece of new linen. The expressed juice is then, by brisk agitation, mingled with an equal part by weight of alcohol. This mixture is allowed to stand eight days in a well-stoppered bottle, in a dark, cool place, and then filtered.

Drug power of tincture, $\frac{1}{2}$.

Dilutions must be prepared as directed under Class I.

PHELLANDRIUM AQUATICUM, *Linn.*

Synonyms, Œnanthe Phellandrium, *Lamarck.* Œnanthe Sarmentosa. Fœniculum Aquaticum. Fœniculum Caballinum.

Nat. Ord., Umbelliferæ.

Common Names, Phellandrium. Five-leaved Water-Hemlock.

This is a biennial plant found growing in Europe and Northern Asia, in swamps and on river banks. The submersed leaves are narrow, linear, others are pinnately divided, leaflets cut-lobed or pinnatifid.

Flowers white, in umbels. Seeds brown, oblong-ovate, about one-eighth of an inch long, furnished with three dorsal ribs and two lateral ones, and having several oil-tubes. The seeds have an acrid, bitter taste, and the odor of caraway with some unpleasantness.

This drug was first proven by Nenning, Germany.

Preparation.—The fresh, carefully dried fruit, is coarsely powdered, covered with five parts by weight of alcohol, and allowed to remain eight days, in a well-stoppered bottle, in a dark, cool place, being shaken twice a day. The tincture is then poured off, strained and filtered.

Drug power of tincture, $\frac{1}{10}$.

Dilutions must be prepared as directed under Class IV.

PHOSPHORUS.

Symbol, P.

Atomic Weight, 31.

Origin and Preparation of Phosphorus.—Phosphorus does not exist free in nature. It is found in combination as phosphate in many minerals as *apatite* (a calcium compound), *pyromorphite* (lead), *Wagnerite* (magnesium), etc.; enormous deposits of calcium phosphate are found in South Carolina and in some of the Caribean Islands. The element was first obtained free in 1669 by evaporating urine and igniting the dried residue, and in 1769 it was found to exist in bones. Phosphorus may be obtained from calcined bones by treating them with sulphuric acid, leaching off the liquid result, evaporating it to dryness and then distilling the residue with charcoal in earthen retorts, each retort being connected with a wide bent tube whose free end is under water. The crude phosphorus so obtained is purified by melting it under water and agitating it with a mixture of sulphuric acid and potassium dichromate, by which means the impurities are oxidized; afterward the melted phosphorus is, while under warm water, run into tubes.

Properties.—Phosphorus comes in commerce in cylindrical sticks which are transparent, colorless or pale yellow, and have a waxy lustre. At ordinary temperatures it has the consistency of wax, but at low temperatures it becomes brittle and crystalline. Its specific gravity is 1.83. Its freshly cut surface emits a garlicky odor, and when nearly covered by a layer of water, a stick of phosphorus oxidizes slowly with the production of phosphorus oxide in white fumes and of ozone, whose characteristic odor is often mistakenly considered to be the odor of phosphorus; this slow oxidation is evidenced by a slight luminosity called phosphorescence, of course only visible in the dark. A trace of naphtha, or oil of turpentine, or a small amount of olefiant gas in the air is sufficient to prevent this phenomenon. Heated in the air to 50° C. (122° F.) it inflames and burns vividly, producing phosphoric oxide. When heated to 290° C. (554° F.) out of contact with the air it distils over unchanged.

Phosphorus is soluble in carbon disulphide, chloroform, the volatile and fixed oils; 100 parts of the following take up of phosphorus: volatile oils about four parts, fixed oils two, ether from one to one and one-third, ordinary commercial sulphuric ether 0.5, and 90 per cent. alcohol 0.3. It is insoluble in water. When kept under water for a long time it becomes covered with a thin white coating from superficial oxidation by the atmospheric air dissolved in the water.

Phosphorus was first proven by Hahnemann.

Preparation for Homœopathic Use.—Strong (95 per cent.) alcohol with an excess of phosphorus is put into an open bottle in a hot-water bath, and after the phosphorus has melted, vigorously shaken till cold, then decanted.

Amount of drug power, $\frac{1}{1000}$.

The above saturated solution corresponds to the third decimal potency. Ten drops of this solution with ninety drops of strong alcohol give the 4x or 2 potency. Further potencies are made after the customary manner. In *Hahnemann's Chronic Diseases* a method is given for preparing phosphorus by trituration; alcoholic solutions are, however, preferable.

A solution of one part of pure phosphorus in 100 of absolute ether will have the strength of the 1st dilution; of this, one part mixed with nine parts of absolute alcohol, will give the 3x dilution, and from this the 2d dilution can be made with alcohol in the regular way; dilute alcohol should not be used until the 6th dilution is reached.

PHOSPHORUS RUBER.

Synonyms, Amorphous Phosphorus. Red Phosphorus.

When ordinary phosphorus is heated to 250° C. (482° F.) for many hours in an atmosphere not containing oxygen, it is converted into a chocolate-red powder, whose properties differ in a remarkable manner from those of the element in its ordinary state. It no longer oxidizes in the air, it has no odor, is not soluble in the ordinary solvents of phosphorus, and it is not poisonous. Its specific gravity is 2.14. When heated to 260° C. (500° F.) it is reconverted into the common phosphorus, and if the heating be done in the air, of course it then inflames.

Amorphous phosphorus may be kept in the air without igniting, and may even be wrapped in paper and handled without fear of ignition. Unless thoroughly purified, it is apt to contain a small amount of unaltered phosphorus; it may be purified by suspending it in a solution of calcium chloride, specific gravity about 2.0, when any common phosphorus present will float and can be removed, the red phosphorus at the same time sinking. The latter is to be removed from the bath surrounding it, well washed in water and dried.

A proving of amorphorus phosphorus was read by Dr. H. Noah Martin at the Am. Inst. of Hom., Session of 1882.

Preparation for Homœopathic Use.—Amorphous phosphorus is triturated as directed under Class VII, but the sugar of milk and the phosphorus must be kept moistened with alcohol. The precaution should be taken of testing amorphous phosphorus for the ordinary kind (*vide supra*); the presence of even a small amount of the latter would lead to ignition from friction in trituration.

PHYSOSTIGMA.

Synonyms, Physostigma Venenosum, *Balfour.* Eseré Nut. Faba Calabarica. Faba Physostigmatis.

Nat. Ord., Leguminosæ.

Common Names, Calabar Bean. Chop Nut. Known among the negroes of Western Africa as the Ordeal Bean of Calabar.

The plant is a perennial which grows near the mouths of the Niger and the Old Calabar river on the Gulf of Guinea. The plant is climbing in habit, and although its stem is woody, it often reaches a height of fifty feet or more. The root is spreading and has many fine rootlets, to which are attached small fleshy tubers. The flowers are purplish in color, are fully an inch across, in shape like those of *Phaseolus,* except that the style is developed backward beyond the stigma, as a broad, flat, hooked appendage, and that the seeds are surrounded by a deeply grooved hilum. The seeds or beans are oblong subreniform in outline, and with one side markedly convex, the other flat or slightly concave. They are from an inch to an inch and a half long, about three quarters of an inch broad, and in thickness from one-half to five-eighths of an inch. The seed is deep chocolate-brown in color, with a dull polish, and the tint becomes lighter on the ridges bordering the remarkable furrow or groove already mentioned. They have scarcely any more taste than an ordinary bean, and in the dry state have no odor; after being boiled, or during the evaporation of their alcoholic tincture, an odor recalling that of cantharides is perceived.

The first systematic proving was by Dr. H. L. Chase, U. S.

Preparation.—The bean is pulverized, weighed, covered with five parts by weight of alcohol, and allowed to remain eight days in a well-stoppered bottle, at the ordinary temperature, in a dark, cool place, being shaken twice a day. The tincture is then poured off, strained and filtered.

Drug power of tincture, $\frac{1}{10}$.

Dilutions must be prepared as directed under Class IV.

PHYTOLACCA.

Synonyms, Phytolacca Decandra, *Linn.*

Nat. Ord., Phytolaccaceæ.

Common Names, Poke. Garget Weed. Pigeon Berry. American Nightshade. Chongras. Cocum. Northern Jalap.

This indigenous perennial plant has a large branching root, brownish externally, and within white, fleshy and fibrous, from which ascends annually a stem an inch or two in diameter, and frequently reaching a height of six or eight feet. The stem is smooth, round and branching, and when mature is purplish in color. The leaves are smooth, entire, on short petioles; they are oblong-ovate, pointed and of a rich green color. The flowers are numerous, small, greenish-white, in terminal racemes. Calyx five parted, corolla-like; corolla of concave, ovate petals; stamens ten, pistils ten. Fruit a dark purple berry, in clusters, containing a purple-red juice.

Preparation.—The fresh root is chopped and pounded to a pulp and weighed. Then two parts by weight of alcohol are taken, the pulp mixed thoroughly with one-sixth part of it, and the rest of the alcohol added. After having stirred the whole well, pour it into a well-stoppered bottle, and let it stand eight days in a dark, cool place. The tincture is then separated by decanting, straining and filtering.

Drug power of tincture, $\frac{1}{6}$.

Dilutions must be prepared as directed under Class III.

PICHURIM.

Synonyms, Nectandra Puchury Major, *Nees.* Faba Pichurim. Nuces Sassafras.

Nat. Ord., Lauraceæ.

Common Names, Pichurim Beans. Sassafras Nut.

These are the separated cotyledons of the seed or "bean" of a tree growing in Brazil. They are ovate-oblong or elliptical, flat on one side, arched on the other, of grayish-brown color externally, chocolate-colored internally, and have an odor and taste as of nutmegs and sassafras mingled. The seeds are about an inch and a half long, and half an inch broad.

Preparation.—The ripe seeds are coarsely powdered, covered with five parts by weight of alcohol, and allowed to remain eight days in a well-stoppered bottle, in a dark, cool place, being shaken twice a day. The tincture is then poured off, strained and filtered.

Drug power of tincture, $\frac{1}{10}$.

Dilutions must be prepared as directed under Class IV.

PILOCARPINUM MURIATICUM.

Synonym, Hydrochlorate of Pilocarpin. Muriate of Pilocarpin.

Origin and Preparation.—This alkaloid was obtained from jaborandi leaves by Byasson (1875). It is soluble in alcohol, ether, chloroform, ammonia and dilute acids. By dissolving in water the alcoholic extract from the leaves, adding an alkali to the solution to liberate the alkaloid, agitating with chloroform to dissolve the latter, removing the chloroformic layer and evaporating, we obtain pilocarpin itself. When this is exactly neutralized with HCl, the so-called muriate is obtained.

Properties.—Muriate of pilocarpin is in colorless, transparent, crystalline laminæ, which are easily soluble in water, and possess a weakly bitter, somewhat astringent taste.

Preparation for Homœopathic Use.—Muriate of pilocarpin is triturated, as directed under Class VII.

PIMPINELLA SAXIFRAGA, *Linn.*

Synonyms, Pimpinella Alba. Pimpinella Hircinæ. Pimpinella Nostratis. Pimpinella Umbelliferæ. Tragoselinum.

Nat. Ord., Umbelliferæ.

Common Names, Bibernell. Small Burnet Saxifrage. Pimpinel.

This is a perennial umbelliferous European plant, growing on sunny hills, and in dry meadows and pastures. Rootstock slender, hot and acrid to the taste. Stem one to three feet high, slender, furrowed, branched. Leaflets four to eight pairs, very variable, serrate-lobed or almost pinnatifid; lobes of cauline leaves much narrower. Umbels flat-topped. Flowers white. Fruit one-eighth inch long, glabrous, broadly ovoid; styles small, short, reflexed. The root is brown yellow or blackish, usually one-headed, not over one-half inch thick, finely annulated above, wrinkled and verrucose below; the bark is very thick, spongy, either white or yellowish, contains numerous resin-cells, and is radially striate, enclosing a yellow wood.

It was first proven by Dr. Schelling, Germany.

Preparation.—The fresh root, gathered in May, is chopped and pounded to a pulp and weighed. Then two parts by weight of alcohol are taken, the pulp mixed thoroughly with one-sixth part of it, and the rest of the alcohol added. After having stirred the whole, pour it into a well-stoppered bottle, and let it stand eight days in a dark, cool place. The tincture is then separated by decanting, straining and filtering.

Amount of drug power, ½.

Dilutions must be prepared as directed under Class III.

PINUS SYLVESTRIS, *Linn.*

Nat. Ord., Coniferæ.

Common Names, Scotch Fir. Scotch Pine. Wild Pine.

This species of Pine is distributed through the plains of Northern and mountains of Southern Europe, Siberia and Mantchooria. Its height is from 50 to 100 feet, the trunk attaining a circumference of 12 feet; wood red or white; bark red-brown, rough. Leaves two to three inches long, acicular, acute, grooved above, convex and glaucous beneath, minutely serrulate, sheath fimbriate. Male catkins one-fourth inch long, spiked, yellow; connective produced. Female cones one to two inches long, one to three together, acute; scales few, ends rhomboid with a transverse keel and deciduous point. Seeds one-half inch long, wing cuneate, much exceeding the nucleus.

It was first proven by Dr. Fielitz, Germany.

Preparation.—The fresh shoots are chopped and pounded to a pulp and weighed. Then two parts by weight of alcohol are taken, the pulp mixed thoroughly with one-sixth part of it, and the rest of the alcohol added. After having stirred the whole well, pour it into a well-stoppered bottle, and let it stand eight days in a dark, cool place. The tincture is then separated by decanting, straining and filtering.

Amount of drug power, $\frac{1}{6}$.
Dilutions must be prepared as directed under Class III.

PIPER METHYSTICUM, *Forster.*

Synonym, Macropiper Methysticum.
Nat. Ord., Piperaceæ.
Common Names, Ava-Ava. Kava-Kava.

This shrub is indigenous to the Sandwich Islands and to other islands in the Pacific. It has a spongy, woody, large root; its odor resembles that of the lilac and its taste is slightly pungent and bitter.

Preparation.—The fresh root is chopped and pounded to a pulp and weighed. Then two parts by weight of alcohol are taken, the pulp mixed thoroughly with one-sixth part of it, and the rest of the alcohol added. After having stirred the whole well, pour it into a well-stoppered bottle, and let it stand eight days in a dark, cool place. The tincture is then separated by decanting, straining and filtering.

Drug power of tincture, $\frac{1}{6}$.
Dilutions must be prepared as directed under Class III.

PIPER NIGRUM, *Linn.*

Nat. Ord., Piperaceæ.
Common Name, Black Pepper.

The pepper plant is a native of Malabar and is cultivated in Sumatra, Java, Borneo and other places in the East Indies. It has also been introduced into the West India Islands. It is a perennial plant with jointed stem, branching dichotomously, and from eight to fifteen feet long. The leaves are entire, broadly ovate, acuminate, five to seven-nerved, leathery and of a dark green color, on petioles. The flowers are small, whitish, in slender spikes. The fruit is small, round and berry-like, from twenty to thirty on a common pendulous fruit-stalk, and when fully ripe is red; the berries are gathered before maturity, and by drying become blackish-gray or brown and wrinkled. After drying they are globular, about the size of a pea, internally whitish and have the pungent taste and peculiar odor of pepper.

It was introduced into our Materia Medica by Dr. Berridge, England.

Preparation.—The unripe dried berries, coarsely powdered, are covered with five parts by weight of alcohol, and allowed to remain eight days in a well-stoppered bottle, in a dark, cool place, being shaken twice a day. The tincture is then poured off, strained and filtered.

Drug power of tincture, $\frac{1}{10}$.
Dilutions must be prepared as directed under Class IV.

PLANTAGO MAJOR, *Linn.*

Nat. Ord., Plantaginaceæ.
Common Names, Greater Plaintain. Rib Grass. Way Bread.

This plant is very common in Europe and North America, often found growing by roadsides and footpaths. From a fibrous root, a round scape rises, varying in height from one to three feet. The leaves are broadly ovate, smooth, entire or somewhat toothed, five to seven-nerved, each of which contains a strong fibre which may be pulled out, and abruptly narrowed into a long channelled petiole. The flowers are white, very small, imbricated, numerous, and densely disposed on a cylindrical spike, from five to twenty inches long. Small plants are frequently found with the spikes only half an inch to two inches long, and the leaves and stalks proportionately small. Stamens and styles long. Seeds numerous.

This drug was first proven by Dr. F. Humphreys, U. S.

Preparation.—The fresh plant, gathered when coming into flower, is chopped and pounded to a pulp and weighed. Then two parts by weight of alcohol are taken, the pulp mixed thoroughly with one-sixth part of it, and the rest of the alcohol added. After having stirred the whole, pour it into a well-stoppered bottle, and let it stand eight days in a dark, cool place. The tincture is then separated by decanting, straining and filtering.

Drug power of tincture, $\frac{1}{6}$.

Dilutions must be prepared as directed under Class III.

PLATINA.

Synonyms, Platinum. Platinum Metallicum.

Symbol, Pt.

Atomic Weight, 195.

Origin and Preparation of Platinum.—Platinum is found in nature in the metallic state in granular rounded masses, and occasionally in octohedrons. The grains are seldom pure platinum, generally being combinations of platinum with gold, iron or copper, together with iridium, osmium, ruthenium and palladium. It occurs in California, in South America, in Russia and in some other countries.

Preparation.—Crude platinum is melted with its own weight of sulphide of lead and half that weight of metallic lead; the platinum dissolves in the melted lead and the other metals are left. The alloy of platinum and lead is melted, and in that state exposed to a current of air in which, at the temperature of the mass, the lead oxidizes and flows off as slag; the platinum is left behind in a porous mass. When the latter is exposed to the blast of the oxyhydrogen blow-pipe it is melted, and is then cast into proper moulds.

Properties.—Platinum is a brilliant metal, white in color yet having a blue tinge. Its specific gravity is 21.5. In tenacity and hardness it is like copper, and it is very malleable and ductile. It is only fusible before the oxyhydrogen flame. It is unalterable in the air, and is not affected by any single acid, only yielding to the action of aqua regia. Precipitated platinum, fit for homœopathic triturations, may be obtained by placing polished steel rods in a dilute solution of platinic chloride upon which the metal will be deposited as a spongy iron-gray mass, without lustre. The precipitate, after being scraped off the rods with wooden scrapers, is to be boiled with hydrochloric acid, then washed well with distilled water and dried.

It was first proven by Hahnemann.

Preparation for Homœopathic Use.—Precipitated metallic platinum is triturated, as directed under Class VII.

PLATINUM MURIATICUM.

Synonyms, Platinic Chloride. Platina Chlorata. Platini Chloridum. Chloras Platinicus.

Common Names, Muriate of Platinum. Chloride of Platinum.

Formula, $Pt\ Cl_4,\ 5H_2O$.

Molecular Weight, 427.

Preparation.—Platinic chloride is obtained by dissolving finely divided platinum in nitro-muriatic acid; when the solution is complete it is to be evaporated to dryness, and there will be left a red or brown residue, which is very deliquescent. The residue is to be re-dissolved in hydrochloric acid and heated to expel any nitric acid remaining. It is then to be evaporated, at a heat not over 120° C. (248° F.), to dryness, a red crystalline mass being the result.

Properties.—Obtained as above directed platinic chloride is a red-brown, crystalline, hygroscopic powder, having a sharp metallic taste; it is easily soluble in water and alcohol, forming transparent, deep yellow solutions, (a dark reddish-brown solution is dependent on presence of iridium or of platinous chloride). By heating, it loses at first its water of crystallization and then a part of its chlorine, and becomes reduced to the platinous state and finally, with the loss of all its chlorine, there remains only the metal.

Tests.—The platinic chloride of commerce contains always some water, but the amount should not exceed five per cent. After heating one gram of platinic chloride for some hours on the water bath there should be a loss in weight of only five per cent. The same amount, heated to redness in a porcelain crucible, should yield at least 55 per cent. of metallic platinum; the residue in the crucible, when digested with pure nitric acid, and the solution diluted with an equal volume of water and filtered through glass-wool, should yield a filtrate which ought to evaporate without residue.

It was first proven by Dr. Höfer, Germany.

Preparation for Homœopathic Use.—One part by weight of pure platinic chloride is dissolved in ninety-nine parts by weight of distilled water.

Amount of drug power, $\frac{1}{100}$.

Dilutions must be prepared as directed under Class V—β.

PLECTRANTHUS FRUCTICOSUS, *L'Heritier.*

Synonym, Germanea Urticæfolia, *Linn.*

Nat. Ord., Labiatæ.

This aromatic shrub is a native of the Cape of Good Hope, and is grown quite extensively in gardens in Germany, where it is used as a domestic remedy for intermittent fever, cramps, etc.

The provings were made by the Austrian Provers' Union.

Preparation.—The dried, powdered herb is covered with five parts by weight of alcohol, and allowed to remain eight days, in a well-stoppered bottle, in a dark, cool place, being shaken twice a day. The tincture is then poured off, strained and filtered.

Drug power of tincture, $\frac{1}{10}$.

Dilutions must be prepared as directed under Class IV.

PLUMBAGO LITTORALIS.

Nat. Ord., Plumbaginaceæ.

Common Name, (in Brazil) Picao de Praia.

This is a creeper, inhabiting the shores of the bay of Rio Janeiro. Its stem is herbaceous, rounded, covered with short and rather stiff hairs. Its leaves are simple, opposite, gradually tapering to a short channeled petiole adhering to that of the opposite side, and forming tufts at certain intervals whence arise adventitious roots. The flowers form little axillary heads, with from fifteen to twenty flowers each, arising from an involucre with five divisions and supported by a somewhat filiform pedicle. Calyx tubulous, monophyllous, with five teeth, and much shorter than the tube of the corolla. The corolla is monopetalous, yellowish-white, tubular, puffed up at its extremity, with five reflexed divisions, and five stamens with bilocular, connivent anthers which are longer than the corolla. Ovary one-celled, flat at the top, whence proceeds a slender style, terminated by a glandular stigma which is longer than the stamens. Fruit monospermous, elongated, with a crustaceous integument covered with a number of stiff hairs that are bent over, and which presents irregular longitudinal furrows. The root is perennial and ramose.

It was introduced into our Materia Medica by Dr. Mure, Brazil.

Preparation.—The fresh leaves are chopped and pounded to a pulp and weighed. Then two parts by weight of alcohol are taken, the pulp mixed thoroughly with one-sixth part of it, and the rest of the alcohol added. After having stirred the whole, pour it into a well-stoppered bottle, and let it stand eight days in a dark, cool place. The tincture is then separated by decanting, straining and filtering.

Drug power of tincture, $\frac{1}{6}$.

Dilutions must be prepared as directed under Class III.

PLUMBUM.

Synonym, Plumbum Metallicum.

Common Name, Lead.

Symbol, Pb

Atomic Weight, 207.

Origin and Preparation of Lead.—Lead does not often occur in nature in the metallic state. While there are upwards of twenty ores of this metal known to the mineralogist, all the lead of commerce may be said to be procured from five minerals, viz.: the carbonate, sulphate, phosphate, arsenate and sulphide, the latter furnishing more of the metal than all the others. The sulphide, known as *galena*, is found in almost every country on the globe. Lead is prepared from galena by first roasting it on the floor of a reverberatory furnace; both its constituents are thereby oxidized, lead oxide and sulphate being produced. The furnace is then tightly closed, and the last named products react upon the undecomposed lead sulphide, forming sulphurous oxide and metallic lead.

Lead is a brilliant metal of a bluish-gray color, and is so soft that it can be readily cut with a knife, and on paper leaves a bluish-gray streak. It is very malleable. Its specific gravity is 11.4. Lead fuses at 325° C. (617° F.), and can be obtained crystallized in regular octohedrons. At a red heat it is somewhat volatile. Its tenacity is very feeble. It is not affected by perfectly dry air or by water free from air, but the ordinary air tarnishes it; so spring and other waters act upon it, especially if they contain nitrates or chlorides. Waters containing CO_2 or sulphates, cause a deposit on the surface of the metal of a film of carbonate or sulphate of lead, and this film prevents any further action by such water. Sulphuric and hydrochloric acids do not attack it, or only feebly, at ordinary temperatures, but in the presence of air and moisture weak acids, such as acetic and other vegetable acids unite with it, forming salts. It dissolves easily in nitric acid.

Plumbum Metallicum Precipitatum.—To obtain pure lead in the form of powder, the galvanic process of reduction by means of rods of zinc is the most convenient. Crystals of acetate of lead are dissolved in one hundred times their quantity of distilled water, and in four or six ounces of this solution, contained in a suitable porcelain dish, a few polished rods of zinc are put. The decomposition takes place immediately, and continues as long as the reduction of the acetate of lead is incomplete. If this process of reduction is to succeed entirely, the following rules should be observed: 1. The leaden crystals which cluster around the rods of zinc should be frequently detached, in order to prevent the formation of thick laminæ which it would be difficult to pulverize. 2. The liquid, which now contains acetate of zinc, should be poured off as soon as the reduction ceases, and a fresh solution of the acetate of lead should be added. 3. As soon as the operation is concluded, the precipitate, which is a dark gray, loose, porous mass, though still cohering in lumps, should be washed with hot distilled water, avoiding every mechanical pressure lest the soft mass should be pressed into firm balls. 4. As soon as the water which is used for washing flows off quite clear, the precipitate should be collected on a filter, and the liquid removed by gently pressing the precipitate between the fingers, after which the metal is to be taken out of the filter and pressed with the hand between several layers of bibulous paper until the metal ceases to adhere to the paper; finally, gently rub the metal in a warmed porcelain mortar, in order to effect its perfect dessication.

The first provers were Bethmann, Hartmann, Hering and Nenning, in Germany.

Preparation for Homœopathic Use.—The precipitated lead is triturated, as directed under Class VII.

PLUMBUM ACETICUM.

Synonyms, Plumbic Acetate. Acetas Plumbicus. Plumbi Acetas. Saccharum Saturni.

Common Names, Acetate of Lead. Sugar of Lead.

Formula, $Pb\ (C_2\ H_3\ O_2)_2,\ 3\ H_2\ O$.

Molecular Weight, 379.

Preparation of Acetate of Lead.—"Take of oxide of lead in fine powder, twenty-four ounces; acetic acid, two pints, or a sufficiency; distilled water, one pint. Mix the acetic acid and the water, add the oxide of lead, and dissolve with the aid of a gentle heat. Filter, evaporate till a pellicle forms, and set aside to crystallize, first adding a little acetic acid should the fluid not have a distinctly acid reaction. Drain and dry the crystals on filtering paper without heat."—Br. P.

Properties.—Pure acetate of lead forms colorless, glistening, transparent, right-rhombic prisms of a weakly acid reaction, an acetous odor and a sweet, metallic taste. They effloresce in the air and become covered with a deposit of carbonate. They are soluble in one and three-quarter parts of cold and in one-half part of boiling water, and in eight parts of alcohol. The aqueous solutions become turbid from the absorption of CO_2 from the atmosphere and the consequent formation of carbonate. Heated to 40° (104° F.) the salt liquefies in its water of crystallization; at a higher temperature it loses this water, and if heated strongly is decomposed with the production of acetone.

Tests.—The impurities likely to be present in this salt are the chloride and nitrate of lead, acetate of sodium, compounds of calcium and copper, and traces of iron. When a solution of lead acetate in distilled water is decomposed with ammonium hydrate in excess, and allowed to stand for some time, the supernatant fluid should be perfectly colorless (a blue coloration indicates the presence of copper). The precipitate produced in this test should be of a pure white color (a yellow tint is due to iron).

One gram of lead acetate is to be dissolved in 10 CC. of distilled water, and after complete solution fifty or sixty drops of dilute sulphuric acid are added and the mixture thoroughly shaken and then filtered. A part of the filtrate on being evaporated and then heated strongly should leave no residue (absence of acetate of sodium or of calcium hydrate). Other portions of the filtrate may be tested with potassium ferrocyanide (a red precipitate means copper), with silver nitrate (chloride), and with a mixture of ferrous sulphate solution and strong sulphuric acid (a purple-brown coloration shows the presence of a nitrate).

Preparation for Homœopathic Use.—One part by weight of pure acetate of lead is dissolved in ninety-nine parts by weight of distilled water.

Amount of drug power, $\frac{1}{100}$.

Dilutions must be prepared as directed under Class V—β.

Triturations are prepared as directed under Class VII.

Note.—The trituration is to be preferred on account of its stability.

PLUMBUM CARBONICUM.

Synonyms, Plumbic Carbonate. Carbonas Plumbicus. Cerussa. Plumbi Carbonas.

Common Name, Carbonate of Lead.

Formula, $Pb\ CO_3$.

Molecular Weight, 267.

Preparation of Carbonate of Lead.—This compound is found native as white lead ore or *cerusite* in crystals of the trimetric system. The salt is readily obtained by precipitating in the cold a solution of the acetate of lead with sodium carbonate. When the lead solution is boiling a basic salt falls, whose formula is $2\,(Pb\ CO_3),\ Pb\ (HO)_2$.

Properties.—The simple carbonate is a heavy, soft, white powder, insoluble in water and in alcohol. With dilute acetic or nitric acid it effervesces from the liberation of CO_2, and forms the corresponding salt of lead which remains in solution.

Tests.—When dissolved in dilute nitric acid the solution should be complete. A residue may be due to lead sulphate, calcium sulphate or barium sulphate. The solution when treated with caustic alkali in excess, should also show complete absence of calcium carbonate, phosphate or barium sulphate.

Preparation for Homœopathic Use.—Pure carbonate of lead is triturated, as directed under Class VII.

PLUMBUM IODATUM.

Synonyms, Plumbic Iodide. Ioduretum Plumbicum. Plumbi Iodidum.

Common Name, Iodide of Lead.

Formula, $Pb\ I_2$.

Molecular Weight, 461.

Preparation of Iodide of Lead.—Take of nitrate of lead, iodide of potassium, each four troy ounces; distilled water a sufficient quantity. Dissolve the nitrate of lead with the aid of heat in a pint and a half, and the iodide of potassium in half a pint of the water, and mix the solutions. Collect the precipitate on a filter, wash it with distilled water, and dry it with a gentle heat.—Br. P.

Properties.—Lead iodide, when prepared by the directions given above, is a yellow powder; when the precipitation takes place in boiling solutions, it is in thin six-sided scales of a golden-yellow color. The powder is without odor or taste, is soluble in 1,300 parts of water at 20° C. (68° F.) and in 200 parts of boiling water: it is slightly soluble in alcohol, ether, and in dilute solution of potassium iodide; it is readily dissolved by solutions of caustic alkali, of alkaline acetates, of ammonium chloride and by concentrated solutions of metallic iodides. It dissolves without color in solution of sodium hyposulphite; at a strong heat it melts, becomes red, and loses a part of its iodine with the evolution of fumes which at first are yellow and finally violet-colored, and there remains behind a basic iodide of lead.

Tests.—When one part of lead iodide is rubbed up in a mortar with two of ammonium chloride, and the mixture added to two parts of water, the color is rapidly discharged; otherwise the presence of lead chromate may be assumed.

Preparation for Homœopathic Use.—Pure iodide of lead is triturated, as directed under Class VII.

PODOPHYLLUM.

Synonyms, Podophyllum Peltatum, *Linn.* Aconitifolius Humilis. Anapodophyllum Canadense.

Nat. Ord., Berberidaceæ.

Common Names, May-Apple. Mandrake. Indian Apple. Ground Lemons. Duck's Foot.

This is a perennial herbaceous plant found growing plentifully in the Middle and Western States and southward. It has a creeping root-stock several feet in length, and in thickness about a fourth of an inch. The root-stock is jointed, smooth and of a brown color externally; at the joints rootlets are given off. Stem round, erect; about a foot high, sheathed at the base, dividing at the top into two round petioles, between which is a peduncle bearing a solitary drooping flower. Each petiole bears a large broadly-cordate leaf with from five to seven lobes, each lobe bifid and dentate towards its apex. Sepals three, oval, concave, obtuse, deciduous; petals six to nine, obovate, obtuse, concave. Stamens nine to eighteen; anthers linear. Fruit a large yellow, ovoid, one-celled berry, crowned with the solitary stigma.

Introduced into our Materia Medica by Dr. W. Williamson, U. S.

Preparation.—The fresh root, gathered before the fruit is ripe, is chopped and pounded to a pulp and weighed. Then two parts by weight of alcohol are taken, the pulp mixed thoroughly with one-sixth part of it, and the rest of the alcohol added. After having stirred the whole, pour it into a well-stoppered bottle, and let it stand eight days in a dark, cool place. The tincture is then separated by decanting, straining and filtering.

Drug power of tincture, $\frac{1}{6}$.

Dilutions must be prepared as directed under Class III.

POLYGONUM HYDROPIPEROIDES, *Michaux.*

Synonym, Polygonum Mite, *Persoon* (not of *Schrank*).

Nat. Ord., Polygonaceæ.

Common Name, Mild Water Pepper.

This indigenous perennial, grows in ditches and wet places, and is common southward. Stem smooth, branching one to three feet high; sheaths narrow, hairy-bristly. Leaves linear-lanceolate, tapering each way. Flowers white-roseate, on two or more slender spikes; stamens eight; style three-cleft. Achenium three-cornered, smooth. Flowers in August and September.

It was first proven by Dr. W. E Payne, U. S.

Preparation.—The fresh plant is chopped and pounded to a pulp and weighed. Then two parts by weight of alcohol are taken, the pulp mixed thoroughly with one-sixth part of it, and the rest of the alcohol added. After having stirred the whole, pour it into a well-stoppered bottle, and let it stand eight days in a dark, cool place. The tincture is then separated by decanting, straining and filtering.

Drug power of tincture, $\frac{1}{6}$.

Dilutions must be prepared as directed under Class III.

POLYGONUM PUNCTATUM, *Elliott.*

Synonyms, Polygonum Acre, *Humboldt, Bonpland* and *Kunth.* Polygonum Hydropiperoides, *Pursh* (not of *Michaux*).

Nat. Ord., Polygonaceæ.

Common Names, Water Smartweed. Biting Persicaria. Knotweed. Wild Smartweed.

This perennial plant is of the same habit as is *P. hydropiperoides.* Its nearly smooth stem is from two to five feet high. Leaves lanceolate, tapering. Spikes erect, bearing whitish or flesh-colored flowers. Stamens eight; style three-parted; achenia three-cornered, shining, smooth. Flowers from July to September.

Preparation.—The fresh plant is chopped and pounded to a pulp and weighed. Then two parts by weight of alcohol are taken, the pulp mixed thoroughly with one-sixth part of it, and the rest of the alcohol added. After having stirred the whole well, pour it into a well-stoppered bottle, and let it stand eight days in a dark, cool place. The tincture is then separated by decanting, straining and filtering.

Amount of drug power, $\frac{1}{6}$.

Dilutions must be prepared as directed under Class III.

POPULUS.

Synonym, Populus Tremuloides, *Michaux.*

Nat. Ord., Salicaceæ.

Common Names, American Aspen. Quaking Aspen. Quiver Leaf. Trembling Poplar.

This indigenous tree is abundant in the Eastern and Middle States, growing in woods chiefly. It reaches a height of from twenty-five to forty feet. The bark is smooth and greenish-white. Leaves small, on long petioles laterally compressed, so that the leaves respond to the motion of the slightest breeze. Leaves orbicular-heart-shaped, short-acuminate, sharp-serrate and with downy margins. Aments furnished with silky hairs.

It was introduced into our Materia Medica by Dr. E. M. Hale, U. S.

Preparation.—The fresh inner bark is chopped and pounded to a pulp and weighed. Then two parts by weight of alcohol are taken, and having mixed the pulp thoroughly with one-sixth part of it, the rest of the alcohol is added. After having stirred the whole, pour it into a well-stoppered bottle, and let it stand eight days in a dark, cool place. The tincture is then separated by decanting, straining and filtering.

Amount of drug power, $\frac{1}{6}$.
Dilutions must be prepared as directed under Class III.

PROPYLAMINUM.

Synonyms, Propylamin. Trimethylamina. Trimethylamine.
Formula, $(CH_3)_3N$.
Molecular Weight, 59.

Origin and Preparation of Trimethylamina.—This body occurs ready formed in many organic substances, especially as a product of decomposition. It has been found in herring-pickle, in the plant *Chenopodium vulvaria*, in the flowers of *Crataegus oxycantha*, *Pyrus acuparia*, *Pyrus communis*, *Arnica montana*, in ergot of rye, in guano, in putrefying yeast, etc.; it is also produced by heating narcotin with potassium hydrate.

Preparation.—Trimethylamine may be readily and cheaply obtained by distilling a mixture of undiluted herring-brine, with its own volume of a mixture composed of 150 parts of calcium hydrate, 200 of potash and 1700 of water, in a large glass flask. The distillate is neutralized with hydrochloric acid, evaporated to dryness, the saline residue extracted with alcohol and the alcohol distilled off. The residue is mixed with lime and water and again distilled.

Properties.—Trimethylamine is an oily alkaline liquid, colorless and mobile and having an odor which resembles that of stale herring-brine and of ammonia; it boils at 9° C. (48.2° F.); at temperatures higher than this it is a colorless gas which inflames readily. It mixes with water and alcohol in all proportions. It forms with acids crystallizable salts, soluble in water. The officinal German trimethylamine is a twenty per cent. solution in water When this body was first obtained from herring-brine it was called propylamine; later researches have shown that although the two bodies are isomeric they are entirely different.

Preparation for Homœopathic Use.—One part by weight of pure trimethylamina is dissolved in ninety-nine parts by weight of distilled water.

Amount of drug power, $\frac{1}{100}$.
Dilutions must be prepared as directed under Class V—β.

PRUNUS PADUS, *Linn.*

Synonyms, Cerasus Padus, *D C.* Padus Avium. Prunus Racemosa, *Lam.* Padus Vulgaris.
Nat. Ord., Rosaceæ.
Common Name, Bird Cherry.

This tree is distributed through Europe, Northern Africa, Siberia and Western Asia to the Himalayas. It is from ten to twenty feet in height, growing in copses and woods, and is found at an elevation of 1,500 feet in England. Leaves are from two to four inches long, elliptical or obovate, acutely doubly serrate, unequally cordate at the base, axils of the nerves pubescent; stipules linear-subulate, glandular-serrate. Racemes three to five inches long, from short lateral buds, lax-flowered. Flowers half an inch to three-quarters of an inch in diameter, white, erect, then pendulous; pedicels a quarter inch long, erect in fruit; bracts deciduous, linear. Calyx-lobes obtuse, glandular-serrate. Petals erose. Drupe one-third inch in diameter, ovoid, black, bitter; stone globose, rugose. Flowers appear in May.

It was first proven by Lembke, Germany.

Preparation.—The fresh bark of the young twigs gathered in spring is chopped and pounded to a pulp and weighed. Then two parts by weight of alcohol are taken, the pulp mixed thoroughly with one-sixth part of it, and the rest of the alcohol added. After having stirred the whole, pour it into a well-stoppered bottle and let it stand eight days in a dark, cool place. The tincture is then separated by decanting, straining and filtering.

Amount of drug power, $\frac{1}{6}$.

Dilutions must be prepared as directed under Class III.

PRUNUS SPINOSA, *Linn.*

Synonyms, Acacia Germanica. Prunus Communis. Prunus Insititia.

Nat. Ord., Rosaceæ.

Common Names, Sloe. Blackthorn.

This tree is a native of Europe, but has been introduced to this country, where it is found growing as a shrub twelve to fifteen feet high along roadsides and waste places in New England and southward to Pennsylvania. Bark black; branches spiny; leaves obovate elliptical or ovate-elliptical, sharply dentate, at length glabrous; pedicels glabrous; fruit small, globular, black with a bloom, the stone turgid, acute on one edge. Flowers solitary, campanulate, with obtuse lobes, precede the leaves.

It was first proven by Dr. Wahle, Germany.

Preparation.—The fresh flower-buds, just opening, are chopped and pounded to a pulp and weighed, then mixed thoroughly with two-thirds by weight of alcohol, and the whole pressed out through a piece of new linen. The tincture thus obtained is allowed to stand eight days in a well-stoppered bottle, in a dark, cool place and then filtered.

Amount of drug power, $\frac{1}{2}$.

Dilutions must be prepared as directed under Class II.

PSORINUM, *Hering.*

A Nosode.

Dr. Constantine Hering gives the following account of its procurement on page 366, Vol. II. of the *North American Journal of Homœopathy:*

"In the autumn of 1830, I collected the pus from the itch pustule of a young and otherwise healthy negro. He had been handling some stuff from Germany, and had thus been infected (Dr. H. at that time resided in Surinam), but whether by means of *acari* or not I cannot say. The pustules were full, large and yellow, particularly between the fingers, on the hands and forearms. I opened all the mature, unscratched pustules for several days in succession, and collected the pus in a vial with alcohol. After shaking it well and allowing it to stand, I commenced my provings with the tincture on the healthy. Its effects were striking and decided. I administered it to the sick with good results, and sometimes witnessed aggravations. I called this preparation *Psorinum.*"

"When this alcohol is placed in a watch-glass and allowed to evaporate, small, needle-shaped and transparent crystals of a cooling, pungent taste will be left behind. I have always been of the opinion that this salt, contained in the morbid product, was the cause of its peculiar effects."

Preparation.—From the tincture obtained as described above, attenuations are prepared according to Class VI.—β.

PTELEA TRIFOLIATA, *Linn.*

Synonyms, Amyris Elemifera. Ptelea Viticifolia.

Nat. Ord., Rutaceæ.

Common Names, Wafer Ash. Wingseed. Shrubby Trefoil. Hop Tree.

This shrub is indigenous, growing abundantly west of the Alleghanies, in shady, moist hedges, and in rocky places. It is from six to eight feet high, with leaves trifoliate, and marked with pellucid dots; the leaflets are sessile, ovate, short, acuminate, downy beneath when young, crenulate or obscurely toothed; lateral ones inequilateral, terminal ones cuneate at base, from three to four and a half inches long, by from one and one-fourth to one and one-half inches wide. The flowers are polygamous, greenish-white, nearly half an inch in diameter, have a disagreeable odor, and are disposed in terminal corymbose cymes. Stamens mostly four; style short; fruit a two-celled and two-seeded samara, nearly one inch in diameter, winged all round, nearly orbicular.

It was first proven by Prof. Th. Nichol, United States.

Preparation.—The fresh bark of the root is chopped and pounded to a pulp and weighed. Then two parts by weight of alcohol are taken, the pulp mixed thoroughly with one-sixth part of it, and the rest of the alcohol added. After having stirred the whole, pour it into a well-stoppered bottle, and let it stand eight days in a dark, cool place. The tincture is then separated by decanting, straining and filtering.

Drug power of tincture, $\frac{1}{6}$.

Dilutions must be prepared as directed under Class III.

PULSATILLA.

Synonyms, Pulsatilla Nigricans. Pulsatilla Pratensis, *Miller.* Anemone Pratensis, *Linn.* Herba Venti.

Nat. Ord., Ranunculaceæ.

Common Names, Meadow Anemone. Pasque-Flower. Wind-Flower.

The small or true meadow anemone is found on sunny elevated places and pasture-grounds where the soil is sandy, and also in clear pine-forests, in Central and Northern Europe. The leaves, only imperfectly developed before the flowering-time, are radical, petiolate, bipinnate; from the crown of leaves lying upon the ground rises the round flower-scape, which is three to six inches long, straight and leafless, at the top of which the beautiful campanulate, very dark violet-brown flower appears, whose six petals are a little narrowed at the points and are then revolute; it is pendulous during the flowering-time. The sessile involucre consists of three, many-fold linear-lanceolate, pinnate-cleft leaflets, at first close to the flower, later, by elongation of the peduncle, remote; the whole plant is beset with soft, silky-like, white hairs, and has a woolly, lax appearance. It is odorless, but emits when bruised, a most acrid vapor, causing lachrymation. The *Anemone Pulsatilla* to which it is very similar, distinguishes itself by being hairy, by its more shaggy scape, curved above, by its flower which is *only half as large* and of a much darker color and with petals bent backwards at the point.

It was first proven by Hahnemann.

Preparation.—The fresh plant, gathered when in flower, is chopped and pounded to a pulp and weighed. Then two parts by weight of alcohol are taken, the pulp mixed thoroughly with one-sixth part of it, and the rest of the alcohol added. After having stirred the whole, pour it into a well-stoppered bottle, and let it stand eight days in a dark, cool place. The tincture is then separated by decanting, straining and filtering.

Drug power of tincture, $\frac{1}{6}$.

Dilutions must be prepared as directed under Class III.

PULSATILLA NUTTALLIANA, *De Candolle.*

Synonyms, Anemone Ludoviciana, *Nuttall.* Anemone Flavescens. Clematis Hirsutissima. Anemone Patens, *Linn*, v. Nuttalliana, *Gray.*

Nat. Ord., Ranunculaceæ.

Common Names, American Pulsatilla. Pasque-Flower.

This plant is found in North America, from Illinois and Wisconsin west to the Rocky Mountains, and south to Louisiana. Its character is as follows: Villous, with long silken hairs. Stem erect; in flower, very short; in fruit, eight to twelve inches high. Leaves long-stalked, ternately divided, the lateral divisions two-parted, the middle one stalked and three-parted, the segments once or twice cleft into narrowly linear and acute lobes. Involucres lobed like the leaves, sessile, subulately dissected, concave or cup-shaped in arrangement. Sepals five to seven, purplish, spreading, about one inch long, silky outside. Flowers single, appearing before the leaves, pale purple, cup-shaped. Carpels 50 to 75, with plumous tails, one to two inches in length, collected into a roundish head. Flowers appear in early spring.

It was first proven by Dr. W. H. Burt, U. S.

Preparation.—The fresh plant, gathered when in flower, is chopped and pounded to a pulp and weighed. Then two parts by weight of alcohol are taken, the pulp mixed thoroughly with one-sixth part of it, and the rest of the alcohol added. After having stirred the whole pour it into a well-stoppered bottle and let it stand eight days in a dark, cool place. The tincture is then separated by decanting, straining and filtering.

Drug power of tincture, $\frac{1}{6}$.

Dilutions must be prepared as directed under Class III.

PYCNANTHEMUM LINIFOLIUM, *Pursh.*

Nat. Ord., Labiatæ.

Common Name, Virginia Thyme.

This is an indigenous perennial herb found in dry situations from Massachusetts westward to Iowa, and southward. It is from one to two feet high, with sessile, entire, rigid, linear leaves. The flowers are clustered in terminal compact heads, with ciliate bracts. Flowers whitish. The taste of the plant is bitter and resinous. Flowers in August.

Preparation.—The fresh plant is chopped and pounded to a pulp and weighed. Then two parts by weight of alcohol are taken, and having mixed the pulp thoroughly with one-sixth part of it, the rest of the alcohol is added. After having stirred the whole, pour it into a well-stoppered bottle, and let it stand eight days in a dark, cool place. The tincture is then separated by decanting, straining and filtering.

Amount of drug power, $\frac{1}{6}$.

Dilutions must be prepared as directed under Class III.

PYRUS AMERICANA, *DC.*

Nat. Ord., Rosaceæ.

Common Name, American Mountain Ash.

This is a small indigenous tree found growing in mountain woods throughout the Middle and Eastern States. It reaches a height of from fifteen to twenty feet; the trunk is covered with bark of a reddish-brown color. The leaves are often a foot long, odd-pinnate, leaflets thirteen to fifteen, two to three inches long, lanceolate, taper-pointed, sharp-serrate, bright green. Flowers small, white, in large, terminal, flat cymes. Fruit a scarlet globose berry, as large as or larger than a pea.

It was proven by Dr. H. P. Gatchell, U. S.

Preparation.—The fresh bark is chopped and pounded to a pulp and weighed. Then two parts by weight of alcohol are taken, the pulp mixed thoroughly with one-sixth part of it, and the rest of the alcohol added. After having stirred the whole well, and poured it into a well-stoppered bottle, it is allowed to stand eight days in a dark, cool place. The tincture is then separated by decanting, straining and filtering.

Drug power of tincture, $\frac{1}{6}$.

Dilutions must be prepared as directed under Class III.

QUASSIA.

Synonyms, Quassia Amara, *Linn.* Picrænia Excelsa, *Lindl.* Picrasma Excelsa, *Planchon.* Simaruba Excelsa, *DC.*

Nat. Ord., Simarubaceæ.

Common Names, Quassia. Surinam Quassia. Bitter Ash. Bitter Wood.

This tree is common on elevated lands in Jamaica, and is also found in the Islands of Antigua and St. Vincent. The tree resembles the ash, is from fifty to sixty feet high, with alternate, pinnatifid leaves; leaflets elliptical, acuminate, without petioles, deep green above, paler beneath. The flowers are inconspicuous and greenish, and the fruit is a black shining drupe the size of a pea. The quassia from the Jamaica tree is not officinal in the Germanica Pharmacopœia, and the edition of 1872 forbids the use of it.

The Surinam Quassia, officinal in Germany and used also in France, is from *Quassia amara*, a shrub or small tree, with pinnatifid leaves and with bright red flowers. The fruit is a two-celled capsule. Surinam quassia is in cylindrical, or at times bent, branching pieces varying in thickness from that of a finger to that of an arm; in length from a foot to a yard, and frequently covered with the thin whitish-gray bark, which is easily removable. The wood is yellow, without odor, and has a very bitter taste. It is light and finely fibrous. The Jamaica quassia has a wrinkled, thicker, rougher bark than has the Surinam variety, and the bark is not readily separable; the Jamaica wood is paler in color and denser.

It was proven by Dr. J. O. Müller, Austria.

Preparation.—The dried wood, of the branches and trunk of the tree, is coarsely powdered, covered with five parts by weight of alcohol, and allowed to remain eight days in a well-stoppered bottle, in a dark, cool place, being shaken twice a day. The tincture is then poured off, strained and filtered.

Drug power of tincture, $\frac{1}{10}$.

Dilutions must be prepared as directed under Class IV.

QUILLAIA SAPONARIA, *Molina.*

Nat. Ord., Rosaceæ.

Common Names, Quillaya. Soapbark.

Q. saponaria is an evergreen tree found growing in Peru and Chili. The bark is used in medicine and contains the active principle, *Saponin.* The bark comes in commerce in pieces two or three feet long, by several inches in width. The pieces are flat and about one-fourth of an inch thick. The external corky layer is generally removed, leaving a pale, brownish-colored, smooth inner layer. The bark has considerable toughness, is dense, and on fracture, splinters. It is without odor, and its taste is at first merely mucilaginous, but afterward is sharp and acrid. The dust from the powdered bark provokes sneezing; an infusion of the bark produces a lather like that of soap.

Preparation.—The dry bark is coarsely powdered, covered with five parts by weight of alcohol, and allowed to remain eight days in a well-stoppered bottle, in a dark, cool place, being shaken twice a day. The tincture is then poured off, strained and filtered.

Drug power of tincture, $\frac{1}{10}$.

Dilutions must be prepared as directed under Class IV.

RANUNCULUS ACRIS, *Linn.*

Synonyms, Ranunculus Californicus. Ranunculus Canus. Ranunculus Delphinifolius.

Nat. Ord., Ranunculaceæ.

Common Names, Tall Crowfoot. Tall Buttercup.

The tall buttercup is found as a common plant in fields in New England and Canada. Its stem is two or three feet high, erect. Leaves pubescent, deeply trifid, divisions three-parted, sessile, and their segments in lanceolate or linear, crowded lobes. Flowers yellow, rather large. Calyx of five ovate sepals. Corolla of five roundish petals, shining; achenium with a short, recurved beak. Flowers from June to September.

It was first proven by Dr. Franz, Germany.

Preparation.—The fresh herb, gathered in October, is chopped and pounded to a pulp and pressed out in a piece of new linen. The expressed juice is then, by brisk agitation, mingled with an equal part by weight of alcohol, allowed to stand eight days in a well-stoppered bottle, in a dark, cool place, and then filtered.

Amount of drug power, $\frac{1}{2}$.

Dilutions must be prepared as directed under Class I.

RANUNCULUS BULBOSUS, *Linn.*

Synonym, Ranunculus Tuberosus.

Nat. Ord., Ranunculaceæ.

Common Name, Crowfoot. Bulbous-rooted Buttercup.

This buttercup is common in New England. Its stem arises from a bulb-like root, and is from six to eighteen inches high. Radical leaves, three-cleft, the lateral divisions sessile, the terminal one petiolate and ternate, all wedge-shaped, cleft and dentate. Flowers of a rich, glossy yellow, over an inch broad; sepals five, reflexed; petals six to seven. Peduncles furrowed. Achenia short-beaked.

This drug was first proven by Dr. C. G. Franz, Germany.

Preparation.—The fresh, blooming plant is gathered in June, the herb separated from the bulbs, and the juice pressed out; the bulbs, with the addition of a little alcohol, are pounded to a viscid pulp, and also expressed. The juices thus obtained are mixed together and to the mixture is added its own weight of alcohol. Two parts by weight of alcohol are poured upon the residuum of the expressed bulbs, which is subjected to maceration for three days, and then submitted to pressure. This essence is mixed with that from the herb and bulbs, and the whole is allowed to stand eight days in a well-stoppered bottle, in a dark, cool place, and then filtered.

Drug power of tincture, ¼.

Dilutions must be prepared as directed under Class I., except that forty drops of tincture to sixty drops of dilute alcohol are used for the first decimal, and four drops of tincture to ninety-six drops of dilute alcohol for the first centesimal dilution.

RANUNCULUS FLAMMULA, *Linn.*

Synonym, Ranunculus Lingua.

Nat. Ord., Ranunculaceæ.

Common Names, Small or Burning Crowfoot. Marsh Buttercup. Spearwort.

This herb is aquatic in habit, growing in ditches and swamps from Canada southward as far as North Carolina. Stem reclining at base, erect above. Leaves lanceolate; lower ones on petioles, upper ones linear. Flowers bright yellow, solitary. Petals five to seven, much longer than the sepals. Achenia roundish, short-mucronate.

It was introduced into our Materia Medica by Dr. Franz, Germany.

Preparation.—The fresh herb (without the root), gathered while in bloom, is chopped and pounded to a pulp, enclosed in a piece of new linen and subjected to pressure. The expressed juice is then, by brisk agitation, mingled with an equal part by weight of alcohol. This mixture is allowed to stand eight days in a well-stoppered bottle, in a dark, cool place, and then filtered.

Drug power of tincture, ½.

Dilutions must be prepared as directed under Class I.

RANUNCULUS REPENS, *Linn.*

Synonyms, Ranunculus Lanuginosis. Ranunculus Tomentosus.

Nat. Ord., Ranunculaceæ.

Common Names, Creeping Crowfoot. Creeping Buttercup.

This species has a fibrous root, and grows in moist and shady places. Stems ascending, sometimes sending out long runners. Leaves three-parted, divisions petiolate, three-cleft, unequally incised. Flowers medium sized, bright yellow; peduncles furrowed. Fruit broadly margined and pointed. A very variable species.

It was introduced into our Materia Medica by Dr. Franz, Germany.

Preparation.—The fresh herb, gathered in October, is chopped and pounded to a pulp, enclosed in a piece of new linen and subjected to pressure. The expressed juice is then, by brisk agitation, mingled with an equal part by weight of alcohol, and allowed to stand eight days in a well-stoppered bottle, in a dark, cool place, and then filtered.

Amount of drug power, ½.

Dilutions must be prepared as directed under Class I.

RANUNCULUS SCELERATUS, *Linn.*

Synonyms, Ranunculus Palustris. Herba Sardoa.
Nat. Ord., Ranunculaceæ.
Common Names, Celery-leaved Crowfoot. Cursed Crowfoot. Marsh Crowfoot.

This buttercup is found growing in wet places from Canada to Georgia. It is smooth and glabrous; stem twelve to eighteen inches high, thick and hollow. Radical leaves, three-parted, with rounded lobes. Lower stem-leaves, three-parted, the divisions obtusely incised and serrate. Upper stem-leaves nearly sessile, lobes oblong-linear, almost entire. Flowers small, pale yellow. Fruit barely mucronulate.

It was first proven by Dr. Franz, Germany.

Preparation.—The fresh herb, gathered in October, is chopped and pounded to a pulp and weighed. Then two parts by weight of alcohol are taken, the pulp mixed thoroughly with one-sixth part of it, and the rest of the alcohol added. After having stirred the whole, pour it into a well-stoppered bottle, and let it stand eight days in a dark, cool place. The tincture is then separated by decanting, straining and filtering.

Drug power of tincture, $\frac{1}{6}$.

Dilutions must be prepared as directed under Class III.

RAPHANUS SATIVUS NIGER, *Linn.*

Synonyms, Raphanus Hortensis. Raphanus Nigrum.
Nat. Ord., Cruciferæ.
Common Names, Black Garden Radish. Spanish Black Radish.

This radish is a native of China, but has been cultivated all over Europe from time immemorial, and is somewhat cultivated in this country. The very large, roundish, turnip-shaped root, attaining a weight of more than one pound, has a black or black-gray cuticular investment, a white, compact, very juicy flesh and an especially pungent taste and smell.

It was proven by Dr. Nusser, France.

Preparation.—In the month of July, the fresh roots of medium size (hollow or juiceless roots are to be rejected), are chopped and pounded to a pulp and weighed. Then two parts by weight of alcohol are taken, and having mixed the pulp thoroughly with one-sixth part of it, the rest of the alcohol is added. After having stirred the whole, pour it into a well-stoppered bottle, and let it stand eight days in a dark, cool place. The tincture is then separated by decanting, straining and filtering.

Drug power of tincture, $\frac{1}{6}$.

Dilutions must be prepared as directed under Class III.

RESINA ITU.

Synonym, Itu.

This is a resin spoken of in Mure's Materia Medica of the Brazilian

Empire, as coming from the province of St. Paul, and as being used empirically for hernia.

Preparation.—The resin is triturated, as directed under Class VII.

RHEUM.

Synonyms, Rheum Officinale, *Baillon.* Rhabarbarum.

Nat. Ord., Polygonaceæ.

Common Name, Rhubarb.

The botanical source of Rhubarb has not been positively determined. For a long time it was supposed to be *R. palmatum,* but this has been strenuously denied by observers, especially Flückiger and Hanbury, who declare that *R. officinale* is the only species yielding a root-stock which agrees with the drug. The plant or plants which yield rhubarb are inhabitants of China, and they are spread over a vast area. From the little that is known concerning the origin of the drug and its preparation for market, we are only able to say that the root is dug up in the beginning of autumn, is then cleaned, its cortical part cut off, and the root divided into pieces for drying. This is done either by exposure to the sun and air, or by the aid of artificial heat.

Rhubarb comes in commerce either direct from Shanghai, and is then known as Chinese rhubarb, or from China *via* India, in the latter case being called East India rhubarb; it is of the same origin in either circumstance. What was formerly imported under the name of Russian rhubarb was that which was brought overland into Siberia and thence into Russia proper. Turkey rhubarb was the name given to the article brought from China through Persia into Turkey.

China rhubarb comes in sections of a massive root, in various forms, barrel-shaped, conical, plano-convex or irregular; the forms are generally kept assorted by their shapes and classed as round or flat rhubarb. The pieces are often perforated; the outer surface is somewhat shrivelled, with an attached portion of unremoved bark. In well developed pieces, China rhubarb appears, in cross section, to be made up of medullary rays irregularly curved and forming irregularly grouped whorls, radio-stellate in appearance. The general aspect is a whitish or yellowish background, on which the medullary rays appear reddish-yellow or reddish-brown. The fracture of rhubarb is uneven, its odor is peculiar and aromatic, but not agreeable; between the teeth it gives rise to a "gritty" sensation from the crystals of calcium oxalate which it contains; it has a bitter, astringent, nauseous taste.

It was first proven by Hahnemann.

Preparation.—The root in coarse powder is covered with five parts by weight of alcohol, and allowed to remain eight days in a well-stoppered bottle, in a dark, cool place, being shaken twice a day. The tincture is then poured off, strained and filtered.

Drug power of tincture, $\frac{1}{10}$.

Dilutions must be prepared as directed under Class IV.

Triturations of the powdered root are prepared as directed under Class VII.

RHODIUM.

Symbol, Rh.

Atomic Weight, 104.

Origin and Preparation of Rhodium.—The solution from which platinum and palladium have been separated, in the manner already described (see article Iridium), is mixed with hydrochloric acid, and evaporated to dryness. The residue is treated with alcohol of specific gravity 0.837, which dissolves everything except the double chloride of rhodium and sodium. This is well washed with spirit, dried, heated to whiteness and then boiled with water, whereby sodium chloride is dissolved out, and metallic rhodium remains.

Properties.—Thus obtained, rhodium is a white, coherent, spongy mass, more infusible and less capable of being welded than platinum. Its specific gravity varies from 10.6 to 11. Rhodium is very brittle; reduced to powder and heated in the air, it becomes oxidized, and the same alteration occurs to a greater extent when it is fused with nitrate or bisulphate of potassium. None of the acids, singly or conjoined, dissolves this metal, unless it be in the state of alloy, as with platinum, in which state it is attacked by nitro-muriatic acid.

Preparation for Homœopathic Use.—Pure rhodium is triturated, as directed under Class VII.

RHODODENDRON.

Synonym, Rhododendron Chrysanthemum, *Linn.*

Nat. Ord., Ericaceæ.

Common Names, Yellow-flowered Rhododendron. Rosebay.

This is an evergreen shrub found growing in Siberia upon mountain heights. Stem about a foot high, branched. Leaves thick, obtuse, large, oblong, petiolate, rugged and veined on the upper surface, lighter beneath. Flowers yellow, corolla rotate. The leaves smell slightly like rhubarb. The absence of this odor and a rusty color of the under surface of the leaves indicate the substitution of *R. ferrugineum.*

Flowers in July.

It was introduced into our Materia Medica by Dr. E. Seidel, Germany.

Preparation.—The carefully dried leaves, powdered, are covered with five parts by weight of alcohol, and allowed to remain eight days in a well-stoppered bottle, in a dark, cool place, being shaken twice a day. The tincture is then poured off, strained and filtered.

Drug power of tincture, $\frac{1}{6}$.

Dilutions must be prepared as directed under Class IV.

RHUS AROMATICA, *Aiton.*

Nat. Ord., Anacardiaceæ.

Common Names, Fragrant Sumach. Sweet Sumach.

This indigenous small shrub is found growing in dry rocky soil, from Vermont westward and southward. Leaves pubescent when young, thickish when old; leaflets three, rhombic-ovate, unequally cut-toothed, the middle one wedge-shaped at the base; the crushed leaves are sweet-scented.

Flowers yellow, appear in April and May.

Preparation.—The fresh bark of the root is chopped and pounded to a pulp and weighed. Then two parts by weight of alcohol are taken, the pulp mixed thoroughly with one-sixth part of it, and the rest of the alcohol added. After having stirred the whole, pour it into a well-stoppered bottle and let it stand eight days in a dark, cool place. The tincture is then separated by decanting, straining and filtering.

Amount of drug power, $\frac{1}{6}$.

Dilutions must be prepared as directed under Class III.

RHUS GLABRA, *Linn.*

Synonyms, Rhus Carolinense. Rhus Elegans.

Nat. Ord., Anacardiaceæ.

Common Names, Sumach. Smooth or Upland Sumach.

This is an indigenous shrub from six to fifteen feet high and somewhat straggling. The bark is light gray in color with a tinge of red. Leaves and branches glabrous. Leaves, on smooth petioles, are compound; leaflets in pairs, sessile, except the odd one at the end, are from 11 to 31 in number, lanceolate, pointed, sharply serrate, green above, whitish beneath. Flowers greenish-red in color, in terminal, thyrsoid panicles, and are followed by clusters of small red berries, covered with crimson hair. The fruit is acid and astringent.

Flowers in June and July.

It was first proven by Dr. A. V. Marshall, United States.

Preparation.—The fresh bark is chopped and pounded to a pulp and weighed. Then two parts by weight of alcohol are taken, the pulp mixed thoroughly with one-sixth part of it, and the rest of the alcohol added. After having stirred the whole well, it is poured into a well-stoppered bottle, and allowed to remain eight days in a dark, cool place, being shaken twice a day. The tincture is then poured off, strained and filtered.

Drug power of tincture, $\frac{1}{6}$.

Dilutions must be prepared as directed under Class III.

RHUS RADICANS, *Linn.*

Nat. Ord., Anacardiaceæ.

Common Names, Poison Ivy. Poison Vine.

It seems still a disputed question whether this differs from Rhus

Toxicodendron in anything but habit, Rhus Tox. being a dwarf, erect shrub, while Rhus Rad. is a climber, with stem five to forty feet long, furnished with numerous radicles by which it adheres to trees and climbs up them like ivy. The leaves of Rhus Rad. are almost entire and glabrous.

Since Rhus Tox. and Rhus Rad. have been separately proved, and each proving contains symptoms peculiar to itself, it is much the better plan to make tinctures of each and keep them separate.

It was first proved by Dr. B. F. Joslin, United States.

Preparation.—The fresh leaves, collected after sunset on cloudy, sultry days, from shady places, in May and June, before the period of flowering, are chopped and pounded to a pulp and weighed. Then two parts by weight of alcohol are added, the whole poured into a well-stoppered bottle, and allowed to stand eight days in a dark, cool place. The tincture is then separated by decanting, straining and filtering.

Drug power of tincture, ⅙.

Dilutions must be prepared as directed under Class III.

RHUS TOXICODENDRON, *Linn.*

Synonyms, Rhus Humile. Rhus Pubescens. Rhus Toxicarium. Rhus Verrucosa. Vitis Canadensis.

Nat. Ord., Anacardiaceæ.

Common Names, Mercury Vine. Poison Ash. Poison Oak. Poison Vine.

This shrub grows in fields, woods and along fences, all over North America, and has been introduced into Europe; it is one to three feet high, with leaflets angularly indented, and pubescent beneath; roots reddish, branchy; stems erect, bark striated, of a gray-brown color, and full of numerous papillæ of a deep brown; leaves pinnated, long petioled, yellowish-green, veined; folioles almost three inches long, oval, incised, shining, and of a deep green color above, pale green and pubescent beneath; flowers small, yellowish-green, in axillary spikes; fruit monospermous, oval, whitish-gray, marked with five furrows. The plant when wounded emits a milky juice, which becomes black on exposure to the air. The plant, being very poisonous, should be handled with great caution.

It was introduced into our Materia Medica by Hahnemann.

Preparation.—The fresh leaves, collected after sunset on cloudy, sultry days, from shady places, in May and June, before the period of flowering, are chopped and pounded to a pulp and weighed. Then two parts by weight of alcohol are added, the whole poured into a well-stoppered bottle, and allowed to stand eight days in a dark, cool place. The tincture is then separated by decanting, straining and filtering.

Drug power of tincture, ⅙.

Dilutions must be prepared as directed under Class III.

RHUS VENENATA, *De Candolle.*

Synonyms, Rhus Vernicifera. Rhus Vernix, *Linn.*
Nat. Ord., Anacardiaceæ.
Common Names, Poison Sumach. Poison Dogwood. Poison Elder. Poison Wood. Swamp Sumach. Varnish Tree.

This species grows in swamps in the United States and in Canada. It is a shrub six to eighteen feet high, is glabrous; leaves with from seven to thirteen oval or obovate-oblong, abruptly acuminate, entire leaflets. The fruit is yellowish, globular.

It was first proven by Dr. Bute, United States.

Preparation.—The fresh leaves and bark are chopped and pounded to a pulp and weighed. Then two parts by weight of alcohol are added, the whole poured into a well-stoppered bottle and allowed to stand eight days in a dark, cool place. The tincture is then separated by decanting, straining and filtering.

Amount of drug power, ⅙.

Dilutions must be prepared as directed under Class III.

RICINUS COMMUNIS, *Linn.*

Synonyms, Ricinus Africanus. Ricinus Europæus. Ricinus Lividus. Ricinus Viridis. Palma Christi.
Nat. Ord, Euphorbiaceæ.
Common Name, Castor Oil Plant.

For general description of the castor oil plant see article Oleum Ricini. The seeds are about the size of a bean, compressed, ellipsoid in form, from three-tenths to six-tenths of an inch long, and their greatest width is about four-tenths of an inch. The apex of the seed is prolonged into a short beak, on whose inner side is a large tumid caruncle; from the latter extends a raphe to the lower end of the ventral surface. The epidermis is shining, gray in color, and prettily marked with brownish bands and spots, the color and form of the markings varying greatly; it is not separable by rubbing, but after softening in water comes off in leathery strips. Within is a black testa, quite thin, and filled out with the kernel or nucleus, white and oily. The kernel is easily split into halves; unless the seed is rancid, its taste is bland with but slight acridity.

Preparation.—The ripe seeds are coarsely powdered, covered with five parts by weight of alcohol, and the whole is allowed to remain eight days in a well-stoppered bottle, in a dark, cool place, being shaken twice a day. The tincture is then poured off, strained and filtered.

Drug power of tincture, $\frac{1}{10}$

Dilutions must be prepared as directed under Class IV.

ROBINIA.

Synonyms, Robinia Pseud-acacia, *Linn.* Pseud-acacia Odorata.
Nat. Ord., Leguminosæ.
Common Names, Locust Tree. False Acacia. Yellow Locust.

The locust is a well known indigenous tree common in the Middle and Southern States; it is cultivated much farther north and also in Europe. Under favorable conditions it often reaches a height of eighty feet, and the diameter of the trunk three or four feet. The bark is rather smooth, grayish-brown externally, yellowish within. Leaves odd-pinnate; leaflets in from eight to twelve pairs with an odd terminal one, all oval, thin, nearly sessile and smooth. The flowers are showy, white and fragrant, in clustered, hanging, axillary racemes. The pod is narrow, flat, three or four inches long, and contains five or six small blackish-brown hard seeds. The thorns with which the young tree is armed disappear at maturity.

It was first proven by Dr. W. H. Burt, United States.

Preparation.—The fresh bark of the young twigs is chopped and pounded to a pulp and weighed. Then two parts by weight of alcohol are taken, the pulp mixed thoroughly with one-sixth part of it, and the rest of the alcohol added. After having stirred the whole well, pour it into a well-stoppered bottle and let it stand eight days in a dark, cool place. The tincture is then separated by decanting, straining and filtering.

Amount of drug power, ⅙.

Dilutions must be prepared as directed under Class III.

ROSA CENTIFOLIA, *Linn.*

Synonyms, Rosa Mucosa. Rosa Provincialis.

Nat. Ord., Rosaceæ.

Common Names, Hundred-Leaved Rose. Cabbage Rose. Pale Rose.

This widely cultivated and varying rose is a native of Southern Europe and Western Asia. It is a shrub, two to four feet high, very prickly, the prickles being straight and scarcely dilated at the base. Leaflets five to seven in number, ovate or elliptic-ovate, margins glandular hairy, sub-pilose beneath. Petals are usually pinkish, mostly round-obovate, of a peculiar well known fragrance. Their taste is sweetish, with some bitterness and slight astringency. Upon drying they become brownish in color and their odor is in great part dissipated.

Preparation.—The fresh petals are pounded to a pulp, weighed, mixed well with two-thirds their weight of alcohol, and pressed out in a piece of new linen. The tincture thus obtained is allowed to stand eight days in a well-stoppered bottle, in a dark, cool place, and then filtered.

Amount of drug power, ½.

Dilutions must be prepared as directed under Class II.

ROSMARINUS.

Synonyms, Rosmarinus Officinalis, *Linn.* Herba Anthos. Libanotis.

Nat. Ord., Labiatæ.

Common Names, Rosemary. Sea-dew.

This evergreen shrub is a native of Southern Europe. It has an erect stem three or four feet high, much branched. Leaves sessile, opposite, linear-oblong, obtuse, entire, dark green and shining above, downy, and at times whitish, beneath. Flowers axillary and terminal, pale blue or white. The flowers and leaves have a balsamic, camphoraceous odor and taste.

Preparation.—The fresh leaves and blossoms are chopped and pounded to a pulp and weighed. Then two parts by weight of alcohol are taken, the pulp mixed thoroughly with one-sixth part of it, and the rest of the alcohol added. After having stirred the whole, pour it into a well-stoppered bottle, and let it stand eight days in a dark, cool place. The tincture is then separated by decanting, straining and filtering.

Drug power of tincture, $\frac{1}{6}$.

Dilutions must be prepared as directed under Class III.

RUDBECKIA HIRTA, *Linn.*

Nat. Ord., Compositæ.

Common Names, Cone-Flower. Great Hairy Rudbeckia.

This is a rough, bristly-hairy plant from one to two feet high, found growing in dry soil from New York to Wisconsin and southward. It is from one to two feet high; stem simple or branched near the base. Leaves almost entire, the upper ones sessile, lanceolate or oblong, lower ones on petioles, three-nerved, spatulate. Flowers in single large heads with about fourteen rays longer than the involucre and bright yellow in color. The disk is conical, bearing dark purplish-brown chaff and flowers. Flowers from June to August.

Preparation.—The fresh herb, in flower, is chopped and pounded to a pulp and weighed. Then two parts by weight of alcohol are taken, the pulp mixed with one-sixth part of it, and the rest of the alcohol added. After having stirred the whole, pour it into a well-stoppered bottle, and let it stand eight days, in a dark, cool place. The tincture is then separated by decanting, straining and filtering.

Amount of drug power, $\frac{1}{6}$.

Dilutions must be prepared as directed under Class III.

RUMEX.

Synonym, Rumex Crispus, *Linn.*

Nat. Ord., Polygonaceæ.

Common Names, Curled Dock. Garden Patience. Yellow Dock.

This plant is a native of Europe, introduced into this country, where it grows wild in pastures, dry fields, waste grounds, etc. From a deep spindle-shaped yellow root, its stem, which is quite smooth, rises three to four feet high. Leaves with strongly wavy-curled margins, lanceolate, acute, the lower truncate or scarcely heart-shaped at the base;

whorls crowded in prolonged wand-like racemes, leafless above; valves round-heart-shaped, obscurely denticulate or entire, mostly all of them grain-bearing.

It was first proved by Dr. Henry A. Houghton, Inaug. Diss., Phila. Hom. Med. Coll., 1852.

Preparation.—The fresh root, gathered at time of flowering, is chopped and pounded to a pulp and weighed. Then two parts by weight of alcohol are taken, the pulp mixed with one-sixth part of it, and the rest of the alcohol added. After having stirred the whole, pour it into a well-stoppered bottle, and let it stand eight days in a dark, cool place. The tincture is then separated by decanting, straining and filtering.

Drug power of tincture, $\frac{1}{6}$.

Dilutions must be prepared as directed under Class III.

RUTA.

Synonyms, Ruta Graveolens, *Linn.* Ruta Latifolia.

Nat. Ord., Rutaceæ.

Common Names, Rue. Bitter Herb. Countryman's Treacle.

This plant is widely cultivated in gardens; it is indigenous to Southern Europe. It is shrub-like in aspect, and near the base is woody and rough externally, above nearly glabrous. Leaves twice to thrice-pinnate and glaucous; segments oblong, obtuse, terminal ones obovate-cuneate, all entire or irregularly incised. The flowers are in terminal corymbs, yellow. Corolla of four to five petals, obovate and distinct. Calyx of four or five sepals united at base. Stamens mostly ten. The odor of the leaves is strong and disagreeable, and the fresh, vigorous plant should be handled with care, as the recent juice inflames the skin upon contact.

It was first proven by Hahnemann.

Preparation.—The fresh herb, gathered shortly before blooming, is chopped and pounded to a fine pulp, enclosed in a piece of new linen and subjected to pressure. The expressed juice is then, by brisk agitation, mingled with an equal part by weight of alcohol. The mixture is allowed to stand eight days in a well-stoppered bottle, in a dark, cool place, and then filtered.

Drug power of tincture, $\frac{1}{2}$.

Dilutions must be prepared as directed under Class I.

SABADILLA.

Synonyms, Sabadilla Officinarum, *Brandt.* Veratrum Sabadilla, *Schlecht.* Asagræa Officinalis, *Lindley.* Schœnocaulon Officinale, *Gray.* Hordeum Causticum. Melanthium Sabadilla.

Nat. Ord., Liliaceæ. (Melanthaceæ.)

Common Names, Sabadilla. Cevadilla. Indian Caustic Barley.

This is a bulbous plant indigenous to Mexico and countries south of it. It is found growing in grassy places on the eastern slopes of volcanic ranges. The plant is bulbous, having a slender scape bearing a narrow spiked raceme of greenish-yellow flowers. The fruit consists of three oblong, pointed follicles on a short pedicel and surrounded by the remains of the six-parted calyx. They are light brown in color and of a paper-like substance. Each contains two pointed, narrow, black seeds nearly four lines in length, shining, rugose and angular, or concave from mutual pressure. Within the compact testa lies the oily albumen, including in its base the small embryo. The seeds are without odor, have a bitter, acrid taste; its powder has active sternutatory powers.

It was first proven by Hahnemann.

Preparation.—The seeds, taken out of the capsules, are coarsely powdered, covered with five parts by weight of alcohol, and allowed to remain eight days in a well-stoppered bottle, in a dark, cool place, being shaken twice a day. The tincture is then poured off, strained and filtered.

Drug power of tincture, $\frac{1}{10}$.

Dilutions must be prepared as directed under Class IV.

SABINA.

Synonyms, Juniperus Sabina, *Linn.* Sabina Officinalis, *Garcke.*
Nat. Ord., Coniferæ.
Common Name, Savine.

Juniperus Sabina is a woody, evergreen shrub, occurring in the Southern Alps in Austria and Switzerland, extending into France, into Italy, and eastward to the Caspian Sea. It has also been found in Newfoundland. In favorable situations it becomes tree-like in character. The bark of the older stems is reddish-brown and rough; on the young branches it is light green. The young shoots are clothed with small, adpressed leaves, which are scale-like, opposite in pairs, rhomboidal in outline, centrally glandular and dark green. As the shoots grow older the leaves become erect and somewhat acuminate. The shrub is diœcious. The fruit is berry-like, blackish-purple, more or less oval, and has three or four bony seeds. The leaves have a disagreeable, balsamic odor and bitter and acrid taste.

It was first proven by Hahnemann.

Preparation.—The fresh tops, collected of the younger branches in April, are chopped and pounded to a pulp and weighed. Then two parts by weight of alcohol are taken, the pulp thoroughly mixed with one-sixth part of it, and the rest of the alcohol added. After stirring the whole well, pour it into a well-stoppered bottle, and let it stand eight days in a dark, cool place. The tincture is then separated by decanting, straining and filtering.

Drug power of tincture, $\frac{1}{6}$.

Dilutions must be prepared as directed under Class III.

SACCHARUM OFFICINARUM, *Linn.*

Synonym, Saccharum Album.
Nat. Ord., Gramineæ.

Common Names, Sugar Cane. White Sugar.

Origin.—This well-known plant is probably a native of Southern Asia, and was undoubtedly cultivated for centuries; its now all but indispensable product seems to have been known in Europe since the time of Alexander the Great, but did not come into general use until after the introduction of the cane into America. At present it is wholly a cultivated plant, not being permitted to flower and being propagated by cuttings of the root-stock. The culm or stem is from eight to sixteen feet high, one to two inches thick, cylindrical, jointed, and contains a central juicy pith. The leaves are broad, flat, linear-lanceolate, four to five feet long and about two inches wide. The flowers are in panicles, from one to two feet in length, composed of numerous, loose, erect, spreading racemes. The juice of the stem contains about twenty per cent. of sucrose or pure cane-sugar.

Preparation.—The ripened stems are chopped and pounded to a pulp and weighed. Then two parts by weight of dilute alcohol are taken, the pulp mixed thoroughly with one-sixth part of it, and the rest of the alcohol added. After having stirred the whole, and having poured it into a well-stoppered bottle, it is allowed to stand eight days in a dark, cool place. The tincture is then separated by decanting, straining and filtering.

Drug power, $\frac{1}{6}$.

Dilutions must be prepared as directed under Class III.

SALIX ALBA, *Linn.*

Nat. Ord., Salicaceæ.

Common Name, White Willow.

The white willow is a native of Europe, but has been naturalized to some extent in the United States. It grows to a height of about thirty feet. The bark of the trunk is brownish and cracked; that of the young branches is greenish and smooth. Its leaves are lanceolate, pointed, dentate, silky-hairy, especially beneath. The bark is bitter. Flowers in terminal cylindrical aments.

Preparation.—The fresh bark is chopped and pounded to a pulp and weighed. Then two parts by weight of alcohol are taken, the pulp mixed thoroughly with one-sixth part of it, and the rest of the alcohol added. After having stirred the whole, pour it into a well-stoppered bottle, and let it stand eight days in a dark, cool place. The tincture is then separated by decanting, straining and filtering.

Amount of drug power, $\frac{1}{6}$.

Dilutions must be prepared as directed under Class III.

SALIX NIGRA, *Marsh.*

Nat. Ord., Salicaceæ.

Common Name, Black Willow.

This tree grows from fifteen to twenty feet high, frequently along streams, especially southward. It has a rough, black bark. Leaves lanceolate and lance-linear, pointed and tapering at each end, serrate, smooth (except on the petioles and midrib), and green on both sides; stipules small, deciduous; scales short and rounded, villous; stamens three to six; pods mostly short-ovate.

It was proven by Dr. E. D. Wright, United States.

Preparation.—The fresh bark is chopped and pounded to a pulp and weighed. Then two parts by weight of alcohol are taken, the pulp mixed thoroughly with one-sixth part of it, and the rest of the alcohol added. After having stirred the whole, pour it into a well-stoppered bottle, and let it stand eight days in a dark, cool place. The tincture is then separated by decanting, straining and filtering.

Amount of drug power, $\frac{1}{6}$.

Dilutions must be prepared as directed under Class III.

SALIX PURPUREA, *Linn.*

Nat. Ord., Salicaceæ.

Common Name, Purple Willow.

This species is a native of Europe, where it grows in low grounds. Its twigs are olive-colored, long and smooth. Leaves obovate-lanceolate, pointed, smooth, serrulate above; catkins cylindrical; scales round and concave, very black; stigmas nearly sessile; ovary sessile.

It was proven by Dr. T. C. Duncan, United States.

Preparation.—The fresh bark is chopped and pounded to a pulp and weighed. Then two parts by weight of alcohol are taken, the pulp mixed thoroughly with one-sixth part of it, and the rest of the alcohol added. After having stirred the whole, pour it into a well-stoppered bottle, and let it stand eight days in a dark, cool place. The tincture is then separated by decanting, straining and filtering.

Amount of drug power, $\frac{1}{6}$.

Dilutions must be prepared as directed under Class III.

SALVIA OFFICINALIS, *Linn.*

Nat. Ord., Labiatæ.

Common Name, Sage.

This is a perennial plant, indigenous to Southern Europe, but widely cultivated elsewhere. The plant's stem is woody at the base, is much branched and is one or two feet high; like the Labiatæ in general its stem is square. The leaves are opposite, on petioles, oblong-lanceolate, crenulate, rugose, grayish-green in color, hairy beneath; lower leaves at times auriculate, upper ones nearly sessile. Flowers in whorled arrangement, forming spikes. Calyx mucronate, striate, bilabiate, brownish. Corolla ringent, bilabiate, upper lip straight or falcate, lower spreading three-lobed, blue. The plant has a peculiar aromatic odor and an aromatic bitter taste.

Preparation.—The fresh leaves are chopped and pounded to a pulp and weighed. Then two parts by weight of alcohol are taken, the pulp thoroughly mixed with one-sixth part of it, and the rest of the alcohol added. After having stirred the whole, pour it into a well-stoppered bottle, and let it stand eight days in a dark, cool place. The tincture is then separated by decanting, straining and filtering.

Amount of drug power, $\frac{1}{6}$.

Dilutions must be prepared as directed under Class III.

SAMBUCUS.

Synonym, Sambucus Nigra, *Linn.*

Nat. Ord., Caprifoliaceæ.

Common Names, European Elder. Bore Tree.

This plant is a large deciduous shrub or small tree, found growing in Central Europe and southward, and extending into the Caucasus and Southern Siberia. Leaves compound, leaflets in several pairs with an odd terminal one, all oblong-oval, acuminate. Flowers in flattened umbellate cymes without bracts. Calyx adherent, four or five-toothed. Corolla rotate, deeply five-lobed, creamy white in color. Fruit a globous, purple berry.

It was first proven by Hahnemann.

Preparation.—Equal parts of the fresh leaves and flowers are chopped and pounded to a pulp, enclosed in a piece of new linen and subjected to pressure. The expressed juice is then, by brisk agitation, mingled with an equal part by weight of alcohol. This mixture is allowed to stand eight days, in a well-stoppered bottle, in a dark, cool place, and then filtered.

Amount of drug power, $\frac{1}{2}$.

Dilutions must be prepared as directed under Class I.

SAMBUCUS CANADENSIS, *Linn.*

Nat. Ord., Caprifoliaceæ.

Common Name, Elder.

This is an indigenous shrub, woody at the base, common in thickets and waste grounds in the United States. Its height is from six to ten feet. Leaflets seven to eleven, oblong, mostly smooth, serrate, the lower ones often binate or trifoliate. Petioles smooth. Flowers numerous in flat-topped cymes. Calyx five-parted. Corolla rotate, five-cleft with obtuse segments, cream-colored or white. Fruit a dark purple berry. The plant has a strong disagreeable odor when bruised, but after drying, the odor is pleasant.

Preparation.—Equal parts of the fresh leaves and flowers are chopped and pounded to a pulp and weighed. Then two parts by weight of alcohol are taken, the pulp mixed thoroughly with one-sixth part of it, and the rest of the alcohol added. After having stirred the whole, pour it into a well-stoppered bottle, and let it stand eight days in a dark, cool place. The tincture is then separated by decanting, straining and filtering.

Amount of drug power, $\frac{1}{6}$.

Dilutions must be prepared as directed under Class III.

SAMBUCUS NIGRA e CORTICE.

Bark of Sambucus Nigra (European Elder).

Preparation.—The fresh inner bark of the young twigs is chopped and pounded to a pulp and weighed. Then two-thirds by weight of alcohol are taken, mixed well with the pulp, and the mixture strained through a piece of new linen. The tincture thus obtained is allowed to stand eight days in a well-stoppered bottle, in a dark, cool place, and then filtered.

Amount of drug power, $\frac{1}{2}$.

Dilutions must be prepared as directed under Class II.

SANGUINARIA.

Synonyms, Sanguinaria Canadensis, *Linn.* Sanguinaria Acaulis. Sanguinaria Vernalis.

Nat. Ord., Papaveraceæ.

Common Names, Bloodroot. Indian Paint. Pauson. Tetter-wort. Turmeric. Puccoon.

This is an indigenous perennial, acaulescent plant. It has a horizontal abrupt root-stalk, fleshy, about three inches long, of a finger's thickness, fleshy, externally reddish-brown in color, bright red within, and sending forth many fine rootlets. From each bud of the root-stalk arises a large smooth leaf and a scape six inches high, bearing a single flower. The leaf is on a channeled petiole, is kidney-shaped, with roundish lobes separated by rounded sinuses, is yellow-green above, paler beneath and marked with an orange-colored venation. The flower is quadrangular in outline, is of short duration, without odor and is white in color. Sepals two, caducous; petals eight to twelve in two or three rows, the outer ones longer. Stamens numerous, anthers orange-colored. Stigma sessile. Fruit a two-valved, oblong capsule, acute at each end, many seeded. All parts of the plant when wounded exude an orange-colored sap, but the tint is deepest in the juice of the root. Flowers in March and April.

The first systematic proving was by Dr. Bute, United States.

Preparation.—The fresh root is chopped and pounded to a pulp and weighed. Then two parts by weight of alcohol are taken, the pulp mixed thoroughly with one-sixth part of it, and the rest of the alcohol added. After having stirred the whole, pour it into a well-stoppered bottle and let it stand eight days in a dark, cool place. The tincture is then separated by decanting, straining and filtering.

Drug power of tincture, $\frac{1}{6}$.

Dilutions must be prepared as directed under Class III.

SANTONINUM.

Synonyms, Santonin. Santonine. Santoninic Anhydride.

Formula, $C_{15}H_{18}O_3$.

Molecular Weight, 246.

Origin.—Santonine is the active principle of santonica, which is the officinal name for the unexpanded flower heads of *Artemisia Maritima* var. *Stechmanniana*. Besser. According to Wilkomm, *Artemisia Cina* (see article Cina) is the mother plant of A. Maritima. Good samples of the drug Santonica are described as being almost exclusively of the unopened flower heads, which are so minute that ninety of them weigh only a grain. It yields from one to two per cent. of essential oil having the peculiar odor and taste of the drug itself, and about one and a half or two per cent. of santonine; as the flowers open, the percentage of santonine decreases. The latter, although not an acid, is readily extracted from the flower heads by milk of lime, as in the presence of bases and H_2O, it takes up water and then unites with the base, forming a santonate. The resulting santonate of calcium is easily soluble in water, and when the aqueous solution is treated with hydrochloric acid, santoninic acid, $C_{15}H_{20}O_4$, at once separates, but immediately giving up one molecule of water is reconverted into santonine, $C_{15}H_{18}O_3$.

Preparation.—Four troy ounces of santonica in moderately coarse powder, are to be digested with an ounce and a half, troy, of recently slaked lime in fine powder, in a pint of dilute alcohol for twenty-four hours, and the mixture is then to be expressed. The residue is to be digested with a pint of dilute alcohol in the same way and again expressed, and this double procedure of digestion and expression is to be done a third time. The resulting alcoholic solutions are to be mixed and distilled down to one-third. This residue is, after filtering, to be evaporated to one-half its volume, and is then to be treated with acetic acid, added gradually until the acid is slightly in excess; the mixture is then to be set aside for forty-eight hours, with repeated stirring. At the end of the time stated, a crystalline mass will have been obtained, which is to be placed upon a loosely stopped funnel, thoroughly washed with water and dried. The dried product is to be dissolved in ten times its weight of alcohol, digested for several hours with animal charcoal, filtered while hot, the charcoal thoroughly washed on the filter with hot alcohol, and the filtrate set aside in the dark. The crystals are to be collected and dried on bibulous paper, both operations being done in the dark, and are then to be placed in a well-stoppered bottle and completely protected from light.

Properties.—Santonine crystallizes from its alcoholic solutions in right rhombic prisms which are permanent in the air, colorless and of a pearly lustre; under the influence of daylight they become yellow. They are without odor, and their taste is bitter. Their specific gravity is 1.217. Santonine requires for its solution 5,000 parts of cold, and 250 of boiling water, 42 of cold, and 3 of boiling 90 per cent. alcohol, between 70 and 80 parts of ether, and 4 of chloroform; it is more or less soluble in the volatile and fatty oils. Its solutions are neutral in reaction and have a bitter taste. When heated to 170° C. (338° F.), the crystals melt, giving off an aromatic odor, and when cooled slowly solidify to a crystalline mass; when cooled rapidly, an amorphous mass is left; by stronger heating, the crystals sublime without more than slight decomposition. When santonine is in contact with alkalies in excess, its color changes to red, but the original color is restored in a short time. As has been already stated, santonine is colored yellow by daylight, but in the direct sunlight the crystals become disrupted into smaller pieces, which form a yellow solution with alcohol, and from which solution may be obtained colorless crystals of photosantonic acid (Sestini). Santonine is properly the anhydride of santoninic acid.

Tests.—Santonine has been found adulterated with gum arabic in laminæ, with boracic acid, salicin, strychnia and brucia—the last three probably by admixture through carelessness. Dissolve a small portion of santonine in chloroform, with shaking; gum, boracic acid and salicin will remain, if present, as undissolved residue. When santonin is heated on platinum foil to redness, there should be no residue left (borax remains as a glassy mass, having an alkaline reaction to turmeric paper); if the alcoholic solution of santonine be ignited, the flame will be of a green color if boracic acid be present. Santonine is to be shaken with twenty volumes of water, to which a few drops of acetic acid have been added, repeatedly agitated for half an hour and then filtered. The filtrate is to be treated with tannin and with picric acid solution; a white precipitate or turbidity in either case indicates the presence of an alkaloid.

Preparation for Homœopathic Use.—One part by weight of pure santonin is dissolved in ninety-nine parts by weight of alcohol.

Amount of drug power, $\frac{1}{100}$.

Dilutions must be prepared as directed under Class VI—β.

Triturations are prepared, as directed under Class VII.

SAPO DOMESTICUS.

Synonym, Sapo Animalis.

Common Name, Curd Soap.

It is made with soda and a purified animal fat, consisting principally of stearin. See article Glycerinum.

When it is dissolved in eight parts of boiling alcohol, the solution, after cooling, forms a translucent, jelly-like mass.

Preparation for Homœopathic Use.—One part by weight of curd soap is dissolved in fifty parts by weight of alcohol.

Amount of drug power, $\frac{1}{100}$.

Dilutions must be prepared as directed under Class VI—β.

Triturations may be prepared as directed under Class VII.

SARRACENIA PURPUREA, *Linn.*

Synonyms, Sarazina Gibbosa. Sarracenia Heterophylla.

Nat. Ord., Sarraceniaceæ.

Common Names, Eve's Cup. Fly Trap. Pitcher Plant. Side-saddle Flower. Huntsman's Cup.

This plant is found in boggy places throughout Canada and the United States. Its rhizome, about an inch long, is conical, oblique, reddish-brown externally and pale brownish within, and is furnished with numerous fibrous prolongations. The leaves are radical, pitcher-shaped, ascending, curved, broadly-winged; the hood erect, open, round-cordate. Their capacity, when of ordinary size, is nearly two ounces, and usually they are partly filled with water and drowned insects. Flower deep purple, nodding, upon a scape fourteen to twenty inches high. Petals fiddle-shaped, arching over a greenish-yellow style. Flowers in June.

It was first proven by Dr. T. C. Duncan, U. S.

Preparation.—The fresh plant, gathered when coming into flower, is chopped and pounded to a pulp and weighed. Then two parts by weight of alcohol are taken, the pulp mixed thoroughly with one-sixth part of it, and the rest of the alcohol added. After having stirred the whole, pour it into a well-stoppered bottle, and let it stand eight days in a dark, cool place. The tincture is then separated by decanting, straining and filtering.

Drug power of tincture, $\frac{1}{6}$.

Dilutions must be prepared as directed under Class III.

SARSAPARILLA.

Synonyms, Smilax Officinalis, *Humboldt*, *Bonpland* and *Kunth*. Smilax Medica, *Schlecht.* Sarsa.

Nat. Ord., Smilaceæ.

Sarsaparilla is the name used for the root of several species of *Smilax* indigenous to Mexico and the countries southward as far as the Northern part of South America. The botanical sources of the drug are not scientifically determined, as the different species inhabit swampy forests which are difficult and dangerous to explore. Besides this, the plants are climbers as well as diœcious, so that the flowers and fruit, produced too at different seasons, are difficult of access, and the leaves vary very greatly in outline. The best known species to which the drug has been ascribed are *S. officinalis* H. B. K., and *S. medica*, Schl. et Cham. Sarsaparilla is classed as either *mealy*, in which starch is shown upon fracture of the bark, or *non-mealy*. The mealy varieties include the Honduras, Guatemala and Brazilian sarsaparillas, and the *non-mealy* are the Jamaican and Mexican kinds. Although this classification is held in commerce it is remarkable that the British Pharmacopœia admits only the Jamaican variety, while in the United States the Honduras sarsaparilla is preferred.

Description.—From a thick, short, knotty rhizome grow horizontally, long fleshy roots of the thickness of a quill or slightly larger. The roots are simple, forked only near the extremities and are furnished with thread-like fibres. In the dried state the roots are more or less furrowed longitudinally. The whole mass of roots with the rhizome attached is brought into the market. The Honduras variety comes in bundles made by folding up the rootlets in lengths of two or three feet and held together by a few turns of the long roots. Its color externally is earthy or grayish-brown. It has no odor, and its taste is mucilaginous with some slight bitterness and acridity.

The drug was first proven by Hahnemann.

Preparation.—The dried root of the Honduras variety is coarsely powdered and covered with five parts by weight of alcohol, and allowed to remain eight days in a well-stoppered bottle, in a dark, cool place, being shaken twice a day. The tincture is then poured off, strained and filtered.

Drug power of tincture, $\frac{1}{10}$.

Dilutions must be prepared as directed under Class IV.

Triturations of the dried root-bark, as directed under Class VII, are to be preferred.

SASSAFRAS.

Synonyms, Sassafras Officinale, *Nees.* Laurus Sassafras, *Linn.*
Nat. Ord., Lauraceæ.
Common Name, Sassafras.

This tree is indigenous to North America north of the Gulf of Mexico. In the Middle and Eastern States it becomes a shrub; its height is from ten to twenty feet, but in Southern and more favorable situations it often reaches fifty feet. The bark of the trunk is gray, rough and furrowed, but upon the young branches it is brown and smoother. Leaves on petioles, alternate, entire and ovate, some of them three-lobed, bright green in color, glabrous above, the young leaves downy beneath. Flowers greenish-yellow, in clustered racemes, diœcious. Fruit a dark blue drupe. All parts of the tree are fragrant and have a sweetish aromatic taste; the bark of the root is of a somewhat stronger and different flavor. When the gray, corky layer is removed the inner bark is found to be nearly white in the recent state, but as seen in commerce is rusty-brown in color, is soft and easily breaks, the fracture being short and cork-like. On cross section it shows radiating striæ.

Preparation.—The dried root-bark, powdered, is covered with five parts by weight of alcohol, and allowed to remain eight days in a well-stoppered bottle, in a dark, cool place, being shaken twice a day. The tincture is then poured off, strained and filtered.

Drug power of tincture, $\frac{1}{10}$.

Dilutions must be prepared as directed under Class IV.

SCILLA.

Synonyms, Scilla Maritima, *Linn.* Cepa Marina. Ornithogalum Maritinum. Squilla Hispanica. Urginea Maritima, *Baker.*
Nat. Ord., Liliaceæ.
Common Names, Squill. Sea Onion.

Scilla maritima is a perennial plant, found generally in countries bordering on the Mediterranean. From a pear-shaped bulb as large as a man's fist, or larger, proceed fibrous roots. Above, the bulb sends forth shining, deep green leaves, lanceolate in shape and pointed, long, and undulate on the margins. From amid the leaves arises a scape from one to three feet high, round and smooth, bearing above, a spike of white flowers, each flower on a purple pedicel. Perianth six-parted, spreading, deciduous; filaments six, filiform. There are two varieties of squill, one possessing colorless bulb-scales, the other having the latter roseate or reddish. The so-called red squills is used in homœopathic pharmacy.

It was first proved by Hahnemann.

Preparation.—The fresh bulb, of which we select the most fleshy, is chopped and pounded to a pulp and weighed. Then two parts of alcohol are taken, the pulp mixed thoroughly with one-sixth part of it, and the rest of the alcohol added. After having stirred the whole, pour it into a well-stoppered bottle, and let it stand eight days in a dark, cool place, being shaken twice a day. The tincture is then poured off, strained and filtered.

Drug power of tincture, ⅙.

Dilutions must be prepared as directed under Class III, except that dilute alcohol be used for the 2x and 1 dilutions.

SCROPHULARIA NODOSA, *Linn.*

Synonyms, Galiopsis. Ocimastrum.

Nat. Ord., Scrophulariaceæ.

Common Names, Carpenter's Square. Figwort. Heal All. Scrofula Plant.

This is a perennial herbaceous plant, found growing in damp woods in Canada and the United States, and in Europe. *Scrophularia Marilandica, Linn.*, was formerly considered a distinct species, but the individual plant of American growth, and to which this name was given is now held to be nearly identical with *Scrophularia nodosa.* Stem four to six feet high, four-sided, opposite branched above. Leaves smooth, three to seven inches long, opposite, petiolate, ovate, ovate-oblong, or upper ones lanceolate, acute, serrate; base broadly cordate, roundish or tapering. Flowers olive-colored in pedunculate cymes. Calyx in five acute segments. Corolla sub-globous, five-lobed, sub-bilabiate. Fruit a two-celled capsule, many seeded. Flowers June to August.

The drug was proven by Dr. Franz, Germany.

Preparation.—The fresh plant, gathered before the development of the blossoms, is chopped and pounded to a pulp and weighed. Then two parts by weight of alcohol are taken, the pulp mixed thoroughly with one-sixth part of it, and the rest of the alcohol added. After having stirred the whole, pour it into a well-stoppered bottle and let it stand eight days in a dark, cool place. The tincture is then separated by decanting, straining and filtering.

Drug power of tincture, ⅙.

Dilutions must be prepared as directed under Class III.

SCUTELLARIA.

Synonym, Scutellaria Lateriflora, *Linn.*

Nat. Ord., Labiatæ.

Common Names, Scullcap. Blue Pimpernel. Hood Wort.

This indigenous perennial plant is a foot or two high, has an erect, smooth, four-angled, much branching stem. Leaves opposite, on long petioles, ovate, acute, serrate. Flowers small, pale blue in color, in long leafy racemes. Corolla tube elongated, upper lip entire and concave, lower in three lobes. The plant grows in all parts of the United States in wet situations near ponds, ditches, etc. Flowers in July and August.

It was first proven by Dr. F. W. Gordon, United States.

Preparation.—The whole fresh plant is chopped and pounded to a pulp and weighed. Then two parts by weight of alcohol are taken, the pulp thoroughly mixed with one-sixth part of it, and the rest of the alcohol added. After having stirred the whole, pour it into a well-stoppered bottle, and let it stand eight days in a dark, cool place. The tincture is then separated by decanting, straining and filtering.

Drug power of tincture, $\frac{1}{6}$.

Dilutions must be prepared as directed under Class III.

SECALE CORNUTUM.

Synonyms, Ergota. Acinula Clavus. Claviceps Purpurea. Spermoedia Clavus.

Nat. Ord., Fungi.

Common Names, Cockspur. Ergot. Horned Rye. Spurred Rye.

This morbid alteration of the seed-bud of rye (and several other cereals) has been attributed to various causes.

According to De Candolle, who calls it *Sclerotium clavus*, this alteration is caused by a fungus which prevents the development of the grain from the commencement, and grows up in its stead. This opinion is supported by the circumstances attending the appearance and growth of the morbid grain; it occurs principally in fertile years when hot weather frequently alternates with warm rains. It is seated between the awns as a cylindrical, somewhat curved, angular body, longitudinally rugose, and frequently resembling the fenugreek, from one-half to one-inch long, of a deep brown violet color without, and a yellow-white, and sometimes a violet-white within, viscid, having an offensive, rancid smell, and a flat, sweetish taste.

Preparation.—The fresh ergot, gathered in a moist, warm summer, shortly before harvest, is chopped and pounded to a pulp and weighed. Then two parts by weight of alcohol are taken, the pulp mixed thoroughly with one-sixth part of it, and the rest of the alcohol added. After having stirred the whole, pour it into a well-stoppered bottle, and let it stand eight days in a dark, cool place. The tincture is then separated by decanting, straining and filtering.

Drug power of tincture, $\frac{1}{6}$.

Dilutions must be prepared as directed under Class III.

SEDINHA.

This is an herbaceous plant, with a slender, round and pubescent stem; the leaves are opposite, lanceolate and very sharp; their upper surface is hairy and of a darker green than their lower surface, which is covered with long, silky hairs. This plant is quite common in the neighborhood of Rio Janeiro.

It was introduced into our Materia Medica by Dr. Mure, Brazil.

Preparation.—The fresh leaves are chopped and pounded to a pulp and weighed. Then two parts by weight of alcohol are taken, and having mixed the pulp thoroughly with one-sixth part of it, the rest of the alcohol is added. After having stirred the whole, pour it into a well-stoppered bottle, and let it stand eight days in a dark, cool place. The tincture is then separated by decanting, straining, and filtering.

Amount of drug power, $\frac{1}{6}$.

Dilutions must be prepared as directed under Class III.

SEDUM ACRE, *Linn.*

Synonym, Sempervivum Minoris.

Nat. Ord., Crassulaceæ.

Common Name, Mossy Stone Crop.

This little plant is a native of Europe, but is sparingly naturalized in the United States, having escaped from gardens. It has a procumbent, spreading branching stem. Leaves very small, alternate, crowded, thick, almost clasping, ovate and obtuse. Flowers yellow, in a scorpoid raceme. Sepals four or five, united at base. Petals four or five, spreading. The plant spreads rapidly over walls, rocks, etc.

Preparation.—The fresh plant, in flower, is chopped and pounded to a pulp and weighed. Then two parts by weight of alcohol are taken, the pulp mixed thoroughly with one-sixth part of it, and the rest of the alcohol added. After having stirred the whole, pour it into a well-stoppered bottle, and let it stand eight days in a dark, cool place. The tincture is then separated by decanting, straining and filtering.

Drug power of tincture, $\frac{1}{6}$.

Dilutions must be prepared as directed under Class III.

SELENIUM.

Symbol, Se.

Atomic Weight, 79.

Origin.—This is a very rare element, much resembling sulphur in its chemical relations, and found in association with that substance in some few localities, or replacing it in certain metallic combinations, as in the lead selenide of Clausthal in the Hartz.

Properties.—Selenium is a reddish-brown solid body, somewhat translucent, and having an imperfect metallic lustre. Its specific gravity, when rapidly cooled after fusion, is 4.3. At 100° C. (212° F.), or a little above, it melts and boils. It is insoluble in water, and exhales, when heated in the air, a peculiar and disagreeable odor, which has been compared to that of decaying horse-radish; it is insoluble in alcohol, but dissolves slightly in carbon disulphide, from which solution it crystallizes.

It was first proven by Dr. Hering.

Preparation for Homœopathic Use.—Selenium is triturated, as directed under Class VII.

SEMPERVIVUM TECTORUM, *Linn.*

Nat. Ord., Crassulaceæ.

Common Name, Houseleek.

This well-known plant is said to be indigenous to the Alpine countries, but is now found widely spread throughout Europe, and is cultivated to some extent in this country. Its leaves are radical, thick, fleshy and mucilaginous, about an inch in length, obovate, green, hairy on the margins. Flowers are rose-colored or purplish; when cultivated the plant rarely flowers. The plant spreads by runners.

Preparation.—The fresh leaves, gathered before the development of the blossoms, are chopped and pounded to a pulp and weighed. Then two parts by weight of alcohol are taken, the pulp mixed thoroughly with one-sixth part of it, and the rest of the alcohol added. After having stirred the whole, pour it into a well-stoppered bottle, and let it stand eight days in a dark, cool place. The tincture is then separated by decanting, straining and filtering.

Drug power of tincture, $\frac{1}{6}$.

Dilutions must be prepared as directed under Class III.

SENECIO AUREUS, *Linn.*

Synonym, Var. Senecio Gracilis, *Linn.*

Nat. Ord., Compositæ.

Common Names, Golden Ragwort. Squaw-Weed.

This perennial has an erect, smoothish, striate stem, one or two feet high, floccose-woolly when young, simple or branched above, terminating in a kind of umbellate, simple or compound corymb. The radical leaves are simple and rounded, the larger mostly cordate, crenate-serrate, and long petioled; the lower cauline leaves lyre-shaped; the upper ones few, slender, cut-pinnatifid, dentate, sessile or partly clasping; the terminal segments lanceolate; peduncles sub-umbellate, and thick upwards; corymb umbel-like. Rays from eight to twelve, four or five lines long, spreading. Flowers golden yellow. Scales linear, acute, and purplish at the apex. The root is horizontal, from half an inch to six or eight inches long, and about two lines in diameter, reddish or purplish externally, and white-purplish internally, with an aromatic taste, and having scattered fibres. It is found growing on the banks of creeks and low marshy ground throughout the north and west of the United States. Senecio Gracilis differs only by its being more slender and growing in rocky places.

It was first proven by Dr. A. E. Small, United States.

Preparation.—The entire fresh plant when in bloom, is chopped and pounded to a pulp and weighed. Then two parts by weight of alcohol are taken, the pulp mixed thoroughly with one-sixth part of it, and the rest of the alcohol added. After having stirred the whole, pour it into a well-stoppered bottle, and let it stand eight days in a dark, cool place. The tincture is then separated by decanting, straining and filtering.

Drug power of tincture, $\frac{1}{6}$.

Dilutions must be prepared as directed under Class III.

SENEGA.

Synonym, Polygala Senega, *Linn.*

Nat. Ord., Polygalaceæ.

Common Names, Rattlesnake Milkwort. Seneca. Seneca Snake-root.

This is an indigenous, perennial plant, more commonly found in the Western States of the Union. It has a woody, branching, contorted root, ash-colored, about one-half inch thick. From the root arise several stems eight to fourteen inches high, erect, simple, smooth and leafy, green near the top, but sometimes tinged red or purple below. Leaves from one to two inches long, lanceolate, tapering at each end, alternate, short-petioled, bright green above, paler beneath. Flowers small, white, irregular, in a filiform spike at the top of the stem. Sepals five, two of them wing-shaped and petal-like. Petals three, cohering by their claws to the filaments. Capsules small, obcordate, compressed, two-valved, two seeded.

Preparation.—The dried root, coarsely powdered, is covered with five parts by weight of alcohol, poured into a well-stoppered bottle, and allowed to remain eight days, at a moderate temperature, in a dark place, being shaken twice a day. The tincture is then poured off, strained and filtered.

Drug power of tincture, $\frac{1}{10}$.

Dilutions must be prepared as directed under Class IV.

SENNA.

Synonyms, Cassia Acutifolia, *Delile.* Cassia Lanceolata, *Nectoux.*

Nat. Ord., Leguminosæ.

Common Name, Senna.

This undershrub is indigenous to Northern Africa, and is found in Upper Egypt, Nubia, Senaar and neighboring districts. The stem is straight, woody, whitish, branching, from two to three feet in height. Leaves alternate, pinnate, on petioles without glands, and with narrow stipules. Leaflets in four or five pairs, short-petiolate, oval-lanceolate, lance-oval, or oval, pointed, mucronate, rather thick, and slightly hairy beneath. Flowers yellow, in axillary racemed spikes. Fruit a broadly oblong legume, about two inches in length, containing about six hard, ash-colored, cordate seeds. The leaves from *C. acutifolia* are known in commerce as Alexandria senna.

Preparation.—The dried leaves, coarsely powdered, are covered with five parts by weight of alcohol, poured into a well-stoppered bottle, and allowed to remain eight days in a dark, cool place, being shaken twice a day. The tincture is then poured off, strained and filtered.

Drug power of tincture, $\frac{1}{10}$.

Dilutions must be prepared as directed under Class IV.

SEPIA.

Synonyms, Sepia Octopus. Sepia Succus. Sepia Officinalis, *Linn.*

Class, Mollusca.

Nat. Ord., Dibranchiata.

Family, Sepiadæ.

Common Names, Squid. Cuttle-fish.

Inky juice of the cuttle-fish.

The cuttle-fish is a cephalopodous mollusc, without an external shell, from one to two feet long, soft-gelatinous, of a brown color verging on red, and spotted black; its body is rounded, elliptical, and enclosed in a sac furnished with a fleshy fin on each side along its whole length. The head, separated from the body by a neck, is salient and round, and provided with salient eyes of a lively red color. The mouth is surrounded by ten arms which are pedunculated, very large, and furnished with suckers. The cuttle-fish ink is an excretory liquid, contained in a bag, about the size and shape of a grape, within the abdomen of the sepia; it is blackish-brown, and is used by these animals to darken the water when they wish to catch their prey or escape from their pursuers. The ink-bag is found separate from the liver, and deeper in the abdominal cavity; its external duct ends in a kind of funnel, and opens near that part of the neck where the anus of the animal is situated. In the back of the fish is found an oval-oblong, moveable bone, from five to ten inches long, and from one and a half to three inches broad, somewhat convex, cretaceous and spongy. The cuttle-fish inhabits the seas of Europe, especially the Mediterranean. Sepia in a dry state, as it occurs in trade, appears to be a dark blackish-brown, solid mass, of shining, conchoidal, very brittle fracture, having a faint smell of seafish, nearly without taste and scarcely dyeing the saliva. It is enclosed in little skins and is of the shape of grapes. The artificial sepia (Indian ink) used in drawing, should not be used.

The drug was first proved by Hahnemann.

Preparation.—The pure, powdered sepia is covered with five parts by weight of dilute alcohol, poured into a well-stoppered bottle, and allowed to remain eight days in a dark, cool place, being shaken twice a day. The tincture is then poured off, strained and filtered.

Drug power of tincture, $\frac{1}{10}$.

Dilutions must be prepared as directed under Class IV.

Triturations of genuine sepia are prepared, freed from its cuticular envelope, as directed under Class VII.

Triturations of this remedy are preferable.

SERPENTARIA.

Synonym, Aristolochia Serpentaria, *Linn.*

Nat. Ord., Aristolochiaceæ.

Common Names, Virginia Snakeroot. Serpentaria.

This is an indigenous, perennial, herbaceous plant, found growing in hedges, thickets, and moist woods, from Pennsylvania west to Illinois, and south to Louisiana. The root is a short, horizontal stock, which gives off numerous slender rootlets, and from the same root several stems often arise. Stem nearly a foot high, erect, flexuous, subsimple, jointed, at times reddish or purple at the base. Leaves petiolate, oblong or ovate, cordate, acuminate, thin, and pale yellow-green. Flowers solitary, on long pedicels, nearly radical, slender and bending. Calyx tubular, dull purple, leathery, contracted in the middle, bent like the letter S, limb obscurely two-lipped. Fruit a six-celled, septicidal capsule, many seeded.

Flowers in June and July; earlier south.

It was introduced into our Materia Medica by Jŏrg's provings.

Preparation.—The dried root, coarsely powdered, is covered with five parts by weight of alcohol, and allowed to remain eight days in a well-stoppered bottle, in a dark, cool place, being shaken twice a day. The tincture is then poured off, strained and filtered.

Drug power of tincture, $\frac{1}{10}$.

Dilutions must be prepared as directed under Class IV.

SILICA.

Proper Name, Silicic Oxide.

Synonyms, Silicea. Silicea Terra. Silex. Acidum Silicicum.

Formula, $Si\ O_2$.

Common Names, Pure Flint. Silicious Earth.

Preparation of Silica.—Hahnemann directs this to be prepared as follows: "Take half an ounce of mountain crystal and expose it several times to a red heat, or take pure white sand and wash it with distilled vinegar; when washed mix it with two ounces of powdered natrum, melt the whole in an iron crucible until effervescence has ceased, and the liquefied mass looks clear and smooth, which is then to be poured upon a marble plate. The limpid glass which is thus obtained is to be pulverized while warm, and to be filled in a vial, adding four times its own weight of distilled water (the vial being exactly filled to a level and a stopper being put in immediately). This mixture forms a solution which remains always clear; but upon pouring it into an open vial, which is loosely covered with paper, it becomes decomposed, and the snow white silica separates from the natrum and falls to the bottom of the vial."

The following process, which does not differ in any essential particular from that of Hahnemann, is generally adopted: Take of silica, in powder, one part; dried carbonate of sodium, four parts. Fuse the four parts of dry sodium carbonate in a clay crucible, and gradually add to the fused mass the powdered silica; at each addition an escape of carbonic oxide takes place, so that a roomy crucible should be used.

When the carbonic oxide ceases to come off, pour the fused mass upon a clean marble slab, and while slightly warm break it in a mortar into small pieces and transfer to a wide-mouthed bottle, adding sufficient distilled water to dissolve it; the stopper is to be capped with wet bladder. The following day the solution may be diluted and rapidly filtered through cotton wool to remove particles of dirt, etc.; then add to the filtered liquid hydrochloric acid gradually in small quantities. The hydrated silica is precipitated in the form of a bulky gelatinous white precipitate, which is collected and washed with distilled water upon a square frame filter. The washing must be continued until the filtrate is without taste and no longer precipitates solutions of nitrate of silver. The precipitate, when thoroughly washed, may be advantageously dried upon a porcelain water-bath, when it shrinks to an impalpable powder, which has neither taste nor smell.

It was first proven by Hahnemann.

Preparation for Homœopathic Use.—Pure silica is triturated as directed under Class VII.

SILPHIUM LACINIATUM, *Linn.*

Nat. Ord., Compositæ.

Common Names, Rosin Weed. Compass-Plant. Pilot Weed.

This plant is found growing on the prairies of Illinois and Wisconsin, from thence southward and westward. The plant is rough-bristly; stem stout, three to ten feet high, leafy to the top; leaves pinnately divided, petioled, clasping at the base; segments lanceolate or linear, acute, deeply incised or pinnatifid, rarely entire; heads few, large, somewhat racemed; scales of the involucre ovate, squarrous; achenia broad, winged and deeply notched. The yellow-flowered heads appear in July. The lower and root-leaves are vertical, twelve to thirty inches long, ovate, and on the open prairies tend to present their edges north and south; hence the name *Compass-Plant.*

Preparation.—The fresh herb, in flower, is chopped and pounded to a pulp and weighed. Then two parts by weight of alcohol are taken, the pulp mixed thoroughly with one-sixth part of it, and the rest of the alcohol added. After having stirred the whole, pour into a well-stoppered bottle, and let it stand eight days in a dark, cool place. The tincture is then separated by decanting, straining and filtering.

Drug power of tincture, $\frac{1}{6}$.

Dilutions must be prepared as directed under Class III.

SIMARUBA OFFICINALIS, *De Candolle.*

Synonyms, Simaruba Amara, *Aublet.* Simaruba Guianensis, *Richard.* Quassia Simaruba, *Linn.*
Nat. Ord., Simarubaceæ.
Common Name, Simaruba.

For description of the tree see article Quassia. The bark of the root comes in commerce in pieces several feet in length, an inch or two or three in width and from one-eighth to one-fourth of an inch in thickness. The pieces are either simply curved or are in quills. The outer surface of the bark is rough and much wrinkled, but when the outer, yellow-brownish, corky layer is removed there is seen the middle grayish-brown layer. The liber is thick, coarsely fibrous, of a dull brown color, the inner surface being striated and lighter in tint. The bark is difficult to break transversely, the bast fibres being very tough. A transverse section shows a granular outer layer, and internally, obliquely radiating striæ. The taste of the bark is strongly bitter; has no odor.

Preparation.—The bark of the root is coarsely powdered and covered with five parts by weight of alcohol, poured into a well-stoppered bottle, and allowed to remain eight days in a dark, cool place, being shaken twice a day. The tincture is then poured off, strained and filtered.

Amount of drug power, $\frac{1}{10}$.

Dilutions must be prepared as directed under Class IV.

SINAPIS NIGRA, *Linn.*

Synonyms, Brassica Nigra. Melanosinapis Communis.
Nat. Ord., Cruciferæ.
Common Name, Black Mustard.

This plant is a native of Europe, but has been naturalized to some extent in the United States. It is an annual, herbaceous in habit, from three to six feet high. Stem smooth, round, striate and branching. Leaves all petiolate, lower ones lyrate-pinnate, dentate, upper ones lance-linear, dependent, entire. Flowers small, sepals and petals sulphur-yellow, rather crowded on peduncles near the ends of the branches. Fruit a pod or silique, erect, subterete, short-beaked. Seeds numerous, small, globous, nearly black. Flowers in June and July.

Introduced into our Materia Medica by Dr. Clarence W. Butler, United States.

Preparation.—The ripe seeds, coarsely powdered, are covered with five parts by weight of alcohol, poured into a well-stoppered bottle, and allowed to remain eight days in a dark, cool place, being shaken twice a day. The tincture is then poured off, strained and filtered.

Drug power of tincture, $\frac{1}{10}$.

Dilutions must be prepared as directed under Class IV.

SOLANUM.

Synonym, Solanum Nigrum, *Linn.*
Nat. Ord., Solanaceæ.
Common Names, Common Nightshade. Black Nightshade.

This is a very common homely weed, said to be poisonous, growing in shaded grounds and fields, in Europe, Asia and America. Stem annual, a foot high, much branched and often spreading, four-angled; leaves ovate, crose-toothed; flowers (very small, white) in small and umbel-like lateral clusters, drooping; berries globular, black. Flowers appear from July to September.

The first proving was by Lembke, Germany.

Preparation.—The fresh herb, gathered when coming into bloom, is chopped and pounded to a pulp, and pressed out in a piece of new linen. The expressed juice is then, by brisk agitation, mingled with an equal part by weight of alcohol. This mixture is allowed to stand eight days in a well-stoppered bottle, in a dark, cool place, and then filtered.

Amount of drug power, ½.

Dilutions must be prepared as directed under Class I.

SOLANUM ARREBENTA.

Synonyms, Solanum Rebenta, *Vell.* Solanum Aculeatissimum. Arrebenta Cavallos.
Nat. Ord., Solanaceæ.

This bush grows spontaneously in the province of Rio Janeiro, along roads and in cultivated places. It is from ten to sixteen inches high; its branches, which bifurcate regularly, are, while young, covered with strong thorns growing from above downwards. Leaves slightly pubescent, cordate, with five obtuse lobes; their veins are furnished with a few irregularly distributed thorns. The flowers are supported by peduncles arising from the axils of the leaves in groups of two or three. Calyx five-parted, very prickly on the outside; corolla with five divisions; five stamens; a style. Berry red, fleshy, two-celled, containing a large number of small seeds. Roots fibrous, arising from a common rhizome.

It was introduced into our Materia Medica by Dr. Mure, Brazil.

Preparation.—The fresh leaves are triturated as directed under Class IX.

SOLANUM MAMMOSUM, *Linn.*

Synonym, Mammiform Solanum.
Nat. Ord., Solanaceæ.
Common Name, Nipple Nightshade.

This bush is a native of Virginia, the Carolinas and the West Indies, and grows in hedges and on cultivated places. Stem herbaceous, furnished with prickles and long hairs, erect, branchy, from three to four feet high; leaves large, generally broader than long, cordiform, irregularly-angular, lobed, shaggy on both sides, with yellow nerves on the lower surface, the midrib furnished with dark yellow prickles; flowers scattered, panicled, of a blue-gray color; berries macuniform, yellow.

It was introduced into our Materia Medica by Dr. Hering.

Preparation.—The fresh, ripe berries are pounded to a pulp and pressed out in a piece of new linen. The expressed juice is then, by brisk agitation, mingled with an equal part by weight of alcohol. This mixture is allowed to stand eight days in a well stoppered bottle, in a dark, cool place, and then filtered.

Drug power of tincture, ½.

Dilutions must be prepared as directed under Class I.

SOLANUM OLERACEUM, *Velloz.*

Synonyms, Gyquirioba. Juquerioba.

Nat. Ord., Solanaceæ.

This is an herbaceous plant with a creeping and somewhat ligneous, cylindrical stem, the upper branches being covered with short and crooked thorns. The leaves, of a dark green color, are alternate, irregularly pinnate; the folioles are long, lanceolate, almost sessile on a thorny spike; they are from seven to nine, those at the top being the largest. The flowers are supported by ramose pedicles, which do not grow out of axils; calyx campanulate, with five divisions; corolla greenish-white, monopetalous, with five equal, rotaceous, somewhat reflexed divisions alternating with those of the calyx; stamens five, with erect, converging and bilocular anthers; their filaments are short, with the exception of one, which is longer than the rest; ovary oval, surmounted by a filiform style. Berry spherical, two-celled, of a dark green color, with white spots. This solanum grows on the shores around Rio Janeiro, in damp and shady places.

It was introduced into our Materia Medica by Dr. Muré, Brazil.

Preparation.—The fresh blossoms are triturated as directed under Class IX.

SOLANUM TUBEROSUM ÆGROTANS.

The Diseased Potato.

The potato is a native of Chili, but is very largely cultivated in nearly all countries. It is an herbaceous plant, with a branchy stem about one or two feet high. Its leaves are pinnatifid, with leaflets that are oval, entire, slightly hairy on their lower surface and almost opposite. Smaller folioles sometimes arise between the larger ones. The flowers constitute corymbs either erect or inclined; calyx in five parts; corolla of a white-violet color, with five equal divisions; five stamens attached to the base of the corolla; one style and stigma; fleshy berry with two cells. The roots develop tubers of different sizes, called potatoes. The potato-rot first reveals itself by brown spots irregularly distributed through the interior of the tubers; gradually these spots are transformed into white points of a cottony appearance, which may be compared to the cryptogamic growth termed byssus, found on damp wood. From this plant a general process of decomposition sets in, and the potato then exhales an insupportable nauseous odor.

Introduced into our Materia Medica by Dr. Mure, Brazil.

Preparation.—The potato in such a state of decomposition as to contain brown portions intermingled with the byssus-shaped parts described above, is triturated as directed under Class IX.

SOLIDAGO VIRGA-AUREA, *Linn.*

Nat. Ord., Compositæ.

Common Name, Golden-Rod.

This is a variable species indigenous to Europe, Northern Asia, and on this continent to Canada and the northern portion of the United States. It is from one to three feet high, branched above, pubescent or nearly glabrous; leaves lanceolate or oblanceolate, or the lower elliptical-obovate or nearly spatulate, petioled, serrate with small appressed teeth or nearly entire; racemes thyrsoid or simple, narrow; scales of the involucre lanceolate or linear, acute. The flower-heads contain eight or ten ligulate and several tubular disc-florets of a yellow color. The herb has an aromatic odor, and a bitterish and somewhat astringent taste.

Preparation.—The fresh blossoms are chopped and pounded to a pulp and weighed. Then two parts by weight of alcohol are taken, the pulp mixed thoroughly with one-sixth part of it, and the rest of the alcohol added. After having stirred the whole, pour it into a well-stoppered bottle, and let it stand eight days in a dark, cool place. The tincture is then separated by decanting, straining and filtering.

Drug power of tincture, $\frac{1}{6}$.

Dilutions must be prepared as directed under Class III.

SPARTIUM SCOPARIUM, *Linn.*

Synonyms, Cytisus Scoparius, *Link.* Sarothamnus Scoparius, *Koch.* Sarothamnus Vulgaris, *Wimmer.* Genista Scoparia, *Lamarck.*

Nat. Ord., Leguminosæ.

Common Names, Broom. Broom Tops.

The broom is a woody shrub from three to six feet high. It is found in Central and Southern Russia; in Southern Europe its place is supplied by other species. It is found plentifully in the valley of the Rhine in Southern Germany and Silesia, but is most abundant in Great Britain and throughout the more temperate portions of Western and Northern Europe; it is occasionally found in the Middle and Southern United States. It has numerous straight ascending branches, which are sharply five-angled. Leaves tri-foliate, petiolate, leaflets obovate or elliptic-lanceolate. Towards the extremities of the branches the leaves are generally represented by one nearly sessile ovate leaflet.

Leaves, when young, are reddish-hairy. Flowers papilionaceous, bright yellow, odorous, solitary and axillary. Legume oblong, one and a half to two inches long, compressed, dark brown and fringed with hair on its edge. Seeds ten to twelve, olive-colored.

Preparation.—The fresh blossoms are pounded to a pulp and weighed. Then two parts by weight of alcohol are taken, the pulp mixed thoroughly with one-sixth part of it, and the rest of the alcohol added. After having stirred the whole, pour it into a well-stoppered bottle, and let it stand eight days in a dark, cool place. The tincture is then separated by decanting, straining and filtering.

Amount of drug power, $\frac{1}{6}$.

Dilutions must be prepared as directed under Class III.

SPIGELIA.

Synonyms, Spigelia Anthelmia, *Linn.* Anthelmia Quadriphylla.
Nat. Ord., Loganiaceæ.
Common Names, Pinkroot. Wormgrass.

This is an annual plant of the West Indies and South America. Its root is short and divided into numerous long, thin, blackish and internally whitish branches. Its stem is herbaceous, twelve to eighteen inches high, channeled and branched. Leaves opposite in pairs, those which terminate the branches four together in the form of a cross, ovate, pointed. The flowers stand in short spikes, and are pale reddish or purple, not over one-half inch long. The dried plant is of a grayish-green color, and has a faint odor and a bitter taste. Its flowers appear in July.

It was first proven by Hahnemann.

Preparation.—The freshly dried herb, having been gathered when bearing flowers and seeds, is finely powdered, covered with five parts by weight of alcohol, and allowed to remain eight days in a well-stoppered bottle, in a dark, cool place, being shaken twice a day. The tincture is then poured off, strained and filtered.

Drug power of tincture, $\frac{1}{10}$.

Dilutions must be prepared as directed under Class IV.

SPIGGURUS MARTINI.

Synonyms, Sphingurus Martini. Chætomys Subspinosus.
Class, Mammalia.
Order, Glires.
Family, Hystrichina.
Common Name, Porcupine.

The porcupine is common in Brazil, where it lives on trees and secures itself by means of its hind feet; it uses its tail, which is pretty long, as a means of descending. Its length, from the muzzle to the tip of the tail, is about a foot; the tail is almost as long as the trunk. The upper parts of the body are covered with sharp prickles about an inch and a half long, and attached to the skin by means of a very thin pedicle. The head-prickles are white at the base, black in the middle and yellowish-brown at the top, the dorsal-prickles are of a sulphur yellow color at their base. The prickles on the rump and the first third of the tail, are black at their extremity. All the prickles are very close together, mingled with a few long and fine hairs. The lower limbs are covered with a grayish fur, interspersed with little prickles; the tail is furnished with prickles at its upper part, and is covered with stiff and black hairs; the extremity of the tail is bare.

It was proven by Dr. J. Vincente Martins, Brazil.

Preparation.—The prickles taken from the sides of the animal, are triturated according to Class IX.

SPONGIA.

Synonyms, Spongia Tosta. Spongia Officinalis, *Linn.*

Class, Poriphera.

Order, Ceratospongiæ.

Common Name, Sponge.

Origin and Description.—Sponges are among the lowest class of animal organisms. They inhabit both the sea and fresh water, and grow from a broad attachment to rocks or other hard substances. From the attachment a mass of tissue arises which branches or interlaces in various modes. The whole mass is traversed by anastomosing canals, opening on the outside and appearing then as different sized pores. The skeleton in some kinds is formed in great part of splinter-shaped masses made up of lime and silica; in others there is no skeletal part, the whole body consisting of proliferations of a gelatinous or semi-cartilaginous consistency. Sponges are gathered by divers, who descend to the rock bearing the growths, and tear the latter away from their attachments. This industry is carried on largely in the Mediterranean near Syria and Greece; also in the waters surrounding the West India Islands and in the Pacific Ocean. The kind prescribed in homœopathic practice is that known in commerce as Turkey sponge. It is soft, compressible and elastic, and is in various sized pieces, generally oblong and hollowed out or cup-shaped.

The drug was first proven by Hahnemann.

Preparation for Homœopathic Use.—Turkey sponge roasted brown (but not burnt) in a roaster kept turning over burning charcoal, is covered with five parts by weight of alcohol, and allowed to remain eight days in a well-stoppered bottle, in a dark, cool place, being shaken twice a day. The tincture is then poured off, strained and filtered.

Amount of drug power, $\frac{1}{10}$.

Dilutions must be prepared as directed under Class IV.

Triturations prepared as directed under Class VII are also officinal.

STANNUM.

Synonym, Stannum Metallicum.

Common Names, Tin. Metallic Tin. Pure Tin.

Symbol, Sn.

Atomic Weight, 118.

Origin and Preparation of Tin.—Tin is found in nature in the metallic state in small amount only; it more frequently occurs as disulphide in tin pyrites and most abundantly as dioxide in the ore known as *tinstone* or *cassiterite*. The metal has been known from the remotest times; it is mentioned by Moses in Numbers XXXI., 22, and Homer speaks of it in the Iliad. The largest deposits of the ore are in Cornwall and Devonshire in England, in the Island of Banca and in Malacca; it has also been found in other countries, among them Australia, and California in the United States.

Preparation.—The tinstone is crushed, roasted and washed, then mixed with charcoal and reduced in a peculiar form of reverberatory furnace. It is refined by melting it and thrusting into the bath of melted metal billets of green wood; the disengagement of gas from the wood produces a constant ebullition in the melted tin and causes a froth on the surface, which consists chiefly of the oxides of other metals, together with some oxide of tin; this scum is skimmed off and the tin is ladled into moulds. The purest tin comes in granular fragments, and is known as *grain-tin*, a less pure form in ingots being known as *block-tin*. The purest quality of tin comes from the Island of Banca, and is termed *strait-tin*.

Properties.—Tin is a soft, brilliant white metal, with a faint tinge of blue. When warmed it emits a characteristic odor, and when bent it gives forth a peculiar crackling sound known as the cry of tin; this sound is caused by the interior crystals breaking against each other. Its specific gravity is 7.29; it crystallizes in two forms belonging to the isometric and quadratic systems respectively. It is extremely malleable, and at the temperature of boiling water can be readily drawn into wire; its tenacity is, however, but slight. When heated to about 200° C. (392° F.), or when cooled to a low temperature it becomes brittle and can then be easily powdered. At about 230° C. (446° F.) it melts, and at a white heat volatilizes. The metal takes a fine polish and has then but little radiating power. It does not oxidize in the air even when moist, at ordinary temperatures, and but very slightly in water. When fused in the air, however, its surface becomes covered with a thin gray film consisting of both the stannous and stannic oxides. Tin is not attacked by strong nitric acid, specific gravity 1.5, the metal even preserving its characteristic brilliancy, but when the acid is diluted it attacks the metal with great violence and converts it to metastannic acid. Dilute sulphuric acid attacks tin slowly with the evolution of hydrogen, the hot concentrated acid acts very energetically with the production of sulphurous acid. Tin forms with other metals many valuable alloys; among these may be mentioned gun-metal, bronze, bell metal, speculum metal, type metal, pewter and britannia.

Stannum Precipitatum.—For medicinal purposes we first reduce tin by melting it and pouring it into a deep vessel filled with pure water when it assumes the form of thin laminæ.

One part of such laminated tin is covered, in a suitable vessel, with pure concentrated muriatic acid, and set aside at a moderate warmth for solution. Without fear of contamination a polished copper vessel may be advantageously employed for this purpose as long as care is taken to have tin always in excess. By adding the muriatic acid gradually, perfect solution is effected. This solution, filtered, is diluted with fourteen parts of distilled water. After having slightly acidulated the solution with pure muriatic acid, if necessary, the galvanic reduction of the metal is effected by the addition of zinc, and the whole process is followed up as given under Plumbum. In this way a subtile and quite pure metallic powder is obtained, of a light yellowish-gray color, dull, which assumes a metallic brilliancy under the burnishing-steel.

It was first proven by Hahnemann.

Preparation for Homœopathic Use.—The precipitated metal is triturated, as directed under Class VII.

STAPHISAGRIA.

Synonyms, Delphinium Staphisagria, *Linn.* Staphydis Agria. Staphisagria Pedicularis.

Nat. Ord., Ranunculaceæ.

Common Names, Staves Acre. Lark-spur.

This is an annual or biennial plant found growing in Southern Europe in poor soils. Its stem is simple, erect, downy and grows to a height of a foot or more. Leaves palmately, five to seven-lobed, on hairy petioles. Flowers are in terminal racemes on long pedicels. Sepals five, irregular, the upper one spurred behind Petals four, very irregular, the two upper ones protracted into two tubular nectariferous spurs enclosed in the spur of the calyx. Fruit a straight, oblong capsule; seeds irregularly triangular, as large as wheat grains, externally brown and wrinkled, internally pale and oily. The seeds have a faint disagreeable odor and a bitter followed by a burning taste.

It was first proven by Hahnemann.

Preparation.—The ripe seed, coarsely powdered, is covered with five parts by weight of alcohol, and allowed to remain eight days in a well stoppered bottle, in a dark, cool place, being shaken twice a day. The tincture is poured off, strained and filtered.

Drug power of tincture, $\frac{1}{10}$.

Dilutions must be prepared as directed under Class IV.

STICTA.

Synonyms, Sticta Pulmonaria, *Linn.* Laboria Pulmonaria. Lichen Pulmonarius. Pulmonaria Reticulata.

Nat. Ord., Lichenes.

Common Names, Lungwort Lichen. Tree Lungwort. Oak-lungs. Lung Moss.

This lichen is found growing on the trunks of large trees in the northern and mountainous counties of England, and in New England, New York, Pennsylvania and Carolina in the United States. It is leafy, laciniated, obtuse, smooth; green above, and pitted, somewhat reticulated; downy beneath; shields mostly marginal.

It was first proven by Dr. S. P. Burdick, United States.

Preparation.—The fresh lichen, grown on the sugar-maple, is finely chopped, covered with five parts by weight of dilute alcohol, the mixture poured into a well-stoppered bottle, and allowed to remain eight days in a dark, cool place, being shaken twice a day. The tincture is then poured off, strained and filtered.

Amount of drug power, $\frac{1}{10}$.

Dilutions must be prepared as directed under Class IV.

STILLINGIA.

Synonyms, Stillingia Sylvatica, *Linn.* Sapium Sylvaticum, *Torrey.*

Nat. Ord., Euphorbiaceæ.

Common Names, Cock-up-hat. Queen's Root. Queen's Delight. Yaw Root.

This indigenous, perennial plant is found growing in pine barrens and sandy soils, from Virginia to Florida and Louisiana. The stem is herbaceous, simple, two or three feet high. Leaves alternate, sub-sessile, cuneate at base, serrulate and obtuse at apex. The plant is monœcious. Flowers yellowish, in a simple spike. Male flowers have a cup-shaped calyx, lobed and crenulate. Female flowers have a three-lobed calyx and trifid style. Fertile flowers at base of spike. Capsules three-lobed, three-celled, three-seeded. The plant, like most of the Euphorbiaceæ, emits a milky juice when wounded.

It was first proven by Dr. A. B. Nichols, United States.

Preparation.—The fresh root is chopped and pounded to a pulp and weighed. Then two parts by weight of alcohol are taken, and after thoroughly mixing the pulp with one-sixth part of it, the rest of the alcohol is added. After having stirred the whole, pour it into a well-stoppered bottle, and let it stand eight days in a dark, cool place. The tincture is then separated by decanting, straining and filtering.

Drug power of tincture, $\frac{1}{6}$.

Dilutions must be prepared as directed under Class III.

STRAMONIUM.

Synonyms, Datura Stramonium, *Linn.* Solanum Maniacum.

Nat. Ord., Solanaceæ.

Common Names, Jamestown or "jimson" Weed. Thornapple.

This plant is found in many parts of the world, but is believed to be a native of Asia. In the United States it is widely distributed and is found near towns and villages, on roadsides, near dung-heaps or rubbish. The plant is an annual; its root is large, whitish, furnished with many fine rootlets. The stem is about three feet high, smooth, hollow, dichotomously branched above. Leaves are short-petiolate, at the base of the dichotomous branches, five or six inches long, of a general ovate-triangular form with large irregular teeth and sinuses, dark green above, paler beneath. Flowers large, solitary, axillary on peduncles. Corolla infundibuliform, with a long tube and a plaited five-toothed border, color creamy white. Fruit a two-celled, four-valved capsule, the cells two to three parted. Seeds small, reniform, flattened, nearly black in color, without odor unless crushed and of a nauseous, bitter taste with some acridity. The whole plant has a rank, offensive odor. Flowers from June to August according to its locality.

The drug was first proven by Hahnemann.

Preparation.—The ripe seed, powdered, is covered with five parts by weight of alcohol, poured into a well-stoppered bottle and allowed to remain eight days in a dark, cool place, being shaken twice a day. The tincture is then poured off, strained and filtered.

Drug power of tincture, $\frac{1}{10}$.

Dilutions must be prepared as directed under Class IV.

STRONTIANA CARBONICA.

Synonyms, Strontium Carbonate. Strontianite. Carbonas Stronticus. Strontianæ Carbonas.

Mineral, $Sr\,CO_3$.

Common Name, Carbonate of Strontium.

This salt occurs native as the mineral *strontianite* in Strontian, in Argyleshire, where it was first observed. It is also found in the Hartz, in Saxony, and in other places.

Properties.—The crystals of carbonate of strontium are right rhombic prisms, with lateral cleavage nearly perfect; also fibrous granular. Green, white, gray, yellow, brown, usually light colors; vitreous, transparent, translucent; brittle, with white streak. It puffs by heat, fuses on the edges, emitting a brilliant light, and gives a reddish color to the reducing flame; it is soluble in acids with effervescence. It requires for solution over 18,000 parts of cold water (Fresenius), and 833 parts of water saturated with CO_2 at 10° C. (50° F.), and in this state it occurs in some mineral waters from which by evaporation it appears in needle-shaped crystals. When heated in close vessels it does not part with its CO_2 at any temperature less than that of a forge fire, but in a stream of aqueous vapor or moist air it is decomposed with the formation of the hydrate. It is not decomposed by solutions of the alkaline sulphates at any temperature.

It was first proven by Nenning, Germany.

Preparation.—For homœopathic purposes we dissolve carbonate of strontium in muriatic acid and set aside to crystallize. It is purified by repeated recrystallization. Of this pure strontium chloride one part is dissolved in ten parts of distilled water, and from this the carbonate is reprecipitated by a solution of carbonate of sodium. The precipitate is washed repeatedly and carefully dried. It is a white, light, fine powder, similar in appearance to carbonate of magnesium.

Preparation for Homœopathic Use.—The pure strontiana carbonica is triturated as directed under Class VII.

STRYCHNINUM.

Synonyms, Strychninum Purum. Strychnia.
Common Name, Strychnine.
Formula, $C_{21} H_{22} N_2 O_2$.
Molecular Weight, 334.

Preparation of Strychnia.—One part of Nux Vomica, finely comminuted by rasping, is to be macerated for twenty-four hours in 43 parts of very dilute hydrochloric acid ($\frac{1}{200}$ in strength); at the end of the time the whole is to be boiled for two hours and expressed through linen. The residue is to be submitted to the same procedure twice, successively, using each time the same amount of the dilute acid. The resulting decoctions are to be mixed and evaporated to a thin syrupy consistence and there is to be added a milk of lime made by slaking lime to the amount of one-sixth of the weight of the Nux Vomica taken, in three parts of water; the mixture is to be boiled for ten minutes with constant stirring and is then to be transferred to a double linen bag in which the precipitate is to be thoroughly washed with distilled water. The precipitate is now to be pressed and dried, and then powdered. The powder, which contains brucia, is to be treated repeatedly with dilute alcohol to remove the latter until the washings are no longer, or but faintly, reddened when tested with nitric acid. The residue is to be repeatedly boiled with alcohol until a portion of the former no longer tastes bitter; the resulting alcoholic solutions are to be mixed, placed on a water-bath and the alcohol distilled off. The residue after being washed is to be mixed with three parts of water, heated gently and treated with gradual additions of sulphuric acid until the reaction is neutral and the alkaloid dissolved. Purified animal charcoal is now to be added, the mixture boiled for a few minutes, filtered, partly evaporated and set aside to crystallize. The crystals of the sulphate of strychnia thus obtained, are to be dissolved in water, and water of ammonia added gradually until the strychnia is entirely precipitated. This precipitate of pure strychnia is to be dried on bibulous paper and transferred to a well-stoppered bottle.

Properties—Strychnia crystallizes from its alcoholic solutions in small colorless four-sided prisms. It is without odor and has a very bitter taste. It is slightly soluble in water, and the solution is intensely bitter; it requires for solution about 7,000 parts of cold, 2,500 of boiling water, 200 of cold and 20 of boiling 90 per cent. alcohol, 1,250 of ether, about 300 of glycerine and 5 of chloroform. In absolute alcohol it is almost insoluble; it is soluble in the fixed and volatile oils. In dilute acid solutions it is dissolved with the formation of neutral salts. It is precipitated from its solutions by the alkalies, tannin, potassium iodide and potassium sulphocyanate (white) and by platinic and gold chlorides (yellow).

Tests.—For its identification a few crystals of strychnia are to be dissolved in a few drops of pure concentrated sulphuric acid in the cold; when the solution is touched by a crystal of potassium dichromate there occurs a blue or violet coloration which soon passes into red and then into green. A test to determine whether a specimen be mixed with morphia, or be entirely the latter, is the following: A solution of the substance is made in dilute alcohol and then treated with weak potash solution; a precipitate insoluble in excess of the alkali is dependent upon the presence of strychnia as between the two alkaloids, morphia being soluble in the reagent. If morphia be present with strychnia the test given above for the identification of strychnia will show a distinctly brown coloration. When a few crystals of strychnia are boiled in water with a few drops of silver nitrate solution, or of an alkaline copper solution, a precipitate of the reduced metal will show the presence of morphia. Strychnia or its salts should dissolve in a 25 per cent. nitric acid without color, and when heated to 50° C. (122° F.) the solution will remain colorless; a red color shows the presence of brucia. As it is difficult to free strychnia entirely from brucia a slight reddening by this test may be allowed. When strychnia or its salts are dissolved in water with the aid of few drops of sulphuric acid, the solution should show no turbidity when treated with potassium carbonate solution, otherwise the presence of other alkaloids may be assumed. A portion of the alkaloid when incinerated upon platinum foil should be consumed without residue (absence of inorganic impurities).

Preparation for Homœopathic Use.—Pure strychnia is triturated as directed under Class VII.

STRYCHNINUM MURIATICUM.

Synonym, Strychniæ Hydrochloras.
Common Name, Muriate of Strychnia.
Formula, 2 (C_{21} H_{22} N_2 O_2 HCl), $3H_2O$.
Molecular Weight, 795.

Preparation and Properties of Muriate of Strychnia.—By carefully neutralizing warm dilute hydrochloric acid with strychnia until the reaction is neutral; the solution is then to be set aside to crystallize. The salt crystallizes in colorless, silky needles which effloresce in the air; they are soluble in about fifty parts of cold water.

Tests.—Those given in the article strychninum are applicable to the salts of strychnia generally.

Preparation for Homœopathic Use.—Pure muriate of strychnia is triturated as directed under Class VII.

STRYCHNINUM NITRICUM.

Synonym, Strychniæ Nitras.
Common Name, Nitrate of Strychnia.
Formula, C_{21} H_{22} N_2 O_2, HNO_3.
Molecular Weight, 397.

Preparation.—One hundred parts of strychnia are to be exactly neutralized with pure nitric acid, specific gravity 1.185, diluted with twice its volume of water. About sixty-three parts of the strong acid will be required. The use of the acid insufficiently diluted will result in the formation of an acid salt. The solution is to be set aside to crystallize.

Properties.—Nitrate of strychnia crystallizes in tufts of permanent, colorless, fine, flexible, silky needles, which are neutral in reaction, without odor, and possess a very bitter taste. They are soluble slowly in ninety parts of cold, and in from two to three of boiling water, in seventy of cold, and in five of boiling 90 per cent. alcohol, in thirty of glycerine. They are insoluble in ether. When heated they swell up, turn yellow, and emit puffs of nitrogen gas or its lower oxides and a carbonaceous residue is left which is at last completely consumed. For tests see article Strychninum.

Preparation for Homœopathic Use.—Pure nitrate of strychnia is triturated, as directed under Class VII.

STRYCHNINUM PHOSPHORICUM.

Synonym, Strychniæ Phosphas.

Common Name, Phosphate of Strychnia.

Preparation.—By exactly neutralizing warm, dilute, phosphoric acid with strychnia and setting aside the solution to crystallize, the crystals appear as silky needles.

Preparation for Homœopathic Use.—Pure phosphate of strychnia is triturated, as directed under Class VII.

STRYCHNINUM SULPHURICUM.

Synonym, Strychniæ Sulphas.

Common Name, Sulphate of Strychnia.

Formula, $(C_{21} H_{22} N_2 O_2)_2 H_2 SO_4, 7H_2 O$.

Molecular Weight, 892.

Preparation of Sulphate of Strychnia.—This salt may be prepared by neutralizing a boiling mixture of ten parts of concentrated sulphuric acid, 100 of distilled water, and 100 of alcohol, with sixty-seven parts of strychnia. The solution is to be set aside in a cool place to crystallize. As the crystals are deliquescent they should be dried in a warm place.

Properties.—Sulphate of strychnia is in small, four-sided, orthorhombic prisms, which are perfectly neutral in reaction, are soluble in about ten parts of cold water, and easily so in aqueous alcohol. When heated to 135° C. (275° F.) the crystals melt and part with their water of crystallization.

Tests.—See article Strychninum.

Preparation for Homœopathic Use.—Pure sulphate of strychnia is triturated, as directed under Class VII.

SUCCINUM.

Synonym, Amber.

Origin.—Amber is considered to be a fossil resin, and according to Goeppert is the exudation of an extinct coniferous tree *Pinites succinifer;* the chemical properties and mode of occurrence of the substance leave scarcely a doubt of its having some such origin. It has been found encrusting or penetrating fossil wood, just as resin does at the present day, and enclosing the cones and leaves of the trees; numerous insects, the inhabitants of ancient forests, are often found embalmed in it. Amber occurs plentifully in regular veins in some parts of Prussia; it has also been found in Southern Germany, France, Italy, Spain, Sweden and Norway, on the shores of the Caspian Sea, in Siberia, China, India, North America and Greenland.

Properties.—Amber is a hard, brittle, tasteless substance, sometimes perfectly transparent, but oftener opaque or nearly so; it is of all colors, but generally yellow or orange. Its specific gravity varies from 1.065 to 1.070. It is slightly brittle and its fracture is conchoidal; it takes a fine polish, becomes electrified by friction, and at the same time, as also when heated, it emits a peculiar odor. Amber is insoluble in water and alcohol, but the latter, when nearly water-free, extracts from it a reddish colored substance. It is soluble in sulphuric acid, causing a reddish-purple solution, but is reprecipitated on the addition of water; it is not soluble without decomposition in other acids nor in the fatty or volatile oils; pure alkalies dissolve it.

Tests.—Amber is sometimes falsified with rosin or colophony, or similar bodies; these being soluble in alcohol, the fraud is readily detected. From copal it is distinguished by its greater specific gravity, by its higher melting point, by its less solubility in cajeput oil and by the blue color which its powder gives to the alcohol flame when projected into the latter (copal powder colors the flame yellow). Amber becomes soft when heated to about 215° C. (419° F.), and at about 290° C. (554° F.) it melts with the production of the vapors of succinic acid, leaving a brownish resin, the so-called *colophonium succini.*

Preparation for Homœopathic Use.—Amber is triturated, as directed under Class VII.

SULPHUR.

Synonyms, Sulphur Sublimatum Lotum. Flores Sulphuris.

Common Names, Brimstone. Washed Sublimed Sulphur. Flowers of Sulphur.

Symbol, S.

Atomic Weight, 32.

Origin.—This element has been known from the earliest times. It occurs native either as transparent, amber-colored crystals or in opaque lemon-yellow masses. It is found principally in Sicily, in beds of a blue clay formation, and similar beds containing sulphur exist in other parts of Europe and in Mexico. It also occurs in combination with different metals as sulphide, as in iron-pyrites, copper-pyrites, galena, cinnabar, gray antimony and realgar. In combination with hydrogen, as hydrogen sulphide, it occurs in many mineral waters and in the products of animal decomposition. It exists as an essential constituent in many animal tissues and its compounds are in many vegetables, especially cruciferous and alliaceous plants, as mustard and garlic.

Preparation.—Native sulphur is found mixed with many earthy impurities; to free it from these it is subjected to a rough process of distillation in two rows of pots connected at the bottom by tubes. The sulphur is converted into vapor by heat, passes through the tubes into the second row of vessels, acting as receivers, is there condensed to a liquid and is run out into wooden vessels filled with water placed beneath. The sulphur thus prepared contains enough foreign substances to render further purification necessary. This is done by another distillation in cylinders of iron, in which it is converted into vapor, and the vapor entering a brick chamber is there condensed as a fine powder when the walls of the chamber are cold; afterward, when the walls become hot, the sulphur condenses to a liquid, which collects on the floor, and is then ladled into moulds. The sulphur condensed in the form of powder is known as flowers of sulphur, that which is moulded being known as roll brimstone. Sulphur is also obtained from pyrites by piling the mineral in a conical heap, surrounding the heap with wood and applying fire. The sulphur is set free from its combination and collects as a liquid in cavities arranged in different parts of the conical mass; it has then to be purified.

Properties.—Sulphur exists in three forms, one ordinary variety as it exists in nature and two allotropic forms. The ordinary variety of sulphur is a lemon-yellow solid made up of octohedral crystals, quite brittle, having specific gravity of 2.05. It is readily soluble in carbon disulphide, disulphide of chlorine, turpentine, petroleum, etc.; it is slightly soluble in alcohol and ether. This is often called the octohedral variety.

The second modification may be obtained by the slow cooling of melted sulphur or by heating octohedral sulphur for some time, at a temperature of 105° to 115° C. (221° to 239° F.). Upon heating a quantity of sulphur and allowing it to cool until a crust is formed, there will be found upon breaking the crust and pouring out the still liquid sulphur within, an arrangement of transparent yellowish-brown needles belonging to the monoclinic system. Their specific gravity is 1.98. This variety is called the monoclinic variety; it is soluble in carbon disulphide.

The third kind of sulphur is produced by heating sulphur to 250° C. (482° F.) and then suddenly cooling it by pouring it in a thin stream into cold water. It is thus obtained as a soft, yellowish-brown, semi-transparent mass, which is capable of being drawn out into threads possessing considerable elasticity and tenacity. Its specific gravity is 1.95. Both the latter forms of sulphur become changed into the first variety slowly at ordinary temperatures. Roll sulphur of commerce, when fresh, is made up of oblique prismatic crystals, but after being kept for some time the mass is found to consist of octohedra, although it generally retains the specific gravity proper to the prismatic form. When heated in the air to 260° C. (500° F.) it takes fire and burns with a pale blue flame, and at the same time produces sulphurous oxide, whose odor is known as that of burning sulphur. Heated to 440° C. (824° F.) out of contact of air, sulphur boils evolving a dense reddish-brown vapor. In the state of vapor sulphur combines with many metals, and if slips of metallic foil or wire be introduced into the vapor of sulphur, combustion takes place with the production of a sulphide of the metal.

Flowers of sulphur do not present a crystalline structure, but are made up of round granules composed of insoluble sulphur enclosing the soluble variety. What is known as milk of sulphur is produced when an acid is added to a solution of an alkaline polysulphide; this also consists of minute granules similar to those of sublimed sulphur; it has a greenish-white color.

Tests.—Sulphur should be completely dissipated by heat; fixed impurities are left behind as a residue. Milk of sulphur, if precipitated by sulphuric acid, mixes more readily with water than pure precipitated sulphur, and leaves on ignition a large amount of fixed residue. Sulphur obtained from pyrites often contains arsenic, which may be detected, if present in more than minute quantities, by digesting it with ammonium hydrate, filtering and then adding hydrochloric acid, when yellow sulphide of arsenic will be thrown down. For minute quantities of arsenic, Marsh's test may be used. Selenium, if present, may be detected by heating with nitro-muriatic acid, diluting with water, filtering, and concentrating the filtrate; the latter will contain selenious acid, and yields, on the addition of sulphite of sodium, a bright red or nearly brown precipitate of selenium. This may be removed, dried and ignited on platinum foil, when it will burn with a flame similar to that of sulphur, but the odor given off is like that of decaying horse-radish.

Sulphur was first proven by Hahnemann.

Preparation for Homœopathic Use.—Washed sublimed sulphur is triturated as directed under Class VII.

Sulphuris Tinctura.—One part by weight of washed sublimed sulphur is covered with ten parts by weight of 95 per cent. alcohol, the mixture poured into a well-stoppered bottle, and allowed to remain eight days, being shaken twice a day. The tincture is then poured off, and filtered.

This preparation was considered by Hahnemann to equal the 1 potency ($\frac{1}{100}$).

Dilutions must be prepared as directed under Class VI—β.

SULPHUR IODATUM.

Synonyms, Sulphuris Iodidum. Ioduretum Sulfuris.

Common Name, Iodide of Sulphur.

Preparation of Iodide of Sulphur.—One part of sublimed

sulphur is to be intimately mixed with four parts of iodine. The mixture is to be placed in a flask, the latter loosely corked and warmed at a gentle heat upon a sand-bath until the color of the mixture has become uniformly dark. The heat is to be then increased until the mixture melts, and the flask is to be inclined in various directions that the liquid may take up any iodine which may have condensed upon the inner surface of the vessel. The heat is to be removed, and after the iodide has become solid by cooling, the flask is to be broken and the iodide removed and broken into pieces, which should be kept in well-stoppered bottles.

Properties.—Prepared as directed above, iodide of sulphur is a grayish-black, radio-crystalline mass, having a metallic lustre. It gives off iodine on exposure to the air, and consequently has the odor of that substance. It is insoluble in water; boiling water decomposes it into iodine and sulphur. Alcohol, ether, and solutions of potassium hydrate and of potassium iodide dissolve out the iodine from the combination. It is soluble in less than one part of carbon disulphide and in about sixty parts of glycerine.

It was proven by Dr. H. Kelsall, Month. Hom. Rev., 2, 155.

Preparation for Homœopathic Use.—Iodide of sulphur is triturated as directed under Class VII.

SUMBUL.

Synonyms, Sumbulus Moschatus, *Reinsch.* Ferula Sumbul, *Hook, f.* Jatamansi.

Nat. Ord., Umbelliferæ.

Common Name, Musk-root.

The sumbul plant is found in the elevated lands of Central Asia. Its root had been introduced into Russia about 1835, as a substitute for musk, but the botanical source of the drug was not positively known until 1869, when Fedschenko, a Russian traveller, discovered the plant itself in the northern portion of the province of Bokhara, in Turkestan. The plant is perennial, grows to a height of about eight feet. Radical leaves are large, tri-pinnate; cauline leaves small, gradually decreasing in size towards the top of the plant. The root is brought into commerce by way of Russia, but a root which comes *via* Bombay and which is called Bombay Sumbul, is really the root of Dorema ammoniacum. The root is found in commerce in slices about an inch in thickness, and from one to two inches in diameter, although specimens are occasionally seen measuring five inches across. Externally the root is covered with a thin, dark bark, and both annularly and longitudinally wrinkled. On section the root exhibits a farinaceous-looking parenchyma, dotted with yellowish-brown resinous points, and having a somewhat irregular arrangement of pale brown fibro-vascular bundles.

The root has a strong musk-like odor and a bitter, aromatic taste.

It was first proven by Lembke, Germany.

Preparation.—The dried root, coarsely powdered, is covered with five parts by weight of alcohol, and allowed to remain eight days, in a well-stoppered bottle, in a dark, cool place, being shaken twice a day. The tincture is then poured off, strained and filtered.

Drug power of tincture, $\frac{1}{10}$.

Dilutions must be prepared as directed under Class IV.

SYMPHORICARPUS.

Synonym, Symphoricarpus Racemosus, *Michaux.*

Nat. Ord., Caprifoliaceæ.

Common Name, Snow Berry.

This is an indigenous shrub from two to three feet high, found growing from Canada and the New England States westward. Stem smooth; leaves opposite, oval or oblong, wavy-margined, pale beneath, short-petiolate. Flowers in an interrupted, leafy spike. Corolla monopetalous, small, rose-colored, throat filled with hairs. Fruit a globous, four-celled, two-seeded berry, snow-white in color.

It was introduced into our Materia Medica by Dr. S. P. Burdick, United States.

Preparation.—The fresh, ripe berries are gently crushed to a pulp and weighed. Then two parts by weight of alcohol are taken, and the pulp mixed thoroughly with one-sixth part of it, and the rest of the alcohol added. After stirring the whole well, and pouring it into a well-stoppered bottle, it is allowed to stand eight days in a dark, cool place. The tincture is then separated by decanting, straining and filtering.

Drug power of tincture, $\frac{1}{6}$.

Dilutions must be prepared as directed under Class III.

SYMPHYTUM.

Synonyms, Symphytum Officinale, *Linn.* Consolida Majoris.

Nat. Ord., Borraginaceæ.

Common Names, Comfrey. Gum Plant. Healing Herb.

This is a large, coarse-looking, perennial plant, native of Europe, and found growing on the banks of streams and in wet meadows and low grounds throughout the Middle States of the Union. Stem hairy-bristly, branching above, two or three feet high. Leaves alternate, decurrent; lower ones petiolate, ovate-lanceolate; upper lanceolate. Flowers yellowish-white, rarely purplish, in nodding raceme-like clusters. Corolla tubular-campanulate, the limb with five recurved teeth, the orifice closed with five linear-awl-shaped scales. The root is about six inches long, about one inch thick at top, tapering, few-branched. It is mucilaginous, and has a sweetish, slightly astringent taste.

Flowers in June.

Preparation.—The fresh root, gathered before the plant blooms, is chopped and pounded to a pulp and weighed. Then two parts by weight of alcohol are taken, the pulp mixed thoroughly with one-sixth part of it and the rest of the alcohol added. After having stirred the whole, pour it into a well-stoppered bottle, and let it stand eight days in a dark, cool place. The tincture is then separated by decanting, straining and filtering.

Drug power of tincture, $\frac{1}{6}$.

Dilutions must be prepared as directed under Class III.

TABACUM.

Synonym, Nicotiana Tabacum, *Linn.*

Nat. Ord., Solanaceæ.

Common Name, Tobacco.

This widely cultivated plant is probably a native of Central America. It was first exported to Europe in 1586, from the island of Tabago. The wild plant is at present unknown. It is an annual plant; root large, fibrous. Stem round, erect, viscid-pubescent, branching near the top, four to six feet high. Leaves entire, alternate, sessile, decurrent, from one to two feet long and from six inches to a foot wide, oval-lanceolate and pointed. Flowers rose-colored, in loose, terminal panicles. Calyx urceolate, five-cleft. Corolla funnel-shaped, regular limb, five-lobed, plaited on the border.

The whole plant is viscid, fetid, and has an acrid, bitter, nauseous taste. Flowers in July.

It was first proven by Nenning, Germany.

Preparation.—The dried leaves of the genuine Havana tobacco, cut up, are covered with five parts by weight of alcohol, and allowed to remain eight days in a well-stoppered bottle, in a dark, cool place, being shaken twice a day. The tincture is then poured off, strained and filtered.

Drug power of tincture, $\frac{1}{10}$.

Dilutions must be prepared as directed under Class IV.

TAMUS COMMUNIS, *Linn.*

Nat. Ord., Dioscoreaceæ.

Common Name, Black Bryony.

This plant, a native of Southern Europe, Northern Africa and Western Asia, is found growing in copses and hedges. Rootstock ovoid, black, fleshy, subterranean. Stem many feet long, very slender, angular, branched. Leaves two to three inches long, ovate-cordate, acuminate, long-petioled, obscurely laterally lobed, five to seven-nerved, tip setaceous; stipules reflexed. Flowers one-sixth inch in diameter; males solitary or fascicled on slender racemes which are branched at the base; female racemes one inch shorter, recurved, few flowered; bracts minute. Berry one-half inch, oblong, red.

Flowers appear in May and June.

Preparation.—The fresh root is chopped and pounded to a pulp, enclosed in a piece of new linen and subjected to pressure. The expressed juice is then, by brisk agitation, mingled with an equal part by weight of alcohol. This mixture is allowed to stand eight days in a well-stoppered bottle, in a dark, cool place, and then filtered.

Amount of drug power, $\frac{1}{2}$.

Dilutions must be prepared as directed under Class I.

TANACETUM VULGARE, *Linn.*

Synonym, Athanasia.
Nat. Ord., Compositæ.
Common Name, Tansy.

This plant is a native of Europe and Central Asia. It is naturalized in many parts of the United States, where it is found growing in old fields, on roadsides, etc. From its perennial, stout, many-headed root arise a cluster of stems two to three feet high, obscurely angular, often purple at the base. Leaves alternate, almost sessile, from five or six to ten inches long, pinnately divided; segments oblong-lanceolate, pinnatifid, incisely-serrate, glandular-punctate. Flowers yellow, in a dense corymb; heads many-flowered, nearly discoid, all fertile; ray florets terete, tubular, three-toothed. Achenia obovate, with a large epigynous disk. The whole plant has a strong, disagreeable odor, and a bitter, aromatic taste.

Flowers in July and August.

Preparation.—Equal parts of the fresh leaves and blossoms are chopped and pounded to a pulp and weighed. Then two parts by weight of alcohol are taken, the pulp mixed thoroughly with one-sixth part of it, and the rest of the alcohol added. After having stirred the whole, pour it into a well-stoppered bottle, and let it stand eight days in a dark, cool place. The tincture is then separated by decanting, straining and filtering.

Amount of drug power, $\frac{1}{6}$.

Dilutions must be prepared as directed under Class III.

TARAXACUM.

Synonyms, Taraxacum Dens-leonis, *Desfontaines.* Taraxacum Officinale, *Wiggers.* Leontodon Taraxacum, *Linn.*
Nat. Ord., Compositæ.
Common Names, Dandelion. Puff Ball.

This is a perennial herb found growing in the greater portion of the Northern Hemisphere. Root six inches long or longer, one-half to one inch thick, almost cylindrical, few branched below. Leaves all radical, with teeth and lobes turned backward. Scape hollow, surmounted by a head of yellow flowers, involucre double, outer scales reflexed. Flowers all ligulate; achenia produced into a long beak. After the flower-head has closed and decayed, the hollow scape rises higher, carrying a globular airy head of fruit, each achenium being crowned with a white capillary pappus. The plant flowers from April to November.

It was first proven by Hahnemann.

Preparation.—The whole plant, with the root, gathered in April and May, before the flower is opened, is chopped and pounded to a pulp and pressed out in a piece of new linen. The expressed juice is then, by brisk agitation, mingled with an equal part by weight of alcohol. This mixture is allowed to stand in a well-stoppered bottle for eight days, in a dark, cool place, and then filtered.

Drug power of tincture, $\frac{1}{2}$.

Dilutions must be prepared as directed under Class I.

TARENTULA CUBENSIS.

Synonym, Tarantula.
Class, Arachnida.
Nat. Ord., Araneidea.
Family, Lycosidæ.
Common Name, Cuban Spider.

The *Tarentula Cubensis*, found in Cuba and Mexico, belongs to the same family as the *Tarentula Hispana.*

"Although apparently alike, these species differ widely in their pathogenetic and therapeutical effects. The Tarantula Hispana is a nervous remedy, acting deeply and powerfully on the cerebro-spinal system, and many cases of chorea, hysteria, etc., have been cured by this precious agent."

"The *Tarantula Cubensis*, on the other hand, seems to be a toxæmic remedy, acting directly on the blood, and being in this way an analogue of crotalus, apis, arsenicum, etc. It seems to be especially useful in maglignant ulcers and abscesses, anthrax and the like."—From *Dr. J. Navarro's article, read before the Hom. Med. Soc. of N. Y. Co., N. Y. Med. Times*, 1880.

Preparation.—Dr. Navarro put the live spiders into a glass jar, and by irritating them caused them to throw off their virus on the sides of the jar, whereupon strong alcohol was poured in, and from this tincture dilutions were made according to class VI—β.

TARENTULA HISPANA.

Synonym, Lycosa Tarantula.
Class, Arachnida.
Nat. Ord., Araneidea.
Family, Lycosidæ.

This hairy spider, frequently found in Spain, is a native of South America. The specimen used by Marquis Dr. Nunez, who first instituted provings in 1864, were collected at Pardo, Spain. [See *N. A. Jour. of Hom.*, Feb., 1872.] No appreciable difference seems to exist between the virus of the male or that of the female spider.

Preparation.—Dr. Nunez triturated the live spider with sugar of milk to dryness. From this further triturations were made according to Class VII.

TAXUS BACCATA *Linn.*

Nat. Ord., Coniferæ.
Common Names, Yew. Ground Hemlock.

The yew tree is believed to be indigenous to Central and Southern Asia, and extends into the Northern part of Africa and throughout the greater portion of Europe. It is an evergreen tree or shrub, and lives to a very great age. It has linear or spatulate-linear leaves, alternate, imbricated around the young branches; they are bright green and glossy above, paler beneath. Fruit an oblong-oval, bell-shaped ovule, becoming at maturity a seed nearly enclosed in a scarlet arillus which is open above. The leaves have the odor of turpentine and their taste is unpleasant, bitter and acrid.

The first provings of the drug were by Dr. Gastier, France.

Preparation.—The fresh leaves are chopped and pounded to a pulp and weighed. Then take two-thirds by weight of alcohol, add it to the pulp, stirring and mixing well, and strain through a piece of new linen. The tincture thus obtained is allowed to stand eight days in a well-stoppered bottle, in a dark, cool place, and then filtered.

Drug power of tincture, ½.

Dilutions must be prepared as directed under Class II.

TECOMA RADICANS, *Jussieu.*

Synonym, Bignonia Radicans, *Linn.*

Nat. Ord., Bignoniaceæ.

Common Name, Trumpet Creeper.

This is a climbing plant, growing in rich soil, from Pennsylvania to Illinois and southward, but is also cultivated farther north. It climbs by radical tendrils; leaves unequally pinnate; leaflets four to five pairs, ovate-acuminate, toothed; flowers in terminal corymbs; calyx campanulate, five-toothed; corolla infundibuliform, five-lobed, slightly irregular, two to three inches long, bright scarlet, very showy; stamens four, included. Pod six inches long; seeds transversely winged. Flowers from July to September.

Preparation.—The fresh root is chopped and pounded to a pulp and weighed. Then two parts by weight of alcohol are taken, the pulp mixed thoroughly with one-sixth part of it, and the rest of the alcohol added. After having stirred the whole well, pour it into a well-stoppered bottle and let it stand eight days in a dark, cool place. The tincture is then separated by decanting, straining and filtering.

Amount of drug power, ⅙.

Dilutions must be prepared as directed under Class III.

TELA ARANEÆ.

Common Names, Spider's Web. Cobweb.

This is the web of the common house spider, *Tegeneria domestica.* The web of *T. medicinalis* has been used in this country. The spider inhabits dark places in dwellings, barns, etc.; it is brown or blackish in color. The web found in cellars of houses is believed by many to possess greater medicinal powers than that of the field spider.

Preparation.—The recently spun web, free from dust, is triturated as directed under Class VII.

TELLURIUM.

Symbol, Te.

Atomic Weight, 64.

Origin and Preparation of Tellurium.—This element possesses many of the characters of a metal, but it bears so close a resemblance to selenium, both in its physical properties and its chemical relations, that it is most appropriately placed in the same group with that body. Tellurium is found in a few scarce minerals in association with gold, silver, lead and bismuth, apparently replacing sulphur, and is most easily extracted from the bismuth sulpho-telluride of Chemnitz in Saxony. The finely powdered ore is mixed with an equal weight of dry sodium carbonate, the mixture made into a paste with oil, and heated to whiteness in a closely covered crucible. Sodium telluride and sulphide are thereby produced, and metallic bismuth is set free. The fused mass is dissolved in water, and the solution freely exposed to the air, when the sodium and sulphur oxidize to sodium hydrate and hyposulphite, while the tellurium separates in the metallic state.

Properties.—Tellurium has the color and lustre of silver; by fusion and slow cooling it may be made to exhibit the form of rhombohedral crystals similar to those of antimony and arsenic. It is brittle, and is a comparatively bad conductor of heat and electricity; it has a density of 6.26, melts at a little below red heat, and volatilizes at a higher temperature. Tellurium burns when heated in the air, and is oxidized by nitric acid.

It was first proven by Dr. J. W. Metcalf, U. S.

Preparation for Homœopathic Use.—Tellurium is triturated, as directed under Class VII.

TEREBINTHINA.

Synonym, Oleum Terebinthinæ.

Common Name, Oil of Turpentine.

Origin.—Crude turpentine is an oleo-resin existing in the resin-ducts of many species of Pinus, and procured by making peculiarly shaped excavations called "pockets," in the trunk of the tree. When crude turpentine is distilled with water, nearly the whole of its oil passes over, and there is left in the still a resinous body known as Colophony or *rosin;* the distillate is purified by repeated rectification with water.

Properties.—Oil of turpentine is a colorless, mobile liquid possessing a peculiar aromatic and rather disagreeable odor. It is soluble in ten or twelve parts of 90 per cent. alcohol and is insoluble in water. Its specific gravity is from 0.860 to 0.89. It boils at 180° C. (356° F.). Pure turpentine oil is a mixture of several hydrocarbons having the general formula $C_{10} H_{16}$. It mixes in all proportions with absolute alcohol, ether and carbon disulphide. It dissolves iodine, sulphur, phosphorus, and many organic substances insoluble in water, such as fixed oils, resins, etc.; upon exposure to the air, turpentine absorbs oxygen, becomes thicker, and at last resinous. From the gradual oxidation, carbonic, acetic and formic acids are produced, and at the same time a part of the absorbed oxygen is converted into ozone; hence, oil of turpentine after prolonged exposure to the air, always contains oxygen and ozone in solution, together with an oxidation compound.

Chlorine, bromine and powdered iodine act upon it with great violence; nitric acid attacks it rapidly, and if the acid be concentrated, the turpentine takes fire.

Tests.—Pure turpentine oil, when shaken with one-twentieth of its weight of caustic ammonia, should not become either viscid or gelatinous. A layer of the oil, about one millimeter in thickness, in a flat porcelain dish should be completely evaporated at the heat of the water-bath. When adulterated with benzine, the specific gravity is lessened and the specimen is not completely soluble in twelve volumes of 90 per cent. alcohol. An oil which has become thick by keeping, can be purified by distilling 200 parts of it with 1,000 or 1,200 of water to which has been added one of caustic lime.

It was first proved by Dr. E. Seidel, Germany.

Preparation for Homœopathic Use.—One part by weight of purified oil of turpentine is dissolved in ninety-nine parts by weight of alcohol.

Amount of drug power, $\frac{1}{100}$.

Dilutions must be prepared as directed under Class VI—β.

TEUCRIUM.

Synonyms, Teucrium Marum, *Linn.* Marum Verum. Herba Cyriaci. Marjorana Syriaca.

Nat. Ord., Labiatæ.

Common Names, Syrian Herb Mastich. Cat Thyme.

This plant is indigenous to Southern Europe and Africa, but is often cultivated in more northern countries, growing about one foot high. The shrubby stem is hard, thin, erect, fine-tomentose and much branched. Leaves small, vivid green above, downy beneath, oval, entire, on long petioles. Flowers red, small, in one-sided terminal racemes. The flowers have taste and odor similar to camphor and valerian, which are lost by careless treatment in drying. Flowers in June and July.

It was first proven by Dr. Stapf, Germany.

Preparation.—The fresh plant, gathered shortly before the plant comes into bloom, is chopped and pounded to a pulp and pressed out in a piece of new linen. The expressed juice is then, by brisk agitation, mingled with an equal part by weight of alcohol. This mixture is allowed to stand eight days in a well-stoppered bottle in a dark, cool place and then filtered.

Drug power of tincture, $\frac{1}{2}$.

Dilutions must be prepared as directed under Class I.

THASPIUM AUREUM, *Nuttall.*

Synonyms, Zizia Aurea, *Koch.* Smyrnium Aureum, *Linn.* Sium Trifoliatum. Sison Aureus.

Nat. Ord., Umbelliferæ.

Common Names, Golden Alexanders. Meadow Parsnip.

This plant is indigenous to the United States and Canada, growing along moist river-banks and in meadows. Stems from one to two feet high, somewhat branching above, rather slender, erect, hollow, angular-furrowed, smooth as is every other part of the plant, and furnished with few leaves. Leaves one to two ternate; leaflets oval-lanceolate cut serrate. The lower leaves are long-petiolate. The umbels are about two inches broad, of ten to fifteen rays, the umbellets half an inch broad, dense. Flowers numerous, orange-yellow, appear in June. Fruit oval, brown, with strong and sharp ribs.

The drug was first proven by Dr. E. E. Marcy, United States.

Preparation.—The fresh plant is chopped and pounded to a pulp and weighed. Then two parts by weight of alcohol are taken, the pulp mixed thoroughly with one-sixth part of it, and the rest of the alcohol added. After having stirred the whole, pour it into a well-stoppered bottle and let it stand eight days, in a dark, cool place. The tincture is then separated by decanting, straining and filtering.

Amount of drug power, $\frac{1}{6}$.

Dilutions must be prepared as directed under Class III.

THEA CHINENSIS.

Synonym, Camellia Thea, *Link.*

Nat. Ord., Cammelliaceæ.

Common Name, Tea.

The tea-plant is a shrub indigenous to Southern and Eastern Asia. It is cultivated largely in China, Japan and India. Leaves lance-oval, or obovate, generally pointed, at the base sharp-sinuate, becoming serrate towards the point, green and shining above, paler beneath. They vary in size, but average two to three inches in length and from one-half to one inch broad; they are on short petioles. Flowers white, solitary or in axillary clusters of two or three.

Preparation.—Pekoe-tea is powdered and covered with five parts by weight of alcohol. Having poured it into a well-stoppered bottle, it is allowed to remain eight days in a dark, cool place, being shaken twice a day. The tincture is then poured off, strained and filtered.

Amount of drug power, $\frac{1}{10}$.

Dilutions must be prepared as directed under Class IV.

THEIN.

Synonyms, Theina. Theine.

Origin.—Oudry discovered, in 1827, in tea a crystalline substance which he named *thein,* and in 1838 both Jobst and Mulder showed this substance to be identical with *caffein.* The percentage of theine in tea varies with the quality and origin of the leaves. Stenhouse obtained from a sample of tea coming from the Himalaya region, 2.13 per cent. According to Peligot, hyson tea contains from 2.2 to 3.4 per cent., and gunpowder tea from 2.2 to 4.1 per cent. of theine.

For its properties see article Caffeinum.

Preparation.—Where it is desired to obtain the alkaloid from tea leaves the following simple process is offered: The finely powdered tea leaves are heated for a few minutes with three times their quantity of chloroform, and the liquid when cold is filtered off. The chloroform is then removed by distillation, the residue well washed with hot water and filtered; the filtrate on evaporation leaves a crystalline mass of caffeine (theine); or it may be obtained in larger proportion by macerating in four parts of water, one part of the finely powdered leaves with one of slaked lime; the water is to be evaporated and the dried residue extracted with chloroform. The chloroform is then to be distilled off, the residue treated with boiling water and the whole thrown upon a moistened filter. The filtrate after being partly evaporated is set aside to crystallize.

Preparation for Homœopathic Use.—Thein is triturated as directed under Class VII.

THERIDION CURASSAVICUM, *Walk.*

Synonym, Aranya.
Class, Arachnida.
Order, Araneidea.
Common Names, Black Spider of Curaçoa. Orange Spider.

This spider is about the size of a cherry-stone, and is found on orange trees in the West Indies. When young, it is velvety-black in appearance, marked with antero-posterior lines composed of white dots. At the posterior part of the body there are three orange-red spots, while upon the belly there is a large, square, yellow spot.

It was proven by Dr. Hering.

Preparation.—The live spider is crushed and covered with five parts by weight of alcohol. Having poured it into a well-stoppered bottle, it is allowed to remain eight days in a dark, cool place, being shaken twice a day. The tincture is then poured off, strained and filtered.

Amount of drug power, $\frac{1}{10}$.

Dilutions must be prepared as directed under Class IV.

THLASPI BURSA PASTORIS, *Linn.*

Synonym, Capsella Bursa Pastoris, *Mœnch.*
Nat. Ord., Cruciferæ.
Common Name, Shepherd's Purse.

This common plant is a native of Europe, but is now found widely spread in fields, pastures and on roadsides in this country. Stem six inches to a foot high, nearly smooth above, hairy below, striate and branching. Radical leaves two to eight inches long, incised. Stem leaves smaller, narrow, auricled at base, semi-clasping. Flowers very small, white in terminal corymbs. Fruit an obcordate trangular silicle containing many brown seeds. Flowers from April to September.

Preparation.—The fresh plant, gathered when in flower, is chopped and pounded to a pulp and weighed. Then take two-thirds by weight of alcohol, add it to the pulp, stirring and mixing well together, and strain through a piece of new linen. The tincture thus obtained is allowed to stand eight days in a well-stoppered bottle, in a dark, cool place, and then filtered.

Drug power of tincture, ½.

Dilutions must be prepared as directed under Class II.

THUJA.

Synonyms, Thuja Occidentalis, *Linn.* Cedrus Lycea.

Nat. Ord., Coniferæ.

Common Names, Arbor Vitæ. Tree of Life. White Cedar.

This indigenous evergreen tree grows wild in the Northern States and Canada, and is also cultivated for ornament in our gardens. It is a branchy tree from its root, sometimes rising thirty feet in height; the branches are flat, compressed and imbricated; leaves short, evergreen, overlapping like tiles, with obtuse scales, disposed in four ranks; flowers mostly monœcious on different branches, in very small terminal ovoid catkins. Stamens with a scale-like filament or connective, bearing four anther-cells. Fertile catkins of few imbricated scales, fixed by the base, each bearing two erect ovules, dry and spreading at maturity. Cotyledons two. Scales of the cones pointless; seeds broadly winged all round. The flowers appear in May and June, and are of a brownish-yellow color. The leaves when rubbed between the hands give off a pungent aromatic resinous odor.

It was first proven by Hahnemann.

Preparation.—The fresh leaves, gathered when the plant is just flowering, are chopped and pounded to a pulp and weighed. Then take two-thirds by weight of alcohol, mix it with the pulp, strain through a piece of new linen, and allow the mixture to stand eight days in a well-stoppered bottle, in a dark, cool place and then filter.

Drug power of tincture, ½.

Dilutions must be prepared as directed under Class II.

THYMUS.

Synonym, Thymus Serpyllum, *Linn.*

Nat. Ord., Labiatæ.

Common Name, Wild Thyme.

This perennial little plant is very common in France and Germany, and grows on sunny hills, pasture-grounds, along roads and ditches. Root ligneous, branchy; stems, some erect, others creeping, downy, thin, ligneous, quadrangular; leaves oblong-oval, glabrous or hairy, on short peduncles, blunt or rounded, dark green on the upper surface, paler and spotted on the lower, veined. Flowers purplish, in capitate verticils at the end of the stems; calyx ovate, two-lipped, thirteen-nerved, hairy in the throat; the upper lip three-toothed, spreading; the lower two-cleft, with the awl-shaped divisions ciliate. Corolla short, slightly two-lipped; the upper lip straight and thick, notched at the apex; the lower three-cleft. Stamens four, straight and distinct, usually exserted.

Preparation.—The fresh plant, in flower, is chopped and pounded to a pulp and weighed. Then add two-thirds by weight of alcohol, mix with pulp, strain through a piece of new linen, and allow the mixture to stand eight days in a well-stoppered bottle, in a dark, cool place, and then filter.

Drug power of tincture, $\frac{1}{2}$.

Dilutions must be prepared as directed under Class II.

TILIA.

Synonym, Tilia Europæa, *Linn.*

Nat. Ord., Tiliaceæ.

Common Name, Lime or Linden Tree.

This is a handsome tree, indigenous to Europe, sometimes 120 feet in height, but generally not above half that size. Leaves stalked, broadly heart-shaped or nearly orbicular, often oblique, and always pointed, serrate on the edge, glabrous above and more or less downy underneath, especially in the angles of the principal veins. Peduncles hanging amongst the leaves, bordered or winged half way up by the long, narrow, leaf-like bract. Flowers sweet-scented, pale whitish-green. Nut woody, globular, becoming one-celled and one or two-seeded.

It was first proven by Dr. J. O. Müller and Dr. Fröhlich, Austria.

Preparation.—The fresh blossoms, freed from the peduncle, are pounded to a pulp and weighed. Then two parts by weight of alcohol are taken, the pulp mixed thoroughly with one-sixth part of it, and the rest of the alcohol added. After having stirred the whole, pour it into a well-stoppered bottle, and let it stand eight days in a dark, cool place. The tincture is then separated by decanting, straining and filtering.

Drug power of tincture, $\frac{1}{6}$.

Dilutions must be prepared as directed under Class III.

TITANIUM.

Symbol, Ti.

Atomic Weight, 50.

Origin and Preparation of Titanium.—This is one of the rarer metals, and is never found in the metallic state. The most important titanium minerals are *rutile, brookite,* and *anatase,* which are different forms of titanic oxide, and the several varieties of titaniferous iron, consisting of ferrous titanate, sometimes alone, but more generally mixed with ferric or ferroso-ferric oxide. Occasionally in the slag adhering to the bottom of blast-furnaces in which iron ore is reduced, small, brilliant copper-colored cubes, hard enough to scratch glass, and in the highest degree infusible, are found. This substance, of which a single smelting furnace in the Hartz produced as much as eighty pounds, was formerly believed to be metallic titanium. Recent researches of Wöhler, however, have shown it to be a combination of titanium cyanide with titanium nitride. When these crystals are powdered, mixed with potassium hydrate and fused, ammonia is evolved, and potassium titanate is formed. Metallic titanium in a finely divided state may be obtained by heating titanium and potassium fluoride with potassium. This element is remarkable for its affinity for nitrogen; when heated in the air, it simultaneously absorbs oxygen and nitrogen.

Preparation for Homœopathic Use.—Metallic titanium is triturated as directed under Class VII.

TRADESCANTIA DIURETICA, *Martius.*

Synonym, Tradescantia Commelina.
Nat. Ord., Commelyneæ. (Liliaceæ).
Common Name, Spiderwort.

This herbaceous plant is pretty common in Brazil. Its ramose and cylindrical stems are erect or a little inclined; the leaves are alternate, sheathed, somewhat lanceolate, and forming at the extremity of the branches, tufts, whence arise long pedicels, each of which carries from four to six flowers; perianth double, three-leaved, the outer one having sharp, herbaceous divisions, and the inner one being petaloid and blue-colored. Stamens six; a free tri-locular ovary, surmounted by a simple style.

Introduced into our Materia Medica by Dr. Mure, Brazil.

Preparation.—The fresh leaves, gathered at time of flowering are chopped and pounded to a pulp and weighed. Then two parts by weight of alcohol are taken, the pulp mixed with one-sixth part of it, and the rest of the alcohol added. After having stirred the whole pour it into a well-stoppered bottle, and let it stand eight days in a dark, cool place. The tincture is then separated by decanting, straining and filtering.

Drug power of tincture, $\frac{1}{6}$.

Dilutions must be prepared as directed under Class III.

TRIFOLIUM.

Synonym, Trifolium Pratense, *Linn.*
Nat. Ord., Leguminosæ.
Common Name, Red Clover.

This is a biennial plant, common throughout the United States. Stems ascending, thinly hirsute; leaflets oval or obovate, often notched at the end and with a pale spot above; stipules broad, bristle-pointed; heads ovate, sessile.

It was first proven by Dr. T. C. Duncan, U. S.

Preparation.—The fresh blossoms are pounded to a pulp and weighed. Then two parts by weight of alcohol are taken, the pulp mixed thoroughly with one-sixth part of it, and the rest of the alcohol added. After having stirred the whole, pour it into a well-stoppered bottle, and let it stand eight days in a dark, cool place. The tincture is then separated by decanting, straining and filtering.

Drug power of tincture, $\frac{1}{6}$.

Dilutions must be prepared as directed under Class III.

TRIFOLIUM ARVENSE, *Linn.*

Nat. Ord., Leguminosæ.

Common Names, Rabbit Foot. Stone Clover.

This species is a native of Europe and Central Asia, and has been introduced into America, where it is found growing in old fields. Stems are from five to ten inches high, silky and branching; leaflets oblanceolate; heads becoming very soft-downy and grayish, oblong or cylindrical; calyx-teeth silky-plumose, longer than the whitish corolla; root annual.

Preparation.—The fresh plant, gathered in July and freed from all ligneous stalks, is chopped and pounded to a pulp and weighed. Then two parts by weight of alcohol are taken, the pulp mixed thoroughly with one-sixth part of it, and the rest of the alcohol added. After having stirred the whole well, pour it into a well-stoppered bottle, and let it stand eight days in a dark, cool place. The tincture is then separated by decanting, straining and filtering.

Amount of drug power, $\frac{1}{6}$.

Dilutions must be prepared as directed under Class III.

TRILLIUM.

Synonyms, Trillium Pendulum, *Aiton* and *Muhlenberg.* Trillium Album.

Nat. Ord., Smilaceæ.

Common Name, White Beth-Root.

This is an indigenous plant, common in the Middle and Western States, growing in rich soils, in damp, rocky and shady woods. Root oblong, tuberous, from which arises a slender stem, from ten to fifteen inches in height. Leaves three, whorled at the top of the stem, sub-orbicular rhomboidal, abruptly acuminate, from three to five inches in diameter, on petioles about a line in length. Flowers white, solitary, terminal, cernuous, on a recurved peduncle, from one to two and a half inches long. Sepals green, oblong-lanceolate, acuminate, an inch long. Petals white, oblong-ovate, acute, one and a quarter inches in length, by half an inch broad. Styles three, erect, with curved stigma.

Preparation.—The fresh root is chopped and pounded to a pulp and weighed. Then two parts by weight of alcohol are taken, and having mixed the pulp thoroughly with one-sixth part of it, the rest of the alcohol is added. After having stirred the whole, pour it into a well-stoppered bottle, and let it stand eight days in a dark, cool place. The tincture is then separated by decanting, straining and filtering.

Drug power of tincture, $\frac{1}{6}$.
Dilutions must be prepared as directed under Class III.

TRIOSTEUM PERFOLIATUM, *Linn.*

Nat. Ord., Caprifoliaceæ.
Common Names, Fever-Wort. Horse Gentian.
This perennial herb is indigenous, found in rich woodlands. Its stems are from two to four feet high, softly hairy; leaves oval, abruptly narrowed below, downy beneath. Flowers sessile, in clusters, brownish-purple, appearing in June. Calyx five-parted; segments linear-lanceolate, leaf-like, persistent. Corolla tubular, gibbous at the base, sub-equally five-lobed, scarcely longer than the calyx; stamens five. Ovary mostly three-celled, in fruit forming a rather dry drupe, orange-colored, half an inch long, containing three, angled and ribbed, one-seeded, bony nutlets.
It was proven by Dr. W. Williamson, U. S.
Preparation.—The fresh root is chopped and pounded to a pulp and weighed. Then two parts by weight of alcohol are taken, the pulp mixed thoroughly with one-sixth part of it, and the rest of the alcohol added. After having stirred the whole, pour it into a well-stoppered bottle, and let it stand eight days in a dark, cool place. The tincture is then separated by decanting, straining and filtering.
Amount of drug power, $\frac{1}{6}$.
Dilutions must be prepared as directed under Class III.

TROMBIDIUM MUSCÆ DOMESTICÆ.

Synonyms, Trombidium Holosericeum. Leptus Auctumnalis.
Class, Arachnida.
Order, Acaridea.
A minute bright red acarus, found under the wings of the common house-fly in Philadelphia, the provings of which were made by Dr. J. P. Harvey.
Preparation.—The entire acarus is crushed and covered with fifty parts by weight of alcohol. Having poured it into a well-stoppered bottle, it is allowed to remain eight days in a dark, cool place, being shaken twice a day. The tincture is then poured off, strained and filtered.
Amount of drug power, $\frac{1}{100}$.
Dilutions must be prepared as directed under Class VI—β.

TUSSILAGO PETASITES, *Linn.*

Synonym, Petasites Vulgaris, *Desf.*
Nat. Ord., Compositæ.
Common Names, Butter-Bur. Pestilence Wort.
This plant is a native of Europe. Leaves, the small ones or scales

numerous, oblong or linear, entire and erect; the radical ones appearing much later than the flower stems, angular and toothed, covered underneath with a loose, white, cottony wool, of which there is a little also on the upper side. Flowering stems not in tufts, as in the *common Coltsfoot*, often a foot high when full grown, with many flower-heads of a dull pinkish-purple, in a narrow, oblong, terminal panicle, and almost diœcious. The male plant has a looser panicle of smaller heads, the florets either all tubular and male (the pistil, although apparently perfect, having no ovule and forming no seed), or with a few filiform female ones on the outside; the female panicle more compact, the heads larger, the florets all filiform, or with a few tubular male ones in the centre.

It was proven by Dr. Küchenmeister, Germany.

Preparation.—The fresh plant is chopped and pounded to a pulp and weighed. Then two parts by weight of alcohol are taken, the pulp mixed thoroughly with one-sixth part of it, and the rest of the alcohol added. After having stirred the whole, pour it into a well-stoppered bottle, and let it stand eight days in a dark cool place. The tincture is then separated by decanting, straining and filtering.

Amount of drug power, $\frac{1}{6}$.

Dilutions must be prepared as directed under Class III.

UPAS TIEUTE.

Synonym, Strychnos Tieuté, *Leschenault.*

Nat. Ord., Loganiaceæ.

Common Name, Upas Tree.

Upas is a term used in the Malay tongue for arrow poison. In the Celebes and Borneo the word *ipo* is employed with the same meaning.. Commonly, however, the term "Upas" is applied to two special arrow poisons used in the East Indies, viz., *Upas Antiar*, and *Upas Radja* or *Upas Tieuté.* Upas Antiar is prepared from the milky juice of *Antiaris toxicaria*, the poison tree of Macassar.

Upas Radja, or Upas Tieuté, also called Upas Tjettik, and far in the interior of India *Sung-sig* (dagger-poison), is prepared from the younger roots and the bark of the older roots of Strychnos Tieuté, a climbing woody plant growing in Java. The parts named are boiled for an hour with the addition of various non-essential ingredients as garlic, pepper, etc. The substance so obtained is evaporated to a viscid mass. It is brownish-black in the fresh state, but when dry resembles opium in appearance. Its taste is bitter, it is in great part soluble in alcohol, and its poisonous constituents are, according to Pelletier and Caventou, strychnia and brucia.

It was first proven by Dr. Pitet, France.

Preparation for Homœopathic Use.—One part by weight of upas tieuté is dissolved in fifty parts weight of alcohol.

Amount of drug power, $\frac{1}{100}$.

Dilutions must be prepared as directed under Class VI—β.

URANIUM NITRICUM.

Proper Name, Uranyl Nitrate.
Synonyms, Uranic Nitrate. Uranii Nitras.
Common Name, Nitrate of Uranium.
Formula, $(U_2O_2)(NO_3)_2, 6H_2O$.
Molecular Weight, 504.

Origin.—Uranium is a rare metal; its principal ore consists of impure uranoso-uranic oxide (pitchblende) containing sulphur, arsenic, lead, iron and several other metals. It occurs in other mineral forms, as carbonate, sulphate, etc. The nitrate is used in medicine.

Preparation.—Ebelmann's method is to digest pulverized pitchblende with hydrochloric acid to dissolve oxides of calcium, magnesium, manganese and other metals; the residue is to be washed, dried and then roasted with charcoal. The cooled mass is to be exhausted with strong hydrochloric acid to remove iron, copper and lead as completely as possible; again the washed residue is to be roasted and dissolved in nitric acid. The solution thus obtained is to be evaporated to dryness and again treated with water which leaves arseniate of iron undissolved; the filtrate is to be treated with hydrogen sulphide and evaporated until crystallization begins; the resulting crystals are to be purified by recrystallization. A perfectly pure uranium nitrate may be obtained by dissolving the ordinary nitrate, prepared as directed above, in water and precipitating with oxalic acid; the resulting oxalate of uranium is to be washed, dried and heated to full redness, when uranous oxide remains as the sole residue. This is to be dissolved in nitric acid and crystallized out.

Properties.—Uranium nitrate forms trimetric prisms which are yellow in color when viewed by direct light; when the light falls obliquely to the observer the crystals have a green fluorescence. The crystals deliquesce superficially in the air; when heated they melt in their water of crystallization, and if more strongly heated give up their nitric acid and become converted into uranic and finally into uranoso-uranic oxide. They are soluble in water, alcohol and ether. The salt is decomposed under the influence of light, hence the crystals should be kept in bottles securely protected therefrom.

It was proven by E. S. Blake, M. B., England.

Preparation for Homœopathic Use.—The pure nitrate of uranium is triturated as directed under Class VII.

URTICA.

Synonyms, Urtica Urens, *Linn.* Urtica Minora.
Nat. Ord., Urticaceæ.
Common Names, Common Nettle. Dwarf Stinging Nettle.

The small or dwarf nettle is widely distributed in North America, although but sparingly in the northern portion. It is found also in both Europe and Asia. It is an annual, stem a foot to a foot and a half high, covered with venomous stinging hairs, and branching. Leaves opposite, petiolate, stipulate, from one to two inches long, broad-elliptic or ovate, three-veined, deeply acute-serrate. Flowers green, in drooping axilliary clusters, in pairs.

The stinging power of nettles is due, according to Saladin, to acid ammonium carbonate contained in glands beneath their epidermis. When the herb is distilled with water the distillate contains formic acid (Gorup-Besanez).

It was first proven by Dr. John Redman Coxe, Jr., U. S.

Preparation.—The entire fresh plant, gathered when in flower, is chopped and pounded to a pulp and weighed. Then two parts by weight of alcohol are taken, the pulp mixed thoroughly with one-sixth part of it, and the rest of the alcohol added. After having stirred the whole pour it into a well-stoppered bottle, and let it stand eight days in a dark, cool place. The tincture is then separated by decanting, straining and filtering.

Drug power of tincture, $\frac{1}{6}$.

Dilutions must be prepared as directed under Class III.

URTICA DIOICA, *Linn.*

Nat. Ord., Urticaceæ.

Common Name, Great or Large Nettle.

This nettle is like the preceding as to its origin and distribution, except that it is more abundant in North America than U. urens. Stem two to four feet high, obtusely four-angled, branching, hispid with stinging hairs. Leaves opposite, stipulate on petioles. Leaves cordate, lance-ovate, coarsely serrate, two to three inches long, conspicuously pointed. Flowers small, greenish, generally diœcious, in branching panicled spikes.

Preparation.—The fresh herb, gathered when coming into flower, is chopped and pounded to a pulp and weighed. Then two parts by weight of alcohol are taken, the pulp mixed thoroughly with one-sixth part of it, and the rest of the alcohol added. After having stirred the whole, pour it into a well-stoppered bottle, and let it stand eight days in a dark, cool place. The tincture is then separated by decanting, straining and filtering.

Drug power of tincture, $\frac{1}{6}$.

Dilutions must be prepared as directed under Class III.

USNEA BARBATA, *Fries.*

Nat. Ord., Lichenes.

U. barbata is a very common lichen found growing in pendulous masses on the bark of trees, in large forests. The genus Usnea is characterized as follows; apothecia sub-terminal, rounded, peltate; the open disk placed upon the filamentous, medullary stratum, the margin generally radiate-ciliate. Thallus cartilagineous, at first erect, suffructiculose, becoming more or less filamentous or pendulous with age, the medullary layer somewhat separated from the crustaceous cortical stratum. The species *U. barbata* has an irregularly branched, terete thallus, at length annulate-cracked, glaucous; apothecia almost inmarginate, radiate; disk pale. It has a number of forms or varieties, viz., var. *florida*, v. *strigosa*, v. *rubigenea*, v. *hirta*, v. *plicata* and v. *darypoga*, the latter being also termed *U. barbata*, Hoffm. and *Lichen barbatus*, Linn.

Preparation.—The fresh lichen finely chopped, is covered with five parts by weight of dilute alcohol, the whole poured into a well-stoppered bottle, and allowed to remain eight days in a dark, cool place, being shaken twice a day. The tincture is then poured off, strained and filtered.

Drug power of tincture, $\frac{1}{10}$.

Dilutions must be prepared as directed under Class IV.

USTILAGO MAIDIS, *Corda*.

Nat. Ord., Fungi.

Common Names, Maize Smut. Corn Smut.

This is a fungus found growing on the Indian corn, *Zea mays*.

It is often as large, sometimes larger than an orange. It is covered with a dark gray or brown epidermis, which bursts when ripe. The spores are spherical, minute, their surface covered with echinulate warts like prickles; they are deep-seated, nearly black and pulverulent, having the appearance of soot under the naked eye.

It was introduced into our Materia Medica by Dr. W. H. Burt, U. S.

Preparation.—The fresh, just ripe fungus, is powdered and covered with five parts by weight of alcohol, and allowed to remain eight days in a well-steppered bottle, in a dark, cool place, being shaken twice a day. The tincture is then poured off, strained and filtered.

Amount of drug power, $\frac{1}{10}$.

Dilutions must be prepared as directed under Class IV.

Triturations of the ripe fungus are prepared as directed under Class VII.

UVA URSI.

Synonyms, Arctostaphylos Uva-ursi, *Sprengel*. Arbutus Uva-ursi, *Linn.*

Nat. Ord., Ericaceæ.

Common Name, Bearberry.

This is a small evergreen shrub, procumbent in habit, found growing in Europe, North America and Northern Asia, in fact over the greater portion of the Northern Hemisphere. It prefers dry, sandy, or even rocky situations. Stem much branched; leaves almost sessile, obovate, about an inch long, and from one-quarter to three-eighths of an inch wide, entire, with margins somewhat reflexed. The leaves are slightly pubescent when young, afterward smooth, shining above, and leathery, paler and minutely reticulated beneath. Flowers urceolate, whitish, in short pendent racemes. Fruit a drupe, bright red in color, with five flat nutlets, each one seeded.

Flowers in May.

The drug was first proven by Hahnemann.

Preparation.—The fresh leaves, gathered in autumn, are chopped and pounded to a pulp and weighed. Then take two-thirds by weight of alcohol, add it to the pulp, stir and mix well, and strain through a piece of new linen. The tincture thus obtained is allowed to stand eight days in a well-stoppered bottle, in a dark, cool place, and then filtered.

Drug power of tincture, $\frac{1}{2}$.

Dilutions must be prepared as directed under Class II.

VACCININUM.

Common Names, Vaccine Virus. Bovine Virus.

Preparation for Homœopathic Use.—The genuine vaccine matter, taken fresh from a healthy young heifer, is triturated as directed under Class VIII.

VALERIANA OFFICINALIS, *Linn.*

Synonym, Phu Germanicum.

Nat. Ord., Valerianaceæ.

Common Name, Great Wild Valerian.

V. officinalis is an herbaceous perennial plant of handsome aspect, found growing in almost the whole of Europe north of Spain, and in Asia, from the Crimea to Manchuria and northward. It grows on plains and uplands, and has been found at an elevation of 1200 feet above the sea-level. In the wild state the plant varies greatly according to its situation, as many as eight varieties having been noticed by botanists. It is cultivated in Germany, England and Holland, and to some extent in the United States. The stem is from two to four feet high, erect, round, furrowed, branching at the top. Radical leaves large, lanceolate, on lengthened petioles. Stem leaves on short, sheathing petioles, elliptical, with deep serrations. Flowers small, white or tinged with rose-color, in crowded, compound cymes. Fruit a one-celled, one-seeded capsule.

The root is used in medicine. It is seen in commerce as an upright rhizome as thick as the little finger, giving off many slender rootlets and a few horizontal branches. The root has a peculiar odor, somewhat terebinthinate and camphoraceous, and its taste is bitter and aromatic.

It was first proven by Hahnemann.

Preparation.—The dried root, coarsely powdered, is covered with five parts by weight of alcohol, and allowed to remain eight days in a well-stoppered bottle, in a dark, cool place, being shaken twice a day. The tincture is then poured off, strained and filtered.

Drug power of tincture, $\frac{1}{10}$.

Dilutions must be prepared as directed under Class IV.

VARIOLINUM.

Common Name, Small Pox Virus.

Preparation for Homœopathic Use.—The contents of a ripe small pox pustule are triturated, as directed under Class VIII.

VERATRUM ALBUM, *Linn.*

Synonyms, Elleborum Album. Helleborus Albus.

Nat. Ord., Liliaceæ.

Common Names, White Hellebore. European Hellebore.

This is a perennial, herbaceous plant, growing in moist grassy spots, in the mountainous portions of middle Europe, and extending eastward through Asiatic Russia. Stem from two to four feet high; leaves alternate, broad-oval or elliptical, nearly six inches long, entire, sheathing at base, strongly veined and plaited. Flowers in large racemose-panicles; perianth, of six petaloid segments, united at the base, yellowish-white within, green without. Fruit a three-lobed capsule, many seeded. The root is used in medicine; the rootstock is cylindrical, fleshy, about an inch in diameter with stoutish long rootlets; in the fresh state it has a garlicky odor.

In commerce the root is found cylindrical or sub-conical in shape, dull earthy black in color, and roughened in surface below by the scars left by old roots. Its top is crowned by leaf-bases. On transverse section of the root is seen a broad white ring, within which is a pale buff centre. Its taste is bitter and acrid, followed by a sensation of numbness and tingling. Its powder acts as a violent sternutatory.

It was first proven by Hahnemann.

Preparation.—The dried root, coarsely powdered, is covered with five parts by weight of alcohol and allowed to remain eight days in a well-stoppered bottle, in a dark, cool place, being shaken twice a day. The tincture is then poured off, strained and filtered.

Drug power of tincture, $\frac{1}{10}$.

Dilutions must be prepared as directed under Class IV.

VERATRUM VIRIDE, *Aiton.*

Synonym, Helonias Viridis.

Nat. Ord., Liliaceæ.

Common Names, American Hellebore. Swamp Hellebore.

Recent writers consider this plant as merely a variety of the preceding. Flückiger and Hanbury say, that the green colored variety, *Veratrum Lobelianum* found in Alpine mountain meadows, is indistinguishable from *Veratrum viride,* Ait. Regel describes (*Tentamen Floræ Ussur,* St. Petersburg, 1861, 153, quoted by F. and H.), four varieties of *Veratrum album* occurring in the Amoor region in Siberia and identified one with *Veratrum viride.* Gray considers *Veratrum viride* "much too near Veratrum album of Europe." Sims, 1808, quoted by F. and H, says that the flowers of *Veratrum viride* "are more inclined to a yellow-green" than those of *Veratrum album,* the petals broader and more erect, the margins, especially about claw, covered with a white mealiness.

The American white hellebore is a coarse plant found growing in wet meadows and swamps from Canada to Georgia. Leaves large, nearly a foot long and half as wide, sheathing at the base. Stem striate, pubescent, two to four feet high. Flowers in pyramidal panicles, made up of dense, spreading, spike-like racemes. In commerce the rhizome is found dried with the roots attached, the latter being pale brown in color, and towards their ends giving out slender fibrous rootlets. For convenience in drying, the rootstocks are quartered lengthwise. The rhizome is also sent into market deprived of its roots, cut into transverse slices and dried. The slices are about an inch in the average diameter, curled and shrunken by drying and in color whitish, buff or brownish.

Preparation.—The fresh root, gathered in autumn, is chopped and pounded to a pulp and weighed. Then two parts by weight of dilute alcohol are taken, the pulp mixed thoroughly with one-sixth part of it, and the rest of the alcohol added. After having stirred the whole, pour into a well-stoppered bottle, and let it stand eight days in a dark, cool place. The tincture is then separated by decanting, straining and filtering.

Amount of drug power, $\frac{1}{6}$.

Dilutions must be prepared as directed under Class III, except that dilute alcohol is to be used until the 2 and 4x are reached.

VERBASCUM.

Synonyms, Verbascum Thapsus, *Linn.* Thapsus Barbatus.

Nat. Ord., Scrophulariaceæ.

Common Names, Mullein. Blattaria. Flannel Plant.

This plant is a native of Europe, but has become naturalized in North America, where it is found very frequently in fields, etc. The whole plant is densely tomentous throughout; stem erect, three to five feet high, stout, simple, angles winged by the decurrent bases of the oblong acute leaves; flowers (yellow, very rarely white) in a prolonged and very dense club-shaped spike; lower stamens usually beardless; pod globular, many-seeded.

It was first proven by Hahnemann.

Preparation.—The fresh plant, gathered when coming into bloom, is chopped and pounded to a pulp and weighed. Then two parts by weight of alcohol are taken, the pulp mixed thoroughly with one-sixth part of it, and the rest of the alcohol added. After having stirred the whole, pour it into a well-stoppered bottle, and let it stand eight days in a dark, cool place. The tincture is then separated by decanting, straining and filtering.

Amount of drug power, $\frac{1}{2}$.

Dilutions must be prepared as directed under Class III.

VERBENA HASTATA, *Linn.*

Nat. Ord., Verbenaceæ.

Common Names, Blue Vervain. Purvain. Wild Hyssop.

This plant is indigenous to this country, where it is found very frequently on low and waste grounds. It is tall, from four to six feet high; leaves lanceolate or oblong-lanceolate, acuminate, incisely-serrate, on petioles, the lower often lobed and sometimes hastate at the base; spikes slender, erect, densely flowered, panicled or corymbed. Flowers from July to September.

Preparation.—The fresh plant, in flower, is chopped and pounded to a pulp and weighed. Then two parts by weight of alcohol are taken, the pulp mixed thoroughly with one-sixth part of it, and the rest of the alcohol added. After having stirred the whole, pour it into a well-stoppered bottle, and let it stand eight days in a dark, cool place. The tincture is then separated by decanting, straining and filtering.

Amount of drug power, $\frac{1}{6}$

Dilutions must be prepared as directed under Class III.

VERBENA OFFICINALIS, *Linn.*

Synonym, Verbena Maris.

Nat. Ord., Verbenaceæ.

Common Names, Vervain. Verbena. White Vervain.

This plant grows in Germany and the south of Europe, in sandy places, along roads, hedges, and on heaps of rubbish. Stem is erect, from one to three feet high, loosely branched; leaves pinnatifid or three-cleft, oblong-lanceolate, sessile, smooth above, the lobes cut and toothed; spikes panicled, very slender; bracts small, much shorter than the very small purplish flowers. Flowers appear all summer.

Preparation.—The fresh herb, in flower, is chopped and pounded to a pulp and weighed. Then add two-thirds by weight of alcohol, stir well, and strain through a piece of new linen. The tincture thus obtained is allowed to stand eight days in a well-stoppered bottle in a dark, cool place, and then filtered.

Amount of drug power, $\frac{1}{2}$.

Dilutions must be prepared as directed under Class II.

VERBENA URTICÆFOLIA, *Linn.*

Nat. Ord., Verbenaceæ.

Common Name, Nettle-Leaved or White Vervain.

This plant is found growing in old fields and roadsides in Mexico, West Indies and in other portions of America. The stems are rather tall, sub-pubescent; leaves ovate or ovate-lanceolate, acute, coarsely serrate, petiolate; spikes very slender, at length much elongated, with the flowers separate, loosely panicled, very small, white.

Preparation. —The fresh plant, in flower, is chopped and pounded to a pulp and weighed. Then two-thirds by weight of alcohol are taken, mixed well with the pulp, and the whole is pressed out in a piece of new linen. This tincture is allowed to stand eight days in a well-stoppered bottle, in a dark, cool place and then filtered.

Amount of drug power, $\frac{1}{2}$.

Dilutions must be prepared as directed under Class II.

VERONICA BECCABUNGA.

Synonym, Veronica Americana, *Schweinitz.*

Nat. Ord., Scrophulariaceæ.

Common Name, Brooklime.

This plant is found in Europe and Asia, growing near springs and in running waters. Stem smooth, decumbent below, erect above, twelve to eighteen inches long. Leaves opposite, on short petioles, oval, serrate, obtuse; they are about an inch and a half long and smooth. Flowers pale blue, veined, in loose axillary racemes. Fruit a roundish-turgid capsule, two-celled, few-seeded.

Preparation.—The fresh plant, gathered when in bloom, is chopped and pounded to a pulp and weighed. Then add two-thirds by weight of alcohol to the pulp, stirring and mixing well, and strain through a piece of new linen. The tincture thus obtained is allowed to stand eight days in a well-stoppered bottle, in a dark, cool place, and then filtered.

Drug power of tincture, $\frac{1}{2}$.

Dilutions must be prepared as directed under Class II.

VESPA CRABRO.

Class, Insecta.

Order, Hymenoptera.

Family, Vesparia.

Common Name, Wasp.

The common wasp of Europe.

Preparation.—Live wasps are put into a bottle, and after being aggravated by shaking, are covered with five times their weight of strong alcohol, and the whole allowed to remain eight days, in a dark, cool place, being shaken twice a day. The tincture is then poured off, strained and filtered.

Amount of drug power, $\frac{1}{10}$.

Dilutions must be prepared as directed under Class IV.

VIBURNUM OPULUS, *Linn.*

Synonyms, Viburnum Edule. Viburnum Oxycoccus.

Nat. Ord., Caprifoliaceæ.

Common Names, High Cranberry. Sheep's Berry. Snowball.

This shrub has nearly smooth, upright stems from five to ten feet high; leaves three to five-veined, three-lobed, broadly wedge-shaped or truncate at the base, the divaricate lobes pointed, mostly crenate-toothed on the sides, entire in the sinuses; petioles bearing two glands at the apex, cymes pedunculate. Fruit spherical, pleasantly acid, bright red, resembling the common cranberry in flavor, the stone very flat, nearly orbicular; leaf-buds enclosed in one or two pairs of scales. It grows in low grounds, along streams; common in the Alleghanies as far South as the borders of Maryland.

Preparation.—The fresh bark of the root is pounded to a fine pulp and weighed. Then two parts by weight of alcohol are taken, and after thoroughly mixing the pulp with one-sixth part of it, the rest of the alcohol is added. After having stirred the whole, pour it into a well-stoppered bottle, and let it stand eight days in a dark, cool place. The tincture is then separated by decanting, straining and filtering.

Drug power of tincture, $\frac{1}{6}$.

Dilutions must be prepared as directed under Class III.

VIBURNUM PRUNIFOLIUM, *Linn.*

Nat. Ord., Caprifoliaceæ.

Common Names, Black Haw. Plum-leaved Viburnum.

This is a shrub or small tree, in height from ten to twenty feet, found growing in woods and thickets from New York southward to Georgia and westward to the Mississippi. Leaves opposite, from two to three inches long and nearly half as wide, on slightly margined petioles; they are smooth, shining above, oval or roundish-obovate, sharply serrulate. Flowers white, in terminal, nearly sessile, large cymes; corolla rotate, five-parted. Fruit an oval bluish-black berry, containing a smooth, flattened putamen. The berry is sweet and eatable.

Preparation.—The fresh ripe fruit is pounded to a pulp and weighed. Then two parts by weight of alcohol are taken, the pulp mixed thoroughly with one-sixth part of it, and the rest of the alcohol added. After having stirred the whole, pour it into a well-stoppered bottle, and let it stand eight days in a dark, cool place. The tincture is then separated by decanting, straining and filtering.

Drug power of tincture, $\frac{1}{6}$.

Dilutions must be prepared as directed under Class III.

VINCA MINOR, *Linn.*

Synonym, Vinca Pervinca.

Nat. Ord., Apocynaceæ.

Common Name, Lesser Periwinkle.

This evergreen is a native of Europe, and is found in shaded woods and stony slopes or hedges, and is also frequently reared in gardens for ornament. It has a creeping root-stock, long, trailing, barren shoots, with short, erect, flowering stems about six inches high. Leaves are narrow-ovate or oblong, evergreen, shining, and perfectly glabrous, opposite and entire. Pedicels shorter than the leaves. Corolla small, blue, the tube broad, almost bell-shaped, with a flat spreading limb, with five broad oblique segments twisted in the bud; stamens five, enclosed in the tube. It differs from *Vinca major* in its smaller size, more trailing habit, narrower leaves, which are perfectly glabrous, and shorter and broader segments to the calyx, without any hairs on their edges. The flowers appear in April and May.

It was introduced into our Materia Medica by Dr. Rosenberg, Germany.

Preparation.—The fresh plant, gathered at the beginning of flowering, is chopped and pounded to a pulp and weighed. Then add two-thirds by weight of alcohol to the pulp, stir and mix well together, and strain through a piece of new linen. The tincture thus obtained is allowed to stand eight days in a well-stoppered bottle, in a dark, cool place, and then filtered.

Drug power of tincture, $\frac{1}{2}$.

Dilutions must be prepared as directed under Class II.

VIOLA ODORATA, *Linn.*

Synonyms, Viola Imberis. Viola Suavis.

Nat. Ord., Violaceæ.

Common Name, Sweet-scented Violet.

This delightfully scented plant is found growing in Europe and Northern Asia, but has become naturalized to some extent in the United States. It is characterized by its long filiform, trailing runners. Leaves cordate, crenate, nearly smooth. Flowers small, fragrant, dark-blue, solitary, on a recurved angular pedicel. Petals five, irregular, the broadest spurred at the base, lateral ones having a hairy line. The flowers appear in April and May.

It was first proven by Hahnemann.

Preparation.—The fresh plant, gathered when in flower, is chopped and pounded to a pulp and weighed. Then two parts by weight of alcohol are taken, the pulp mixed thoroughly with one-sixth part of it, and the rest of the alcohol added. After having stirred the whole, pour it into a well-stoppered bottle and let it stand eight days in a dark, cool place. The tincture is then separated by decanting, straining and filtering.

Drug power of tincture, $\frac{1}{6}$.

Dilutions must be prepared as directed under Class III.

VIOLA TRICOLOR, *Linn.*

Synonyms, Viola Trinitatis. Jacea.

Nat. Ord., Violaceæ.

Common Names, Pansy. Heart's Ease.

The pansy is a well known flower, much cultivated in all civilized countries. It is indigenous to Europe and Northern Asia. Stem angular, erect or ascending, diffusely branched. Leaves oblong-ovate, lower ones ovate-cordate, deeply crenate; the stipules nearly as large as the leaves and lyrate-pinnatifid. Flowers on long peduncles, are five-parted, variable in size. Petals, the two upper purple, lateral ones white, lower one striated, all yellow at the base.

It was first proven by Hahnemann.

Preparation.—The fresh plants, gathered when in flower (those bearing yellow and blue flowers are preferable), are chopped and pounded to a pulp and weighed. Then two parts by weight of alcohol are taken, the pulp mixed thoroughly with one-sixth part of it, and the rest of the alcohol added. After having stirred the whole, pour it into a well-stoppered bottle, and let it stand eight days in a dark, cool place. The tincture is then separated by decanting, straining and filtering.

Drug power of tincture, $\frac{1}{6}$.

Dilutions must be prepared as directed under Class III.

VIPERA REDI.

Class, Reptilia.
Order, Ophidia.
Family, Viperidæ.
Common Name, Italian Viper.

Short provings of the virus of this reptile are given in Jahr's Symptomen Codex.

Preparation.—The fresh poison is triturated as directed under Class VIII.

VIPERA TORVA.

Class, Reptilia.
Order, Ophidia.
Family, Viperidæ.
Common Name, German Viper.

Short provings of the virus of this reptile are given in Jahr's Symptomen Codex.

Preparation.—The fresh poison is triturated as directed under Class VIII.

VISCUM ALBUM, *Linn.*

Synonym, Viscum Flavescens.
Nat. Ord., Loranthaceæ.
Common Name, Mistletoe.

This is a shrubby evergreen, parasitic plant, found growing upon the oak, elm, apple and other fruit trees, by whose juices they are sustained through the medium of simple roots which pierce the bark and the sap-vessels. The plant is indigenous to Europe, and is somewhat celebrated in English song and story. It is yellow-green, branched and jointed, and reaches a length of nearly two feet, forming a pendent bush. Leaves opposite, thick, without stipules, obtuse, narrow, oblong or oval, entire. Flowers generally diœcious, in spikes or clusters. Fruit, a berry white, nearly transparent, with a viscid pulp, imbedded in which is a single seed.

Preparation.—Equal parts of the fresh berries and leaves are chopped and pounded to a pulp and weighed. Then two parts by weight of alcohol are taken, the pulp mixed thoroughly with one-sixth part of it, and the rest of the alcohol added. After having stirred the whole, pour it into a well-stoppered bottle, and let it stand eight days in a dark, cool place. The tincture is then separated by decanting, straining and filtering.

Drug power of tincture, $\frac{1}{6}$.

Dilutions must be prepared as directed under Class III.

VITIS VINIFERA, *Linn.*

Nat. Ord., Vitaceæ.

Common Name, Common Grape Vine.

The common grape vine is a native of Central Asia, but has become naturalized in nearly all temperate climates. Leaves cordate, sinuately five-lobed, glabrous or tomentose; flowers all perfect. By cultivation it sports into endless varieties, which differ in the form, color, size and flavor of the fruit and in respect to the hardiness of constitution. In New England its cultivation is chiefly confined to the garden as a dessert fruit; but there are extensive vineyards in the Middle and Western States for the production of wine. The vine is propagated by cuttings. Varieties without end may be raised from the seed, which will bear fruit the fourth or fifth year. A vineyard, it is said, will continue to produce fruit for two hundred years.

Preparation.—The fresh leaves are chopped and pounded to a pulp and pressed out in a piece of new linen. The expressed juice is then, by brisk agitation, mingled with an equal part by weight of alcohol. The mixture is allowed to stand eight days in a dark, cool place, in a well-stoppered bottle and then filtered.

Amount of drug power, $\frac{1}{2}$.

Dilutions must be prepared as directed under Class I.

VULPIS FEL.

From Canis Vulpes.

Class, Mammalia.

Order, Carnivora.

Family, Canina.

Common Name, Fox-gall.

Preparation.—The fresh gall is triturated as directed under Class IX.

VULPIS HEPAR.

From Canis Vulpes.

Class, Mammalia.

Order, Carnivora.

Family, Canina.

Common Name, Fox-liver.

Preparation.—The carefully dried liver is triturated as directed under Class VII.

VULPIS PULMO.

Synonym, Pulmo Vulpis. From Canis Vulpes.
Class, Mammalia.
Order, Carnivora.
Family, Canina.
Common Name, Fox-lungs.
Preparation.—The carefully dried lungs are triturated as directed under Class VII.

WYETHIA HELENIOIDES, *Nuttall.*

Synonyms, Alarçonia Helenioides, *De Candolle.* Melarhiza Inuloides, *Kellogg.*
Nat. Ord., Compositæ.
Soft-tomentose, or becoming with age nearly glabrous, a foot or two high; leaves oblong or ovate; radical ones a foot or more long, four to six inches wide; cauline about half the size, all contracted at base into a short petiole; heads mostly leafy at base; outer scales of the involucre ovate-lanceolate or ovate, sometimes toothed; achenia more or less pubescent at top when young. This perennial inhabits hillsides; common near San Francisco and through the valley of the Sacramento.
Preparation.—The fresh root is chopped and pounded to a pulp and weighed. Then two parts by weight of alcohol are taken, the pulp mixed with one-sixth part of it, and the rest of the alcohol added. After having stirred the whole well, pour it into a well-stoppered bottle, and let it stand eight days in a dark, cool place. The tincture is then separated by decanting, straining and filtering.
Drug power of tincture, $\frac{1}{6}$.
Dilutions must be prepared as directed under Class III.

XANTHIUM SPINOSUM, *Linn.*

Nat. Ord., Compositæ.
Common Name, Spiny Clotbur.
This plant is a native of Southern Europe, but is found growing in the United States from Massachusetts to Georgia, on roadsides and in fields. The plant is white-tomentose, a foot or two high, and is armed with straw-colored spines, arranged triply at the base of the leaves. Leaves on petioles, ovate-lanceolate, entire, or three-lobed, or dentate. Flower heads sessile, axillary, lower ones fertile, upper ones sterile. Fertile involucre closed, ovoid, coriaceous, and clothed with rough prickles forming a rough burr.
Preparation.—The fresh herb, in flower, is chopped and pounded to a pulp and weighed. Then two parts by weight of alcohol are taken, the pulp mixed thoroughly with one-sixth part of it, and the rest of the

alcohol added. After having stirred the whole, pour it into a well-stoppered bottle, and let it stand eight days in a dark, cool place. The tincture is then separated by decanting, straining and filtering.

Amount of drug power, $\frac{1}{6}$.

Dilutions must be prepared as directed under Class III.

XANTHOXYLUM FRAXINEUM, *Willdenow.*

Synonyms, Xanthoxylon Americanum, *Miller.* Hylax Fraxineum.

Nat. Ord., Rutaceæ.

Common Names, Prickly Ash. Pellitory. Suterberry. Yellow Wood.

This is an indigenous shrub found growing in the greater portion of the United States. It is often ten or twelve feet high, and prefers woods and shady places. The branches are armed with strong, conical, brown prickles. Leaves alternate, pinnate; leaflets about five pairs, with an odd one terminal, attached to a common petiole, either prickly or not. The leaflets are sessile, ovate, sub-entire, smooth above, downy beneath. Flowers small, greenish, in dense, axillary umbels, and appear before the leaves. Some individuals bear both male and female flowers, others only female. Calyx none; petals five. In the fruitful flower, pistils three to five. Fruit an oval capsule, two-valved, one to two-seeded, greenish-red.

Flowers in April and May.

The bark is used in medicine. It is found in commerce in quills varying in diameter from one-twelfth inch to one inch, and in lengths of two inches or less. The bark is about one-sixteenth of an inch thick, is grayish-brown externally, nearly smooth, with faint longitudinal furrows, occasionally marked by wart-like growths and irregularly splashed with white, and is sparsely spinous. Beneath the external layer is a green one, and below that is the yellowish inner bark. The bark is without odor and has a bitter, aromatic taste.

It was introduced into the Homœopathic Materia Medica by Dr. Charles Cullis, United States.

Preparation.—The fresh bark, in coarse powder, is covered with two parts by weight of alcohol, and allowed to remain eight days in a well-stoppered bottle, in a dark, cool place, being shaken twice a day. The tincture is then poured off, strained and filtered.

Drug power of tincture, $\frac{1}{6}$.

Dilutions must be prepared as directed under Class III.

YUCCA.

Synonym, Yucca Filamentosa, *Linn.*

Nat. Ord., Liliaceæ.

Common Names, Bear Grass. Adam's Needle.

This plant is found growing in sandy soil, in East Virginia and southward, where it is called *Spanish Bayonet.* Its trunk, rising from a running rootstalk to a height of a foot or less above the ground, is covered with the lanceolate, unarmed, coriaceous leaves, bearing filaments on their margins; the leaves are from one to two feet long. The scape-like flower-stem is from six to eight feet high, erect, and terminated by an ample pyramidal panicle of simple racemes. Perianth of six petaloid (white) oval or oblong, acute flat sepals, withering-persistent, the three inner broader, longer than the six stamens. Stigmas three, sessile. Capsule oblong, somewhat hexagonal, three-celled; cells imperfectly divided by a partition from the back, fleshy, loculicidally three-valved from the apex. Seeds numerous in each cell, depressed.

Flowers appear in July.

It was first proved by Dr. Charles E. Rowell, United States.

Preparation.—The fresh roots and leaves are chopped and pounded to a pulp and weighed. Then two parts by weight of alcohol are taken, the pulp mixed thoroughly with one-sixth part of it, and the rest of the alcohol added. After having stirred the whole, pour it into a well-stoppered bottle, and let it stand eight days in a dark, cool place. The tincture is then separated by decanting, straining and filtering.

Amount of drug power, $\frac{1}{6}$.

Dilutions must be prepared as directed under Class III.

ZINCUM.

Synonyms, Zincum Metallicum. Stannum Indicum.

Common Names, Zinc. Metallic Zinc.

Symbol, Zn.

Atomic Weight, 65.

Origin.—Zinc has been found in the metallic state in Australia, but commonly it is obtained only in combination. Zinc occurs in considerable abundance as *calamine*, a silicate of the metal; as *Smithsonite* formerly termed *calamine*, a carbonate; as *blende*, a sulphide, and as red zinc ore, an oxide. Small quantities of aluminate, arsenate, phosphate and sulphate of the metal are also found.

The extraction of the metal from its ores is done on a large scale in Silesia, Belgium, England, and to some extent in the United States. The first four named ores of zinc are calcined before being smelted. The roasted ore is then mixed with half its weight of powdered charcoal, coke or anthracite coal, and subjected to distillation in closed iron or earthen vessels, at a very high temperature. The carbon of the charcoal or other coal unites with the oxygen of the oxide into which the ore had been converted by roasting, and the metal being volatile at the temperature of the distillation, is carried into suitable receivers by means of apparatus which varies in its character in different countries. The zinc so obtained is remelted, cast into ingots and comes in commerce under the name of spelter. Commercial zinc is contaminated with lead and iron, and in a less degree with tin and cadmium; and occasionally it contains traces of arsenic and copper. The metal may be obtained perfectly pure by passing sulphuretted hydrogen through a strong and somewhat acid solution of zinc sulphate, filtering off any precipitate, boiling the solution to expel the sulphuretted hydrogen, and then precipitating the zinc as carbonate by means of sodium carbonate. The carbonate is to be washed, redissolved in pure sulphuric acid, dried, mixed with charcoal prepared from loaf sugar, and the mixture distilled in a porcelain retort.

Properties.—Zinc is a bluish-white metal, ordinarily hard and brittle, whose fracture exhibits a crystalline structure. It readily takes a high polish, but this is lost upon exposure for a time to the air. Its specific gravity is about 7.0. Absolutely pure zinc is malleable at ordinary temperatures, and may be hammered into thin leaves. Commercial zinc which is impure and brittle at low temperatures becomes malleable between 100° and 150° C. (212°–302° F.); at 210° C. (410° F.) it again becomes brittle, and may be pulverized in a mortar kept at that temperature. Zinc melts at 412° C. (773.6° F.) and at 1040° C. (1904° F.), it boils and volatilizes, and in the presence of oxygen burns with a greenish flame, forming the oxide. Commercial zinc dissolves easily in dilute sulphuric, hydrochloric and other acids, with the formation of the respective zinc salts and the evolution of hydrogen. This is due to the presence of other metals, and the consequent formation of a galvanic couple with displacement and liberation of the hydrogen of the acid as above stated. Pure zinc is acted upon by the same acids very slowly, but if another and more negative metal be present the electro-decomposition takes place. On bending a rod or bar of zinc, it emits a slight crepitating noise, similar to but weaker than that of tin.

The metal was first proven by Hahnemann.

Preparation for Homœopathic Use.—The pure metal, heated to 410° F. and finely powdered is triturated, as directed under Class VII.

ZINCUM ACETICUM.

Synonyms, Zinc Acetate. Zinci Acetas.
Common Name, Acetate of Zinc.
Formula, $Zn(C_2H_3O_2)_2, 3H_2O$.
Molecular Weight, 237.

Preparation of Acetate of Zinc.—One hundred parts of commercial zinc oxide, free from iron oxide, are to be mixed with 250 parts of distilled water and 530 parts of dilute acetic acid of specific gravity 1.040, and about 15 parts of pure metallic zinc, in small pieces, are to be dropped into the mixture. The whole is to be heated for half a day on the water-bath. The fluid is to be filtered while boiling and the filtrate set aside to crystallize. After the lapse of a day, a second crop of crystals may be obtained by adding to the mother liquor a small quantity of acetic acid, evaporating to one-half and again setting aside to crystallize; the crystals are to be dried upon bibulous paper.

Properties.—Acetate of zinc crystallizes in six-sided, colorless, transparent, pearly, rhombic tables or plates. They feel greasy to the touch, and possess a weak acetous odor and a nauseating metallic taste. In the air the crystals become efflorescent from loss of some of their acid and water of crystallization; they are soluble in three parts of cold, in one and a half of boiling water, in thirty of cold and in two of boiling 90 per cent. alcohol. The crystals melt when heated to 100° C (212° F.) with a loss of a small portion of their acid, and become then solid, and when further heated to 195° C. (383° F.) they again become fluid, and sublimed zinc acetate is produced in squamous forms.

Tests.—These are chiefly for the presence of lead, cadmium and magnesia. A solution of zinc salt is to be treated with caustic alkali; the resulting precipitate should dissolve in an excess of the reagent (any undissolved portion means cadmium oxide or magnesia). The alkaline solution, when treated with hydrogen sulphide, gives a white precipitate of zinc sulphide (if lead oxide is present the precipitate is dark brown or blackish). When zinc acetate solution is treated with ammonium carbonate a voluminous whitish precipitate of zinc carbonate occurs, which is redissolved in excess of the precipitant (an undissolved portion is due to cadmium oxide or lead oxide). When a few drops of phosphoric acid are added to the ammoniacal solution, a white precipitate, falling immediately or in a very short time, denotes the presence of a magnesium salt.

It was first proven by Hahnemann.

Preparation for Homœopathic Use.—Pure acetate of zinc is triturated as directed under Class VII.

ZINCUM BROMATUM.

Synonym, Zinc Bromide. Zinci Bromidum.

Common Name, Bromide of Zinc.

Formula, $Zn\ Br_2$.

Molecular Weight, 225.

Preparation.—This compound may be prepared by digesting pure granulated zinc in hydrobromic acid; some slips of platinum foil are to be placed in the liquid, so that they shall touch the zinc fragments; a galvanic action is immediately set up with the formation of zinc bromide and the evolution of hydrogen. The zinc is to be kept in contact with the platinum and in excess. As soon as the evolution of hydrogen has ceased, the solution is to be filtered, concentrated and evaporated to dryness upon a water-bath.

Properties.—The hydrated bromide of zinc, prepared as directed above, is an indistinctly crystalline, very deliquescent mass. When heated the mass yields a sublimate of zinc bromide in white needles, whose specific gravity is 3.643. Zinc bromide has a styptic, sweetish taste, dissolves freely in water and is soluble in alcohol and ether.

Preparation for Homœopathic Use.—Bromide of zinc is triturated, as directed under Class VII, but owing to the deliquescence of the salt, the first decimal will not keep well.

ZINCUM CARBONICUM.

Synonyms, Zinc Carbonate. Zinci Carbonas Præcipitata.

Common Names, Carbonate of Zinc. Precipitated Carbonate of Zinc.

Formula, Zn CO_3, Zn H_2 O_2.

Molecular Weight, 224.

Preparation of Carbonate of Zinc.—One hundred parts of pure crystallized zinc sulphate, free from iron, are dissolved in 2,000 parts of distilled water, and while boiling, filtered; the boiling-hot filtrate is to be mixed gradually and with constant stirring, with a filtered and hot solution of 115 parts of crystallized sodium carbonate in 2,000 parts of distilled water. After the precipitate has subsided it is to be collected on a muslin strainer, and washed with hot distilled water until the washings are no longer rendered turbid by barium chloride solution; it is then to be dried at a gentle heat.

Properties.—The preparation made by the directions given above consists of the carbonate and hydrate of zinc; it is a soft, very white powder, insoluble in water, but readily dissolves in dilute acids with effervescence and the formation of zinc salts of the acids used. The officinal carbonate is without taste or odor. When heated to redness it parts with its CO_2 and H_2O, and there is left oxide of zinc to the amount of about 70 per cent.

Tests.—When the compound is dissolved in dilute nitric acid the solution should show no change on being treated with barium nitrate (sulphate), and silver nitrate (chloride). The same solution, when treated with ammonium carbonate in excess, should be clear, the precipitate first appearing being redissolved in excess of the reagent (absence of calcium), and when to the clear ammoniacal solution a drop or two of phosphoric acid are added no precipitate should occur (magnesia); with hydrogen sulphide the zinc salts in alkaline or neutral solution are precipitated as a white sulphide.

Preparation for Homœopathic Use.—Pure carbonate of zinc is triturated, as directed under Class VII.

ZINCUM MURIATICUM.

Synonyms, Zinc Chloride. Zinci Chloridum. Zincum Muriaticum.

Common Name, Chloride of Zinc.

Formula, Zn Cl_2.

Molecular Weight, 136.

Preparation of Chloride of Zinc.—Dissolve 120 parts of pure carbonate of zinc in as much pure hydrochloric acid as may be required to form a clear solution; the acid is to be added gradually, about 300 parts being needed. The solution is to be placed in a cylindrical glass vessel and allowed to stand until any undissolved residue has settled; the clear solution is then decanted and usually needs no filtration; if such seem necessary it is to be done through glass-wool, paper not being suitable. The solution is to be transferred to a porcelain dish and evaporated at a gentle heat with frequent stirring, in a place free from dust. As soon as a somewhat thick mass is obtained it is to be placed on the water-bath and evaporated to dryness quickly to prevent as far as possible the loss of chlorine. The dry, hot, hygroscopic mass is to be fused in a covered porcelain casserole, the liquid poured on a heated flat stone, and when it has solidified it is to be broken into pieces and the fragments immediately transferred to a well-stoppered bottle.

Properties.—Chloride of zinc is a white crystalline powder, or is in white opaque masses or sticks. It has a caustic, metallic, nauseating saline taste, is without odor, and has an acid reaction. It absorbs water readily from the air and soon becomes converted into a clear fluid. Heated to 115° C. (239° F.) it melts to a clear liquid, which, upon cooling, becomes a grayish-white mass; at a full red heat it volatilizes in thick white fumes, leaving a yellowish-white residue consisting of zinc oxide and chloride, a part of the zinc chloride subliming in white needles. Chloride of zinc is easily soluble in water, and in alcohol, less readily in ether. Solutions of the officinal preparation are generally somewhat turbid from the presence of the oxychloride. From an aqueous solution of syrupy consistence, zinc chloride separates out in small deliquescent octohedral crystals containing one molecule of water.

Tests.—Its complete solubility in alcohol rendered acid with HCl evidences the absence of impurities which are insoluble in alcohol. A clear solution in water acidulated with HCl, becomes precipitated at first when ammonium carbonate is added; when the alkali is added in excess, with shaking, the precipitate first formed is redissolved (a permanent precipitate under these conditions is dependent upon the presence of calcium compounds). A precipitate formed in the alkaline solution upon the addition of ammonium phosphate, and which does not disappear upon further treatment with ammonium carbonate, is due to the presence of magnesia or a magnesium compound. Lastly, when the alkaline solution is saturated with hydrogen sulphide, a precipitate which is not perfectly white shows contamination with other metals.

Preparation for Homœopathic Use.—Pure chloride of zinc is triturated, as directed under Class VII, but owing to the deliquescence of the salt, the lower triturations will not keep well.

ZINCUM FERROCYANATUM.

Synonym, Zinci Ferrocyanidum.
Common Name, Ferrocyanide of Zinc.
Formula, $Zn_2\ Fe\ (CN)_6,\ 3H_2O$.
Molecular Weight, 396.

Preparation of Ferrocyanide of Zinc.—Six parts of crystallized potassium ferrocyanide are to be dissolved in sixty parts of distilled water, the solution is filtered and then added gradually, with constant stirring, to a filtered solution of eight parts of crystallized sulphate of zinc in 180 parts of water. The mixture is allowed to stand for several hours in a warm place and afterwards in a cold one. The precipitate is to be thrown on a filter and washed thereon as long as the washings give any turbidity with barium chloride solution. The residue is to be dried at a very gentle heat and then rubbed to powder.

Properties.—Officinal ferrocyanide of zinc is a white, tasteless, odorless powder; it is insoluble in water and alcohol, is not attacked by very dilute acids nor by caustic ammonia solution, but dissolves readily in potassium hydrate. When heated to redness on platinum foil there is left a residue consisting of oxides of iron and zinc.

Tests.—Ferrocyanide of zinc, when shaken with dilute acetic acid, should yield nothing to the acid; the filtrate from the mixture should leave no residue upon evaporation from platinum foil, nor should it be colored when saturated with hydrogen sulphide (absence of heavy metals in the latter, of fixed salts in the former experiment).

Preparation for Homœopathic Use.—Ferrocyanide of zinc is triturated as directed under Class VII.

ZINCUM CYANATUM.

Synonyms, Zinci Cyanidum. Zincum Cyanuretum.

Common Name, Cyanide of Zinc.

Formula, $Zn\ (C\ N)_2$.

Preparation.—A solution of ten parts of dry chloride of zinc is to be mixed with a solution of ten parts of potassium cyanide in 100 of distilled water, and to the mixture are to be added three parts of dilute acetic acid. The precipitate is to be washed upon a filter, at first with 100 parts of water acidulated with three parts of dilute acetic acid, afterward with distilled water only. The washed precipitate is to be pressed between folds of bibulous paper to remove as much moisture as possible and then dried quickly at a temperature of about 30° C. (86° F.)

Properties.—Zinc cyanide is a white, soft, amorphous powder almost without taste or odor. It is insoluble in water and alcohol, but dissolves readily in strong acids with the formation of a zinc salt of the acid used, and the liberation of cyanogen, the solution giving the reaction for hydrocyanic acid. When heated to redness on platinum foil a residue of zinc oxide is left, which when dissolved in hydrochloric acid and then treated with potassium ferrocyanide solution does not give a blue precipitate (distinguishing from the ferrocyanide of zinc.)

Tests.—The tests to be applied are those described in the article Zincum muriaticum.

Preparation for Homœopathic Use.—Pure cyanide of zinc is triturated as directed under Class VII.

ZINCUM IODATUM.

Synonyms, Zinc Iodide. Zinci Iodidum.

Common Name, Iodide of Zinc.

Formula, ZnI_2.
Molecular Weight,, 319.
Preparation of Iodide of Zinc.—In a glass flask, whose capacity is about 100 CC., are to be placed ten parts of pure iodine and twenty of distilled water, and then are to be gradually added three parts of pure granulated zinc. The bottom of the flask is to be heated to between 30° and 40° C. (86°–104° F.), and its mouth covered with a glass funnel. After all the zinc has been taken up, the mixture is to be digested for some hours, the colorless solution filtered through glass-wool, and evaporated in a flat porcelain dish at a gentle heat to dryness. The dried mass is to be at once transferred to small glass bottles carefully closed with cork-stoppers.
Properties.—Zinc iodide forms a colorless saline mass without odor and possessing a sharp metallic taste. It is easily soluble in water and alcohol; when heated it melts, and at a higher temperature gives off iodine vapor until at last only zinc oxide remains. When carefully heated it may be sublimed and condensed in needles, and from its aqueous solutions it may by careful evaporation be obtained in regular octohedrons or cubo-octohedrons.
Tests.—A small quantity of the iodide of zinc when treated with a few drops of ammonium sulphide should show only a white turbidity (a coloration indicates the presence of other metals). Towards ammonium carbonate solution and phosphoric acid it behaves precisely as does zinc chloride. 0.5 gram of dry zinc iodide when shaken with five grams of alcohol should dissolve almost completely, and from the somewhat turbid solution there should not separate out any crystalline substance. To this fluid is to be added a solution of 0.6 gram of silver nitrate in 30 CC. of distilled water. After violent shaking the fluid is allowed to stand that the precipitate may settle, and there are to be added to it five grams of pure caustic ammonia solution, and the mixture strongly agitated. The precipitate is to be thrown upon a tared filter which has been washed with a not too dilute nitric acid. The filtrate when treated with nitric acid in excess should yield no precipitate (absence of zinc chloride or bromide). A slight turbidity which does not materially impair the transparency of the filtrate is permissible and may be due to a trace of silver iodide. The yellowish-white precipitate is to be washed with distilled water, dried upon a water-bath and weighed, and should weigh at least 0.7 gram.
Preparation.—Iodide of zinc is triturated as directed under Class VII.

ZINCUM OXYDATUM.

Synonyms, Zinc Oxide. Zincum Oxydatum Purum. Zinci Oxidum. Calx Zinci. Lana Philosophica. Nihilum Album. Pompholyx.
Common Name, Oxide of Zinc.
Formula, ZnO.
Molecular Weight, 81.
Preparation of Oxide of Zinc.—Take of precipitated carbonate

of zinc, twelve troy ounces. Place it in a shallow vessel and expose to a low red heat until the water and carbonic acid are entirely expelled. This may be known by removing a portion from the centre of the mass upon a warmed glass rod, adding to it a little water and a few drops of hydrochloric acid; should no effervescence ensue the operation is completed.

Properties.—Pure oxide of zinc is a soft, odorless, tasteless, white powder. It absorbs CO_2 as well as moisture upon exposure to the air. It is not readily fusible, becomes citron yellow on heating, but upon cooling resumes its original color. After being heated to redness it emits light in the dark for about half an hour. At a white heat it melts to a yellowish glass. It is insoluble in water but dissolves readily in dilute sulphuric, hydrochloric, nitric and acetic acids, forming the corresponding salts. From its combination with any of these acids it is reprecipitated as a hydrate by caustic alkali.

Tests.—One part of pure zinc oxide placed in a test-tube with ten parts of distilled water and the mixture thoroughly shaken, should yield a filtrate which is indifferent to test-paper, or at most barely alkaline, and a few drops when evaporated on a watch-glass should leave no residue; the purest Swedish filter paper should be used in this test. A portion of the damp zinc oxide is to be placed in a test-tube and treated with a 25 per cent. nitric acid; there should be no effervescence perceptible to the eye. If reddish-yellow fumes are observable the presence of particles of metallic zinc or of zinc sub-oxide is indicated, and such specimens should be rejected. If the nitric acid solution be clear it may be further tested with silver nitrate (for zinc chloride), with barium nitrate (for sulphate), and a third part is to be treated gradually with ammonium carbonate solution until the latter is strongly in excess. The precipitate of zinc oxide which at first falls, is afterward redissolved in excess of the precipitant and the fluid becomes clear and colorless. Should it be turbid cadmium, lead or calcium compounds may be present; if clear a few drops of ammonium phosphate solution are to be added; usually there falls a slight precipitate which redissolves on the further addition of caustic ammonia, a precipitate not redissolving being due to magnesia. The ammoniacal solution when treated with hydrogen sulphide should show only a white precipitate.

Preparation for Homœopathic Use.—Pure oxide of zinc is triturated as directed under Class VII.

ZINCUM PHOSPHORATUM.

Synonym, Zinc Phosphide. Zinci Phosphidum.
Common Names, Phosphide of Zinc. Phosphuret of Zinc.
Formula, $Zn_3 P_2$.
Molecular Weight, 257.

Preparation of Phosphide of Zinc.—Phosphide of zinc has been prepared in a number of different ways. Some not unattended with danger to the operator, others giving results not always identical.

The following method of Proust gives a product which is tolerably constant. Nitrogen gas is liberated from ammonium nitrate by heating the latter, and the gas is led through a bottle containing dilute hydrochloric acid and into which calcium phosphide is introduced by means of a wide tube. Phosphoretted hydrogen is evolved and it, together with the nitrogen, are washed by passing through a wash-bottle; the mixed gases are then led into a porcelain tube in which granulated zinc is kept at a red heat. The whole apparatus is to be filled with nitrogen gas before the generation of hydrogen phosphide is begun. When the mixed gases come in contact with the red hot zinc the phosphoretted hydrogen yields its phosphorus to the metal, forming phosphide of zinc, and the liberated hydrogen and the nitrogen gas pass out. After the phosphoretted hydrogen ceases to come off the apparatus may be cooled, but the passing of nitrogen gas must be continued until cooling is complete.

Properties.—Phosphide of zinc is a more or less metallic-looking friable mass, whose surface is strewn with small rhombic prisms; it has the odor of phosphorus, and when powdered resembles iron reduced by hydrogen, or it is a gray, permanent powder having a metallic lustre without any unchanged particles of zinc. Out of contact with the air it is completely volatile by heat and melts at a higher temperature than the fusing point of zinc. Acids decompose it with the evolution of phosphoretted hydrogen and the formation of zinc salts; nitric acid changes it however into zinc oxide and zinc phosphate. It is unaffected by alkalies. By heating in the air it is gradually changed into zinc phosphate.

Tests.—Finely powdered zinc phosphide should upon ocular examination show no particles of metallic zinc. A gram of the finely powdered phosphide when treated with an aqueous solution of ammonium chloride, allowed to stand for a day and then filtered, will give a residue which after washing, first with water, next with alcohol and finally with ether, and then dried, should weigh at least 0.9 gram.

Preparation for Homœopathic Use.—Pure phosphide of zinc is triturated as directed under Class VII.

ZINCUM SULPHURICUM.

Synonyms, Zinc Sulphate. Zinci Sulphas. Vitriolum Album.
Common Names, Sulphate of Zinc. White Vitriol.
Formula, $Zn\,SO_4, 7H_2O$.
Molecular Weight, 287.

Preparation of Sulphate of Zinc.—Take of granulated zinc, sixteen ounces; sulphuric acid, twelve fluid ounces; distilled water, four pints; solution of chlorine, a sufficiency; carbonate of zinc, one-half ounce, or a sufficiency. Pour the sulphuric acid, previously mixed with the water, on the zinc contained in a porcelain basin, and, when effervescence has nearly ceased aid the action by a gentle heat. Filter the fluid into a gallon bottle, and add gradually with constant agitation the solution of chlorine until the fluid acquires a permanent odor of chlorine. Add now with continued agitation the carbonate of zinc until a brown precipitate appears; let it settle, filter the solution, evaporate until a pellicle forms on the surface, and set aside to crystallize. Dry the crystals by exposure to the air on filtering paper placed on porous tiles. More crystals may be obtained by again evaporating the mother liquor.—Br. P.

Properties.—Pure zinc sulphate separates from its solutions at ordinary temperatures in right rhombic prisms isomorphous with the crystals of the analogous magnesian salt, or, when crystallized rapidly with stirring, in small prismatic needles. The crystals are transparent colorless and odorless, but have a sharp, nauseous, saline, metallic taste, and are acid in reaction; they are superficially efflorescent, becoming thereby white and opaque. When heated to 100° C. (212° F.), the crystals melt and part with six molecules of their water; the remaining molecule refuses to leave the sulphuric constituent, and when forced out of the crystals by heat, is accompanied by a portion of the acid. At a red heat the crystals lose all their sulphuric acid, and there is left only zinc oxide. The salt is soluble in one and a quarter parts of cold, and in less than one-half part of boiling water, at the temperature of which, as has been stated, the crystals melt in their own water. When the salt is crystallized from solutions at a temperature above 30° C. (86° F.), it may be obtained in oblique rhombic prisms having a less proportion of water, *i. e.*, two, five and six molecules. The salt is insoluble in absolute alcohol, and dilute alcohol dissolves but little.

Tests.—These are practically the same as those given under the article Zincum Aceticum. The usual impurities are iron and magnesia, and possibly zinc chloride which may be detected by treating the dilute solution with silver nitrate. Zinc sulphate forms crystallizable combinations with sulphates of the alkalies; the presence of these in a specimen of the salt may readily be determined. One part of crystallized zinc sulphate is dissolved in ten times its volume of distilled water, and to the solution is added a solution of one and a quarter parts of crystallized acetate of lead in one hundred parts by weight of distilled water, agitated and filtered. The filtrate is to be completely saturated with hydrogen sulphide, again filtered, and the filtrate evaporated from platinum foil; a residue remaining after heating to redness, depends on the presence of an alkaline sulphate or magnesium sulphate.

Preparation for Homœopathic Use.—Pure sulphate of zinc is triturated, as directed under Class VII.

ZINCUM VALERIANICUM.

Synonyms, Zinc Valerianate. Zinci Valerianas.
Common Names, Valerianate of Zinc.
Formula, $Zn (C_5H_9 O_2)_2, H_2O$.
Molecular Weight, 285.
Preparation of Valerianate of Zinc.—Take of sulphate of

zinc, five and a half ounces (avoird.); valerianate of soda, five ounces; distilled water, a sufficiency. Dissolve the salts separately, each in two pints (imperial) of the water, raise both solutions to near the boiling point, mix them, cool, and skim off the crystals which are porduced. Evaporate the mother-liquor at a heat not exceeding 200° F. to four fluid ounces, cool again, remove the crystals which have formed and add them to those which have been already obtained. Drain the crystals on a paper filter, and wash them with a small quantity of cold distilled water till the washings give but a very feeble precipitate with chloride of barium. Let them now be again drained and dried on filtering paper at ordinary temperatures.—Br. P.

Properties.—Officinal valerianate of zinc forms white crystalline scales, pearly in lustre and greasy to the touch, or a powder made up of small crystalline scales. The salt has a weak odor of valerianic acid and an astringent, sweet, aromatic taste. It is soluble in from 90 to 100 parts of cold, but is far less soluble in hot water, dissolves in 40 parts of 90 per cent. alcohol, and is only slightly taken up by ether. When its aqueous solutions are heated to boiling, it is decomposed with the formation of a basic salt, which dissolves with difficulty, and an acid salt readily soluble. When heated to about 250° C. (482° F.) the salt volatilizes.

Tests.—In a porcelain dish, one gram of the salt is to be well moistened with nitric acid and then dried at a gentle heat; the process of moistening with the acid and of drying are to be repeated and the salt is then brought to a red heat; the residue should not weigh less than .29 gram (29 per cent.). The treatment with nitric acid in the way indicated results in the formation of zinc nitrate, which does not easily volatilize. When .5 gram of the valerianate are shaken with 3 CC. of water in a test tube, and 10 or 15 drops of hydrochloric acid added, valerianic acid is liberated and appears in oily drops upon the surface of the liquid. About .5 gram of the valerianate is to be shaken with boiling hot water and filtered; the filtrate, when treated with a few drops of ferric chloride solution and in its turn filtered, should not be colored red (absence of zinc acetate), nor upon treatment with barium solution should it give any turbidity (absence of zinc sulphate). Falsification of valerianate of zinc with butyrate of the metal may be detected by mixing cold concentrated solutions of the suspected valerianate and of acetate of copper. If butytrate be present, a blue turbidity or precipitate will immediately occur.

Preparation for Homœopathic Use.—Pure valerianate of zinc is triturated, as directed under Class VII.

ZINGIBER OFFICINALE, *Roscoe.*

Synonyms, Amomum Zingiber, *Linn.* Zingiber Album. Zingiber Nigrum.

Nat. Ord., Zingiberaceæ.

Common Name, Ginger.

The ginger plant is reed-like in appearance, having an annual, leafy stem three or four feet high. It is a native of Asia and is extensively cultivated in the warmer portions of that land; it has also been introduced into the West Indies, and the tropical regions of South America, Western Africa and Australia. The stems rise from a rhizome. Leaves sheathing elongated, the blade nearly a foot in length, and becoming lance-linear above. The flowers are in conical spikes on special shorter stems arising from the root-stock. Flowers yellow or variegated. For medicinal use the rhizome is deprived of its epidermis by scraping; it is then washed and dried in the sun. It is found in commerce in pieces rarely exceeding four inches in length, made up of a number of short, laterally compressed knobby shoots, the summit of each shoot indicating by depressions the former attachments of the leafy stems. The rhizome is somewhat palmate in outline; its color is pale buff. It breaks readily, its fracture being short, granular and bristly-fibrous. The terminal or younger portion of the rhizome on section appears pale yellow, soft and starchy; the older portion is resinous and of flinty hardness.

Preparation.—The dried root powdered, is covered with five parts by weight of alcohol, and allowed to remain eight days in a well-stoppered bottle, in a dark, cool place, being shaken twice a day. The tincture is then poured off, strained and filtered.

Drug power of tincture, $\frac{1}{10}$.

Dilutions must be prepared as directed under Class IV.

AMBROSIA.

Synonym, Ambrosia Artemisiæfolia, *Linn.*

Nat. Ord., Compositæ.

Common Names, Rag Weed. Hog Weed.

This is a perennial, indigenous plant, found growing in waste places everywhere from Canada to Georgia. Stem two or three feet high, branching, hairy or rough, pubescent. Leaves alternate, thin, twice-pinnatifid, smooth above, hairy beneath, on ciliate petioles. Flowers in terminal panicled racemes. Barren flowers in cup-shaped groups, made up of from five to twenty funnel-shaped staminate flowers, chaffy. Fertile flowers in heads, grouped one to three together, sessile in the axils of leaves or bracts at the base of the racemed sterile heads. Fruit an ovoid or globular achenium, armed with about six acute teeth or spines.

Preparation.—The fresh leaves and flowers are chopped and pounded to a pulp and weighed. Then two parts by weight of alcohol are taken, the pulp mixed with one-sixth part of it, and the rest of the alcohol added. After having stirred the whole, pour it into a well-stoppered bottle, and let it stand eight days in a dark, cool place. The tincture is separated by decanting, straining and filtering.

Drug power of tincture, $\frac{1}{6}$.

Dilutions must be prepared as directed under Class III.

ANILINUM SULPHURICUM.

Synonyms, Monophenylamine Sulphate. Sulphate of aniline.

Formula, $(C_6 H_7 N)_2 H_2 SO_4$.

Origin.—When nitrobenzol is acted upon by nascent hydrogen, the latter removes the whole of the oxygen from the former and substitutes two atoms of hydrogen; the substance produced is aniline. The reaction is exhibited as follows: $C_6 H_5 (NO_2)$ [nitrobenzol] $+ H_6 = C_6 H_7 N$ [aniline] $+ 2 H_2O$.

Aniline was discovered in 1826, by Unverdorben, who obtained it from indigo. It is produced in a great number of reactions, the most important of which are, the reducing action of ferrous acetate on nitrobenzol, the distillation of coal-tar oil with hydrochloric acid, and treating powdered indigo with potassium hydrate in a retort and distilling, the distillate being separable into a brown resinous residue and a colorless distillate of aniline.

Aniline is a transparent, mobile, colorless, oily liquid, whose odor is faint and resembles that of wine, and whose taste is aromatic and burning. It is slightly soluble in water, and itself dissolves a portion of the latter. It dissolves in all proportions in ether, alcohol, carbon disulphide and the fixed and volatile oils. Aniline ranks as a strong organic base, uniting readily with acids to form salts which generally are crystallizable, but it does not displace their basic hydrogen. It is the source of very many brilliant dyes; it exerts a deleterious effect upon the animal organism.

Preparation and Properties of Aniline Sulphate.—This compound may be readily obtained by exactly neutralizing aniline with pure sulphuric acid. The mixture solidifies to a crystalline pulp; this is to be pressed and then purified by re-crystallization. The salt is readily soluble in water and to a less degree in dilute alcohol. In absolute alcohol it is slightly soluble and not at all in ether. It may be heated to 100° C. (212° F.) without undergoing any change. If cautiously heated to a higher temperature it gives up aniline and water and becomes converted into phenylsulphamic acid. If raised to a still higher temperature, a different decomposition occurs, sulphurous oxide being given off and aniline sulphite formed, some carbonaceous matter remaining. Its alcoholic solution saturated at the boiling point of that liquid becomes solid on cooling.

Tests.—If the materials from which the salt is prepared be pure, the tests to be applied are merely those for identification. When to a dilute solution containing aniline or its salts are added a few drops of solution of chlorinated lime or other hypochlorite, a bright violet-blue color is produced. A solution of the sulphate of aniline when treated with barium chloride solution gives a white precipitate of barium sulphate, insoluble in nitric acid.

It was proven by Dr. J. B. Bell, United States.

Preparation for Homœopathic Use.—Pure sulphate of aniline is triturated, as directed under Class VII.

APPENDIX.

In this place we mention such preparations which, though frequently called for, are not entitled to a place in the Pharmacopœia proper.

ECLECTIC PREPARATIONS OF MEDICINAL PLANTS, SO-CALLED "RESINOIDS," OR "ACTIVE PRINCIPLES."

Under the name of *Resinoids* a line of preparations has been originated and brought into extensive use by eclectic physicians. These consist of precipitates in the form of powder obtained by mixing a strong alcoholic tincture of any given plant or part thereof, with three or four times its bulk of water, by which process all constituents soluble in alcohol only are precipitated. The precipitates are then collected, dried and pulverized, and are known in commerce and to the medical profession under the general name *Resinoids*, it being claimed that these preparations embody and represent the "active principles" of the respective plants. No definite directions or generally adopted rules for the preparation of these products have been published, and every manufacturer seems to be guided by his individual experience.

The use of these eclectic preparations among homœopathic practitioners has greatly diminished of late years, for it has been generally observed that well prepared homœopathic tinctures made from fresh succulent plants, give far better satisfaction than these precipitates which are made, without exception, from dried materials.

Preparation for Homœopathic Use.—We prepare triturations in the usual manner according to Class VII.

Below we give a list of these preparations with the names of the plants from which they are derived.

Aconitin,	derived from	*Aconitum napellus.*
Aletrin,	" "	*Aletris farinosa.*
Alnuin,	" "	*Alnus rubra.*
Ampelopsin,	" "	*Ampelopsis quinquefolia.*
Apocynin,	" "	*Apocynum Cannabinum.*

ATROPIN,	derived from	*Atropa belladonna.*
ASCLEPIN,	" "	*Asclepias tuberosa.*
BAPTISIN,	" "	*Baptisia tinctoria.*
CAULOPHYLLIN,	" "	*Caulophyllum thalictroides.*
CERASIN,	" "	*Cerasus Virginiana.*
CHELONIN,	" "	*Chelone glabra.*
CHIMAPHILIN,	" "	*Chimaphila umbellata.*
CHIONANTHIN,	" "	*Chionanthus Virginica.*
COLLINSONIN,	" "	*Collinsonia Canadensis.*
CORNIN,	" "	*Cornus Florida.*
CORYDALIN,	" "	*Corydalis formosa.*
CYPRIPEDIN,	" "	*Cypripedium pubescens.*
DIGITALIN,	" "	*Digitalis purpurea.*
DIOSCORIN,	" "	*Dioscorea villosa.*
EUONYMIN,	" "	*Euonymus atropurpureus.*
EUPATORIN (Perf.)	" "	*Eupatorium perfoliatum.*
EUPATORIN (Purp.)	" "	*Eupatorium purpureum.*
FRASERIN,	" "	*Frasera Carolinensis.*
GELSEMIN,	" "	*Gelsemium sempervirens.*
GERANIN,	" "	*Geranium maculatum.*
GOSSYPIN,	" "	*Gossypium herbaceum.*
HAMAMELIN,	" "	*Hamamelis Virginica.*
HELONIN,	" "	*Helonias dioica.*
HYDRASTIN,	" "	*Hydrastis Canadensis.*
HYOSCYAMIN,	" "	*Hyoscyamus niger.*
IRISIN,	" "	*Iris versicolor.*
JUGLANDIN,	" "	*Juglans cinerea.*
LEONTODIN,	" "	*Leontodon taraxacum*
LEPTANDRIN,	" "	*Leptandra Virginica.*
LOBELIN,	" "	*Lobelia inflata.*
LYCOPIN,	" "	*Lycopus Virginicus.*
MACROTIN,	" "	*Cimicifuga racemosa.*
MENISPERMIN,	" "	*Menispermum Canadensis.*
MYRICIN,	" "	*Myrica cerifera.*
PHYTOLACCIN,	" "	*Phytolacca decandra.*
POPULIN,	" "	*Populus tremuloides.*
PODOPHYLLIN,	" "	*Podophyllum peltatum.*
PTELEIN,	" "	*Ptelea trifoliata.*
RUMIN,	" "	*Rumex crispus.*
SANGUINARIN,	" "	*Sanguinaria Canadensis.*
SCUTELLARIN,	" "	*Scutellaria laterifolia.*
SENECIN,	" "	*Senecio gracilis.*
STILLINGIN,	" "	*Stillingia sylvatica.*
TRILLIN,	" "	*Trillium pendulum.*
VERATRIN,	" "	*Veratrum viride.*
VIBURNIN,	" "	*Viburnum opulus.*
XANTHOXYLIN,	" "	*Xanthoxylum fraxineum.*

The fact that the manufacturers gave to many of these resinoids names identical with those which had been generally accepted as denoting the *alkaloids* of the respective plants, led to innumerable misunderstandings and annoyances.

Thus *Aconitin, Atropin, Digitalin, Hyoscyamin*, etc., are identical in name with the well known alkaloids, and when it is considered that there is a great difference in action and dose between these preparations and the real alkaloids, the objections to continuing the use of both are patent. Of late this difficulty was sought to be overcome by changing the ending of the names of alkaloids to *ia* as in Aconitia, Atropia, Digitalia, etc., but the difference is so small that only the absolute discontinuance of the eclectic preparations mentioned will prevent what may, under certain circumstances, prove to be serious mistakes.

CERATES AND OINTMENTS.

These may be prepared in various ways, as will be seen by the following formulas:

Spermaceti Ointment.

Take of Spermaceti,	5	parts.
White Wax,	2	"
Almond Oil,	16	"

Melt by a gentle heat, remove the mixture, and stir constantly until cool.

Simple Cerate.

Should a firmer cerate be required, the following will be preferable.

Take of Spermaceti,	3	parts.
White Wax,	6	"
Olive Oil,	14	"

Melt the spermaceti and wax, add the oil, and stir until cool.

Another simple cerate is prepared by taking:

Petrolatum, ...	16	parts.
Paraffin, ...	3	"

Melt, remove the mixture, and stir constantly until cool.

Of late a new solid preparation of Petroleum has been introduced, the melting point of which is 115° F., while Petrolatum or Vaseline melts at 95° F. This can be used without any admixture. The Petroleum preparations have this great advantage over all other compositions, that they never become rancid, but seem to keep unchanged for any length of time.

With either of above cerates any given tincture intended for external use may be incorporated in the proportion of one part of tincture to twenty parts of cerate, with the exception of Cantharis and Rhus tox. which should not be made stronger than one part of the tincture to forty of the cerate.

The *modus operandi* is as follows:

Melt a given quantity of the cerate on the water-bath, in a porcelain dish, add the requisite amount of tincture by degrees, and continue the heat until all the fluid has evaporated.

Graphites Cerate is prepared by carefully rubbing together in a mortar one part of pure graphites in the finest powder with forty parts of cerate.

ARNICA OIL.

Preparation.—Take of recently gathered arnica root in coarse powder, one part, and of the finest olive oil, ten parts, put the ingredients into a well-stoppered, wide-mouthed bottle, and macerate in a warm place for two weeks, then express and filter.

This most excellent preparation is worthy of more extended use; its healing properties are marvelous, and it can be used with most beneficial effect on raw and cut surfaces, where arnica tincture, even largely diluted, cannot be borne.

GLYCERINUM AMYLI.

A very suitable form of ointment having for its constituents GLYCERINE AND STARCH is prepared as follows:

Take of Starch,	1 ounce.
Glycerine,	8 fluid ounces.

Rub them together until they are intimately mixed, then transfer the mixture to a porcelain dish, and apply a heat gradually raised to 240° F., stirring it constantly until the starch particles are completely broken and a translucent jelly is formed.—Br. P.

In medicating, the same proportions may be taken as with the ointments.

GLYCEROLES.

These consist of the medicine mixed with glycerine, and the proportions usually employed are the same as in the case of ointments. They form very convenient preparations, and, being soluble in all proportions in water and alcohol, can be diluted to form both liniments, lotions and injections.

LOTIONS.

Lotions are prepared in the following ways:

1. By simply diluting the medicine with distilled water in the pro-

portion of 1 in 10 or 1 in 100; in the latter case 1½ fluid drachms to the pint is very nearly the correct proportion.

2. By diluting a glycerole of the medicine with 4 or 9 times its measure of distilled water.

TINCTURE TRITURATIONS.

These preparations are vegetable remedies in the form of triturations. One ounce of a given mother tincture prepared from the fresh plant is triturated with ten ounces of sugar of milk for one full hour, when volatilization is complete, and a perfectly dry and stable powder results, the characteristic odor and medicinal property of the mother tincture used being retained. From this 1x trituration the 2x is made by taking one ounce and triturating it as usual for one hour with nine ounces of sugar of milk, and from this 2x trituration the 3x is made by a similar process.

This form of preparation has been found very convenient for dispensing low potencies of vegetable medicines.

TABLET TRITURATES.

These are made of any trituration (with a few exceptions); they are round, flat, one-quarter of an inch in diameter by one-eighth of an inch thick, and average two grains in weight. They are very convenient for dispensing, as each tablet constitutes a dose. These tablets, from their ready solubility or diffusibility, are destined to come into general use. Their advantage can be appreciated at once when they are allowed to dissolve in the mouth or in a teaspoonful of water, in which way they are readily administered.

TABLE OF WEIGHTS AND MEASURES.

Apothecaries' Weight, U. S.

One pound,	℔ =	12 Troy ounces	= 5,760 grs.	= 13 ounces avoird.	72.5 grs.
One Troy ounce,	℥ =	8 drachms	= 480 "	= 1 ounce "	42.5 "
One drachm,	ʒ =	3 scruples	= 60 "		
One scruple,	℈		= 20 "		
One grain,	gr.		= 1 grain.		

	Cubic In.	Troy Grs.
1 minim, ♏	0.00376	0.949
60 " = 1 fl. dr., f ʒ	0.2256	56.96
480 " = 8 " = 1 fl. oz., f ℥	1.8047	455.69
7680 " = 128 " = 16 " = 1 pint, O. . .	28.875	7291.11
61440 " = 1024 fl. drs. = 128 fl. ozs. = 8 pts. = 1 gal.	231.	58328.88

Avoirdupois Weight, Br.

One pound, ℔ = 16 ounces = 7000 Troy grains = ℔ i ℥ij ʒiv gr. xl.
One ounce, oz. = 437.5 " = ʒvij gr. xvijss.
One grain, gr. = 1 grain.

The weights ordered in the British Pharmacopœia are the pound, ounce and grain avoirdupois as given above. The same authority, however, leaves it optional with physicians to use in *prescribing* the symbols ℈ and ʒ, the former representing 20, and the latter 60 grains.

In the measurement of liquids by the same Pharmacopœia, Imperial measure is used for the higher denominations and the fluid-ounce and its subdivisions fluid-drachm and minim, for the lower denomination of volume.

It is to be observed that the fluid-ounce, Br., is the volume occupied by 437.5 grains of distilled water at 60° F. (15.5° C.), hence the fluid-ounce Br. P. weighs exactly one ounce avoirdupois.

Liquid Measure, Br. (See explanation above.)

	Troy grains.	Avoirdupois.
1 minim, *min.*	0.91	
60 minims = 1 fl. dr., *fl. dr.*	54.68	
480 " = 8 fl. drs. = 1 fl. oz. *fl. oz.*	437.5 =	1 ounce.
9600 " = 160 " = 20 fl. ozs. = 1 pint, O.	8750. =	1.25 pound.
76800 " = 1280 " = 160 " = 8 pints =	70000. =	10 pounds.

Relative Value of Wine or Apothecaries' and Imperial Measures.

Wine measure.	Imperial measure. Pints.	Fl oz.	Fl dr.	Minims.
1 minim	.	.	.	1.04
1 fluidrachm	.	.	1	2.5
1 fluidounce	.	1	0	20.
1 pint	.	16	5	19.
1 gallon	6	13	2	32.02

Imperial measure.	Wine measure. Galls.	Pints.	f℥.	fʒ.	Minims.
1 minim	.	.	.	.	0.96
1 fluidrachm	.	.	.	.	58
1 fluidounce	.	.	.	7	41
1 pint	.	1	3	1	37
1 gallon	1	1	9	4	53.6

24 fluidounces wine measure plus 1 grain = 25 fluidounces imperial measure.

French Metric Weights and Measures.

In the metric system of weights and measures the standard of length is the meter (mètre), which is the ten-millionth of the distance from the equator to the pole, *i. e.*, of a quadrant of a great circle on the earth's surface. The meter is divided into $\frac{1}{10}$ths, called decimeters, these again into $\frac{1}{10}$ths called centimeters, and these into $\frac{1}{10}$ths called millimeters. The meter is also multiplied by 10, making a decameter, this is again multiplied by 10, making a hectometer, and continuing through kilometre to myriometre. The cube of a $\frac{1}{10}$th of a meter or decimeter gives the standard of capacity and is called a litre; this is sub-divided by 10 successively, the third sub-division being a millilitre, *i. e.*, the cube of a centimetre, called cubic centimetre and expressed CC.

The weight of 1 CC of distilled water at its greatest density (4° C.), is the unit of weight, and is called one gram (gramme).

The mutual relation of the French weights and measures are given in the table:

Metric Weights.

1 milligram = 0.001 gram.
10 milligrams = 1 centigram = 0.010 gram.
100 " = 10 centigrams = 1 decigram = 0.100 gram.
1000 " = 100 " = 10 decigrams = 1.000 "

1 gram (the weight of 1 cubic centimeter of water at 4° C.).
10 grams = 1 dekagram.
100 " = 10 dekagrams = 1 hektogram.
1000 " = 100 " = 10 hektograms = 1 kilogram.

Metric Measures.

1 milliliter (or 1 cubic centimeter, abbreviated into CC.) = 0.001 liter.
10 milliliters = 1 centiliter = 0.010 liter.
100 " = 10 centiliters = 1 deciliter = 0.100 liter.
1000 " = 100 " = 10 deciliters = 1.000 liter.

1 liter (or 1 cubic decimeter).
10 liters = 1 dekaliter.
100 " = 10 dekaliters = 1 hektoliter.
1000 " = 100 " = 10 hektoliters = 1 kiloliter.

---

1 litre = 1 cubic decimeter = 1.0567 quarts.
1 gram = 15.432 grains.
1 cubic inch = 16.38617 CC.
1 gallon (Imp.) = 4.54346 litres.
1 ounce, Troy = 31.1035 grams.
1 pound (avoir.) = 0.45359 kilogram.
1 grain = 0.0647989 gram.

Value of Apothecaries' or Troy Weights in Metric Weights.

GRAIN.	MILLIGRAMS.	GRAINS.	GRAMS.	APOTHECARIES' WEIGHT.	GRAMS.
1/64 =	1.012	i =	0.06479895	ʒi =	3.888
1/60 =	1.080	ij =	0.1295	ʒij =	7.775
1/50 =	1.296	iij =	0.1943	ʒiij =	11.663
1/48 =	1.350	iv =	0.2591	ʒiv =	15.550
1/40 =	1.620	v =	0.3239	ʒv =	19.439
1/36 =	1.800	vi =	0.3887	ʒvi =	23.327
1/32 =	2.025	vij =	0.4535	ʒvij =	27.215
1/30 =	2.160	viij =	0.5183	℥i =	31.103
1/25 =	2.592	ix =	0.5831	℥ij =	62.207
1/24 =	2.670	x =	0.6479	℥iij =	93.310
1/20 =	3.240	xij =	0.7775	℥iv =	124.414
1/16 =	4.050	xv =	0.9719	℥v =	155.516
1/15 =	4.320	xvi =	1.036	℥vi =	186.620
1/12 =	5.540	xviij =	1.166	℥vij =	217.723
1/10 =	6.480	xx =	1.295	℥viij =	248.826
1/8 =	8.099	xxiv =	1.555	℥ix =	279.930
1/6 =	10.799	xxv =	1.620	℥x =	311.032
1/5 =	12.959	xxx =	1.944	℥xi =	342.136
1/4 =	16.199	xl =	2.592	lbi =	373.242
1/3 =	21.599	l =	3.240	lbij =	746.487
1/2 =	32.399	lx =	3.888	lbiij =	1119.726

Table Comparing Apothecaries' Weights and Measures and Gram Weights.

The gram values herein given are calculated to approximate correctness. The column for liquids lighter than water refers to preparations (tinctures) made with strong alcohol, as well as to ethereal and fatty oils whose specific gravity does not exceed 0.95. The column for liquids of the specific gravity of water, includes preparations made with dilute alcohol. The column for liquids heavier than water, refers to syrups and preparations made from glycerine (certain fluid extracts).

TROY WEIGHT.	GRAMS.	APOTHECARIES' MEASURE.	GRAMS.		
			Liquids Lighter than Water.	Liquids Specific gravity of Water.	Liquids heavier than Water.
Grain 1/16	.004	Minim 1	.055	.06	.08
1/12	.005	2	.11	.12	.16
1/10	.006	3	.16	.18	.24
1/8	.008	4	.22	.24	.32
1/6	.010	5	.28	.3	.40
1/4	.016	6	.33	.36	.48
1/3	.02	7	.38	.42	.56
1/2	.03	8	.45	.48	.64
3/4	.05	9	.50	.54	.72
1	.064	10	.55	.6	.80
2	.13	12	.65	.72	.96
3	.19	14	.77	.84	1.12
4	.26	15	.80	.9	1.20
5	.32	16	.88	.96	1.28
6	.39	20	1.11	1.20	1.60
7	.45	25	1.40	1.50	2.00
8	.52	30	1.70	1.80	2.50
9	.58	35	2.00	2.10	2.90
10 (℈ss)	.65	40	2.20	2.40	3.30
12	.78	48	2.70	2.88	4.00
14	.90	50	2.80	3.00	4.15
15	.97	60 (fʒi)	3.40	3.69	5.00
16	1.04	65	3.60	3.90	5.30
18	1.18	72	4.05	4.32	6.00
20 (℈i)	1.3	80	4.50	4.8	6.65
24	1.5	90 (fʒiss)	5.10	5.4	7.50
30 (ʒss)	1.94	96	5.40	5.76	8.00
32	2.1	100	5.60	6.00	8.30
36	2.3	120 (fʒii)	6.75	7.20	10.00
40 (℈ii)	2.6	150 (fʒiiss)	8.50	9.00	12.50
45	2.91	160	9.00	9.60	13.30
50 (℈iiss)	3.2	180 (fʒiii)	10.10	10.80	15.00
60 (ʒi)	3.88	210 (fʒiiiss)	11.80	12.60	17.50
70	4.55	240 (fʒiv)	13.50	14.40	20.00
80 (℈iv)	5.2	fʒv	16.90	18.00	25.00
90 (ʒiss)	5.9	fʒvss	18.60	19.80	27.50
100 (℈v)	6.5	fʒvi	20.25	21.60	30.00
110 (℈vss)	7.1	fʒvii	23.60	25.40	35.00
120 (ʒii)	7.78	fʒviii (f℥i)	27.00	28.80	40.00
150 (ʒiiss)	9.72	fʒix	30.40	32.40	45.00
180 (ʒiii)	11.66	fʒx	33.75	36.0	50.00
240 (℥ss)	15.5	fʒxii (f℥iss)	40.50	43.2	60.00
300 (ʒv)	19.4	fʒxiv	47.25	50.4	70.00
360 (ʒvi)	23.3	f℥ii	54.00	57.6	80.00
420 (ʒvii)	27.2	f℥iiss	67.50	74.0	100.00
480 (℥i)	31.1	f℥iii	81.00	86.4	120.00
℥ii	62.2	f℥iiiss	94.50	100.8	140.00
℥iv	124.4	f℥iv	108.00	115.2	160.00

LIST OF AUTHORITIES.

Encyclopedia of Pure Materia Medica (Allen.)
Jahr and Grüner's Pharmacopœia (Hempel's Trans.)
British Homœopathic Pharmacopœia.
Altschul's Real-Lexicon.
Buchner's Homœopathische Arzneibereitungslehre.
Gruner's Homöopathische Pharmacopoe.
Hale's New Remedies. Ed. 1867.
Hale's New Remedies. " 1882.
Mure's Materia Medica.
Kleinert's Quellen-Nachweis der physiologischen Arzneiprüfungen.
Flückinger and Hanbury, Pharmacographia.
British Pharmacopœia, with additions, 1874. Ed. 1880.
United States Pharmacopœia.
Squire's Companion to the British Pharmacopœia.
Hager's Commentar zur Pharmacopœa Germanica.
Hager's Handbuch der Pharmaceutischen Praxis.
Homöopathisches Real Lexicon.
Hahnemann's Chronic Diseases (Hempel 's Trans.)
Hahnemann's Reine Arzneimittellehre.
Watts' Dictionary of Chemistry, 5 vols., with supplements.
Bloxam's Chemistry,
Fowne's Chemistry.
Fresenius' Qualitative Analysis.
Galloway's " "
Wagner's Die Chemie.
Heppe's Die Chemischen Reactionen.
Köhler's Physiologischen Therapeutik.
Brush's Determinative Mineralogy.
Genera Plantarum (Bentham et Hooker.)
Cooke's Handbook of British Fungi.
Gray's Manual of Botany.
Wood's Class Book of Botany.
The Hahnemannian Monthly.
Foster's Physiology.

INDEX.

F. E. BOERICKE'S

(LATE BOERICKE & TAFEL)

Homœopathic Publications,

PHILADELPHIA.

ALLEN, DR. TIMOTHY F. The Encyclopedia of Pure Materia Medica; a Record of the Positive Effects of Drugs upon the Healthy Human Organism. With contributions from Dr. Richard Hughes, of England; Dr. C. Hering, of Philadelphia; Dr. Carroll Dunham, of New York; Dr. Adolph Lippe, of Philadelphia, and others. Ten volumes. Price bound in cloth, $60.00; in half morocco or sheep, $70.00

This is the most complete and extensive work on Materia Medica ever attempted in the history of medicine—a work to which the homœopathic practitioner may turn with the certainty of finding the whole pathogenetic record of any remedy ever used in homœopathy, the record of which being published either in book form or in journals.

"With the Volumes IX. and X. now before us—ALLEN'S ENCYCLOPEDIA OF PURE MATERIA MEDICA—is completed. It comprises all remedies proved or applied by Homœopaths. With truly wonderful diligence everything has been carefully collated from the whole medical literature that could be put under contribution to Homœopathy, thus enabling anyone who wants to make a thorough study of Materia Medica, or who wants to read up a special remedy to find what he needs and where to look for it. . . . As regards printing, paper, and general get-up, the house of Boericke & Tafel has fully upheld its old established reputation."—*From the Allgemeine Homœopathische Zeitung.*

ALLEN, DR. TIMOTHY F. A General Symptom Register of the Homœopathic Materia Medica.—1,331 pages. Large 8vo.

Cloth, ... $12.00
Half morocco or sheep, ... $14.00

This valuable work was eagerly welcomed by the homœopathic profession, and a large portion of the edition has already been disposed of. The work can be obtained through every homœopathic pharmacy, and those desiring to secure a copy should send in their orders without delay, as but a limited number of copies remain available.

"The long hoped for 'Index' has come, and now lies before us in all the glory of a comely volume of 1,331 pages, beautifully printed on good, clear paper, and bound in cloth.

"Every scientific practitioner in the world will heartily thank the indefatigable author for crowning his pharmaco-encyclopedic edifice so promptly with a workable repertorial index. The thing we are most thankful for is that *the arrangement is strictly alphabetical.* FIRST, THE PART AFFECTED; SECOND, THE SENSATION, *conditioned or modified.* No fads or fancies, theories or hypotheses. Of course everybody has a copy of the 'Encyclopedia,' and now everybody will get a copy of the Index. We cannot pretend to review such a work. It bears every mark of care, capability and conscientiousness, and to hunt about for specks of dirt on such a grand picture is not the kind of work for us. The only piece of advice we offer to intending purchasers is that they ask for it bound in leather, for common cloth binding, no matter how nice to the eye, soon begins to tear at the back, and becomes the source of endless annoyance. This applies, of course, to a work for frequent reference, and Allen's 'Index' is practically a dictionary to his 'Encyclopedia,' and as such will be used many times a day."—*From the Homœopathic World.*

ALLEN AND NORTON. Ophthalmic Therapeutics. See Norton's Ophthalmic Therapeutics.

ALLEN, WILLIAM A. Repertory of the Symptoms of Intermittent Fever. Arranged by WILLIAM A. ALLEN. 107 pages. 12mo. Cloth. Price, ... $1.00

We give a letter of Timothy F. Allen, M.D., recommending the publication of this little work:

"I have carefully examined the repertory of Dr. Wm. Allen, of Flushing, and assure you that it is exceedingly valuable. It should be printed in pocket form. I should use it constantly. Dr. Allen has a large experience in the treatment of intermittents, and his own observations are entitled to great respect."

BAEHR, DR. B. The Science of Therapeutics according to the Principles of Homœopathy. Translated and enriched with numerous additions from Kafka and other sources, by C. J. HEMPEL, M.D. Two volumes. 1387 pages. Half morocco, ... $9.00

"The descriptions of disease—no easy thing to write—are always clear and full, sometimes felicitous. The style is easy and readable, and not too prolix. Above all, the relations of maladies to medicines are studied no less philosophically than experimentally, with an avoidance of abstract theorizing on one side, and of mere empiricism on the other, which is most satisfactory."—*From the British Journal of Homœopathy.*

BELL and LAIRD, DRS. The Homœopathic Therapeutics of Diarrhœa, Dysentery, Cholera, Cholera Morbus, Cholera Infantum, and all other Loose Evacuations of the Bowels; by JAMES B. BELL, M.D. Second edition. 275 pages. 12mo. Cloth, ... $1.50

"This little book, issued in 1869, by Dr. Bell, has long been a standard work in Homœopathic Therapeutics. We feel quite within bounds in asserting that it has been the means under our law, of saving thousands of lives. Than this no greater commendation could be penned. . . . In this second edition, Dr. Bell has been assisted by Dr. Laird, of Maine; also by Drs. Lippe, William P. Wesselhoeft and E. A. Farrington. Thirty-eight new remedies are given; the old text largely re-written; many rubrics added to the repertory; a new feature, the 'black type,' for especially characteristic symptoms, introduced.

"This is a typical homœopathic work, which no homœopathic physician can afford to be without. The typographical setting is worthy of the book."—*From the Homœopathic Physician.*

BERJEAU, J. PH. The Homœopathic Treatment of Syphilis, Gonorrhœa, Spermatorrhœa, and Urinary Diseases. Revised, with numerous additions, by J. H. P. FROST, M.D. 256 pages. 12mo. Cloth, ... $1.50

"This work is unmistakably the production of a practical man. It is short, pithy, and contains a vast deal of sound practical instruction. The diseases are briefly described; the directions for treatment are succinct and summary. It is a book which might with profit be consulted by all practitioners of homœopathy."—*North American Journal.*

BREYFOGLE, DR. W. L. Epitome of Homœopathic Medicines. 383 pages, ... $1.25

We quote from the author's preface:

"It has been my aim, throughout, to arrange in as concise form as possible, the leading symptoms of all well-established provings. To accomplish this, I have compared Lippe's Mat. Med.; the Symtomen-Codex; Jahr's Epitome; Bœnninghausen's Therapeutic Pocket-Book, and Hale's New Remedies.

BRIGHAM, DR. GERSHAM N. Phthisis Pulmonalis, or Tubercular Consumption. Pp. 224. 8vo. Cloth. Price, . . $2.00

This interesting work on a subject which has been the "Opprobrium Medicorum" for generations past, has met with a favorable reception at the hands of the profession. It is a scholarly work and treats its subject from the standpoint of pure homœopathy.

"Just now a fresh move of interest in consumption is passing over the world, and hence we may say Dr. Brigham's monograph comes apropos; but on the other hand it comes too early, as the parasitic nature of phthisis is now the great phthisiological question which belittles and dwarfs every other.

"Our author's work must be pronounced as decidedly able, and its principal defects are those of the subject itself in its present state of development. In our opinion the whole question is still involved in too much doubt and difficulty to admit of its being handled very lucidly at present. Dr. Brigham tries very hard to clear the deck of all notions that might be in the way of handling the subject scientifically, but he does not quite succeed even in defining clearly one single form of phthisis. Why? because in the present state of the subject it is impossible for any man to do so, and we question whether a much better book on phthisis is possible at present."—*From The Homœopathic World*, for October, 1882.

BRYANT, DR. J. A Pocket Manual, or Repertory of Homœopathic Medicine, Alphabetically and Nosologically arranged, which may be used as the Physicians' *Vade-mecum*, the Travellers' Medical Companion, or the Family Physician. Containing the Principal Remedies for the most important Diseases; Symptoms, Sensations, Characteristics of Diseases, etc.; with the principal Pathogenetic Effects of the Medicines on the most important Organs and Functions of the Body, together with Diagnosis, Explanation of Technical Terms, Directions for the Selection and Exhibition of Remedies, Rules of Diet, etc. Compiled from the best Homœopathic authorities. Third edition. 352 pages. 18mo. Cloth, $1.50

DR. BURNETT'S ESSAYS. Ecce Medicus; Natrum Muriaticum; Gold; The Causes of Cataract; Curability of Cataract; Diseases of the Veins; Supersalinity of the Blood. Pp. 296. 8vo. Cloth. Price, ... $2.50

Dr. Burnett's essays were so favorably received in this country, that they would undoubtedly have commanded a very large sale, had they not been so high in price. As it was the six essays would have cost over five dollars, and in order to bring them within reach of the many we reprinted them, by special arrangement with the author, who contributed a new essay, "The Causes of Cataract," not hitherto published, and a general introduction to the volume.

The book is printed in good style on heavy toned paper and well bound, and we are able to furnish it at less than half the price of the imported volumes.

We feel sure that these suggestive and sprightly monographs will be highly appreciated by the profession at large.

BUTLER, DR. JOHN. A Text-Book of Electro-Therapeutics and Electro-Surgery; FOR THE USE OF STUDENTS AND GENERAL PRACTITIONERS. By JOHN BUTLER, M.D., L.R.C.P.E., L.R.C.S.I., etc., etc. Second edition, revised and enlarged. 350 pages. 8vo. Cloth, $3.00

"Among the many works extant on Medical Electricity, we have seen nothing that comes so near 'filling the bill' as this. The book is sufficiently comprehensive for the student or the practitioner. The fact that it is written by an enthusiastic and very intelligent homœopathist, gives to it additional value. It places electricity on the same basis as other drugs, and points out by specific symptoms when the agent is indicated. The use of electricity is therefore clearly no longer an exception to the law of *similia*, but acts curatively only when used in accordance with that law. We are not left to conjecture and doubt, but can clearly see the specific indications of the agent, in the disease we have under observation. The author has done the profession an invaluable service in thus making plain the pathogenesis of this wonderful agent. The reader will find no difficulty in following both the pathology and treatment of the cases described. Electricity is not held up as the cure-all of disease, but is shown to be one of the most important and valuable of remedial agents, when used in an intelligent manner. We have seen no work which we can so heartily recommend as this."—*Cincinnati Medical Advance.*

BUTLER, DR. JOHN. Electricity in Surgery. Pp. 111. 12mo. Cloth. Price, ... $1 00

This interesting little volume treats on the application of Electricity to Surgery. The following are some of the subjects treated of: ENLARGEMENT OF THE PROSTATE; STRICTURE; OVARIAN CYSTS; ANEURISM; NAEVUS; TUMORS; ULCERS; HIP DISEASE; SPRAINS; BURNS; GALVANO-CAUTERY; HÆMORRHOIDS; FISTULÆ; PROLAPSUS OF RECTUM; HERNIA, ETC., ETC. The directions given under each operation are most explicit and will be heartily welcomed by the practitioner.

DUNHAM, CARROLL, A.M., M.D. Homœopathy the Science of Therapeutics. A collection of papers elucidating and illustrating the principles of homœopathy. 529 pages. 8vo. Cloth, . . . $3.00
Half morocco, ... $4.00

"More than one-half of this volume is devoted to a careful analysis of various drug-provings. It teaches us Materia Medica after a new fashion, so that a fool can understand, not only the full measure of usefulness, but also the limitations which surround the drug. . . We ought to give an illustration of his method of analysis, but space forbids. We not only urge the thoughtful and studious to obtain the book, which they will esteem as second only to the *Organon* in its philosophy and learning."—*The American Homœopathist.*

DUNHAM, CARROLL, A.M., M.D. Lectures on Materia Medica. 858 pages. 8vo. Cloth, ... $5.00
Half morocco, ... $6.00

"Vol. I. is adorned with a most perfect likeness of Dr. Dunham, upon which stranger and friend will gaze with pleasure. To one skilled in the science of physiognomy there will be seen the unmistakable impress of the great soul that looked so long and steadfastly out of its fair windows. But our readers will be chiefly concerned with the contents of these two books. They are even better than their embellishments. They are chiefly such lectures on Materia Medica as Dr. Dunham alone knew how to write. They are preceded quite naturally by introductory lectures, which he was accustomed to deliver to his classes on general therapeutics, on rules which should guide us in studying drugs, and on the therapeutic law. At the close of Vol. II. we have several papers of great interest, but the most important fact of all is that we have over fifty of our leading remedies presented in a method which belonged peculiarly to the author, as one of the most successful teachers our school has yet produced. . . . Blessed will be the library they adorn, and the wise man or woman into whose mind their light shall shine."—*Cincinnati Medical Advance.*

EDMONDS on Diseases Peculiar to Infants and Children. By W. A. EDMONDS, M.D., Professor of Pædology in the St. Louis Homœopathic College of Physicians and Surgeons, etc., etc., etc. 1881. Pp. 300. 8vo. Cloth, ... $2.50

This work meets with rapid sales, and was accorded a flattering reception by the homœopathic press.

"This is a good, sound book, by an evidently competent man. The preface is as manly as it is unusual, and engages one to go on and read the entire work. In the chapter on the examination of sick children we read that 'no physician will ever have full and comfortable success as a pædologist who has a brusque, reticent, undemonstrative manner. It is indispensable that a physician having children in charge should convince them by his manner that he likes them, and sympathizes with them in their whims, foibles and peculiarities. Their intuitions as to whom they ought to like and ought not to like are marked and wonderfully accurate at a very tender age.' The physician who writes thus is a born pædologist, and most assuredly a very successful practitioner. . . . .

"After the examination of children has been dwelt upon, our author proceeds to discuss of the hygiene of children in a very able and sensible manner. He then discourses upon the various diseases of children in an easy and yet didactic manner, and any one can soon discover that he knows whereof he writes."—*From the Homœopathic World.*

EGGERT, DR. W. The Homœopathic Therapeutics of Uterine and Vaginal Discharges. 543 pages. 8vo. Half morocco, $3.50

The author here brought together in an admirable and comprehensive arrangement everything published to date on the subject in the whole homœopathic literature, besides embodying his own abundant personal experience. The contents, divided into eight parts, are arranged as follows:—PART I. Treats of *Menstruation and Dysmenorrhœa.* PART II. *Menorrhagia.* PART III. *Amenorrhœa.* PART IV. *Abortion and Miscarriage.* PART V. *Metrorrhagia.* PART VI. *Fluor albus.* PART VII. *Lochia,* and PART VIII. *General Concomitants.* No work as complete as this, on the subject, was ever before attempted, and we feel assured that it will meet with great favor by the profession.

GUERNSEY, DR. H. N. The Application of the Principles and Practice of Homœopathy to Obstetrics and the Disorders Peculiar to Women and Young Children. By HENRY N. GUERNSEY, M.D., Professor of Obstetrics and Diseases of Women and Children in the Homœopathic Medical College of Pennsylvania, etc., etc. With numerous Illustrations. Third edition, revised, enlarged, and greatly improved. Pp. 1004. 8vo. Half morocco, ... $8.00

In 1869 this sterling work was first published, and was at once adopted as a text-book at all homœopathic colleges. In 1873 a second edition, considerably enlarged, was issued; in 1878 a third edition was rendered necessary. The wealth of indications for the remedies used in the treatment, tersely and succinctly expressed, giving the gist of the author's immense experience at the bedside, forms a prominent and well appreciated feature of the volume.

"This standard work is a credit to the author and publishers. * * * * * The instructions in the manual and mechanical means employed by the accoucheur are fully up to the latest reliable ideas, while the stand that is taken that all derangements incidental to gestation, parturition and post partum are not purely mechanical, but will in the majority of cases, if not all, succumb to the action of the properly selected homœopathic remedy, shows that Prof. Guernsey has not fallen into the rut of methodical ideas and treatment. . . . . The appendix contains additional suggestions in the treatment of suspended animation of newly-born children, hysteria, ovarian tumors, sterility, etc., suggestions as to diet during sickness of any kind, etc., etc. After the index is a glossary, a useful appendix in itself. Every practitioner should have a copy of this excellent work, even if he has two or three copies of old school text-books on obstetrics and diseases of women."—*From the Cincinnati Medical Advance.*

GUERNSEY, DR. E. Homœopathic Domestic Practice. With full Descriptions of the Dose to each single Case. Containing also Chapters on Anatomy, Physiology, Hygiene, and abridged Materia Medica. Tenth enlarged, revised, and improved edition. Pp. 653. Half leather, $2.50

HAGEN, DR. R. A Guide to the Clinical Examination of Patients and the Diagnosis of Disease. By RICHARD HAGEN, M.D., Privat docent to the University of Leipzig. Translated from the second revised and enlarged edition, by G. E. GRAMM, M.D. Pp. 223. 12mo. Cloth, $1.25

"This is the most perfect guide in the examination of patients that we have ever seen. The author designs it only for the use of students of medicine before attending clinics, but we have looked it carefully through, and do not know of 223 pages of printed matter anywhere of more importance to a physician in his daily bedside examinations. It is simply invaluable."—*From the St. Louis Clinical Review.*

HAHNEMANN, DR. S. Organon of the Art of Healing. By SAMUEL HAHNEMANN, M.D. Aude Sapere. Fifth American edition. Translated from the fifth German edition, by C. WESSELHOEFT, M.D. Pp. 244. 8vo. Cloth, ... $1.75

"To insure a correct rendition of the text of the author, they (the publishers) selected as his translator Dr. Conrad Wesselhoeft, of Boston, an educated physician in every respect, and from his youth up perfectly familiar with the English and German languages, than whom no better selection could have been made." "That he has made, as he himself declares, 'an entirely new and independent translation of the whole work,' a careful comparison of the various paragraphs, notes, etc., with those contained in previous editions, gives abundant evidence; and while he has, so far as possible, adhered strictly to the letter of Hahnemann's text, he has at the same time given a pleasantly flowing rendition that avoids the harshness of a strictly literal translation."—*Hahnemannian Monthly.*

HAHNEMANN, DR. S. The Lesser Writings of. Collected and Translated by R. E. DUDGEON, M.D. With a Preface and Notes by E. MARCY, M.D. With a Steel Engraving of Hahnemann from the statue of Steinhauser. Pp. 784. Half morocco, ... $3.00

This valuable work contains a large number of Essays of great interest to laymen as well as medical men, upon Diet, the Prevention of Diseases, Ventilation of Dwellings, etc. As many of these papers were written before the discovery of the homœopathic theory of cure, the reader will be enabled to peruse in this volume the ideas of a gigantic intellect when directed to subjects of general and practical interest.

HALE, DR. E. M. Lectures on Diseases of the Heart. In three parts. Part. I. Functional Disorders of the Heart. Part II. Inflammatory Affections of the Heart. Part III. Organic Diseases of the Heart. Second enlarged edition. Pp. 248. Cloth, ... $1.75

"After giving a thorough overhauling to the lectures of Dr. Hale, with the full intention of a close criticism, I acknowledge myself conquered. True there are text books on the same subject of thrice the number of pages—more voluminous, *but not so concise;* and in this very conciseness lies the merit of the work. Students will find there everything they need at the bedside of their patients. It fills just a want long felt by the profession, and we can only congratulate Dr. Hale to have found in Messrs. Boericke & Tafel, publishers who have done their work equally well."—*North American Journal of Homœopathy.*

HALE, DR. E. M. Materia Medica and Special Therapeutics of the New Remedies. By EDWIN M. HALE, M.D., Professor of Materia Medica and Therapeutics of the New Remedies in Hahnemann Medical College, Chicago, etc., etc. Fifth edition, revised and enlarged. In two volumes—Vol. I. Special Symptomatology. With new Botanical and Pharmacological Notes. Pp. 770. 1882. Cloth, ... $5.00
Half morocco, ... $6.00

"Dr Hale's work on *New Remedies,* is one both well known and much appreciated on this side of the Atlantic. For many medicines of considerable value we are indebted to his researches. In the present edition, the symptoms produced by the drug investigated, and those which they have been observed to cure, are separated from the clinical observations, by which the former have been confirmed. That this volume contains a very large amount of invaluable information is incontestable, and that every effort has been made to secure both fulness of detail and accuracy of statement, is apparent throughout. For these reasons we can confidently commend Dr. Hale's fourth edition of his well known work on the *New Remedies* to our homœopathic colleagues."—*From the Monthly Homœopathic Review.*

HALE, DR. E. M. Materia Medica and Special Therapeutics of the New Remedies. By EDWIN M. HALE, M.D. Late Professor of Materia Medica and Therapeutics of the New Remedies in Hahnemann Medical College, Chicago; Professor of Materia Medica in the Chicago Homœopathic College, etc. Fifth edition, revised and enlarged (thirty-seven new remedies), in two volumes. Vol. II. Special Therapeutics. With illustrative cases. Pp. 901. 8vo. Cloth, ... $5.00
Half morocco, ... $6.00

"Hale's *New Remedies* is one of the few works which *every* physician, no matter how poor he may be, ought to own. Many other books are very nice to have, and very desirable, but this is indispensable. This volume before us is an elegant specimen of the printers' and binders' art, and equally enjoyable when we consider its contents, which are not only thoroughly scientific, but also as interesting as a novel. Thirty-seven new drugs are added in this edition, besides numerous additions to the effects of drugs, previously discussed. * * * * * We must say and reiterate if necessary, that Dr. Hale has hit the nail on the head in his plan for presenting the new remedies. It does well enough to tabulate and catalogue, for reference in looking up cases, barren lists of symptoms, but for real enjoyable study, for the means of clinching our information and making it stand by us, give us volumes planned and executed like that now under consideration."—*From the New England Medical Gazette.*

HALE, DR. E. M. Medical and Surgical Treatment of the Diseases of Women, especially those causing Sterility. Second edition. Pp. 378. 8vo. Cloth, ... $2.50

"This work is the outcome of a quarter of a century of practical gynæcological experience, and on every page we are struck with its *realness.* It is one of those books that will be kept on a low shelf in the libraries of its possessors, so that it may be found readily at hand in case of need. It is a work that soon will be well-thumbed by the busy practitioner who owns it, because in many a difficult obstetric case he will pace his study, tug at the favorite button a little nervously, and suddenly pause and exclaim, 'Let us see what Hale says about it!' and in seeing what Hale does say about it he will feel strengthened and comforted, as one does after a consultation with a *hülfreicher* colleague in a difficult or dangerous case, in which the enormous responsibility had threatened to crush one.

"In many obstinate uterine cases we shall reach this book down to read again and again what this clinical genius has to say on the subject. We have never seen Professor Hale in the flesh, but we have had scores of consultations with him in the pages of his *New Remedies*, and he has thus feelessly helped us cure many an obstinate case of disease.

"When we get a good book we mentally shake hands with the author, and think gratefully of him for giving us of his great riches. This is a good book, and thus we act and feel towards its gifted author, Professor Hale.'—*From the Homœopathic World, London.*

HART, DR. C. P. Diseases of the Nervous System. Being a Treatise on Spasmodic, Paralytic, Neuralgic and Mental Affections. For the use of Students and Practitioners of Medicine. By CHAS. PORTER HART, M.D., Honorary Member of the College of Physicians and Surgeons of Michigan, etc., etc., etc. Pp. 409. 8vo. Cloth, . $3.00

"This work supplies a need keenly felt in our school—a work which will be useful alike to the general practitioner and specialist; containing, as it does, not only a condensed compilation of the views of the best authorities on the subject treated, but also the author's own clinical experience; to which is appended the appropriate homœopathic treatment of each disease. It is written in an easy, flowing style, at the same time there is no waste of words. * * * * * We consider the work a highly valuable one, bearing the evidence of hard work, considerable research and experience."—*Medico-Chirurgical Quarterly.*

"We feel proud that in Hart's 'Diseases of the Nervous System' we have a work up to date, a work which we need not feel ashamed to put in the hands of the neurologist or alienist for critical examination, a work for which we predict a rapid sale."—*North American Journal of Homœopathy.*

HELMUTH, DR. W. T. A System of Surgery. Illustrated with 568 Engravings on Wood. By WM. TOD HELMUTH, M.D. Third edition. Pp. 1000. Sheep, ... $8.50

This standard work, for many years used as a text-book in all homœopathic colleges, still maintains its rank as the best work ever brought out by our school on the subject. Ever since it was issued the necessity, for the student or practitioner, to invest in allopathic works on the subject ceased to exist. It is up to date, and abounds in valuable hints, for it gives the results of the author's ripe and extensive experience with homœopathic medication in connection with surgical operations. In elegance of diction our author has never been approached.

. . . . "We have in this work a condensed compendium of almost all that is known in practical surgery, written in a terse, forcible, though pleasing style, the author evidently having the rare gift of saying a great deal in a few words, and of saying these few words in a graceful, easy manner. Almost every subject is illustrated with cases from the doctor's own practice; nor has he neglected to put before us the great advantage of homœopathic treatment in surgical diseases. The work is in every respect up to the requirements of the times. . . . .

"Taken altogether, we have no book in our literature that we are more proud of.

"One word of commendation to the publishers is naturally drawn from us as we compare this handsome, clearly-printed, neatly-bound volume with the last edition. The difference is so palpable that there is no necessity of making further comparisons."—*Homœopathic Times.*

HELMUTH, DR. W. T. Supra-Pubic Lithotomy. The High Operation for Stone—Epicystotomy—Hypogastric Lithotomy—"The High Apparatus." By WM. TOD HELMUTH, M.D., Professor of Surgery in the N. Y. Hom. Med. College; Surgeon to the Hahnemann Hospital and to Wards Island Homœopathic Hospital, N. Y. 98 quarto pp. 8 lithographic plates. Cloth. Price, ... $4.00

A superb quarto edition, with lithographic plates, printed in five colors, and illustrated by charts and numerous wood-cuts.

HEINIGKE, DR. CARL. Pathogenetic Outlines of Homœopathic Drugs. By DR. CARL HEINIGKE, of Leipzig. Translated from the German by EMIL TIETZE, M.D., of Philadelphia. Pp. 576. 8vo. Cloth, ... $3.50

"The reader of this work will gain more practical knowledge of a given drug from its pages in the same space of time than from any other book on the same subject.

"The publishers' part of the work has been executed with the usual elegance, neatness and durability which characterizes all their publications which we have seen.

"To the English reading portion of our colleagues, this book will be a boon to be appreciated, in proportion that it is consulted, and will save them many weary researches when in doubt of the true homœopathic remedy."—*American Homœopath.*

HEMPEL, DR. C. J., and DR. J. BEAKLEY. Homœopathic Theory and Practice. With the Homœopathic Treatment of Surgical Diseases. Designed for Students and Practitioners of Medicine, and as a Guide for an intelligent public generally. Fourth edition. Pp. 1100. $3.00

HERING, DR. CONSTANTINE. Condensed Materia Medica. Second edition, more Condensed, Revised, Enlarged and Improved. 806 pages, large 8vo. Half morocco, ... $7.00

This, the most complete work issued from the pen of the late illustrious author, has a very large sale, having been adopted from its first appearance as Text-book in all Homœopathic Colleges in the United States.

"This work, the author tells us, is made up from the manuscript prepared for the 'Guiding Symptoms,' and is intended to give the student an idea of the main features of each drug in as narrow a compass as possible. It is, in fact, the 'Guiding Symptoms' boiled down. It has therefore a value of its own in enabling the student or practitioner to see quickly the chief symptoms of each medicine. Its name indicates its nature exactly, the condensation being more valuable from the hands of Dr. Hering than it might be from others of smaller experience. To those who wish to have such an aid to the Materia Medica beside them, we can recommend it."—*Monthly Homœopathic Review* for September, 1880.

"The favor with which this work has been received, and the rapidity with which it has been adopted as a text-book in all the homœopathic medical colleges, attests most fully its value. Embracing the rich experience and the extensive learning of the author, its authority is unquestioned. The relationship of the drugs is peculiarly valuable, and can be found nowhere else outside of Bœnninghausen. The schema is according to Hahnemann, similarity in symptoms being clearly indicated. Hering's Materia Medica has now become the leading work of its kind in our school. Its broad pages lie invitingly before you. You read over the symptomatology of each drug with the consciousness that each and every line has been well considered before incorporation, and that it is a storehouse of wealth from which every worker can draw his supplies. The appearance of the work reflects credit upon the publishers, who have already gained their reputation as book publishers of the first rank."—*Homœopathic News.*

HERING, DR. CONSTANTINE. Domestic Physician. Seventh American Edition. 464 Pp. $2.50

The present editor, Claude R. Norton, M.D., a former assistant of Dr. Hering, undertook, at his desire, the task of superintending the publication of the work. Some additions to the text have been made, a few remedies introduced, and, at times, slight alterations in the arrangement effected, but the well-known views of the author have been respected in whatever has been done; but for unavoidable reasons, the issue of the present edition has been delayed until this time.

HOMŒOPATHIC POULTRY PHYSICIAN (Poultry Veterinarian); or, Plain Directions for the Homœopathic Treatment of the most Common Ailments of Fowls, Ducks, Geese, Turkeys, and Pigeons, based on the author's large experience, and compiled from the most reliable sources, by Dr. Fr. Schröter. Translated from the German. 84 pages, 12mo. Cloth, ... $0.50

We imported hundreds of copies of this work in the original German for our customers, and as it gave good satisfaction, we thought it advisable to give it an English dress, so as to make it available to the public generally. The little work sells very fast, and our readers will doubtless often have an opportunity to draw the attention of their patrons to it.

HOMŒOPATHIC COOKERY. Second edition. With additions by a Lady of an American Homœopathic Physician. Designed chiefly for the Use of such Persons as are under Homœopathic Treatment. 176 pages. $0.50

HULL'S JAHR. A New Manual of Homœopathic Practice. Edited, with Annotations and Additions, by F. G. Snelling, M.D. Sixth American edition. With an Appendix of the New Remedies, by C. J. Hempel, M.D. 2 vols. 2076 pages, ... $9.00

This first volume, containing the symptomatology, gives the complete pathogenesis of two hundred and eighty-seven remedies, besides a large number of new remedies added by Dr. Hempel, in the appendix. The second volume contains an admirably arranged Repertory. Each chapter is accompanied by copious clinical remarks and the concomitant symptoms of the chief remedies for the malady treated of, thus imparting a mass of information, rendering the work indispensable to every student and practitioner of medicine.

JAHR, DR. G. H. G. Therapeutic Guide; the most Important results of more than Forty Years Practice. With Personal Observations regarding the truly reliable and practically verified Curative Indications in actual cases of disease. Translated, with Notes and New Remedies, by C. J. Hempel, M.D. 546 pages, ... $3.00

"With this characteristically long title, the veteran and indefatigable Jahr gives us another volume of homœopathics. Besides the explanation of its purport contained in the title itself, the author's preface still further sets forth its distinctive aim. It is intended, he says, as a 'guide to beginners, where I only indicate the most important and decisive points for the selection of a remedy, and where I do not offer anything but what my own individual experience, during a practice of forty years, has enabled me to verify as *absolutely decisive* in choosing the proper remedy.' The reader will easily comprehend that, in carrying out this plan, I had rigidly to exclude all cases concerning which I had no experience *of my own* to offer. . . . . We are bound to say that the book itself is agreeable, chatty, and full of practical observation. It may be read straight through with interest, and referred to in the treatment of particular cases with advantage."—*British Journal of Homœopathy.*

JAHR, DR. G. H. G. The Homœopathic Treatment of Diseases of Females and Infants at the Breast. Translated from the French by C. J. Hempel, M.D. 422 pages. Half leather, . . . $2.00

This work deserves the most careful attention on the part of homœopathic practitioners. The diseases to which the female organism is subject are described, with the most minute correctness, and the treatment is likewise indicated with a care that would seem to defy criticism. No one can fail to study this work but with profit and pleasure.

JONES, DR. SAMUEL A. The Grounds of a Homœopaths Faith. Three Lectures, delivered at the request of Matriculates of the Department of Medicine and Surgery (Old School) of the University of Michigan. By Samuel A. Jones, M.D., Professor of Materia Medica, Therapeutics, and Experimental Pathogenesy in the Homœopathic Medical College of the University of Michigan, etc., etc. 92 Pages. 12mo. Cloth (per dozen, $3), ... $0.30

The first Lecture is on *The Law of Similars; its Claim to be a Science in that it Enables Perversion.* The second Lecture, *The Single Remedy a Necessity of Science.* The third Lecture, *The Minimum Dose an Inevitable Sequence.* A fourth Lecture, on *The Dynamization Theory,* was to have finished the course, but was prevented by the approach of final examinations, the preparation for which left no time for hearing evening lectures. The *Lectures* are issued in a convenient size for the coat-pocket; and as an earnest testimony to the truth, we believe they will find their way into many a homœopathic household.

JOHNSON, DR. I. D. Therapeutic Key; or Practical Guide for the Homœopathic Treatment of Acute Diseases. Tenth edition. 347 pages.
Bound in linen, ... $1.75
Bound in flexible leather cover, ... 2.25

The same including twelve insets properly lined and headed for daily visits, $3.25, or the insets separately at $1 per set of twelve. Each inset will be found sufficient for a month's visits in ordinary practice and well supplies the usual visiting list, and this without a perceptible increase in bulk.

This has been one of the best selling works on our shelves; more copies being in circulation of this than of any two other professional works put together. It is safe to say that there are but few homœopathic practitioners in this country but have one or more copies of this little remembrancer in their possession.

"This is a wonderful little book, that seems to contain nearly everything pertaining to the practice of physic, and all neatly epitomized, so that the book may be carried very comfortably in the pocket, to serve as a source for a refresher in a case of need.

"It is a marvel to us how the author has contrived to put into 347 pages such a vast amount of information, and all of the very kind that is needed. No wonder it is in its tenth edition.

"Right in the middle of the book, under P, we find a most useful little chapter, or article, on 'Poisonings,' telling the reader what to do in such cases.—*Homœopathic World, London.*

JOHNSON, DR. I. D. A Guide to Homœopathic Practice. Designed for the Use of Families and Private Individuals. 494 pages. Cloth, ... $2.00

This is the latest work on Domestic Practice issued, and the well and favorably known author has surpassed himself. In this book fifty-six remedies are introduced for internal application, and four for external use. The work consists of two parts. Part I is subdivided into seventeen chapters, each being devoted to a special part of the body, or to a peculiar class of disease. Part II contains a short and concise Materia Medica. The whole is carefully written with a view of avoiding technical terms as much as possible, thus insuring its comprehension by any person of ordinary intelligence.

"Family Guides are often of great service, not only in enabling individuals to relieve the trifling maladies of such frequent occurrence in every family, but in the graver forms of disease, by prompt action to prepare the way for the riper intelligence of the physician.

"The work under notice seems to have been carefully prepared by an intelligent physician, and is one of the handsomest specimens of book-making we have seen from the house of Boericke & Tafel, its publishers."—*Homœopathic Times.*

LAURIE and McCLATCHEY. The Homœopathic Domestic Medicine. By JOSEPH LAURIE, M.D., *Ninth American*, from the Twenty-first English edition. Edited and revised, with numerous and important additions, and the introduction of the new remedies. By R. J. McCLATCHEY, M.D. 1044 pages. 8vo. Half morocco, . . . $5.00

"We do not hesitate to endorse the claims made by the publishers, that this is the most complete, clear, and comprehensive treatise on the domestic homœopathic treatment of disease extant. This handsome volume of nearly eleven hundred pages is divided into six parts. Part I is introductory, and is almost faultless. It gives the most complete and exact directions for the maintenance of health, and of the method of investigating the condition of the sick, and of discriminating between different diseases. It is written in the most lucid style, and is above all things wonderfully free from technicalities. Part II. treats of symptoms, character, distinctions, and treatment of general diseases, together with a chapter on casualties. Part III. takes up diseases peculiar to women. Part IV. is devoted to the disorders of infancy and childhood. Part V. gives the characteristic symptoms of the medicines referred to in the body of the work, while part VI. introduces the repertory."—*Hahnemannian Monthly.*

"Of the usefulness of this work in cases where no educated homœopathic physician is within reach, there can be no question. There is no doubt that domestic homœopathy has done much to make the science known; it has also saved lives in emergencies. The practice has never been so well presented to the public as in this excellent volume."—*New. Eng. Med. Gazette.*

LILIENTHAL, DR. S. Homœopathic Therapeutics. By S. LILIENTHAL, M.D., Editor of North American Journal of Homœopathy, Professor of Clinical Medicine and Psychology in the New York Homœopathic Medical College, and Professor of Theory and Practice in the New York College Hospital for Women, Etc. Second edition. 835 pages. 8vo. Cloth, ... $5.00
Half morocco, ... 6.00

"Certainly no one in our ranks is so well qualified for this work as he who has done it, and in considering the work done, we must have a true conception of the proper sphere of such a work. For the fresh graduate, this book will be invaluable, and to all such we unhesitatingly and very earnestly commend it. To the older one, who says he has no use for this book, we have nothing to say. He is a good one to avoid when well, and to dread when ill. We also hope that he is severely an *unicum*."—*Prof. Samuel A. Jones in American Observer.*

" . . . . It is an extraordinary useful book, and those who add it to their library will never feel regret, for we are not saying too much in pronouncing it the *best work on therapeutics* in homœopathic (or any other) literature. With this under one elbow, and Hering's or Allen's *Materia Medica* under the other, the careful homœopathic practitioner can refute Niemayer's too confident assertion, 'I declare it idle to hope for a time when a medical prescription should be the simple resultant of known quantities.' Doctor, by all means buy Lilienthal's *Homœopathic Therapeutics*. It contains a mine of wealth."—*Prof. Chas. Gatchel in Ibid.*"

LUTZE, DR. A. Manual of Homœopathic Theory and Practice. Designed for the use of Physicians and Families. Translated from the German, with additions by C. J. HEMPEL, M.D. From the sixtieth thousand of the German edition. 750 pp. 8vo. Half leather, $2.50

MALAN, H. Family Guide to the Administration of Homœopathic Remedies. 112 pages. 32mo. Cloth, . . . $0.30

MANUAL OF HOMŒOPATHIC VETERINARY PRACTICE. Designed for all kinds of Domestic Animals and Fowls, prescribing their proper treatment when injured or diseased, and their particular care and general management in health. Second and enlarged edition. 684 pages. 8vo. Half morocco, ... $5.00

" In order to rightly estimate the value and comprehensiveness of this great work, the reader should compare it, as we have done, with the best of those already before the public. In size, fulness, and practical value it is head and shoulders above the very best of them, while in many most important disorders it is far superior to them altogether, containing, as it does, recent forms of disease of which they make no mention."—*Hahnemannian Monthly.*

MARSDEN, DR. J. H. Handbook of Practical Midwifery, WITH FULL INSTRUCTIONS FOR THE HOMŒOPATHIC TREATMENT OF THE DISEASES OF PREGNANCY, AND THE ACCIDENTS AND DISEASES INCIDENT TO LABOR AND THE PUERPERAL STATE. J. H. MARSDEN, A.M., M.D., 315 pages. Cloth, ... $2.25

" It is seldom we have perused a text-book with such entire satisfaction as this. The author has certainly succeeded in his design of furnishing the student and young practitioner, within as narrow limits as possible, all necessary instruction in practical midwifery. The work shows on every page extended research and thorough practical knowledge. The style is clear, the array of facts unique, and the deductions judicious and practical. We are particularly pleased with his discussion of the management of labor, and the management of mother and child immediately after the birth, but much is left open to the common sense and practical judgment of the attendant in peculiar and individual cases."—*Homœopathic Times.*

MORGAN, DR. W. The Text-book for Domestic Practice; being plain and concise directions for the Administration of Homœopathic Medicines in Simple Ailments. 191 pages. 32mo. Cloth, . . . $0.50

This is a concise and short treatise on the most common ailments, printed in convenient size for the pocket; a veritable traveler's companion.

NORTON, DR. GEO. S. Ophthalmic Therapeutics. By GEO. S. NORTON, M.D., Professor of Ophthalmology in the College of the New York Ophthalmic Hospital, Senior Surgeon to the New York Ophthalmic Hospital, etc. With an introduction by PROF. T. F. ALLEN, M.D. Second edition. Re-written and revised, with copious additions. Pp. 342. 8vo. Cloth, ... $2.50

The second edition of Allen & Norton's Ophthalmic Therapeutics has now been issued from the press. It has been re-written, revised and considerably enlarged by Professor Norton, and will, without doubt, be as favorably received as the first edition—out of print since several years. This work embodies the clinical experiences garnered at the N. Y. Ophthalmic Hospital, than which a better appointed and more carefully conducted establishment does not exist in this country. Diseases of the eye are steadily on the increase, and no physician can afford to do without the practical experience as laid down in the sterling work under notice.

RAUE, DR. C. G. Special Pathology and Diagnosis, with Therapeutic Hints. Second edition, re-written and enlarged. Pp. 1,072. Large 8vo. Half morocco or sheep, ... $7.00

This second edition is brought down to date, and, rendered in Dr. Raue's own pregnant, terse style. These thousand pages will be found to be encyclopedic as to the comprehensiveness, and epitomatic as to the condensed form of the information imparted.

" . . . . The first edition has 644 pages; this new has 1,072, and if RAUE has added 428 pages it was because four hundred and twenty-eight pages of *something solid had to find a place in this universe*. . . . . The present edition is written up to date, tersely it is true, but so far as I have read, in consonance with the latest teachings. . . . . I envy the practitioner who can read this second edition without learning something; and I would say to the young graduate, in an expressive Western phrase, '*Tie to it.*' It has become a platitude to compliment publishers, but, really, Boericke & Tafel, and the Globe Printing House, may well be proud of this book."—*S. A. Jones in American Observer.*

REIL, DR. A. ACONITE, Monograph on, its Therapeutic and Physiological Effects, together with its Uses and Accurate Statements, derived from the various Sources of Medical Literature. By A. REIL, M.D. Translated from the German by H. B. Millard, M.D. Prize essay. 168 pages, ... $0.60

"This Monograph, probably the best which has ever been published upon the subject, has been translated and given to the public in English, by Dr. Millard, of New York. Apart from the intrinsic value of the work, which is well known to all medical German scholars, the translation of it has been completed in the most thorough and painstaking way; and all the Latin and Greek quotations have been carefully rendered into English. The book itself is a work of great merit, thoroughly exhausting the whole range of the subject. To obtain a thorough view of the spirit of the action of the drug, we can recommend no better work."—*North American Journal.*

RUSH, DR. JOHN. Veterinary Surgeon. The Hand-book to Veterinary Homœopathy; or, the Homœopathic Treatment of Horses, Cattle, Sheep, Dogs and Swine. From the London edition. With numerous additions from the Seventh German edition of Dr. F. E. Gunther's "Homœopathic Veterinary." Translated by J. F. SHEEK, M.D. 150 pages. 18mo. Cloth, ... $0.50

SCHAEFER, J. C. New Manual of Homœopathic Veterinary Medicine. An easy and comprehensive arrangement of Diseases, adapted to the use of every owner of Domestic Animals, and especially designed for the farmer living out of the reach of medical advice, and showing him the way of treating his sick Horses, Cattle, Sheep, Swine and Dogs, in the most simple, expeditious, safe and cheap manner. Translated from the German, with numerous additions from other veterinary manuals, by C. J. HEMPEL, M.D. 321 pages. 8vo. Cloth, ... $2.00

SHARP'S TRACTS ON HOMŒOPATHY, each, . . . 5
Per hundred, ... $3.00

No. 1. What is Homœopathy?
No. 2. The Defence of Homœopathy.
No. 3. The Truth of "
No. 4. The Small Doses of "
No. 5. The Difficulties of "
No. 6. Advantages of "
No. 7. The Principles of Homœopathy.
No. 8. Controversy on "
No. 9. Remedies of "
No. 10. Provings of "
No. 11. Single Medicines of "
No. 12. Common sense of "

SHARP'S TRACTS, complete set of 12 numbers, $0.50
Bound, ... $0.75

SMALL, DR. A. E. Manual of Homœopathic Practice, for the use of Families and Private Individuals. Fifteenth enlarged edition. 831 pages. 8vo. Half leather, ... $2.50

—— **Manual of Homœopathic Practice.** Translated into German by C. J. HEMPEL, M.D. Eleventh edition. 643 pages. 8vo. Cloth, $2.50

STAPF, DR. E. Additions to the Materia Medica Pura. Translated by C. J. HEMPEL, M.D. 292 pages. 8vo. Cloth, . $1.50

This work is an appendix to Hahnemann's Materia Medica Pura. Every remedy is accompanied with extensive and most interesting clinical remarks, and a variety of cases illustrative of its therapeutical uses.

TESSIER, DR. J. P. Clinical Remarks concerning the Homœopathic Treatment of Pneumonia, preceded by a Retrospective View of the Allopathic Materia Medica, and an Explanation of the Homœopathic Law of Cure. Translated by C. J. HEMPEL, M.D. 131 pages. 8vo. Cloth, ... $0.75

TESTE. A Homœopathic Treatise on the Diseases of Children. By ALPH. TESTE, M.D. Translated from the French by EMMA H. COTE. Fourth edition. 345 pages. 12mo. Cloth, ... $1.50

This sterling work is by no means a new applicant for the favorable consideration of the profession, but is known to the older physicians since many years, and would be as well known to the younger had it not been out of print for nearly eight years. However, as orders for the work were persistently received from all quarters, we concluded to resurrect the book as it were, and purchasing the plates from the quondam publishers, we re-issued it in a much improved form, *i. e.*, well printed on excellent paper. Dr. Teste's work is unique, in that in most cases it recommends for certain affections remedies that are not usually thought of in connection therewith; but, embodying the results of an immense practical experience, they rarely fail to accomplish the desired end.

VERDI, DR. T. S. Maternity, a Popular Treatise for Young Wives and Mothers. By TULLIO SUZZARA VERDI, A.M., M.D., of Washington, D.C. 450 pages. 12mo. Cloth, ... $2.00

"No one needs instruction more than a young mother, and the directions given by Dr. Verdi in this work are such as I should take great pleasure in recommending to all the young mothers, and some of the old ones, in the range of my practice."—*George E. Shipman, M.D., Chicago, Ill.*

"Dr. Verdi's book is replete with useful suggestions for wives and mothers, and his medical instructions for home use accord with the maxims of my best experience in practice."—*John F. Gray, M.D., New York City.*

—— **Mothers and Daughters**: Practical Studies for the Conservation of the Health of Girls. By TULLIO SUZZARA VERDI, A.M, M.D. 287 pages. 12mo. Cloth, ... $1.50

"The people, and especially the women, need enlightening on many points connected with their physical life, and the time is fast approaching when it will no longer be thought singular or 'Yankeeish' that a woman should be instructed in regard to her sexuality, its organs and their functions. . . . . Dr. Verdi is doing a good work in writing such books, and we trust he will continue in the course he has adopted of educating the mother and daughters. The book is handsomely presented. It is printed in good type on fine paper, and is neatly and substantially bound."—*Hahnemannian Monthly.*

VON TAGEN. Biliary Calculi, Perineorrhaphy, Hospital Gangrene, and its Kindred Diseases. 154 pages. 8vo. Cloth, $1.25

"Von Tagen was an industrious worker, a close observer, an able writer. The essays before us bear the marks of this. They are written in an easy, flowing, graceful style, and are full of valuable suggestions. While the essay on perineorrhaphy is mainly of interest to the surgeon, the other essays concern the general practitioner. They are exhaustive and abound in good things. The author is especially emphatic in recommending the use of bromine in the treatment of hospital gangrene, and furnishes striking clinical evidence in support of his recommendation.

"The book forms a neat volume of 150 pages, and is well worthy of careful study."—*Medical Counselor.*

WILLIAMSON, DR. W. Diseases of Females and Children, and their Homœopathic Treatment. Third enlarged edition. 256 pages, ... $1.00

This work contains a short treatise on the homœopathic treatment of the diseases of females and children, the conduct to be observed during pregnancy, labor and confinement, and directions for the management of new-born infants.

WILSON, DR. T. P. Special Indications for Twenty-five Remedies in Intermittent Fever. By T. P. Wilson, M.D., Professor of Theory and Practice, Ophthalmic and Aural Surgery, University of Michigan. 1880. 53 pages. 18mo. Cloth, ... $0.40

This little work gives the characteristic Indications in Intermittent Fever of twenty-five of the mostly used remedies. It is printed on heavy writing paper, and plenty of space is given to make additions.

The name of the drug is printed on the back of the page containing the symptoms, in order that the student may the better exercise his memory.

WINSLOW, DR. W. H. The Human Ear and Its Diseases. A Practical Treatise upon the Examination, Recognition and Treatment of Affections of the Ear and Associate Parts, Prepared for the Instruction of Students and the Guidance of Physicians. By W. H. Winslow, M.D., Ph.D., Oculist and Aurist to the Pittsburg Homœopathic Hospital, etc., etc., with one hundred and thirty-eight illustrations. Pp. 526. 8vo. Cloth. Price, ... $4.50

"It would ill-become a non-specialist to pass judgment upon the intrinsic merits of Dr. Winslow's book, but even a general reader of medicine can see in it an author who has a firm grasp and an intelligent apprehension of his subject. There is about it an air of self-reliant confidence, which, when not offensive, can come only from a consciousness of knowing the matter in hand, and we have never read a medical work which would more quickly lead us to give its author our confidence in his ministrations. This is always the consequence of honest and earnest and inclusive scholarship, and this author is entitled to his meed."—*Dr. S. A. Jones in American Observer.*

WORCESTER, DR. S. Repertory to the Modalities. In their Relations to Temperature, Air, Water, Winds, Weather and Seasons. Based mainly upon Hering's Condensed Materia Medica, with additions from Allen, Lippe and Hale. Compiled and arranged by Samuel Worcester, M.D., Salem, Mass., Lecturer on Insanity and its Jurisprudence at Boston University School of Medicine, etc., etc. 1880. 160 pages. 12mo. Cloth, ... $1.25

"This *Repertory to the Modalities* is indeed a most useful undertaking, and will, without question, be a material aid to rapid and sound prescribing where there *are* prominent modalities. The first chapter treats of the sun and its effects, both beneficial and hurtful, and we see at a glance that *strontium carb.*, *anacardium*, *conium mac.*, and *kali bich.* are likely to be useful to patients who like basking in the sun. No doubt many of these modalities are more or less fanciful; still a great many of them are real and of vast clinical range.

"The book is nicely printed on good paper, and strongly bound. It contains 160 pages. We predict that it will meet with a steady, long-continued sale, and in the course of time be found on the tables of most of those careful and conscientious prescribers who admit the philosophical value of (for instance) lunar aggravations, effects of thunder-storms, etc. And who, being without the priggishness of mere brute science, does not?"—*Homœopathic World*.

WORCESTER, DR. S. Insanity and Its Treatment. Lectures on the Treatment of Insanity and Kindred Nervous Diseases. By SAMUEL WORCESTER, M.D., Salem, Mass. Lecturer on Insanity, Nervous Diseases and Dermatology, at Boston University School of Medicine, etc., etc. 262 pages, ... $3.50

Dr. Worcester was for a number of years assistant physician of the Butler Hospital for the Insane, at Providence, R. I., and was appointed shortly after as Lecturer on Insanity and Nervous Diseases to the Boston University School of Medicine. The work, comprising nearly five hundred pages, will be welcomed by every homœopathic practitioner, for every physician is called upon sooner or later to undertake the treatment of cases of insanity among his patron's families, inasmuch as very many are loth to deliver any afflicted member to a public institution without having first exhausted all means within their power to effect a cure, and the family physician naturally is the first to be put in charge of the case. It is, therefore, of paramount importance that every homœopathic practitioner's library should contain such an indispensable work.

"The basis of Dr. Worcester's work was a course of lectures delivered before the senior students of the Boston University School of Medicine. As now presented with some alterations and additions, it makes a very excellent text-book for students and practitioners. Dr. Worcester has drawn very largely upon standard authorities and his own experience, which has not been small. In the direction of homœopathic treatment, he has received valuable assistance from Drs. Talcott and Butler, of the New York State Asylum. It is not, nor does it pretend to be, an exhaustive work; but as a well-digested summary of our present knowledge of insanity, we feel sure that it will give satisfaction. We cordially recommend it."—*New England Medical Gazette*.

www.ingramcontent.com/pod-product-compliance
Lightning Source LLC
Chambersburg PA
CBHW020856210326
41598CB00018B/1680

* 9 7 8 3 7 4 2 8 1 5 6 5 1 *